MW00784605

Individual Positive Behavior Supports

A Standards-Based Guide to Practices in School and Community Settings

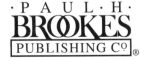

edited by

Fredda Brown, Ph.D.
Queens College
New York, New York

Jacki L. Anderson, Ph.D.
California State University East Bay
Hayward, California

and

Randall L. De Pry, Ph.D.
Portland State University
Portland, Oregon

·P A U L·H·
BROOKES
PUBLISHING C♀.®

Baltimore • London • Sydney

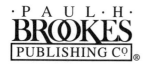

Paul H. Brookes Publishing Co.
Post Office Box 10624
Baltimore, Maryland 21285-0624

www.brookespublishing.com

Typeset by Scribe Inc., Philadelphia, Pennsylvania.
Manufactured in the United States of America by
Sheridan Books, Inc., Chelsea, Michigan.

Photos are used by permission of the individuals pictured and/or their parents/guardians.

Cover image ©istockphoto/Qweek.

The individuals described in this book are composites of the authors' actual experiences or real people. In most instances, names and identifying information have been changed to protect confidentiality. Real names and likenesses are used by permission.

Library of Congress Cataloging-in-Publication Data

The Library of Congress has cataloged the printed edition as follows:
   Individual positive behavior supports : a standards-based guide to practices in school and community settings / [edited by] Fredda Brown, Jacki L. Anderson, Randall L. De Pry.
      p. ; cm.
   Includes bibliographical references and index.
   ISBN 978-1-59857-273-5 (paperback : alk. paper)
   I. Brown, Fredda, editor. II. Anderson, Jacki L., editor. III. De Pry, Randall L., editor.
   [DNLM: 1. Behavior Therapy—methods. 2. Needs Assessment—standards. 3. Early Intervention (Education)—standards. 4. School Health Services. WM 425]

   RJ505.B4
   618.92'89142—dc23   2014019872

British Library Cataloguing in Publication data are available from the British Library.

2018   2017   2016   2015   2014

10   9   8   7   6   5   4   3   2   1

Contents

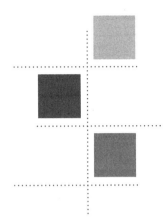

About the Reproducible Materials

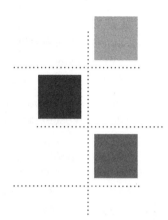

Purchasers of this book may download, print, and/or photocopy Figures 3.3, 10.1, 10.2, 10.3, 20.5, and 24.1 for educational use. These materials are included with the print book and are also available at **http://www.brookespublishing.com/brown/eforms**

Also, for instructors, PowerPoints are available to help you teach a course using *Individual Positive Behavior Supports: A Standards-Based Guide to Practices in School and Community Settings*. Please visit **http://www.brookespublishing.com/brown** to access study questions and customizable PowerPoint presentations for every chapter.

About the Editors

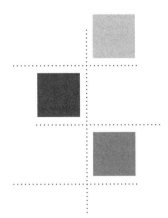

Fredda Brown, Ph.D., received her doctorate in special education from the University of Kansas with a focus on individuals with severe disabilities. Dr. Brown is currently professor of special education at Queens College, the City University of New York. In addition to Dr. Brown's work as a professor and teacher educator, she has spent much of her career providing educational and behavioral consultation to individuals with severe disabilities and their families. She is the editor of several books, and the author of numerous journal articles and book chapters relating to the education of individuals with severe disabilities. Dr. Brown is a former editor in chief of *Research and Practice for Persons with Severe Disabilities (RPSD)* and serves on the editorial boards of *Journal of Positive Behavior Interventions* and *RPSD*. Most recently, her work has focused on professional attitudes regarding behavioral treatment acceptability. She presents her work and ideas nationwide to professionals and families, advocating for positive, dignified, and effective methods of addressing the learning and behavioral needs of individuals with disabilities.

Jacki L. Anderson, Ph.D., received her doctorate from the University of Wisconsin in the areas of communication disorders, child and family studies, and individuals with severe disabilities. She has more than 30 years of experience conducting in-service training activities around the country and has taught for 28 years in the Department of Educational Psychology at California State University East Bay (CSUEB). The education specialist teacher preparation program at CSUEB is a dual-credential program through which students receive both general and special education credentials. Program graduates are known for their excellence in providing effective and innovative educational practices and positive behavior supports. Dr. Anderson's areas of specialization include positive behavior support, teacher training, and inclusive education/life for individuals with severe disabilities. She has been awarded federal funds to pursue these interests via research and training projects; has published the results in textbooks, training manuals, and journal articles; and is on the editorial boards of *Research and Practice for Persons with Severe Disabilities* and *Journal of Positive Behavior Interventions*. Dr. Anderson is actively involved in a variety of professional organizations and policy-making committees, including as a founding member, vice president, and board member of the Association for Positive Behavior Support (APBS); chair of the executive committee and executive vice president of the International TASH organization; former president and current board member of CAL-TASH; president of the board for Casa Allegra Community Services (providing supported living, integrated work, and microenterprise services for individuals with severe disabilities); and a member of several advisory committees to local school districts.

Randall L. De Pry, Ph.D., received his doctorate in special education from the University of Oregon with a focus on individuals with behavioral disabilities. He currently serves as professor of special education and chair of the Department of Special Education at Portland State University. His primary research interests center on positive behavioral interventions and support, including work in social skills instruction, functional behavioral assessment, self-determination, and systemic change models in school and community-based settings. Dr. De Pry served on the board of directors for APBS from 2005 to 2014, including service as secretary, treasurer, and vice president of the board. He is editor of the *APBS Newsletter* and serves on the editorial board of the *Journal of Positive Behavior Interventions* as a consulting editor. Dr. De Pry has presented his work nationally and internationally and works with a variety of schools, agencies, and organizations around disability and behavior support issues.

CONTRIBUTORS

Martin Agran, Ph.D.
Professor
University of Wyoming
1000 E. University Avenue
Laramie, Wyoming 82071

Richard W. Albin, Ph.D.
Senior Research Associate/Associate Professor
1235 University of Oregon
Eugene, Oregon 97405

Sharon Ann Ballard-Krishnan, M.A., RN
Parent and Registered Nurse
Waterford, Michigan

Linda M. Bambara, Ed.D.
Professor of Special Education
Lehigh University
111 Research Drive
Bethlehem, Pennsylvania 18102

Brenda J. Bassingthwaite, Ph.D.
Psychologist
University of Iowa Children's Hospital
100 Hawkins Drive
Iowa City, Iowa 52242

Nila F. Benito
Community Inclusion Coordinator
Florida Center for Inclusive Communities
University of South Florida
13301 Bruce B. Downs Boulevard
Tampa, Florida 33612

Wendy K. Berg, M.A.
Research Manager
University of Iowa
100 Hawkins Drive
Iowa City, Iowa 52242

Chris Borgmeier, Ph.D.
Associate Professor
Portland State University
PO Box 751
Portland, Oregon 97201

Diane M. Browder, Ph.D.
Lake and Edward Snyder Distinguished Professor of Special Education
University of North Carolina at Charlotte
9201 University City Boulevard
Charlotte, North Carolina 28223

Julie Esparza Brown, Ed.D.
Assistant Professor
Portland State University
615 SW Harrison Street
Portland, Oregon 91201

Kaitlin Bundock, M.Ed.
Doctoral Candidate
University of Utah
1721 Campus Center Drive, SAEC 2280
Salt Lake City, Utah 84112

Beth Custer, M.Ed.
Lehigh University
111 Research Drive
Bethlehem, Pennsylvania 18102

Glen Dunlap, Ph.D.
University of Nevada, Reno
College of Education
Reno, Nevada 89557

V. Mark Durand, Ph.D.
Professor
University of South Florida
104 7th Avenue S.
St. Petersburg, Florida 33701

Matt Enyart, M.S.Ed.
Assistant Director of Project Development
Kansas Institute for Positive Behavior Support at the University of Kansas
1000 Sunnyside Avenue
Lawrence, Kansas 66045

Lisa S. Fleisher, Ph.D.
Associate Professor of Educational Psychology
New York University
239 Greene Street #618
New York, New York 10003

Brenda Fossett, M.A., Ph.D.
Instructor
Capilano University
2055 Purcell Way
North Vancouver, British Columbia V7J 3H5

Lise K. Fox, Ph.D.
Professor
University of South Florida
13301 Bruce B. Downs Boulevard
Tampa, Florida 33612

Rachel Freeman, Ph.D.
Associate Research Professor
University of Kansas
1000 Sunnyside Avenue
Lawrence, Kansas 66045

Ann Halvorsen, Ed.D.
Professor of Special Education
California State University, East Bay
25800 Carlos Bee Boulevard
Hayward, California 94542

Leanne S. Hawken, Ph.D.
Professor
University of Utah
1705 E. Campus Center Drive
Salt Lake City, Utah 84112

Meme Hieneman, Ph.D.
Consultant
Positive Behavior Support Applications
Palm Harbor, Florida

Robert H. Horner, Ph.D.
Professor
University of Oregon
1235 University of Oregon
Eugene, Oregon 97403

Kavita V. Kamat, M.S.W., M.Ed., BCBA
Clinical Director
posAbilities: Laurel Behaviour Support Services
101-4664 Lougheed Highway
Burnaby, British Columbia V5C 5T5

Lee Kern, Ph.D.
Professor
Lehigh University
111 Research Drive
Bethlehem, Pennsylvania 18102

Pat Kimbrough, M.S.Ed.
Assistant Director of Operations
Kansas Institute of Positive Behavior Support
University of Kansas
1000 Sunnyside Avenue
Lawrence, Kansas 66049

Todd G. Kopelman, Ph.D., BCBA
Clinical Assistant Professor
University of Iowa
200 Hawkins Drive
Iowa City, Iowa 52242

Catherine Kunsch, Ph.D.
Assistant Professor
Eastern University
1300 Eagle Road
St. David's, Pennsylvania 19087

Angel Lee, ABD
Research Associate
University of North Caroling, Charlotte
9201 University City Boulevard
Charlotte, North Carolina 28223

John F. Lee
Behavior Specialist/Consultant
Center for Disabilities and Development
100 Hawkins Drive
Iowa City, Iowa 52242

Teri Lewis, Ph.D.
Assistant Professor
Oregon State University
2950 SW Jefferson Way
Corvallis, Oregon 97330

Scott D. Lindgren, Ph.D.
Professor
University of Iowa Children's Hospital
100 Hawkins Drive
Iowa City, Iowa 52242

Joseph M. Lucyshyn, Ph.D.
Associate Professor
University of British Columbia
2125 Main Hall
Vancouver, British Columbia V6T1Z4

Sheldon L. Loman, Ph.D.
Assistant Professor
Portland State University
615 SW Harrison Street
Portland, Oregon 97201

Elizabeth R. Lorah, Ph.D.
Assistant Professor
University of Arkansas
Peabody Hall #216
Fayetteville, Arkansas 72701

Kris Matthews, M.S.W., LSCSW
Program Coordinator
University of Kansas
1545 Lilac Lane
Lawrence, Kansas 66045

John McDonnell, Ph.D.
Associate Dean for Faculty Research Support
University of Utah
1720 Campus Center Drive, SAEC 2295
Salt Lake City, Utah 84112

Jennifer McFarland-Whisman, Ph.D., BCBA
Assistant Professor
Marshall University
1 John Marshall Drive
Huntington, West Virginia 25755

Kent McIntosh, Ph.D.
Associate Professor
University of Oregon
1235 University of Oregon
Eugene, Oregon 97403

Ronda Michaelson
File Clerk
North Los Angeles County Regional Center
28415 Industry Drive #502
Valencia, California 91355

Pat Mirenda, Ph.D., BCBA-D
Professor
University of British Columbia
2125 Main Mall
Vancouver, British Columbia V6T124

Tom Neary, M.A.
Special Education Training Specialist
WestEd Center for Prevention and Early Intervention
1107 9th Street
Sacramento, California 95814

Lori Newcomer, Ph.D.
Associate Research Professor
University of Missouri
16 Hill Hall
Columbia, Missouri 65211

Breda V. O'Keefe, Ph.D.
Assistant Professor
University of Utah
1720 Campus Center Drive, SAEC 2294
Salt Lake City, Utah 84112

Robert E. O'Neill, Ph.D.
Professor and Chair of Special Education
University of Utah
1720 Campus Center Drive, SAEC
Salt Lake City, Utah 84112

Yaniz C. Padilla Dalmau, Ph.D.
Outpatient Behavioral Services BCBA Supervisor
Virginia Institute of Autism
1414 Westwood Road
Charlottesville, Virginia 22903

Billie Jo Rodriguez, Ph.D.
Assistant Professor
University of Texas at San Antonio
501 W Cesar E. Chavez Boulevard
San Antonio, Texas 78207

Wayne Sailor, Ph.D.
Professor
University of Kansas
1315 Wakarusa Drive
Lawrence, Kansas 66049

Amanda K. Sanford, Ph.D.
Associate Professor of Special Education
Portland State University
615 SW Harrison Street
Portland, Oregon 97201

Allyson Satter, Ph.D.
Project Coordinator
University of Kansas
1315 Wakarusa Drive
Lawrence, Kansas 66049

Kelly M. Schieltz, Ph.D.
Postdoctoral Psychology Fellow
University of Iowa Children's Hospital
100 Hawkins Drive
Iowa City, Iowa 52242

Kelcey Schmitz, M.S.Ed.
Kansas State Department of Education's Technical
    Assistance System Network
900 SW Jackson Street
Topeka, Kansas 66612

Scott Shepard, M.A.
Director of Avenues Supported Living Services
28415 Industry Drive
Valencia, California 91355

Jeffrey Sprague, Ph.D.
Professor and Codirector
University of Oregon Institute on Violence and
    Destructive Behavior
1265 University of Oregon
Eugene, Oregon 97403

Richard Stock, Ph.D.
Board Certified Behavior Analyst–Doctoral
Capilano University
2055 Purcell Way
North Vancouver, British Columbia V7J 3H5

M. Kathleen Strickland-Cohen, Ph.D.
Assistant Professor
Texas Tech University
PO Box 41071
Lubbock, Texas 79409

Matt Tincani, Ph.D., BCBA-D
Associate Professor
Temple University
1301 Cecil B. Moore Avenue
Philadelphia, Pennsylvania 19380

Anne W. Todd, M.S.
Senior Research Assistant
University of Oregon
1235 University of Oregon
Eugene, Oregon 97401

Bobbie J. Vaughn, Ph.D.
Lead Behavior Analyst
All Children's Hospital Johns Hopkins Medicine
880 6th Street S.
St. Petersburg, Florida 33701

David P. Wacker, Ph.D.
Professor
University of Iowa Children's Hospital
100 Hawkins Drive #251
Iowa City, Iowa 52242

Michael L. Wehmeyer, Ph.D.
Professor of Special Education
University of Kansas
1200 Sunnyside Avenue, Room 3136
Lawrence, Kansas 66213

Deanna Willson-Schafer, M.A.
Inclusion Support Teacher and Program Specialist
Ukiah Unified School District
511 S. Orchard Avenue
Ukiah, California 95482

Nikki Wolf, Ph.D.
Assistant Research Professor
Beach Center on Disability, University of Kansas
1200 Sunnyside Avenue
Lawrence, Kansas 66045

Leah Wood, ABD
Snyder Fellow and Graduate Research Assistant
University of North Carolina at Charlotte
9201 University City Boulevard
Charlotte, North Carolina 28223

Mary Wrenn, M.A.
Speech and Language Therapist
Willard Middle School
2425 Stuart Street
Berkeley, California 94705

Foreword

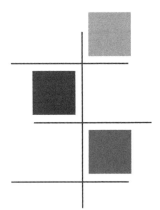

Rud and Ann Turnbull

Personal narratives connect the past with the present by enabling the narrator to explain the "why" and "how" of a drama begun long ago but persisting even now. More than that, the narrative requires the narrator to reflect on the past and to interpret it. Here, then, is a personal narrative that forewords the usual foreword. It is by Rud Turnbull. Ann and Rud then introduce the book with a more formal foreword.

*   *   *

The year is 1973; the place, a science-driven institution for those then known as "the mentally retarded." The setting is a large conference room filled with administrators; psychiatrists; and other physicians, psychologists, social workers, nurses, clergy, and institutionally appointed patient advocates.

I am there because the state's governor asked me, as the father of a child with intellectual disabilities and a lawyer on the faculty of the state's flagship university, to investigate "aversive therapy." The governor had received complaints about it from families of "patients" and was determined to learn what it was and why it spawned concerns.

The presentation about aversive therapy begins. Psychologists explain about baseline data. Being from New York City, I knew

"baseline" was a marker at Ebbetts Field, where my beloved Brooklyn Dodgers played baseball when I was a kid.

The psychologists explained about baselines and about the injury that residents do to themselves and other residents, the risk they pose to staff, and their need to be deterred from these behaviors.

They explain about drug therapy, behavior modification, restraints, and a new technique. It is the "learning to be better box." That device allows them to "correct inappropriate behavior" and then chart subsequent and presumably appropriate behavior against the baseline data.

I ask, "Tell me about the box. What does it do?"

They answer, "When a resident misbehaves, we hold him down, lift his shirt and lower his pants, and use the box on his lower abdomen, where the skin is very sensitive."

I: "What does the box do?"

Answer: "It corrects his behavior."

I: "You are not answering my question. Let me see the box, please."

Answer: "It's in another building."

I: "Please go get it."

Answer: "It's far away."

I: "I am asking you to get it and let me see it and how it works. It seems to me that you are thwarting the governor's request for me to investigate. I am requesting that you get it and show me how it works. Do that now or else I will report to the governor that you refused to cooperate with his personally appointed investigator."

Minutes pass; we all await the courier; he arrives, box in hand.

It is a strange plywood contraption, obviously handmade. It is between 3 and 4 inches square. Two battery nodules protrude from one side, connected by copper wire. A switch on another side is in the usual, switch-down, off position.

I: "Have many of you have used this on yourselves?"

*Answer, with obvious incredulity: "Oh, no! It's for **them**!"*

I remove my blazer, roll up my sleeve, turn on the switch, and apply the copper wire to my bare arm. I am jolted out of a comfortable position in my chair, involuntarily rising some 3 to 4 inches.

And that is how my professional career began. A literally shocking experience impelled me to conduct research on the use of aversive therapy and then to advocate for legal reform.

*   *   *

Neither of us knew at the time that this "aversive therapy" and other such interventions were widely accepted by some members of the scientific community. We soon learned that they were, despite a growing number of professionals, family members, and other advocates who condemned aversives and sought a better way to replace problem behavior with appropriate behavior.

Of the leaders in this reform movement, none was more transformative than Madeleine Will, Assistant Secretary of Education, U.S. Department of Education. Guided by her sensitivities as the parent of a son with intellectual disability, Will determined that there would be a better way: to establish a research and training center to investigate what was referred to at that time as nonaversive behavioral interventions; to fund researchers and

trainers such as Ted Carr, Rob Horner, Glen Dunlap, Wayne Sailor, Bob and Lynn Koegel, and Jacki L. Anderson; and to persuade U.S. Assistant Attorney General William Bradford Reynolds, whose sister was institutionalized, to become personally involved in investigating institutional abuse and aversive interventions.

This book tells the result of approximately 3 decades of positive behavior support (PBS) research. A word or two about those decades enriches the content of this book.

In the early 1980s, the disability rights movement was in its infancy. The right to treatment, manifested in the strategy of deinstitutionalization by repairing institutional conditions, preventing institutional placement, and ensuring release from institutions; the right to education; the right of newborns to receive treatment and not to suffer preventable death because physicians or parents colluded to withhold or withdraw lifesaving medical treatment from them; the right to not experience discrimination solely because of a disability and the search for employment strategies to accompany that right; and the establishment of early intervention and early childhood education—all these initiatives arose within short time frames of each other, were synergistic in their effect, and had scientific bases.

What might be said of this explosion of rights and associated science? At the very least, and perhaps most important of all, it must be said that what passed as acceptable at one time became unacceptable.

Specific to aversive interventions, some scientists defended the intervention on the ground that it was necessary to prevent self-injurious or aggressive behavior. They based their argument solely on science. Their opponents—scientists, lawyers, parents, and other advocates—asserted the contrary proposition that using science as a morally and legally objectionable strategy would not be the only ground for debate.

Indeed, those who relied on ethical and legal challenges to aversive interventions affirmed science's value and the body of scientific knowledge. They demanded, however, that scientists must create a science of positive interventions: "Do no harm; use no 'learning to be better' boxes. Do only what is positive, not punishing; do only evidence-based practices that can withstand ethical and legal muster."

Thus it was that the science of PBS arose out of a sometimes objectionable science. The search for a new science and the marriage of ethics, law, and research focusing on positive, comprehensive lifestyle change, ecological focus, prevention, multidisciplinary partnerships, and systems-level change, were the seeds of PBS. And this science, today, has majestically reformed the lives of people with disabilities (including our beloved son) and their families (including ours).

Our friend and mentor, Ted Carr, one of the fathers of PBS, envisioned PBS as follows, notably combining science with ethics and law that requires system change:

> What are happiness, helpfulness, and hopefulness as they pertain to PBS? Collectively, they represent an empirically driven concern with QOL [quality of life], with support through systems changes, and with linkage to multiple behavioral, social, and biomedical sciences. This is the expanding vision of PBS, a vision that impels us to create meaningful lives and not simply to eliminate psychopathology, a vision that spurs us to change systems and not just people, a vision that motivates us to

seek collaborative possibilities with our colleagues in many different sciences to that we can transcend our superficial differences and focus on deeper commonalities. It is a vision that holds promise for each one of us so that at the end of our lives we can say, "I made a difference." (Carr, 2007, p. 12)

We admonish you to use the accumulated knowledge in this book to become like Ted Carr: a difference maker.

And while you are at it, remember this: "Knowledge itself is power" (Orwell, 1945). That is true, however, only when the powerful use science that rests on morally and legally defensible grounds. The evolution of science results in a revolution of quality of life only when three disciplines inform each other: science, ethics, and law. That is the essential teaching about PBS. It is a science born of many sources. It is the science you will learn by reading and rereading this book. PBS is a science without hidden boxes.

Rud and Ann Turnbull
Distinguished Professors of Special Education
Codirectors, Beach Center on Disability
University of Kansas

REFERENCES

Carr, E.G. (2007). The expanding vision of positive behavior support: Research perspectives on happiness, helpfulness, hopefulness. *Journal of Positive Behavior Interventions, 9,* 3–14.

Orwell, G. (1945). *Animal farm.* London, England: Secker and Warburg.

Preface

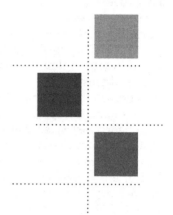

Individual Positive Behavior Supports: A Standards-Based Guide to Practices in School and Community Settings brings together the work of leading scholars to present the foundational knowledge, skills, and dispositions needed to effectively and respectfully support individuals who engage in challenging behaviors. Relying on both the science and the technology of positive behavior support (PBS), this book explores the standard-based competencies that are necessary for individuals, their families, and professionals who work with people who experience challenging behavior across ages, disabilities, and settings.

The book is intended to be comprehensive in scope, and as such, it explores a wide range of topics such as the history of PBS; applied behavior analysis; effective teaming; collaboration with individuals, families, professionals, and other stakeholders; systems-level supports; and examples of the assessment, development, and implementation of multicomponent plans of PBS. The book is organized into the following major sections: I) Foundations of Positive Behavior Support, II) Basic Principles of Behavior, III) Comprehensive Function-Based and Person-Centered Assessments, IV) Function-Driven Interventions, V) Comprehensive Multielement Positive Behavior Support Plans, and VI) Future Directions. The chapters in this book are aligned with the Association for

Positive Behavior Support (APBS) Standards of Practice–Individual Level (SOP-I). These standards were designed to encompass the skills that practitioners of PBS should espouse that underscore both the science *and* values of PBS. To impart these skills, we have invited contributions from leading scholars, researchers, self-advocates, family members, and practitioners in the field of PBS.

POSITIVE BEHAVIOR SUPPORT AS AN APPLIED SCIENCE

To us, PBS is the *zeitgeist* of what we know and believe about supporting people—how they learn, how they thrive, and how they can strive and achieve a personal vision of a good quality of life. Individual PBS brings together values and science. Many in the field of disabilities claim to use PBS, but what does this mean? For people with chronic or persistent challenging behavior, we know that using positive reinforcement in the absence of building skills that will improve quality of life is not sufficient. We know that using person-centered planning without effectively addressing problem behaviors is not sufficient. We know that avoiding the use of aversive interventions without effectively addressing the problem behaviors is not sufficient. We hope that this book will help readers acquire a deep understanding of PBS as an applied science.

POSITIVE BEHAVIOR SUPPORT STANDARDS OF PRACTICE AT THE INDIVIDUAL LEVEL

Since the mid-1980s, PBS has flourished. In 1999, the *Journal of Positive Behavior Interventions* published its first issue, and in 2003, APBS held its first conference. These important activities helped establish the discipline of PBS (Carr, 2007) and moved the discipline to an internationally recognized applied science in a relatively short period of time. In 2005, APBS made the decision to develop standards of practice for PBS. The board recognized the need for standards of practice given the widespread use of PBS, the multiple disciplines that utilize PBS procedures, and the various theoretical perspectives that professionals bring to their respective PBS practices. Drs. Jacki L. Anderson, Fredda Brown, and Brenda Scheuermann were assigned as cochairs of a new committee to organize and coordinate the process of developing and drafting the standards of practice document. This document was developed through a collaborative effort of many individuals who have committed themselves to research and development of PBS over many years. The SOP-I was approved by the APBS board in 2007. Since then, the SOP-I has been a support to the PBS community in a variety of ways, including the following:

- Encouraging dialogue about PBS within the field
- Encouraging dialogue about PBS with professionals of different philosophical orientations
- Developing applied behavior analysis (ABA) and PBS course competencies in higher education
- Developing ABA and PBS course competencies for professional development
- Developing guidelines (for professionals and families) for evaluating the quality of the assessment and program development process provided for any given individual
- Developing guidelines (for professionals and families) for evaluating the quality of the outcomes and associated processes of PBS
- Developing guidelines (for professionals and families) for evaluating the competence of PBS experts/consultants
- Developing guidelines for selection of university or in-service training programs
- Developing guidelines for individuals considering careers as advocates or consultants in the area of PBS
- Developing guidelines for schools, districts, or agencies for developing job descriptions for special education teachers, PBS intervention specialists, or behavior specialists
- Developing guidelines for grant evaluators to assess quality of proposed training/intervention programs for individual-level supports
- Developing guidelines for local, state, and national policy makers relevant to the provision of behavior support in schools, homes, and communities

Our intent is that this book provide the information necessary to ensure the effective implementation of these standards and PBS practices in general wherever PBS can improve lives.

WHO IS THIS BOOK FOR?

This book was written with a variety of audiences in mind. For the higher education audience, we believe that it will support the work of professors as they teach their graduate classes in the subjects of ABA and PBS and meet the complex task of infusing the values and science of the field. Thus this book is appropriate for graduate classes in the following areas: ABA, PBS, special education methods, and behavior management. Furthermore, it is appropriate for training clinical personnel in educational and community-based settings, including adult, vocational, and residential supports. We also believe that this book will be a valuable resource for families. The focus on quality of life across so many of the chapters, the voices of families, and the different ages and types of disabilities that are used to demonstrate the many PBS concepts will be helpful as families face the many changing challenges as their children grow.

REFERENCE

Carr, E.G. (2007). The expanding vision of positive behavior support: Research perspectives on happiness, helpfulness, hopefulness. *Journal of Positive Behavior Interventions, 9,* 3–14.

Acknowledgments

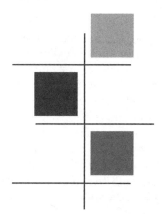

We would like to give our thanks and appreciation to the contributors to this book, to the many contributors to the development of the APBS SOP-I, and to the many families that are working with us to continue to refine and advance the field of positive behavior support. We also would like to express our appreciation to Rebecca Lazo and Steve Plocher from Paul H. Brookes Publishing Co.—without their guidance, support, and nurturance, this book could not have come to fruition. We hope this book helps promote and further the vision of our late friend and mentor of the field, Ted Carr. As he writes,

> Our job is to redesign the counterproductive and unfair environmental contexts that so many people, with and without disabilities, have to contend with every day of their lives. Our job is to give people the skills, the coping strategies, and the desire to deal with the frustration that is an inevitable part of life, particularly the lives of people with disabilities. We must give them and their loved ones the support they need to challenge and reconstruct systems that serve bureaucratic needs rather than human needs. All of these goals reflect the great ideas that are at the heart of PBS, ideas so great that they are worthy of scientific study. (Carr, 2007, p. 3)

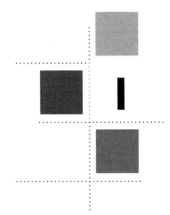

Foundations of
Positive Behavior Support

 STANDARDS ADDRESSED IN THIS SECTION

I. A. Practitioners of positive behavior support (PBS) have the following perspectives on the evolution of PBS and its relationship to applied behavior analysis (ABA) and movements in the disability field:

    1. History of applied behavior analysis and the relationship to PBS

    2. Similarities and unique features of PBS and ABA

    3. Movements in the field of serving people with disabilities that influenced the emergence of PBS practices, including the following:

        a. Deinstitutionalization

        b. Normalization and social role valorization

        c. Community participation

        d. Supported employment

        e. Least restrictive environment and inclusive schooling

        f. Self-determination

I. B. Practitioners applying PBS with individuals adhere to the following basic assumptions about behavior:

    1. Challenging behavior serves a function.

    2. Positive strategies are effective in addressing the most challenging behavior.

    3. When positive behavior intervention strategies fail, additional functional assessment strategies are required to develop more effective PBS strategies.

    4. Features of the environmental context affect behavior.

    5. Reduction of challenging behavior is an important—but not the sole—outcome of successful intervention; effective PBS results in improvements in quality of life, acquisition of valued skills, and access to valued activities.

(continued)

1

I. C. Practitioners applying PBS with individuals include at least 11 key elements in the development of PBS supports:
1. Collaborative team-based decision making
2. Person-centered decision making
3. Self-determination
4. Functional assessment of behavior and functionally derived interventions
5. Identification of outcomes that enhance quality of life and are valued by the individual, their families, and the community
6. Strategies that are acceptable in inclusive community settings
7. Strategies that teach useful and valued skills
8. Strategies that are evidence based and socially and empirically valid to achieve desired outcomes that are at least as effective and efficient as the challenging behavior
9. Techniques that do not cause pain or humiliation or deprive the individual of basic needs
10. Constructive and respectful multicomponent intervention plans that emphasize antecedent interventions, instruction in prosocial behaviors, and environmental modification
11. Ongoing measurement of impact

I. E. Practitioners of PBS understand the following legal and regulatory requirements related to assessment and intervention regarding challenging behavior and behavior change strategies:
1. Requirements of IDEA with respect to PBS
2. State/school/agency regulations and requirements

The four chapters in this first section of the book set a framework for understanding the remaining chapters. The section begins with Chapter 1, "A Historical Perspective on the Evolution of Positive Behavior Support as a Science-Based Discipline." In this chapter, the authors provide us with the historical evolution of positive behavior support (PBS)—from its beginnings in the late 1980s to today. This chapter defines PBS and explores the early movements in the field of disabilities that contributed to the development of PBS, the relationship between applied behavior analysis (ABA) and PBS, and the core features of PBS. In Chapter 2, "Foundational Assumptions About Challenging Behavior and Behavior Interventions," the authors discuss, through the case studies of two individuals, the critical elements that make PBS a unique discipline in its merging of values and science. Chapter 3, "Effective Teaming for Positive Behavior Support," and Chapter 4, "Person-Centered Planning Teams," focus on teaming. In these chapters, we learn about

the importance and the processes involved in developing person-centered behavior support plans that are developed by collaborative teams and aligned with the individual and his or her family's vision of important outcomes. Finally, in Chapter 5, "Supporting Individuals with Challenging Behavior Through Systemic Change," the authors discuss the complex interplay between the environment and the individual's behaviors. Systemic change—such as in the environmental contexts of home, school, community, work, and social systems—is critical for successful and sustainable outcomes for the individuals whom we support.

The chapters in this first section of the book will provide you with a core of information and perspective that will make the chapters that follow more meaningful. It is the synergy of the ideas covered here that will allow you to appreciate the broad impact that PBS has on the lives of individuals with challenging behavior.

Fredda Brown

A Historical Perspective on the Evolution of Positive Behavior Support as a Science-Based Discipline

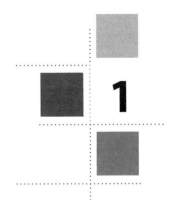

1

Joseph M. Lucyshyn, Glen Dunlap, and Rachel Freeman

The purpose of this chapter is to offer a historical perspective on the development of positive behavior support (PBS) from its beginnings in the late 1980s to its robust state in 2013. We begin with a definition of PBS and a description of its four core features. We then describe the current status of PBS as a scientific discipline. This is followed by an in-depth description of the historical development of PBS as a science-based and values-informed approach to addressing problem behavior and improving the quality of life in both school and community settings.

DEFINITION AND CORE FEATURES

PBS is a practical, science-based approach to understanding and ameliorating problem behavior in individuals across the life span. PBS emphasizes the use of proactive, educative, and reinforcement-based interventions and supports in school and community settings to improve behavior and quality of life

in a manner that is meaningful, durable, and sustainable when implemented by key stakeholders in natural settings (Koegel, Koegel, & Dunlap, 1996; Sailor, Dunlap, Sugai, & Horner, 2009). PBS is a science-based approach in that 1) practices are derived from scientific theory and principles, 2) practices are subjected to formal validation through research, and 3) research is documented and shared in public forums, making it available to all who are interested so that it can be challenged or adopted (Dunlap, Carr, Horner, Zarcone, & Schwartz, 2008; Vaughn & Dammann, 2001). Across settings in which PBS is implemented, four core features stand out: 1) a focus on valued outcomes as defined in collaboration with consumers; 2) the integration of behavioral, biomedical, and social science; 3) the selection and use of empirically validated procedures; and 4) the promotion of systems change as necessary to sustain positive outcomes. These core features are described in the following sections.

Valued Outcomes

PBS promotes changes in behavior, skills, and quality of life that are valued by the individual receiving support and by his or her advocates, such as parents, teachers, and typical support personnel. In addition to preventing and minimizing problem behavior, a PBS process aims to produce substantial and sustainable improvements in the lifestyle of the individual. These outcomes include increasing the person's 1) successful inclusion and competence in school and community settings; 2) ability to appropriately and effectively communicate his or her wants and needs; and 3) quality of life, as defined by their interests and preferences as well as by those of their advocates (Sailor et al., 2009).

Integration of Behavioral, Biomedical, and Social Science

PBS is grounded in the philosophy of contextualism (Morris, 1988) and in the scientific discipline of applied behavior analysis (ABA). ABA, the science of human behavior (Baer, Wolf, & Risley, 1968), provides the primary conceptual and empirical foundation for assessment and intervention design in PBS. The four-part operant model of setting events/establishing operations, antecedent stimuli, target behaviors, and maintaining consequences, validated across a century of behavior research, provides the theoretical backbone for the design of individualized PBS plans. In addition, PBS is informed by other scientific disciplines. For example, biomedical science has contributed to the design of setting event interventions for people with physiological challenges (Carr & Herbert, 2008). Developmental psychology has informed the design of PBS services for young children at risk for behavior problems (Hemmeter, Ostrosky, & Fox, 2006). Principles and processes learned from implementation science[1] have contributed

to the development of systems-level applications of PBS, such as schoolwide positive behavior support (SWPBS) at the school district and state levels (Fixsen, Naoom, Blase, Friedman, & Wallace, 2005; Horner et al., 2009). Cognitive psychology and the new discipline of positive psychology have contributed to an understanding of the importance of self-efficacy and optimism when teaching parents to implement PBS in home settings (Durand, Hieneman, Clarke, Wang, & Rinaldi, 2013).

Empirically Validated Practices

Practitioners of PBS implement interventions that have been validated by empirical research. The applied technologies of behavior change and instruction, developed over 50 years of behavior and educational research with children, youth, and adults, offer a broad range of evidence-based procedures that comprise the components of behavior support plans (Cooper, Heron, & Heward, 2007). In addition, an applied technology of positive behavior intervention, developed over the past 20 years, has added to this evidentiary base (Luiselli, 2006; Scheuermann & Hall, 2012). As evidence-based practitioners, the selection of behavior support strategies is based on three considerations: 1) empirical evidence; 2) clinical expertise and resources available; and 3) the values, preferences, and context of consumers (Spring & Hitchcock, 2009).

Systems Change

PBS practitioners recognize the importance of understanding the natural systems in which interventions are to be implemented and of ensuring that these systems promote rather than hinder plan implementation. Systems theory and its application to families and schools have informed the integration of a systems approach into PBS

---

[1] *Implementation science* is the scientific study of the variables and methods that promote the sustainable adoption and implementation of evidence-based interventions in the fields of health, psychology, and education.

(Lucyshyn, Dunlap, & Albin, 2002; Sugai & Horner, 2002). Practitioners address the family or organizational systems that may need to be strengthened if behavior interventions are to be implemented with fidelity and sustained over time. Family system considerations include the strengths and needs of family subsystems (e.g., marital, sibling, extended family), the quality of family interactions, and the family's position along the life cycle. School system considerations include organizational structures, policies and guiding principles, administrative leadership, resource supports, and professional development opportunities.

CURRENT STATUS AS A SCIENCE-BASED DISCIPLINE

From its beginnings in the late 1980s, PBS has grown into an emerging science-based discipline that has found adherents in the United States, Canada, Australia, and Europe among general and special educators, school administrators, psychologists, social workers, behavior analysts, and families (McIntosh, Bennett, & Price, 2011; Sailor et al., 2009). Features of PBS also have become part of established education law in the United States. In 1997, the U.S. Congress passed into law amendments to the Individual with Disabilities Education Act (IDEA; PL 105-17) that require public school individualized education program (IEP) teams to conduct functional behavioral assessments (FBAs) for children with disabilities who are at risk for out-of-school placement and to consider the use of positive behavior interventions and supports (PBIS) if the children's behaviors impede their learning or that of other students (Turnbull & Turnbull, 2000). These provisions of law were maintained in the 2004 reauthorization of IDEA (PL 108-446), which authorized state and federal funding for preservice and in-service training in whole-school PBS (Von Ravensberg & Tobin, 2008).

To establish PBS as a full-fledged scientific discipline (Vaughn & Dammann, 2001), in the late 1990s and early 2000s, the PBS leadership, inspired by the vision of Dr. Edward Carr, developed venues for the publication of empirical research, dissemination of knowledge, and nurturing of a community of adepts (i.e., skilled practitioners) among researchers and practitioners. A peer-reviewed journal, the *Journal of Positive Behavior Interventions* (*JPBI*), was started (http://pbi.sagepub.com); the Association for Positive Behavior Support (APBS) was founded (http://www.apbs.org); and a yearly international conference was initiated where researchers and practitioners could share current knowledge about the science and practice of PBS in school and community settings (Dunlap & Koegel, 1999; Knoster, Anderson, Carr, Dunlap, & Horner, 2003). In 2007, the APBS Board of Directors, in collaboration with its membership, developed a comprehensive description of PBS standards of practice at the individual level in order to operationalize the concepts and methods essential to the implementation of PBS with people who engage in problem behavior (http://www.apbs.org/standards _of_practice.html; Anderson et al., 2007).

HISTORICAL FOUNDATIONS OF POSITIVE BEHAVIOR SUPPORT

PBS emerged in the late 1980s from three major developments that converged to require a new approach to behavior support: 1) the disability rights movement of the 1960s, 1970s, and 1980s; 2) the emergence of a powerful instructional and intervention technology based on ABA; and 3) the limitations of behavioral technology that relied on *aversive* procedures for controlling challenging behaviors in people with severe disabilities. As advocates succeeded in promoting the rights of people with disabilities to live and participate in the community, a pressing need for effective and socially acceptable strategies of behavior support became increasingly apparent. While advocates pushed for inclusion in school and community settings, the principles and methods of ABA, such as stimulus control and functional analysis, provided the conceptual foundation for procedural solutions to behavior support. This convergence of advocacy and science propelled the establishment of PBS. The factors involved are discussed in more detail in the sections that follow.

Disability Rights Movement

Advocacy for the rights of people with developmental disabilities began in the 1960s and culminated in new U.S. federal laws in the 1970s and 1980s, protecting and advancing the rights of these people. The legal basis for this movement was the 14th Amendment of the U.S. Constitution, with its due process and equal protection clauses that guarantee equal access to life, liberty, and property. It was a movement in three parts: 1) the deinstitutionalization of large aggregate state facilities, 2) the provision of a free and appropriate public school education, and 3) the normalization of adult services in regard to community living and employment.

Deinstitutionalization Strong national discontent with large state institutions for people with developmental disabilities was spurred in the 1960s by the publication of *Christmas in Purgatory* (Blatt & Kaplan, 1966), in which the abject, warehouse-like conditions of the Willowbrook Institution in New York were exposed. In the 1970s, the deinstitutionalization lawsuit, *Halderman v. Pennhurst*—in which a district court ordered the state of Pennsylvania to develop community placements for Pennhurst residents—served to catalyze a national movement to deinstitutionalize large institutions and develop community-based living options (Halderman v. Pennhurst, 1978). At the same time, many of the people who were being moved to community placements were in need of effective and acceptable social and behavior supports.

Right to Education The next advocacy movement helped secure the right to public education for children with disabilities. In the 1970s, lawsuits initiated by parents and their advocates (e.g., *Pennsylvania Association for Retarded Citizens [PARC] v. Commonwealth of Pennsylvania,* 1972; *Mills v. D.C. Board of Education,* 1972) culminated in passage by the U.S. Congress of the landmark federal law, the Education for All Handicapped Children Act of 1975 (PL 94-142, 20 U.S.C. 1401 *et. seq.*). PL 94-142 required public schools to provide equal access to education for school-age children with disabilities in the least restrictive environment (LRE) possible—that is, an educational setting in which school-age children with disabilities have the opportunity to interact with typically developing peers and in which IEPs provide an equal opportunity to learn (Turnbull & Turnbull, 2000). Renewal of the act in 1986 (PL 99-457) extended this right to young children with developmental disabilities, including preschool services for children ages 3 to 5 and early intervention services for infants and children up to age 3. As with the push for deinstitutionalization, the LRE movement brought children with behavioral challenges into direct contact with the broader public, and this carried with it the additional need for effective and acceptable interventions and supports.

Normalization The normalization movement and its advocates sought the right to community living and a valued life for adults with developmental disabilities (Wolfensberger, 1972). Guided by the normalization principle of supporting people with disabilities to achieve a life as culturally normative as possible, through means that are as culturally normative as possible, advocates sought legislation that would establish a right to employment and independent living. These efforts led to the passage of the Rehabilitation Act of 1973 (PL 93-112), which protects individuals with disabilities from discrimination based on their disabilities, authorizes vocational rehabilitation and supported employment for adults, and establishes independent living services throughout the United States. Administrative guidelines emphasize empowerment, self-determination, inclusion in society, and preservation of individual dignity.

Applied Behavior Analysis

Principles of learning, such as operant conditioning, positive and negative reinforcement, and punishment, were first successfully applied to people in the 1950s and early 1960s, after decades of scientific development with nonhuman organisms by early behavioral scientists such as Watson, Thorndike, and Skinner (Cooper et al., 2007). B.F. Skinner, with his elegant experiments that illuminated behavioral principles with precision and his philosophical writings on behaviorism, founded the new science of the experimental analysis of behavior and laid the conceptual and methodological groundwork for ABA. Early applications of operant principles with children and adults in institutional, school, and home settings yielded promising results (Ulrich, Stachnik, & Mabry, 1970) and gave birth to the scientific discipline of ABA (Baer, Wolf, & Risley, 1968). In 1968, the *Journal of Applied Behavior Analysis* was launched to disseminate scientific knowledge about a practical technology of behavior change aimed at improving socially significant behavior in children, youth, and adults.

By the time that the disability rights movement achieved momentum, ABA was recognized as the primary technology for teaching children, youth, and adults with disabilities, including severe disabilities, in school and community settings (Alberto & Troutman, 1986). Given this development, disability rights advocates, behavioral psychologists, and special educators formed a natural alliance that helped advance the deinstitutionalization movement and the inclusion of people with severe disabilities in neighborhood schools and communities. People with severe disabilities were institutionalized because it was widely accepted that they could not be taught. Behavioral researchers and special educators, however, offered empirical evidence that people with severe disabilities could be taught when behavioral principles of learning were effectively applied (Bijou, 1972; Guess, Sailor, & Baer, 1977; Noonan, Brown, Mulligan, & Rettig, 1982). Indeed, by the 1980s, the contributions of ABA to the education and treatment of people with severe disabilities in school and community environments were vast. Behavioral and learning theory played key roles in the development of special education instructional technology, including methods to teach language and communication skills, imitation skills, life skills, academic skills, social skills, and generalized skills (Sailor, Wilcox, & Brown, 1980; Snell, 1987).

In 1974, the American Association for the Education of the Severely/Profoundly Handicapped (AAESPH) was established as an advocacy and scientific organization dedicated to promoting the full inclusion of people with severe and profound disabilities in society and to conducting empirical research that advanced this mission. In 1980, the name of the organization was changed to the Association for the Severely Handicapped (TASH), and in 1983 the organization adopted its current name, The Association for Persons with Severe Handicaps. TASH represented a union of advocacy with advances in behavioral and instructional technology. The organization's flagship journal, the *AAESPH Review* (changed to the *Journal of The Association for Persons with Severe Handicaps* [*JASH*] in 1980 and *Research and Practice for Persons with Severe Disabilities* [*RPSD*] in 2002) contributed empirical knowledge about the use of behavioral principles to effectively teach students with severe handicaps in school and community settings (Horner, Meyer, & Fredericks, 1986). In addition, the TASH leadership advanced the notion that to achieve meaningful and positive outcomes with people with severe disabilities, science and values need to be integrated and have reciprocal influence on each other (Peck, 1991).

Limits of Intervention Technology and Problems with Aversive Consequences

Although ABA provided the behavioral technology that made instruction and inclusion feasible for persons with severe disabilities, the behavior management options that were offered and promoted in the 1970s and 1980s were limited both conceptually and procedurally. Little to no attention was given to procedures that prevented problem behavior. Procedures tended to emphasize behavior management through the influence of contingencies of reinforcement and punishment, including the use of aversive consequences for the most serious problem behavior (Repp & Singh, 1990). Aversive stimuli that were used in the 1970s and 1980s with this population included procedures that caused physical pain (e.g., pinching, slapping, contingent electric shock) or discomfort (e.g., water mist in face, unsweetened lemon juice in mouth) or were considered disrespectful or dehumanizing (e.g., shaving cream in mouth). Such procedures were originally developed in the insulated environment of institutions, where early behavior research with people with severe disabilities was conducted. However, the success of the disability rights movement and the subsequent presence of people with severe disabilities in homes, schools, and workplaces in the community brought these procedures under new and often critical scrutiny.

Opposing Perspectives on Use of Aversives

Opposition to the use of aversive stimulation as a punishment technique was based on several arguments: 1) aversive procedures ran counter to fundamental human values of treating others with respect and dignity; 2) procedures that caused physical pain or tissue damage violated the basic ethical principle of doing no harm to others (Singer, Gert, & Koegel, 1999); 3) aversive stimulation, when implemented without the informed assent or consent of the person or his or her guardians, violated the person's due process and equal protection rights (Turnbull, Stowe, Wilcox, Raper, & Hedges, 2000); and 4) scientific research on the use of punishment showed several side effects, including counteraggression, a decrease in positive behavior, and avoidance of the punishing agent or situation (Newsom, Favell, & Rincover, 1983). Based on these arguments, lawsuits were filed by parents and advocates against school districts and residential programs in which staff used aversive procedures with children and adults with disabilities (Seiden & Zirkel, 1989). In response, human rights committees were set up by school districts and states to monitor and regulate the use of punishment procedures within behavior intervention plans (BIPs; Spreat & Lanzi, 1989). Finally, professional organizations such as TASH and the American Association on Mental Retardation (AAMR; changed to the American Association on Intellectual and Developmental Disabilities [AAIDD] in 2007) put forth position papers that called for the elimination of aversive practices that caused tissue damage or physical pain; were dehumanizing; or evoked extreme discomfort in family members, teachers, or staff (Singh, Lloyd, & Kendall, 1990).

There were other practitioners and researchers, however, who held a different perspective. They viewed the use of aversive stimulation such as contingent electric shock or water mist as acceptable for individuals who engaged in severe problem behavior such as self-injury or physical aggression that put the person with a disability or others at risk for physical harm. They argued that if alternative methods failed, then the person had a right to treatment that included aversive stimulation (Van Houten et al., 1988). In support of this position, professional organizations such as the Association for Behavior Analysis (ABA; changed to the Association for Behavior Analysis International [ABAI] in 1974) and the American Psychological Association (APA) put forth position papers supporting a right to effective treatment, including the use of more aversive procedures, and outlined professional standards for evidence-based assessment and intervention, peer and human rights review, and criteria for success (Singh et al., 1990). In short, a controversy developed regarding the use of aversive procedures, and it became apparent that there was a great need for a technology of behavior management that could be effective in resolving severe problem behavior in a manner that was acceptable to the broader society and that relied on nonaversive techniques.

Initial Steps Toward a Nonaversive Approach In the mid- to late 1980s, these contrasting points of view inspired the first efforts to articulate and develop a nonaversive approach to behavior management. Evans and Meyer (1985) and Lavigna and Donnellan (1986) published the first books to describe an educative approach to treating problem behavior in people with severe disabilities. These were followed by the publication of a seminal case study by Berkman and Meyer (1988) on the successful use of nonaversive strategies to ameliorate severe self-injurious behavior in a 45-year-old man with a severe intellectual disability. In a follow-up book on nonaversive intervention for problem behavior, Meyer and Evans (1989) offered an initial outline of a nonaversive approach that included functional assessment, quality-of-life improvements, functional communication training, positive reinforcement, and mild consequences for problem behavior (e.g., brief withdrawal of positive attention or restricted access to preferred activities).

Given the disability rights laws and their requirements and court litigation on the use of aversive procedures, the U.S. federal government recognized the importance of advancing the science of behavior management toward a more positive and preventive approach. In 1986, the National Institute on Disability and Rehabilitation Research (NIDRR) of the Department of Education put out a Request for Proposals for a "Rehabilitation Research and Training Center (RRTC) on Community-Referenced, Nonaversive Behavior Management." The grant was awarded in 1987 to the University of Oregon and a consortium of collaborating universities, including the State University of New York at Stony Brook, Marshall University (later moving to the University of South Florida in 1988), the University of California at Santa Barbara, San Francisco State University (later moving to the University of Kansas in 1992), and California State University at Hayward. The mission of the consortium, as described in an influential paper (Horner et al., 1990), was to develop a technology of PBS that emphasized the use of preventive and educative strategies and produced rapid, consistent, durable, and generalized changes in problem behavior, while facilitating the development of broad improvements in quality of life. Within this technology, although the judicious use of mild consequence procedures such as withholding the functional reinforcer for problem behavior (i.e., extinction) and brief time-out from reinforcement remained potential components of behavior support plans, consequences that caused tissue damage, physical pain or discomfort, or humiliation or loss of dignity were deemed unacceptable.

Guidance for the Initial Development of Positive Behavior Support

Consortium members along with like-minded scholars and practitioners of PBS (Evans & Meyer, 1985; Gaylord-Ross, 1980; Lavigna & Donnellan, 1986) believed that the solution to the aversive versus nonaversive debate lay in the applied foundations of early ABA as well as new behavioral research. With respect to the early heritage of ABA, Dunlap (2006) pointed to five key features that were conspicuously relevant to the development of the applied science of human behavior: 1) a focus on practical solutions to human problems, 2) a quest for meaningful impact, 3) an emphasis on ecological validity, 4) a commitment to collaboration, and

5) the belief that ideas are more important than ideologies. In addition, five important developments offered important guidance for the design of PBS in light of the effort to preclude the need for aversive procedures in school and community settings. These developments were 1) functional analysis, 2) functional equivalence and functional communication training, 3) antecedent influences on problem behavior, 4) social validity, and 5) collaborative research with consumers.

Functional Analysis By the 1980s, as noted by Mace, Lalli, Lalli, and Shea, a trend in ABA research was "toward the development and evaluation of intervention procedures without analyzing the variables responsible for problem behavior" (1993, p. 76). At that time, few studies that addressed problem behavior utilized functional analysis in the design of interventions (Dietz, 1978). This trend inspired calls by other behavior analysts to return to the field's functional analytic roots (Durand, 1987; Pierce & Epling, 1980). Iwata, Dorsey, Slifer, Bauman, and Richman (1982) contributed to the revival of functional analysis by documenting the use of an elegant, efficient, and effective method for conducting functional analyses. Durand (1987) argued that the use of functional analysis in the design of behavior interventions would contribute to the development of strategies to teach alternatives to severe problem behavior that would diminish the need for aversive procedures.

Functional Equivalence Seminal research in the 1970s and 1980s on the communicative functions of problem behavior in people with severe disabilities showed that problem behaviors were purposeful, achieving the functions of, for example, escape from a difficult task or attention from others (Carr, 1977). Additional research demonstrated the functional equivalence of problem behavior and adaptive communicative behavior—that is, a person with a severe disability will engage in either problem behavior or adaptive communicative behavior, depending on which behavior is more effective and efficient at achieving the desired function (Durand & Crimmins, 1987). These findings led to the development of functional communication training as an effective and efficient procedure for ameliorating severe problem behavior in people with developmental disabilities (Carr & Durand, 1985).

Antecedent Influences on Behavior In the 1980s, applied behavior analytic research began to examine antecedent influences on human behavior, with a focus on proximal antecedent stimuli that occasioned problem behavior or desired behavior (Dunlap & Koegel, 1980; Singer, Singer, & Horner, 1987). These studies provided preliminary evidence, for example, that child-preferred activities, stimulus variation, and high-probability request sequences occasioned desired behavior in children with developmental disabilities. The research offered direction for the empirical development of an antecedent-based technology of problem behavior prevention based on the behavioral principle of stimulus control (Luiselli & Cameron, 1998). In addition, although little to no research existed on the influence of setting events or establishing operations on human behavior, there was growing recognition of the importance of understanding and incorporating these influences into behavioral assessment and intervention (Wahler & Fox, 1981).

Social Validity Beginning in the late 1970s, leaders in the field of behavior analysis recognized that if ABA was to become an integral part of the knowledge of North American society, then the technology would need to be viewed as important and acceptable to consumers. In a seminal paper, Montrose Wolf (1978) coined the term *social validity* and defined it as consumers' assessment of the acceptability, importance, and viability of a behavioral intervention's goals, procedures, and outcomes. He argued that in addition to objective measures of behavior change, behavior analysts also needed to include social validity as a subjective measure when evaluating the effects of an intervention. Schwartz and Baer (1991) reiterated this message and expanded on it, describing methods for designing social validity measures and offering guidelines for their use. In particular, they suggested that the widespread use of social validity assessments might contribute to the successful dissemination of the technology of behavior change.

Collaborative Research with Consumers In 1991, Stephen Fawcett published an influential paper in *JABA* in which he argued that to address more difficult problems at an ecological scale in community settings, applied behavior analysts would do well to embrace a broader set of standards and values that guided research (Fawcett, 1991). Borrowing from the field of community psychology (Rappaport, 1987), these values included 1) developing collaborative relationships with consumers in which research goals and behavioral interventions would be selected and designed together; 2) using ecologically valid research methods such as selecting natural settings for intervention and measuring the extent to which community members are able to implement and sustain interventions and outcomes over long periods of time; and 3) disseminating research results effectively by establishing standards for use to ensure implementation fidelity, providing technical assistance and support to embed interventions in natural environments, and adapting interventions to fit local conditions. This call for collaborative research was also consistent with the views of disability researchers who made a strong case for the use of participatory action research methods to bridge the gap between research and practice for people with disabilities and their families (Bruyere, 1993; Turnbull, Friesen, & Ramirez, 1995).

Defining a Technology of Positive Behavior Support

The special educators and behavioral psychologists who initiated the development of a technology of PBS were enthusiastic about these new directions in the assessment and treatment of severe problem behavior and the dissemination of this knowledge to consumers. These developments led to the creation of an ecological model of ABA based on an expanded framework for functional assessment and intervention design (Horner, Albin, Sprague, & Todd, 2000; Martens & Witt, 1988; O'Neill et al., 1997). The ecological model, based on response class theory and the behavioral principle of stimulus control, included five components: 1) setting events and establishing operations, 2) the value of available consequences, 3) antecedent stimuli, 4) competing behavior response options, and 5) maintaining consequences and their function(s) (Sprague & Horner, 1999). These components were organized into a *competing behavior pathways diagram* that provided a more complete representation of problem behavior and adaptive behavior within the behavioral stream in natural environments (O'Neill et al., 1997). In addition, below the pathways diagram, a table for selecting interventions logically linked to functional assessment results was included to guide the development of multicomponent PBS plans composed of setting event strategies, antecedent strategies, teaching strategies, and consequence strategies.

The competing behavior pathways diagram served to organize the results of a functional assessment in a manner that, in addition to making clear the behavioral structure of problem behavior, also made clear the structure of a solution, characterized by desired behavior and functionally equivalent replacement behavior. This innovation generated new opportunities for the dissemination of ABA to consumers by offering a conceptually rich but visually simple understanding about how the laws of behavior operate in natural, complex environments to maintain problem behavior. Given these qualities, the ecological model was widely adopted by practitioners and researchers in school and community settings in the 1990s and successfully introduced consumers to the elegance and power of the science of behavior change.

The special educators and behavioral psychologists who initiated the development of a technology of PBS, in concert with other scholars, practitioners, and advocates, also sought to integrate values into the emerging science of PBS. They drew these values from those fundamental to civil society and the professions of special education and psychology, as well as those embedded in new special education laws. This effort was aided by the prior and concurrent work of leaders within the TASH organization to define values that would be part of a nonaversive approach to behavior support. These included 1) honoring the dignity of people with disabilities, 2) collaborating with consumers, 3) promoting the full inclusion of people with disabilities, 4) providing training and support to implementers from an empowerment framework (Rappaport, 1987), 5) supporting self-determination in the lives of people with disabilities (Wehmeyer & Schwartz, 1997), and 6) nurturing intellectual humility so that practitioners and researchers remain open and responsive to the perspectives and input of others. Based on this first synthesis of science and values, Horner et al. (1990)

defined the new technology of PBS for people with disabilities who engaged in severe problem behavior as consisting of 10 features (see Table 1.1).

Initial Empirical Development and Dissemination of Positive Behavior Support

The emerging features of PBS (Horner et al., 1990) guided two decades of research and practice aimed at developing, validating, and extending an evidence-based technology of PBS. For the most part, initial studies focused on individual or small groups of children, youth, and adults with developmental disabilities and problem behavior in school and community settings. Concurrent with research, efforts were initiated to disseminate PBS to states throughout the United States. For example, Anderson, Russo, Dunlap, and Albin (1996) developed state training teams to implement a comprehensive PBS training curriculum focused on function-based, individualized behavior support to children and adults with developmental disabilities and severe problem behavior. These teams were composed of representatives of local and state governments, school districts, adult service agencies, and disability advocacy organizations. Following the initial success of these research and dissemination activities, researchers expanded their focus to students

Table 1.1.   Initial features of a technology of positive behavior support

1. Promoting improvements in quality of life

2. Conducting functional analysis and/or assessment

3. Designing multicomponent intervention plans

4. Manipulating setting events and establishing operations

5. Manipulating antecedent stimuli to prevent problem behavior

6. Teaching adaptive behavior, including desire behavior and alternative replacement behavior

7. Using effective consequences that increase reinforcement for positive behavior and diminish or remove reinforcement for problem behavior

8. Minimizing the use of punishers and refraining from use of aversive procedures that bring pain, physical discomfort, humiliation, or a loss of dignity

9. Distinguishing emergency procedures from proactive programming

10. Assessing social validity and ensuring the role of dignity in behavior support

Source: Horner et al. (1990).

at risk for or with behavior disorders. The following is a brief summary of these initial research and dissemination efforts.

Positive Behavior Support Research with Persons with Developmental Disabilities

Three initial lines of research were pursued with children, youth, and adults with developmental disabilities (e.g., autism, intellectual disability, multiple disabilities). First, single-case experimental studies documented the effectiveness of antecedent-based interventions for preventing problem behavior and occasioning positive behavior. These strategies included 1) proximal antecedent strategies such as offering choices, modifying curricular features of instructional activities, and increasing predictability (Dunlap, Foster-Johnson, Clarke, Kern, & Childs, 1995; Flannery & Horner, 1994; Koegel, Dyer, & Bell, 1987) and 2) distal or global setting event strategies such as eliminating the setting event, implementing neutralizing routines, or reducing physical pain (Carr, Smith, Giacin, Whelan, & Pancari, 2003; Horner, Day, & Day, 1997).

Second, single-case experimental studies offered evidence of the acceptability, effectiveness, and durability of functional assessment[2] or functional analysis–based multicomponent behavior support plans implemented by 1) parents in family settings (Buschbacher, Fox, & Clarke, 2004; Clarke, Dunlap, & Vaughn, 1999; Lucyshyn, Albin, & Nixon, 1997), 2) teachers in early childhood education and public school settings (Duda, Dunlap, Fox, Lentini, & Clarke, 2004; Dunlap, Kern-Dunlap, Clarke, & Robbins, 1991), 3) care providers and job coaches in community and work settings (Carr & Carlson, 1993; Kemp & Carr, 1995), and 4) key stakeholders across school and community settings (Carr et al., 1999; Feldman, Condillac, Tough, Hunt, & Griffiths, 2002).

Third, qualitative studies provided insights into the experiences and perspectives of key stakeholders of PBS in school and community settings, such as parents, teachers, adult service providers, and administrators (Fox, Vaughn, Dunlap, & Bucy, 1997; Hieneman & Dunlap, 2000; Turnbull & Ruef, 1997). The knowledge gained from these studies served to inform and improve the relevance, acceptability, and viability of PBS services.

Initial Dissemination of Positive Behavior Support Technology Through State Training Teams

Concurrent with the effort to develop an evidentiary base for a technology of PBS, RRTC consortium members sought to disseminate knowledge about comprehensive, individualized behavior support to practitioners in school and community settings (Anderson et al., 1996; Dunlap et al., 2000). To do so, the consortium invited human service agencies and advocacy organizations in states throughout the United States to apply to form state training teams. Sixteen states were initially selected to participate, and this expanded to 26 state teams by 2002. State training team goals were to improve the quality of life of people with severe disabilities and problem behavior and increase the capacity of local and state agencies to effectively support people with severe disabilities. An in-service training model was developed that used a comprehensive PBS curriculum and a train-the-trainer approach. Training was provided to a broad group of stakeholders, including parents, teachers, adult service providers, university-based educators, administrators, and policy makers. A case study format was used that involved both ongoing coaching of trainers who supported

---

[2] *Functional assessment* (also referred to as *functional behavioral assessment*) is the term used to describe a set of procedures for defining the antecedent and consequent events in the environment that reliably predict and maintain problem behavior. A functional assessment may include interviews; direct observations; rating scales; and systematic, experimental analyses of problem contexts. Functional analysis is a form of experimental analysis in which the functions of behavior are identified by systematically manipulating conditions in the environment and observing the differential effects of these conditions on behavior.

focus individuals in school or community settings and follow-up support of newly trained trainers (Anderson et al., 1996).

Positive Behavior Support Research with Students with Behavior Disorders Given the initial success of research and dissemination efforts focused on people with severe disabilities, researchers sought to extend the emerging evidence-based technology of PBS to children and youth at risk for or with behavior disorders. The high dropout rates and poor postschool outcomes for these children and youth indicated the importance of extending PBS to this population (Walker, Ramsey, & Gresham, 2005). For example, Dunlap and colleagues (Dunlap et al., 1993; Dunlap & Kern, 1993) presented arguments and preliminary empirical evidence for the relevance of functional assessment–based antecedent and multicomponent intervention to improving the behavioral and academic outcomes of children and youth with behavior disorders.

This call to extend the technology of PBS was followed by a cascade of research over the next several years that documented 1) the effectiveness of function-based curricular modifications (e.g., preferred tasks, shorter tasks, choice) for improving the behavior and academic engaged time of students at risk for or with behavior disorders (Kern, Childs, Dunlap, Clarke, & Falk, 1994; Powell & Nelson, 1997) and 2) the effectiveness of function-based multicomponent intervention for improving on-task behavior and/or decreasing disruptive behavior in elementary and secondary schools with children and adolescents at risk for or with behavior disorders (Blair, Umbreit, & Bos, 1999; Ervin, DuPaul, Kern, & Friman, 1998).

Emergence of Positive Behavior Support as a New Science-Based Discipline

The first 15 years (1987–2002) of research and dissemination aimed at developing a practical, effective technology of PBS for use in school and community settings by natural

change agents such as parents, teachers, and adult service providers achieved a remarkable degree of success. These efforts were characterized by 1) empirical research using both quantitative and qualitative methods; 2) dissemination of functional assessment and PBS practices in schools and communities in collaboration with state training teams; and 3) the integration of knowledge from other scientific disciplines such as systems analysis, implementation science, and developmental, clinical, and community psychology.

The focus of PBS researchers and practitioners on the achievement of meaningful, durable, and sustainable outcomes in natural settings had a significant influence on the initial development of PBS as an applied science. This outcomes focus drove the design of PBS research. To achieve such outcomes, a commitment to ecological validity guided the design and conduct of research in natural school and community settings with natural agents of change such as teachers, parents, and adult service providers (Dunlap & Koegel, 1999). Given the logistical challenges of research in natural settings, collaborative research methods were adapted from participatory action research and incorporated into PBS research (Albin, Dunlap, & Lucyshyn, 2002). Researchers also gathered long-term follow-up data to examine the durability and sustainability of PBS outcomes (Carr et al., 1999; Dunlap et al., 2010; Lucyshyn et al., 2007). Doing so contributed to the emergence of a life-span perspective as a central feature of PBS.

This outcomes focus also laid the procedural foundations of PBS. First, professional best practice standards in the fields of special education and psychology guided the use of a collaborative approach to assessment and intervention (Salisbury & Dunst, 1997; Webster-Stratton & Herbert, 1993). Second, the concept of goodness of fit, first used within the field of early intervention with families (Bailey et al., 1986), was adopted as an important consideration in the design of behavior support plans. For consumers to effectively and sustainably implement individualized PBS plans in school or community settings, it was recognized that in addition to designing technically sound plans that were consistent with the laws of behavior, plans also needed to have a good contextual fit with plan implementers (e.g., teachers, parents, job coaches) and with implementation settings (e.g., classrooms, homes, work settings; Albin, Lucyshyn, Horner, & Flannery, 1996). Third, to achieve the core goal of quality-of-life improvement, person-centered planning and wraparound methods were integrated into a process of PBS (Eber, Sugai, Smith, & Scott, 2002; Kincaid & Fox, 2002; O'Brien & O'Brien, 2002). These methods brought together key stakeholders across service settings and provided a strengths-based approach to defining a vision of a successful life for the focus person and an action plan for achieving the vision. Within this context, function-based behavior support plans defined the environmental and behavior supports necessary to achieve this vision.

Given these developments and innovations, Carr et al. (2002) suggested that the features of PBS had broadened and deepened to a point where they represented the emergence of a new applied science. To be sure, PBS maintained philosophical, conceptual, and scientific links to ABA, person-centered values, and normalization/inclusion. However, in a new synthesis, Carr et al. (2002) described the emerging discipline of PBS as composed of 10 defining features. These features are summarized in Table 1.2. This synthesis, in addition to reflecting previous research and practice in PBS up until that time, also served to further guide and define research and practice in PBS over the next 10 years (2003–2012), including the development of SWPBS, the next step in the evolution of PBS.

Table 1.2.   Features of the emerging scientific discipline of positive behavior support

1. Comprehensive lifestyle change and improved quality of life are the goals of intervention and support, and these goals are defined based on the values of those receiving support.

2. Interventions and supports are implemented from a life-span perspective that requires attention to the developmental needs of the focus person and the long-term sustainability of behavior support.

3. Interventions and supports need to be ecological valid—that is, interventions and supports need to relevant, feasible, and effective when used by natural change agents (e.g., teacher, parents, adult service providers) in the real-life settings in which behavior support is being provided.

4. Key stakeholders (i.e., teachers, educational assistants, parents, siblings, friends, job coaches, employers) are empowered to serve as collaborators and partners in the development, implementation, and evaluation of behavior support plans.

5. Social validity—the importance, acceptability, and viability of intervention goals, procedures, and outcomes to key stakeholders—is a primary criterion for the evaluation of the success of a process of behavior intervention and support.

6. When developing interventions and supports, attention to relevant systems variables (e.g., family systems considerations, administrative support in schools) are taken into account, and systems-level supports are put into place to increase the likelihood of implementation fidelity and long-term sustainability.

7. Behavior support plans emphasize the use of strategies that prevent problem behavior, and implementers are empowered to understand and act on the understanding that active and functional intervention occurs primarily when problem behaviors are not present.

8. Behavior support plans are 1) based on a comprehensive assessment of medical, behavioral, and educational variables; 2) guided by principles drawn from behavioral and biomedical science; and 3) evaluated through reliable and valid measurement of behavioral, educational, and quality-of-life outcomes.

9. Researchers and practitioners recognize that knowledge relevant to the successful development and implementation of interventions and supports may be based on multiple research methodologies that aim to develop evidence-based knowledge (e.g., single-case research, group design studies, qualitative methods).

10. The development of practical and effective interventions and supports can be informed by a variety of science-based theoretical perspectives. For example, in addition to applied behavior analysis (ABA), interventions and supports may be informed by biomedical science, developmental psychology, clinical psychology, systems analysis, and implementation science.

Sources: Carr et al. (2002); Dunlap, Carr, Horner, Zarcone, and Schwartz (2008).

Development of Schoolwide Positive Behavior Support

In the late 1990s, PBS researchers began to collaborate with researchers in the area of behavior disorders and with community members to extend the technology of PBS to all students in a school (Sugai & Horner, 1999). Their aim was to prevent problem behavior from developing in young school-age children and to effectively and efficiently ameliorate problem behavior in students at risk for or with behavior disorders. Two concerns and two developments informed this collaboration. First, schools throughout the United States in the 1980s and 1990s were using reactive, punitive strategies in response to discipline problems with students, and these methods were ineffective and counterproductive (Hyman & Perone, 1998). Second, for teachers and other school personnel to sustain the effective use of individualized behavior support plans, a school needed to be a "host environment" for proactive, positive practices with all students (Sugai et al., 2000). In many schools, however, this was not the case, and so individualized behavior support was not sustainable. Third, in the 1990s researchers in the field of behavior disorders articulated positive, proactive models of schoolwide discipline, and initial research that implemented these models showed positive outcomes (Colvin, Kame'enui, & Sugai, 1993; Mayer, 1995). Fourth, Walker et al. (1996) proposed a public health model of behavior support for all students in a school that consisted of primary, secondary, and tertiary tiers of prevention of antisocial behavior. The model offered a compelling way to conceptualize the provision of PBS to all students in a school within a systems approach (Sugai et al., 2000).

The reauthorization in 1997 of IDEA offered an opportunity to extend PBS to all students at a school and district level by integrating PBS with the literature on schoolwide discipline and preventive public health. The reauthorization included grant-based funding for the development of the National Technical Assistance Center for Positive Behavioral Interventions and Supports.

The mission of the center was to develop empirical knowledge and provide technical assistance to schools to create safe school climates and prevent and reduce problem behavior using a whole-school PBS approach. Emphasis was on technical assistance and dissemination that would promote large-scale, effective, and sustainable implementation. The grant was awarded in 1998 to the University of Oregon and consortium partners at the University of Kansas, University of Kentucky, University of Missouri, and University of South Florida, as well as public and private providers of behavior support services.

SWPBS was conceptualized as a three-tiered, public health approach to the prevention of problem behavior in schools. Within the SWPBS framework, organizational systems and a continuum of evidence-based practices are implemented to establish a positive school culture and the individual behavior supports necessary for all students to succeed academically and socially (Sugai et al., 2000; Sugai & Horner, 2006). As noted by Horner and Sugai (2005, October), SWPBS represents the large-scale application of ABA within a systems framework. At Tier 1, primary or universal prevention practices are implemented across the entire school for all students. At Tier 2, students who have not benefited from universal practices are provided with targeted or secondary prevention practices that involve efficient behavior change strategies. Tier 3 is reserved for students who have not responded to primary and secondary prevention. Tertiary support involves intensive, individualized intervention in which a FBA is conducted and an individualized BIP is developed and implemented in collaboration with key stakeholders in the school and community.

Research on Tier 1 and 2 Prevention
Following its conceptualization in the late 1990s and early 2000s, researchers in collaboration with community members initiated

a program of research to develop SWPBS as an evidence-based practice (Horner, Sugai, & Anderson, 2010). Initial quasi-experimental studies provided evidence of an association or functional relation between the implementation of universal prevention strategies and 1) schoolwide improvements in student behavior (Bohanon et al., 2006; Taylor-Green et al., 1997) and 2) improvements in the behavior of targeted groups of students (DePry & Sugai, 2002; Lewis, Sugai, & Colvin, 2000). These studies laid the foundation for large randomized control trials that documented the effectiveness of SWPBS under natural conditions across multiple schools within and across states (Barrett, Bradshaw, & Lewis-Palmer, 2008; Bradshaw, Reinke, Brown, Bevans, & Leaf, 2008; Horner et al., 2009). PBS researchers also established a strong evidentiary base for the effectiveness of secondary (Tier 2) prevention strategies for children or youth at risk for behavior disorders, such as Check In–Check Out (CICO) behavior report card systems (Hawken, MacLeod, & Rawlings, 2007) and First Steps to Success (Walker et al., 2009).

Research on Tier 3 Prevention Concurrent with the empirical development of primary and secondary tiers of prevention within SWPBS, researchers also sought to develop the empirical basis for individualized, function-based intervention with students who were unresponsive to universal or secondary prevention methods. As described earlier in this chapter, multiple studies in school settings documented the effectiveness of function-based, multicomponent PBS for students with developmental disabilities or at risk for or with behavior disorders. However, despite this research, function-based, individualized behavior support had not become common practice in schools (Bambara, Goh, Kern, & Caskie, 2012). Factors hindering widespread adoption included 1) low ecological validity of clinic-based studies in which FBA and BIP were implemented by researchers or school-based studies in

which researchers provided more support for implementation than is naturally available to teachers, 2) scarcity of school personnel who are well trained in FBA and BIP, and 3) poor levels of implementation by teachers and administrators who received short-term in-service training (Ervin et al., 2001; Scott, Liaupsin, Nelson, & McIntyre, 2005).

To address these limitations, PBS researchers worked in collaboration with schools to develop an evidentiary base for FBA and function-based BIP when implemented by typical personnel in school settings. Using single-case experimental designs, researchers documented the efficiency and effectiveness of function-based intervention compared with nonfunction-based intervention when implemented by teachers with students with and without disabilities (Ingram, Lewis-Palmer, & Sugai, 2005; Payne, Scott, & Conroy, 2007). Other researchers developed brief FBA processes and investigated their technical adequacy (McIntosh, Brown, & Borgmeier, 2008). Horner and colleagues, for example, developed a simplified FBA instrument, the Functional Assessment Checklist for Teachers and Staff (FACTS), and documented its reliability, validity, and acceptability through a series of instrument validation and experimental single-case intervention studies (Borgmeier & Horner, 2006; March & Horner, 2002; McIntosh et al., 2008). Dunlap and colleagues (2010) developed a manual-based, standardized model of function-based individualized behavior support in schools: prevent-teach-reinforce (PTR). Preliminary evidence of acceptability and effectiveness was demonstrated in a randomized control trial in five public school districts across two states (Iovannone et al., 2009) and in a single-case experimental study with three children with autism in general education classrooms (Strain, Wilson, & Dunlap, 2011). Although this research on FBA and BIP in schools is promising, as noted by McIntosh et al. (2008), there remains a critical need for additional research to document the effectiveness, feasibility, and sustainability of systems of function-based assessment and behavior support in school settings when implemented by teachers and other school personnel.

Dissemination of SWPBS to State Training Teams

Concurrent with research on the three tiers of SWPBS, members of the PBIS consortium also provided technical assistance to states for the implementation of SWPBS (Sugai & Horner, 2006). Since 1998, SWPBS technical assistance to state training teams has focused on building school, district, and state capacity for SWPBS at the primary, secondary, and tertiary levels of prevention (D. Kincaid, personal communication, September 17, 2012). An implementation blueprint for SWPBS provides guidance for going to scale with SWPBS implementation, including school, district, and state-wide adoption (http://www.pbis.org). Given the accumulated empirical evidence, Horner et al. (2010) concluded that sufficient documentation existed to classify SWPBS as an evidence-based practice, thus warranting large-scale dissemination. As of September 2012, SWPBS was implemented in over 18,000 schools throughout the United States, reaching over 9 million children (R. Horner, personal communication, November 3, 2012).

SWPBS and Students with Severe Disabilities

The rapid rise of SWPBS in schools throughout the United States also raised concerns about the provision of individualized PBS to students with severe disabilities (Bambara & Lohrmann, 2006). Crimmins and Farrell (2006), for example, noted a decrease in research on PBS with individual students in the late 1990s that paralleled an increase in research focused on SWPBS. Given that the original impetus for PBS was the behavior support needs of people with severe disabilities (Horner et al., 1990), researchers in the field of severe disabilities have sought to identify solutions that can ensure that the large-scale dissemination of SWPBS does not leave these students behind. Freeman et al. (2006) suggested that SWPBS provides an infrastructure of positive practices that if utilized can contribute to building an inclusive school culture. Brown and Michaels (2006), challenging the tendency to implement SWPBS vertically (i.e., starting with universal prevention), recommended that the three tiers be implemented simultaneously in schools. Based on these suggestions, Carr (2006) recommended a line of future research that examines the extent to which SWPBS "potentiates the effectiveness" (p. 55) of individualized PBS, such that it becomes more effective compared with individualized PBS absent the infrastructure of SWPBS.

Extensions of Positive Behavior Support

Since 2006, SWPBS has been extended to early childhood education programs, and PBS has been introduced into mental health services for children and families and adapted for the juvenile justice system for adjudicated youth. These developments are described in this section.

Early Childhood Education

Growing concerns about the number of young children entering preschool who lack school readiness and engage in problem behavior have led early childhood educators and researchers to adapt SWPBS to early childhood settings (Benedict, Horner, & Squire, 2007; Fox, Dunlap, Hemmeter, Joseph, & Strain, 2003; Hemmeter, Fox, Jack, & Broyles, 2007). Hemmeter et al. (2007), for example, designed a programwide model of PBS (PWPBS) that is adapted to the philosophy, structure, and resources of early childhood educational settings and to the developmental needs of young children. Implementation of PWPBS in preliminary research using quasi-experimental group designs, 50%–80%, and a randomized waiting-list control trial showed evidence of increases in preschool teachers' use of universal PBS practices (Benedict et al., 2007) and improvements in children's problem behavior and adaptive behavior (Stormont, Covington-Smith, & Lewis, 2007). Taken together, early studies suggest that PWPBS is a promising but still emerging evidence-based practice.

Mental Health System   Enduring challenges faced by the mental health system in the United States to provide children and families with integrated, accessible, effective, family-driven mental health services has spurred an interest in integrating PBS into the mental health care system. Duchnowski and Kutash (2009), for example, proposed the integration of PBS into mental health services within a three-tiered public health model. In this model, a common vision among families, school-based educators and mental health professionals offers universal mental health support to all children and youth, selective interventions to children and youth at risk for more serious problem behavior, and intensive intervention (e.g., behavioral parent training, cognitive behavior therapy) for children and youth with symptoms of a behavior disorder. Frey, Young, Gold, and Trevor (2008), addressing the needs of young children and families in Head Start programs, proposed the integration of mental health services with a PWPBS model of service delivery. Preliminary descriptive and empirical case study research on three-tiered systems of mental health care to families of preschool children with or without disabilities have shown an association among implementation and reductions in parenting stress levels (McCart, Wolf, Sweeney, & Choi, 2009) and improvements in child behavior and family use of positive parenting strategies (Phaneuf & McIntyre, 2011).

Juvenile Justice System   The success of PBS in schools also has led to an interest in adapting this technology for adjudicated youth attending school and residing in secure facilities within the juvenile justice system (Houchins, Jolivette, Wessendorf, McGynn, & Nelson, 2005). This interest has been driven by three factors: 1) the right of adjudicated youth to a free and appropriate public education; 2) national data that show 50%–80% of youth residing in a juvenile justice facility have an educational disability or mental health disorder; and 3) the failure of "get tough" policies that emphasize control and punishment to rehabilitate youth and successfully return them to society.

An effort to adapt PBS to the unique features of secure juvenile facilities was initiated in the early 2000s by the National Technical Assistance Center for PBIS in collaboration with state and local juvenile justice programs and facilities (Nelson, Sugai, & Smith, 2005). Initial efforts focused on defining the general adaptations necessary to educate and support youth who attend school and live within residential programs 24 hours a day (Houchins et al., 2005). Jolivette and Nelson (2010) delineated specific adaptations in regard to establishing a leadership team, providing PBS training, securing staff buy-in, establishing expectations and rules across school and residential programs, and conducting ongoing data monitoring.

PBS has also been adapted and implemented in juvenile homes or youth detention centers in several states (Nelson, Sprague, Jolivette, Smith, & Tobin, 2009). Preliminary descriptive data from a juvenile home in Iowa and a youth detention center in Illinois have been promising, showing substantial reductions in behavior incidents and in the use of restraints. However, as noted by Nelson et al. (2009), PBS in the juvenile justice system remains in its infancy with a significant need for empirical research to investigate its efficacy and acceptability.

CONCLUSION

The evolution of PBS into a science-based discipline that is being widely adopted by educators, psychologists, adult service providers, and families across school and community settings may be attributed to four aspects of its developmental trajectory.

First is the importance that researchers and practitioners in leadership roles have placed on working collaboratively with key stakeholders in natural settings to understand problem behavior from a functional analytic perspective and to develop behavior support plans and supports that are technically sound and contextually appropriate. This commitment to ecological validity paired with an emphasis on empowering stakeholders to serve as partners in assessment and plan design has set the stage for a science-based, collaborative problem-solving model that contributes to the development of prevention-focused environments.

Second, data-based decision making, central to PBS in school and community settings, has established reciprocal feedback loops among PBS researchers and practitioners. Researchers inform practitioners and consumers while practitioners and consumers, in turn, provide researchers with essential information about application in natural settings. This exchange of information has made assessment tools, intervention procedures, and delivery processes increasingly more acceptable, feasible, effective, and sustainable.

A third aspect of the development of PBS that has contributed to its widespread adoption is recognition among the PBS leadership that meaningful, durable, and sustainable improvements in behavior and quality of life require the integration of knowledge across scientific disciplines. In addition to the essential contributions of ABA, other disciplines that inform PBS include developmental and community psychology, systems analysis, and implementation science. This consilience (i.e., integration or unification) of knowledge from different sources is not new, as it has been pursued since the early Greek philosophers (Wilson, 1998). The evolution of PBS represents a contemporary example of the power that lies in a concerted effort among researchers and practitioners to unify knowledge across relevant disciplines

in service to people who engage in problem behavior in school and community settings.

A final aspect of the evolution of PBS into a scientific discipline is the use of multiple research methodologies. This diversity of methodologies has advanced knowledge about PBS in a manner that is holistic and multidimensional, thus establishing a foundation of empirical evidence that more closely conforms to the rich and complex realities inherent in natural settings. As long as those who are active in developing and promoting PBS as a science-based discipline continue to adhere to these key commitments, standards, and values, PBS is likely to continue to grow and prosper. In doing so, researchers and practitioners of PBS may bring significant benefit to an increasingly wider circle of people who engage in problem behavior and to those who care for, educate, and support them.

REFERENCES

Alberto, P.A., & Troutman, A.C. (1986). *Applied behavior analysis for teachers* (2nd ed.). Upper Saddle River, NJ: Merrill/Prentice Hall.

Albin, R.W., Dunlap, G., & Lucyshyn, J.M. (2002). Collaborative research with families on positive behavior support. In J.M. Lucyshyn, G. Dunlap, & R.W. Albin (Eds.), *Positive behavior support with families: Addressing problem behavior in family contexts* (pp. 391–416). Baltimore, MD: Paul H. Brookes Publishing Co.

Albin, R.W., Lucyshyn, J.M., Horner, R.H., & Flannery, K.B. (1996). Contextual fit or behaviour support plans: A model for "goodness of fit." In L. Kern Koegel, R.L. Koegel, & G. Dunlap (Eds.), *Positive behavior support: Including people with difficult behavior in the community* (pp. 81–98). Baltimore, MD: Paul H. Brookes Publishing Co.

Anderson, J.L., Russo, A., Dunlap, G., & Albin, R.W. (1996). A team training model for building the capacity to provide positive behavioral supports in inclusive settings. In L. Koegel, R. Koegel, & G. Dunlap (Eds.), *Positive behavioral support: Including people with difficulty behavior in the community* (pp. 467–490). Baltimore, MD: Paul H. Brookes Publishing Co.

Baer, D.M., Wolf, M.M., & Risley, T.R. (1968). Some current dimensions of applied behavior analysis. *Journal of Applied Behavior Analysis, 1,* 91–97.

Bailey, D.B., Simeonsson, R.J., Winton, P., Huntington, G.S., Comfort, M., Isbell, P., O'Donnell, K., & Helm, J.M. (1986). Family-focused intervention: A functional model for planning, implementing, and evaluating individual family services in early intervention. *Journal of the Division for Early Childhood, 10,* 156–171.

Bambara, L.M., Goh, A., Kern, L., & Caskie, G. (2012). Perceived barriers and enablers to implementing individualized positive behavior interventions and supports in school settings. *Journal of Positive Behavior Interventions, 14,* 228–240.

Bambara, L.M., & Lohrmann, S. (2006). Introduction to special issue on severe disabilities and school-wide positive behavior support. *Research and Practice for Persons with Severe Disabilities, 31,* 1–3.

Barrett, S.B., Bradshaw, C.P., & Lewis-Palmer, T. (2008). Maryland statewide PBIS initiative: Systems, evaluation, and next steps. *Journal of Positive Behavior Interventions, 10,* 105–114.

Benedict, E.A., Horner, R.H., & Squires, J.K. (2007). Assessment and implementation of positive behavior supports in preschools. *Topics in Early Childhood Special Education, 27,* 174–192.

Berkman, K.A., & Meyer, L.H. (1988). Alternative strategies and multiple outcomes in the remediation of severe self-injury: Going "all out" nonaversively. *Journal of The Association for Persons with Severe Handicaps, 13,* 76–86.

Bijou, S.W. (1972). The technology of teaching young handicapped children. In S.W. Bijou & E. Ribes-Inesta (Eds.), *Behavior modification: Issues and extensions* (pp. 27–42). New York, NY: Academic Press.

Blair, K., Umbreit, J., & Bos, C. (1999). Using functional assessment and children's preferences to improve the behavior of your children with behavior disorders. *Behavior Disorders, 24,* 151–166.

Blatt, B., & Kaplan, F. (1986). *Christmas in purgatory.* Newton, MA: Allyn & Bacon.

Borgmeier, C., & Horner, R.H. (2006). An evaluation of the predictive validity of confidence ratings in identifying accurate functional behavioral assessment hypothesis statements. *Journal of Positive Behavior Interventions, 8,* 100–105.

Bradshaw, C.P., Reinke, W.M., Brown, L.D., Bevans, K.B., & Leaf, P.J. (2008). Implementation of school-wide positive behavior interventions and supports (PBIS) in elementary schools: Observations from a randomized trial. *Education and Treatment of Children, 31,* 1–26.

Brown, F., & Michaels, C.A. (2006). School-wide positive behavior support initiatives and students with severe disabilities: A time for reflection. *Research and Practice for Persons with Severe Handicaps, 31,* 57–61.

Bruyere, S.M. (1993). Participatory action research: Overview and implications for family members of persons with disabilities. *Journal of Vocational Rehabilitation, 3,* 62–68.

Buschbacher, P., Fox, L., & Clarke, S. (2004). Recapturing desired family routines: A parent-professional behavioral collaboration. *Research and Practice for Persons with Severe Disabilities, 29,* 25–39.

Carr, E.G. (1977). The motivation of self-injurious behavior: A review of some hypotheses. *Psychological Bulletin, 84,* 800–816.

Carr, E.G. (2006). SWPBS: The greatest good for the greatest number, or the needs of the majority trump the needs of the minority. *Research and Practice for Persons with Severe Handicaps, 31,* 54–56.

Carr, E.G., & Carlson, J.I. (1993). Reduction of severe behavior problems in the community using a multicomponent treatment approach. *Journal of Applied Behavior Analysis, 26,* 157–172.

Carr, E.G., Dunlap, G., Horner, R.H., Koegel, R.L., Turnbull, A.P., Sailor, W., . . . Fox, L. (2002). Positive behavior support: Evolution of an applied science. *Journal of Positive Behavior Interventions, 4,* 4–16.

Carr, E.G., & Durand, V.M. (1985). Reducing behavior problems through functional communication training. *Journal of Applied Behavior Analysis, 18,* 111–126.

Carr, E.G., & Herbert, M.R. (2008). Integrating behavioral and biomedical approaches: A marriage made in heaven. *Autism Advocate, 50,* 46–52.

Carr, E.G., Smith, C.E., Giacin, T.A., Whelan, B.M., & Pancari, J. (2003). Menstrual discomfort as a biological setting event for severe problem behavior: Assessment and intervention. *Mental Retardation, 118,* 117–133.

Clarke, S., Dunlap, G., & Vaughn, B. (1999). Family-centered, assessment-based intervention to improve behavior during an early morning routine. *Journal of Positive Behavior Interventions, 1,* 235–241.

Colvin, G., Kame'enui, E.J., & Sugai, G. (1993). School-wide and classroom management: Reconceptualizing the integration of management of students with behavior problems in general education. *Education and Treatment of Children, 16,* 361–381.

Cooper, J.O., Heron, T.E., & Heward, W.L. (2007). *Applied behavior analysis* (2nd ed.). Upper Saddle River, NJ: Pearson.

Crimmins, D., & Farrell, A.F. (2006). Individualized behavioral support at 15 years: It's still lonely at the top. *Research and Practice for Persons with Severe Disabilities, 31,* 31–44.

DePry, R.L., & Sugai, G. (2002). The effect of active supervision and pre-correction on minor behavioral incidents in a sixth grade general education classroom. *Journal of Behavioral Education, 11,* 255–267.

Dietz, S.M. (1978). Current status of applied behavior analysis: Science vs. technology. *American Psychologist, 33,* 805–814.

Duchnowski, A.J., & Kutash, K. (2009). Integrating PBS, mental health services, and family-driven care. In W. Sailor, G. Dunlap, G. Sugai, & R. Horner (Eds.), *Handbook of positive behavior support* (pp. 203–232). New York, NY: Springer.

Duda, M.A., Dunlap, G., Fox, L., Lentini, R., & Clarke, S. (2004). An experimental evaluation of positive behavior support in a community preschool program. *Topics in Early Childhood Special Education, 24,* 143–155.

Dunlap, G. (2006). The applied behavior analytic heritage of PBS: A dynamic model of action-oriented research. *Journal of Positive Behavior Interventions, 8,* 58–60.

Dunlap, G., Carr, E.G., Horner, R.H., Koegel, R.L., Sailor, W., Clarke, S., . . . Fox, L. (2010). A descriptive, multi-year examination of positive behavior support. *Behavioral Disorders, 35,* 259–293.

Dunlap, G., Carr, E.G., Horner, R.H., Zarcone, J.R., & Schwartz, I. (2008). Positive behavior support and applied behavior analysis: A familial alliance. *Behavior Modification, 32,* 682–698.

Dunlap, G., Foster-Johnson, L., Clarke, S., Kern, L., & Childs, K.E. (1995). Modifying activities to produce functional outcomes: Effects on the problem behaviors of students with disabilities. *Journal of The Association for Persons with Severe Handicaps, 20*, 248–258.

Dunlap, G., Hieneman, M., Knoster, T., Fox, L., Anderson, J., & Albin, R. (2000). Essential elements of inservice training in positive behavior support. *Journal of Positive Behavior Interventions, 2*, 22–32.

Dunlap, G., Iovannone, R., Wilson, K.J., Kincaid, D.K., & Strain, P. (2010). Prevent-teach-reinforce: A standardized model of school-based behavioral intervention. *Journal of Positive Behavior Interventions, 12*, 9–22.

Dunlap, G., & Kern, L. (1993). Assessment and intervention for children within the instructional curriculum. In J. Reichle & D.P. Wacker (Eds.), *Communicative alternatives to challenging behavior* (pp. 177–203). Baltimore, MD: Paul H. Brookes Publishing Co.

Dunlap, G., Kern-Dunlap, L., Clarke, S., & Robbins, F.R. (1991). Functional assessment, curricular revision, and severe behavior problems. *Journal of Applied Behavior Analysis, 24*, 387–397.

Dunlap, G., Kern, L., dePerczel, M., Clarke, S., Wilson, D., Childs, K.E., . . . Falk, G.D. (1993). Functional analysis of classroom variables for students with emotional and behavioral challenges. *Behavioral Disorders, 18*, 275–291.

Dunlap, G., & Koegel, R.L. (1980). Motivating autistic children through stimulus variation. *Journal of Applied Behavior Analysis, 13*, 619–627.

Dunlap, G., & Koegel, R.L. (1999). Welcoming editorial. *Journal of Positive Behavior Interventions, 1*, 2–3.

Durand, V.M. (1987). "Look homeward angel": A call to return to our (functional) roots. *The Behavior Analyst, 10*, 299–302.

Durand, V.M., & Crimmins, D.B. (1988). Identifying the variables maintaining self-injurious behavior. *Journal of Autism and Developmental Disorders, 18*, 99–117.

Durand, V.M., Hieneman, M., Clarke, S., Wang, M., & Rinaldi, M. (2013). Positive family intervention for severe challenging behavior I: A multi-site randomized clinical trial. *Journal of Positive Behavior Interventions.*

Eber, L., Sugai, G., Smith, C.R., & Scott, T.M. (2002). Wraparound and positive behavioral interventions and supports in the schools. *Journal of Emotional and Behavioral Disorders, 10*, 171–180.

Education for All Handicapped Children Act of 1975, PL 94-142, 20 U.S.C. §§ 1400 *et seq.*

Education of the Handicapped Act Amendments of 1986, PL 99-457, 20 U.S.C. §§ 1400 *et seq.*

Ervin, R.A., DuPaul, G.J., Kern, L., & Friman, P.C. (1998). Classroom-based functional and adjunctive assessments: Proactive approaches to intervention selection for adolescents with attention deficit hyperactivity disorder. *Journal of Applied Behavior Analysis, 31*, 65–78.

Ervin, R.A., Radford, P.M., Bertsch, K., Piper, A.L., Erhardt, K.E., & Poling, A. (2001). A descriptive analysis and critique of the empirical literature on school based functional assessment. *School Psychology Review, 30*, 193–210.

Evans, I.M., & Meyer, L.H. (1985). *An educative approach to behavior problems: A practical decision model for interventions with severely handicapped learners.* Baltimore, MD: Paul H. Brookes Publishing Co.

Fawcett, S.B. (1991). Some values guiding community research and action. *Journal of Applied Behavior Analysis, 24*, 621–636.

Feldman, M.A., Condillac, R.A., Tough, S., Hunt, S., & Griffiths, D. (2002). Effectiveness of community positive behavioral intervention for persons with developmental disabilities and severe problem behavior disorders. *Behavior Therapy, 33*, 377–398.

Fixsen, D.L., Naoom, S.F., Blase, K.A., Friedman, R.M., & Wallace, F. (2005). *Implementation research: A synthesis of the literature.* Tampa, FL: University of South Florida, Louis de la Parte Florida Mental Health Institute, The National Implementation Research Network.

Flannery, K.B., & Horner, R.H. (1994). The relationship between predictability and problem behavior for students with severe disabilities. *Journal of Behavioral Education, 4*, 157–176.

Fox, L., Dunlap, G., Hemmeter, M.L., Joseph, G.E., & Strain, P.S. (2003). The teaching pyramid: A model for supporting social competence and preventing challenging behavior in young children. *Young Children, 58*, 48–52.

Fox, L., Vaughn, B., Dunlap, G., & Bucy, M. (1997). Parent-professional partnership: A qualitative analysis of one family's experience. *Journal of The Association for Persons with Severe Handicaps, 22*, 198–207.

Freeman, R., Eber, L., Anderson, C., Irvin, L., Horner, R., Bounds, M., & Roger, B. (2006). Building inclusive school cultures using school-wide positive behavior support: Designing effective, individual support systems for students with significant disabilities. *Research and Practice for Persons with Severe Disabilities, 31*, 4–17.

Frey, A., Young, S., Gold, A., & Trevor, E. (2008). Utilizing a positive behavior support approach to achieve integrated mental health services. *National Head Start Association Dialogue, 11*, 135–156.

Gaylord-Ross, R. (1980). A decision model for the treatment of aberrant behavior in applied settings. In W. Sailor, B. Wilcox, & L. Brown (Eds.), *Methods of instruction for severely handicapped students* (pp. 135–158). Baltimore, MD: Paul H. Brookes Publishing Co.

Guess, D., Sailor, W., & Baer, D.M. (1977). A behavioral-remedial approach to language training for the severely handicapped. In E. Sontag (Ed.), *Educational programming for the severely and profoundly handicapped* (pp. 360–377). Reston, VA: Council for Exceptional Children.

Halderman vs. Pennhurst State School & Hospital, 446 F. Supp. 1295 (E.D. Pa. 1978).

Hawken, L.S., MacLeod, K.S., & Rawlings, L. (2007). Effects of the Behavior Education Program (BEP) on office discipline referrals of elementary school students. *Journal of Positive Behavior Interventions, 9*, 94–101.

Hemmeter, M.L., Fox, L., Jack, S., & Broyles, L. (2007). A program-wide model of positive behavior support in early childhood settings. *Journal of Early Intervention, 29*, 337–355.

Hemmeter, M.L., Ostrosky, M., & Fox, L. (2006). Social and emotional foundations for early learning: A conceptual model for intervention. *School Psychology Review, 35*, 583–601.

Hieneman, M., & Dunlap, G. (2000). Factors affecting the outcomes of community based behavior support: I. Identification and description of factor categories. *Journal of Positive Behavior Interventions, 2*, 161–169.

Horner, R.H., Albin, R.W., Todd, A.W., & Sprague, J. (2000). Positive behavior support for individuals with severe disabilities. In M.E. Snell & F. Brown (Eds.), *Instruction of students with severe disabilities* (6th ed., pp. 206–250). Upper Saddle River, NJ: Pearson.

Horner, R.H., Day, H.M., & Day, J.R. (1997). Using neutralizing routines to reduce problem behavior. *Journal of Applied Behavior Analysis, 30*, 601–614.

Horner, R.H., Dunlap, G., Koegel, R.L., Carr, E.G., Sailor, W., Anderson, J., . . . O'Neill, R. (1990). Toward a technology of "nonaversive" behavioral support. *Journal of The Association for Persons with Severe Handicaps, 15*, 125–132.

Horner, R.H., Meyer, L.H., & Fredericks, H.D.B. (1986). *Education of learners with severe handicaps: Exemplary service strategies.* Baltimore, MD: Paul H. Brookes Publishing Co.

Horner, R.H., & Sugai, G. (2005, October). *School-wide positive behavior support: Implementing ABA at scales of social significance.* Paper presented at the 26th Annual Conference of the Berkshire Association for Behavior Analysis and Therapy, Amherst, MA.

Horner, R.H., Sugai, G., & Anderson, C.M. (2010). Examining the evidence base for school-wide positive behavior support. *Focus on Exceptional Children, 42*, 1–14.

Horner, R.H., Sugai, G., Smolkowski, K., Eber, L., Nakasato, J., Todd, A.W., & Esperanza, J. (2009). A randomized, wait-list controlled effectiveness trial assessing school-wide positive behavior support in elementary schools. *Journal of Positive Behavior Interventions, 11*, 133–144.

Houchins, D.E., Jolivette, S., Wessendorf, S., McGlynn, M., & Nelson, C.M. (2005). Stakeholders' view of implementing positive behavioral support in juvenile justice setting. *Education and Treatment of Children, 28*, 380–399.

Hyman, I.A., & Perone, D.C. (1998). The other side of school violence: Educator policies and practices that may contribute to student misbehavior. *Journal of School Psychology, 36*, 7–27.

Individuals with Disabilities Education Act Amendments (IDEA) of 1997, PL 105-17, 20 U.S.C. §§ 1400 *et seq.*

Individuals with Disabilities Education Improvement Act (IDEA) of 2004, PL 108-446, 20 U.S.C. §§ 1400 *et seq.*

Ingram, K., Lewis-Palmer, T., & Sugai, G. (2005). Function-based intervention planning: Comparing the effectiveness of FBA function-based and non-function-based intervention plans. *Journal of Positive Behavior Interventions, 7*, 224–236.

Iovannone, R., Greenbaum, P.E., Wang, W., Kincaid, D., Dunlap, G., & Strain, P. (2009). Randomized control trial of the prevent-teach-reinforcer (PTR) tertiary intervention for students with problem behavior. *Journal of Emotional and Behavioral Disorders, 17*, 213–225.

Iwata, B.A., Dorsey, M.F., Slifer, K.J., Bauman, K.E., Richman, G.S. (1982). Toward a functional analysis of self-injury. *Analysis and Intervention in Developmental Disabilities, 2*, 3–20.

Jolivette, K., & Nelson, C.M. (2010). Adapting positive behavior interventions and supports for secure juvenile justice settings: Improving facility-wide behavior. *Behavioral Disorders, 36*, 28–42.

Kemp, D.C., & Carr, E.G. (1995). Reduction of severe problem behavior in community employment using a hypothesis-driven multicomponent intervention approach. *Journal of The Association for Persons with Severe Handicaps, 20*, 229–247.

Kern, L., Childs, L.E., Dunlap, G., Clarke, S., & Falk, G.D. (1994). Using assessment-based curricular intervention to improve the classroom behavior of a student with emotional and behavioral challenges. *Journal of Applied Behavior Analysis, 27*, 7–19.

Kincaid, D., & Fox, L. (2002). Person-centered planning and positive behavior support. In S. Holburn & P. Vietze (Eds.), *Person-centered planning: Research, practice, and future directions* (pp. 29–49). Baltimore, MD: Paul H. Brookes Publishing Co.

Knoster, T., Anderson, J., Carr, E.G., Dunlap, G., & Horner, R.H. (2003). Emerging challenges and opportunities: Introducing the Association for Positive Behavior Support. *Journal of Positive Behavior Interventions, 5*, 183–186.

Koegel, R.L., Dyer, K., & Bell, L.K. (1987). The influence of child-preferred activities on autistic children's social behavior. *Journal of Applied Behavior Analysis, 20*, 243–252.

Koegel, L.K., Koegel, R.L., & Dunlap, G. (1996). *Positive behavioral support: Including people with difficult behavior in the community.* Baltimore, MD: Paul H. Brookes Publishing Co.

LaVigna, G.W., & Donnellan, A.M. (1986). *Alternatives to punishment: Nonaversive strategies for solving behavior problems.* New York, NY: Irvington Press.

Lewis, T.J., Sugai, G., & Colvin, G. (2000). The effect of pre-correction and active supervision on the recess behavior of elementary school students. *Education and Treatment of Children, 23*, 109–121.

Lucyshyn, J.M., Albin, R.W., Horner, R., Mann, J., Mann, J., & Wadsworth, G. (2007). Family implementation of positive behavior support with a child with autism: A longitudinal, single case experimental and descriptive replication and extension. *Journal of Positive Behavior Interventions, 9*, 131–150.

Lucyshyn, J.M., Albin, R.W., & Nixon, C.D. (1997). Embedding comprehensive behavioral support in family ecology: An experimental, single-case analysis. *Journal of Consulting and Clinical Psychology, 65*, 241–251.

Lucyshyn, J.M., Dunlap, G., & Albin, R.W. (Eds.). (2002). *Families, and positive behavioral support: Addressing problem behavior in family contexts.* Baltimore, MD: Paul H. Brookes Publishing Co.

Luiselli, J.K. (2006). *Antecedent assessment and intervention: Supporting children and adults with* developmental disabilities in community settings. Baltimore, MD: Paul H. Brookes Publishing Co.

Luiselli, J.K., & Cameron, M.J. (1998). *Antecedent control: Innovative approaches to behavioral support.* Baltimore, MD: Paul H. Brookes Publishing Co.

Mace, F.C., Lalli, J.S., Lalli, B.P., & Shea, M.C. (1993). Functional analysis and treatment of aberrant behavior. In R. Van Houten & S. Axelrod (Eds.), *Behavior analysis and treatment* (pp. 75–99). New York, NY: Plenum Press.

March, R.E., & Horner, R.H. (2002). Feasibility and contributions of functional behavioral assessment in schools. *Journal of Emotional and Behavioral Disorders, 10,* 158–170.

Martens, B.K., & Witt, J.C. (1988). Ecological behavior analysis. In M. Hersen, R.M. Eisler, & P.M. Miller (Eds.), *Progress in behavior modification* (Vol. 22, pp. 115–140). Thousand Oaks, CA: Sage.

Mayer, G. (1995). Preventing antisocial behavior in schools. *Journal of Applied Behavior Analysis, 28,* 467–478.

McCart, A., Wolf, N., Sweeney, H., & Choi, H. (2009). The application of a family-based multi-tiered system of support. *NHSA Dialog: A Research-to-Practice Journal for the Early Intervention Field, 12,* 122–132.

McIntosh, K., Bennett, J.L., & Price, K. (2011). Evaluation of social and academic effects of school-wide positive behaviour support in a Canadian school district. *Exceptionality Education International, 21,* 46–60.

McIntosh, K., Borgmeier, C., Anderson, C.M., Horner, R.H., Rodriquez, B.J., & Tobin, T.J. (2008). Technical adequacy of the functional assessment checklist: Teachers and staff (FACTS) FBA interview measure. *Journal of Positive Behavior Interventions, 10*(1), 33–45.

McIntosh, K., Brown, J.A., & Borgmeier, C.J. (2008). Validity of functional behavior assessment within an RTI framework: Evidence and future directions. *Assessment for Effective Intervention, 34,* 6–14.

Meyer, L.H., & Evans, I.M. (1989). *Nonaversive interventions for behavior problems: A manual for home and community.* Baltimore, MD: Paul H. Brookes Publishing Co.

Mills v. Board of Education, DC. 348 F.Supp. 866 (D. DC 1972).

Morris, E.K. (1988). Contextualism: The world view of behavior analysis. *Journal of Experimental Child Psychology, 46,* 289–323.

Nelson, C.M., Sprague, J.R., Jolivette, K., Smith, C.R., & Tobin, T.J. (2009). Positive behavior support in alternative education, community-based mental health, and juvenile justice settings. In W. Sailor, G. Dunlap, G. Sugai, & R. Horner (Eds.), *Handbook of positive behavior support* (pp. 465–496). New York, NY: Springer.

Nelson, C.M., Sugai, G., & Smith, C. (2005). Positive behavior support offered in juvenile corrections. *Counterpoint, 1,* 6–7.

Newsom, C., Favell, J.E., & Rincover, A. (1983). The side effects of punishment. In S. Axelrod & J. Apsche (Eds.), *The effects of punishment on human behavior* (pp. 285–316). New York, NY: Academic Press.

Noonan, M.J., Brown, F., Mulligan, M., & Rettig, M.A. (1982). Educability of severely handicapped persons:

Both sides of the issue. *The Journal of The Association for the Severely Handicapped, 7,* 3–12.

O'Neill, R.E., Horner, R.H., Albin, R.W., Sprague, J.R., Storey, K., & Newton, J.S. (1997). *Functional assessment and program development for problem behavior: A practical handbook.* Pacific Grove, CA: Brooks/Cole Publishing.

Pennsylvania Association for Retarded Citizens (PARC) v. Commonwealth of Pennsylvania, 334 F.Supp. 1257 (E.D. PA 1972).

Payne, L.D., Scott, T.M., & Conroy, M. (2007). A school-based examination of the efficacy of function-based intervention. *Behavioral Disorders, 32,* 5–17.

Peck, C.A. (1991). Linking values and science in social policy decisions affecting citizens with severe disabilities. In L.H. Meyer, C.A. Peck, & L. Brown (Eds.), *Critical issues in the lives of people with severe disabilities* (pp. 1–16). Baltimore, MD: Paul H. Brookes Publishing Co.

Phaneuf, L.K., & McIntyre, L.L. (2011). The application of a three-tier model of intervention to parent training. *Journal of Positive Behavior Interventions, 13,* 198–207.

Pierce, W.D., & Epling, W.F. (1980). What happened to analysis in applied behavior analysis. *Behavior Analyst, 3,* 1–21.

Powell, S., & Nelson, B. (1997). Effects of choosing academic assignments on a student with attention deficit and hyperactivity disorder. *Journal of Applied Behavior Analysis, 30,* 181–183.

Rappaport, J. (1987). Terms of empowerment/exemplars of prevention: Toward a theory for community psychology. *American Journal of Community Psychology, 15,* 121–148.

Rehabilitation Act of 1973, PL 93-112, 29 U.S.C. §§ 701 et seq.

Repp, A.C., & Singh, N.N. (1990). *Perspectives on the use of nonaversive and aversive interventions for persons with developmental disabilities.* Sycamore, IL: Sycamore Publishing Company.

Sailor, W., Dunlap, G., Sugai, G., & Horner, R. (2009). *Handbook of positive behavior support.* New York, NY: Springer.

Sailor, W., Wilcox, B., & Brown, L. (1980). *Methods of instruction for severely handicapped students.* Baltimore, MD: Paul H. Brookes Publishing Co.

Salisbury, C.L., & Dunst, C.J. (1997). Home, school, and community partnerships: Building inclusive teams. In B. Rainforth & J. York-Barr (Eds.), *Collaborative teams for students with severe disabilities: Integrating therapy and educational services* (2nd ed., pp. 57–87). Baltimore, MD: Paul H. Brookes Publishing Co.

Scheuermann, B.K., & Hall, J.A. (2008). *Positive behavioral supports for the classroom.* Upper Saddle River, NJ: Merrill/Prentice-Hall.

Schwartz, I.S., & Baer, D.M. (1991). Social validity assessments: Is current practice state of the art? *Journal of Applied Behavior Analysis, 24,* 189–204.

Seiden, S.B., & Zirkel, P.A. (1989). Aversive therapy for handicapped students. *Education Law Reporter, 48,* 1029–1044.

Singer, G.H.S., Gert, B., & Koegel, R.L. (1999). A moral framework for analyzing the controversy over aversive behavioral interventions for people with severe mental retardation. *Journal of Positive Behavior Interventions, 1,* 88–100.

Singer, G.H.S., Singer, J., & Horner, R.H. (1987). Using pretask requests to increase the probability of compliance for students with severe disabilities. *Journal of The Association for Persons with Severe Handicaps, 12,* 287–291.

Singh, N.N., Lloyd, J.W., & Kendall, K.A. (1990). Nonaversive and aversive interventions: Introduction. In A.C. Repp & N.N. Singh (Eds.), *Perspectives on the use of nonaversive and aversive interventions for persons with developmental disabilities* (pp. 3–16). Pacific Grove, CA: Brooks/Cole.

Snell, M.E. (1987). *Systematic instruction of persons with severe handicaps* (3rd ed.). Columbus, OH: Charles E. Merrill.

Sprague, J.R., & Horner, R.H. (1999). Low-frequency high-intensity problem behavior: Toward an applied technology of functional assessment and intervention. In A.C. Repp & R.H. Horner (Eds.), *Functional analysis of problem behavior: From effective assessment to effective support* (pp. 98–116). Belmont, CA: Wadsworth.

Spreat, S., & Lanzi, F. (1989). Role of human rights committees in the review of restrictive/aversive behavior modification procedures: A national survey. *Mental Retardation, 27,* 375–382.

Spring, B., & Hitchcock, K. (2009). Evidence-based practice in psychology. In I.B. Weiner & W.E. Craighead (Eds.), *Corsini's encyclopedia of psychology* (4th ed., pp. 603–607). New York, NY: Wiley.

Stormont, M., Covington-Smith, S., & Lewis, T.J. (2007). Teacher implementation of precorrection and praise statements in Head Start classrooms as a component of program-wide positive behavioral support. *Journal of Behavioral Education, 16,* 280–290.

Sugai, G., & Horner, R.H. (1999). Discipline and behavioral support: Practices, pitfalls, & promises. *Effective School Practices, 17,* 10–22.

Sugai, G., & Horner, R. (2002). The evolution of disciplinary practices: School-wide positive behavior supports. *Child and Family Behavior Therapy, 24,* 23–50.

Sugai, G., & Horner, R.H. (2006). A promising approach to expanding and sustaining school-wide positive behavior support. *School Psychology Review, 35,* 245–259.

Sugai, G., Horner, R.H., Dunlap, G., Hieneman, M., Lewis, T.J., Nelson, C.M., . . . Wilcox, B. (2000). Applying positive behavior support and functional behavioral assessment in schools. *Journal of Positive Behavior Interventions, 2*(3), 131–143.

Turnbull, A.P., & Ruef, R. (1997). Family perspectives on problem behavior. *Mental Retardation, 34,* 280–293.

Turnbull, H.R., Stowe, M., Wilcox, B.L., Raper, C., & Hedges, L.P. (2000). The public policy foundations for positive behavioral interventions, strategies and supports. *Journal of Positive Behavior Interventions, 2,* 218–230.

Turnbull, A.P., Friesen, B.J., & Ramirez, C. (1995). *Forging collaborative partnerships with families in the study of disability.* Paper presented at the National Institute on Disability and Rehabilitation Research (NIDRR) Conference on Participatory Action Research, Washington, DC.

Turnbull, H.R., & Turnbull, A.P. (2000). *Free appropriate public education: Law and the education of children with disabilities* (6th ed.). Denver, CO: Love.

Ulrich, R., Stachnik, & Mabry, J. (1970). *Control of human behavior: From cure to prevention* (Vol. 2). Glenview, IL: Scott, Foresman, and Company.

Van Houten, R., Axelrod, S., Bailey, J.S., Favell, J.E., Foxx, R.M., Iwata, B., & Lovaas, O.I. (1988). The right to effective treatment. *Journal of Applied Behavior Analysis, 21,* 381–384.

Vaughn, S., & Dammann, J.E. (2001). Science and sanity in special education. *Behavioral Disorders, 27*(1), 21–29.

Von Ravensberg, H., & Tobin, T. (2008). IDEA 2004: Final regulations and the reauthorized functional behavioral assessment. Retrieved February 18, 2013, from http://papers.ssrn.com/sol3/papers.cfm?abstract_id=1151394

Wahler, R.G., & Fox, J.J. (1981). Setting events in applied behavior analysis: Toward a conceptual and methodological expansion. *Journal of Applied Behavior Analysis, 14,* 327–338.

Walker, H.M., Horner, R.H., Sugai, G., Bullis, M., Sprague, J.R., Bricker, D., & Kaufman, M.J. (1996). Integrated approaches to preventing antisocial behavior patterns among school-age children and youth. *Journal of Emotional and Behavioral Disorders, 4,* 194–209.

Walker, H.M., Ramsey, E., & Gresham, F.M. (2005). *Antisocial behavior in school: Evidence-based practices* (2nd ed.). Belmont, CA: Wadsworth/Thompson Learning.

Walker, H.M., Seeley, J.R., Small, J., Severson, H.H., Feil, E.G., Graham, B.A., . . . Forness, S.R. (2009). A randomized controlled trial of the First Steps to Success early intervention: Demonstration of program efficacy outcomes in a diverse, urban school district. *Journal of Emotional and Behavioral Disorders, 17,* 197–212.

Webster-Stratton, C., & Herbert, M. (1993). "What really happens in parent training?" *Behavior Modification, 17,* 407–456.

Wehmeyer, M.L., & Schwartz, M. (1997). Self-determination and positive adult outcomes: A follow-up study of youth with mental retardation or learning disabilities. *Exceptional Children, 63,* 245–255.

Wilson, E.O. (1998). *Consilience: The unity of knowledge.* New York, NY: Knopf.

Wolf, M.M. (1978). Social validity: The case for subjective measurement or how applied behavior analysis is finding its heart. *Journal of Applied Behavior Analysis, 11,* 203–214.

Wolfensberger, W. (1972). *The principle of normalization in human services.* Toronto, ON: National Institute on Mental Retardation.

Foundational Assumptions About Challenging Behavior and Behavior Interventions

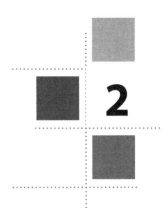

2

Fredda Brown and Jacki L. Anderson

Individualized positive behavior support (PBS) has several foundational assumptions regarding how to support individuals with challenging behaviors; these assumptions influence the development of interventions for increasing appropriate behaviors, decreasing or replacing challenging behaviors, and maintaining a vision for a self-determined quality of life. While we call these foundations *assumptions*, they are more than that. The definition of an assumption is a statement that is accepted as truth without it being verified as such. The behavioral assumptions presented here are indeed assumed, or taken for granted, by those who promote the use of PBS strategies, but they have become assumptions because of their scientific and ethical groundings. There are two types of validity related to science and ethics that support these PBS assumptions.

First, there is *experimental validity*. Experimental validity refers to the unequivocal demonstration that an independent variable (e.g., the behavior support plan, an instructional strategy) is responsible for the change in the dependent variable (e.g., aggressive behavior, greeting responses; Cooper, Heron, & Heward, 2007). Since the early 1990s, there has been an increasing body of literature supporting the PBS methodology. Because of the significant number of research-based articles that have been published, we can also confidently suggest that the strategies promoted by PBS are evidence based. This is particularly important, as the No Child Left Behind Act of 2001 (PL 107-110) requires that evidence-based practices be used to guide classroom practice (Wang & Spillane, 2009). Horner et al. (2005, p. 176) describe criteria for establishing that a practice is evidence based:

> 1) a minimum of five single-subject studies that meet minimally acceptable methodological criteria and document experimental control have been published in peer-reviewed journals, 2) the studies

are conducted by at least three different researchers across at least three different geographical locations, and 3) the five or more studies include a total of at least 20 participants.

There are many evidence-based practices promoted by PBS that will be described throughout the chapters in this book.

The second form of validity is *social validity*. Social validity refers to the significance of the change in behavior to the person's life and is a concept that addresses qualitative aspects of the intervention or program (Brown & Snell, 2011). There are three components to social validity: 1) acceptability of the educational goals, 2) the instructional methods used to achieve the goals, and 3) the importance and social acceptability of the behavior change (Cooper, Heron, & Heward, 2007; Kazdin, 1977; Wolf, 1978). These three components are critical in the development of supports for individuals with challenging behaviors and encourage us to ask the following questions: If the person successfully achieves a goal, will it improve the quality of his or her life? Are the strategies we are using to affect the behavior acceptable to the individual, his or her family, and others in integrated community environments?

It is the rapprochement between experimental validity (concern for scientific demonstration) and social validity (concern for significance of results) that gives PBS its strength and integrity. We may consider experimental validity as the "science" behind PBS and social validity as the "values" behind PBS. Whereas we once focused primarily on experimental validity to determine the value of practices and outcomes, we have moved to a more overarching perspective that additionally includes social validity, especially improvements in quality of life, as a major contributor when evaluating practice and outcomes. Spooner and Brown (2011) suggest the following:

"What works" is only one part of the equation. Scientific evidence for an intervention

must be balanced with its social validity, that is, the treatment acceptability, of the intervention. An intervention might have an evidence-base, but may not be acceptable by the recipients of the intervention and their families. Both standards must be met for our field to incorporate it into our menu of best practices. (p. 512)

This chapter discusses the foundational assumptions of PBS regarding our perspectives on challenging behaviors and the behavior interventions we design to address those behaviors. The Association for Positive Behavior Support's (APBS; 2007) standards of practice for individuals delineates 16 assumptions. Five assumptions apply to how we conceptualize *behavior*, and 11 assumptions apply to the development of PBS *supports*, as shown in Table 2.1.

In this chapter, we first describe two individuals who have very different demographics and characteristics—Sophie and Roberto. We will then demonstrate how the foundations are applied to these individuals and shape how we look at their behavior and how we approach individualized interventions. Sophie's and Roberto's scenarios help us understand the needs of such diverse individuals—many things are very similar yet many things are individualized. These scenarios allow the reader to understand the foundations of PBS; each of these assumptions will then be further developed and demonstrated in the chapters that follow.

MEET SOPHIE

Sophie is a 4-year-old girl from a large urban area. During her pregnancy, Sophie's mother used a variety of substances, including crack cocaine and alcohol. Shortly after her birth, Sophie went to live with her grandmother, who took responsibility for raising her. When Sophie turned 3, her grandmother enrolled her in the local public preschool program available to families with low incomes. (Her state does not provide public preschool for all children.) Sophie appeared to enjoy going to school,

Table 2.1.   Positive behavior support (PBS) assumptions

Assumptions about behavior	Assumptions about the development of PBS supports
1. Problem behavior serves a function.	1. Collaborative, team-based decision making is used.
2. Positive strategies are effective in addressing the most challenging behavior.	2. Decisions are person centered.
	3. Self-determination of the individual is promoted.
3. When positive behavior intervention strategies fail, additional functional assessment strategies are required to develop more effective PBS strategies.	4. Supports are based on functional assessment of behavior.
4. Features of the environmental context affect behavior.	5. Supports include outcomes that enhance quality of life and are valued by individuals, their families, and the community.
5. The reduction of problem behavior is important but not the sole outcome of successful intervention; effective PBS results in improvements in quality of life, acquisition of valued skills, and access to valued activities.	6. Strategies are developed that are acceptable in inclusive community settings.
	7. Strategies are developed that teach useful and valued skills.
	8. All strategies are evidence based and socially and empirically valid to achieve desired outcomes that are at least as effective and efficient as the problem behavior.
	9. Techniques are used that do not cause pain or humiliation or deprive the individual of basic needs.
	10. Constructive and respectful multicomponent intervention plans emphasize antecedent interventions, instruction in prosocial behaviors, and environmental modification.
	11. Plans include ongoing measurement of impact.

but shortly after Sophie began attending the program, her grandmother received a call asking her to come and take Sophie home because her behavior was disruptive to the class. Sophie's grandmother had to leave her work and take public transportation to the school to pick her up and then remain at home with her for the rest of the day. Calls to send Sophie home due to problem behavior continued to occur with increasing frequency until, after 3 months, Sophie was dismissed from the program and referred for an evaluation for special education based on failure to progress in the preschool curriculum and problem behavior such as aggression (e.g., kicking and head-butting other people, cursing, screaming), self-injurious behavior (e.g., pulling her hair, tearing her clothing), and noncompliance. The assessment resulted in a diagnosis of both attention-deficit/hyperactivity disorder (ADHD)

and intellectual disability, and Sophie was placed in a noncategorical special education preschool. The special education preschool teacher had graduate-level credentials in both general and special education—these requirements are more rigorous than the associate's degree required to be a general education early childhood teacher. However, the special education teacher's extensive education did not include training in PBS practices. Thus when a variety of typical punitive measures (e.g., time-out, stern reprimands, loss of privileges, occasional praise for appropriate behavior) did not have an impact on Sophie's problem behavior, her grandmother began once again receiving calls to take her home. After several months, Sophie was once again dismissed from this program.

As what the district considered a "last resort" prior to an out-of-district placement,

Sophie was placed in a newly developed prekindergarten program on a general education preschool site, where a class was cotaught by a preschool teacher and a special education teacher holding credentials in general education and special education in the area of severe disabilities. The teachers' training included extensive preparation in PBS practices. A comprehensive positive behavior support plan (BSP) was developed via a team process and successfully implemented to address issues at school and home.

MEET ROBERTO

Roberto, 32 years old, is from a large urban area. At the age of 18, he was diagnosed as having bipolar disorder. Roberto has had several stays of varying lengths (from 2 to 6 weeks) in psychiatric hospitals. The general goals of his hospital stays included stabilization of mood, medication changes, individual counseling, and participation in group meetings. During his last three hospitalizations, Roberto exhibited several behaviors that were considered disruptive to the unit and dangerous. These behaviors included inappropriate behavior with female staff (e.g., standing and talking too closely, talking about sex), cursing at and instigating arguments and fights with other patients, and disrupting medication dispensing at the nurse's station (e.g., cursing, yelling, breaking in line).

Following a change in hospital administration and oversight by an outside agency, the facility was charged with the mandate to change various components of the medical model that was in use and move toward an approach based on PBS. A PBS team was developed, and Roberto's case was referred to them. Prior to the referral, Roberto's program followed a standard psychiatric hospital approach: psychotropic medication, emergency medication (known as *pro re nata,* or PRN—or medication that is given as needed) and/or restraint for aggressive incidents, points earned for following unit rules (to be turned in for rewards such as

activities, privileges), and points lost for not following unit rules. In addition, he was required to attend individual counseling sessions and group meetings. Nursing staff and psychiatric aides were primarily responsible for the daily routine and implementation of the unit program.

The BSP that was developed for Roberto was intended to bring about many changes, not just for him but for all the patients on the unit, the hospital staff, and the culture of the hospital units. Hospital staff, trained in the traditional medical model, were reluctant to embrace the changes called for in the BSP because these changes focused on more than just Roberto. Contrary to what staff were used to, the indicated changes did not involve the frequency or quality of the reinforcers for appropriate behavior or the type and severity of the negative consequences for displaying inappropriate behaviors. Rather, the changes to Roberto's program would also require changes in the culture of the environment of the psychiatric unit and the roles of some of the hospital staff. The newly designed BSP focused on understanding his challenging behaviors within the context of the unit and the community in which he lived—as opposed to seeing his behaviors just as "bipolar" behaviors. The intent of the plan was to focus on changing some elements of the hospital environment, which was expected to benefit Roberto (as well as many of the other patients), and teaching alternative behaviors in place of the inappropriate behaviors. Roberto's story that follows is a "partial" story. It is partial because, unlike Sophie, Roberto's plan was never implemented. This implementation failure was primarily due to hospital staff's reluctance to change the culture of the hospital; these challenges are embedded in Roberto's story and serve as a vehicle to identify the systems challenges in delivering PBS (see Chapters 3, 5, and 22). PBS depends on the commitment and support of all involved.

Sophie's story is complete in its telling— she has had the benefit of being supported by many stakeholders (e.g., administration, family, teaching staff, peers), who as a team share a vision. Roberto's story, however, reflects only the beginning. Sophie has a developmental disability and attends school. Roberto has mental illness and depends on a variety of departments in the mental health system, many of which have traditionally resisted change and worked within instead of across disciplines. We can learn a lot from Sophie's story about success. And as we follow Roberto's story, we will see the challenges that arise—and from these we can also learn a lot.

In the following sections, we describe the foundational assumptions of PBS and use Sophie and Roberto's stories to demonstrate these assumptions.

POSITIVE BEHAVIOR SUPPORT ASSUMPTIONS ABOUT BEHAVIOR

Problem Behavior Serves a Function for the Person Displaying the Behavior(s)

One of the key concepts to remember when managing problem behavior is that behavior is communicative—that is, it serves a function or purpose for the individual displaying the behavior. Behavior may serve to *get* something for the person (e.g., attention from peers or teacher, materials, sensory stimulation) or serve to have the person *avoid* something (e.g., attention from peers or teacher, difficult or boring activities; O'Neill et al., 1997). Addressing problem behaviors without understanding the purpose, context, or effect of the behavior is not likely to be effective, as the real issue for the individual remains unresolved (Bambara, 2005; Halle, Bambara, & Reichle, 2005). Developing an intervention without understanding the function or purpose of the problem behavior may cause the behavior to become more frequent or severe, leading some interventionists to resort to increasingly intrusive and aversive interventions (Cooper, Heron, & Heward, 2007). Functional behavioral assessment (FBA) is a process used to assess the factors associated with the problem behavior and to understand the function or purpose behind the behavior. (See Chapters 14, 15, and 16 for a comprehensive description and discussion of FBA.) One goal of an FBA is to determine the function of the identified problem behavior. Research has demonstrated that behavior supports that are based on an FBA lead to greater behavior change than supports that are not related to the FBA (Ingram, Lewis-Palmer, & Sugai, 2005; Newcomer & Lewis, 2004).

Sophie

A comprehensive FBA revealed a variety of functions for Sophie's various problem behaviors. Data suggested that Sophie's aggressive behavior toward adults and her cursing and screaming were protests against 1) being told what to do and 2) being denied access to desired objects or activities. Aggressive behavior toward classmates was hypothesized to be attempts at initiating social interactions. Self-injurious behaviors, often accompanied by screaming and crying, were reactions to overstimulation (e.g., the noisy chaos of the full class returning from recess). Instead of coming up with separate intervention strategies for each type of problem behavior (aggression, self-injury, screaming, crying), the team focused on intervention strategies to address the various functions of the behavior (e.g., protesting being told what to do or denied access to preferred activities).

Roberto

When Roberto engaged in cursing or speaking inappropriately to female staff, they talked to him about the rules of the unit and reminded him of the consequences for engaging in those types of behavior (e.g., loss of points). This type of approach focuses on the behavior without regard to *why* it may be happening. Based on observation and data, the new PBS team hypothesized that the function of Roberto's behavior was to gain attention—from both staff and other patients. This hypothesis would drive the development of his BSP.

Positive Strategies Are Effective in Addressing the Most Challenging Behavior

The technology of PBS has developed over the past 3 decades. When comprehensive functional assessments are conducted (see Chapters 14, 15, and 16) and multicomponent behavior intervention plans are developed and implemented with fidelity, we can address even the most severe problem behaviors without resorting to more intrusive measures. Research has demonstrated that with the competent development of a function-driven plan and continued analysis, the most serious problem behaviors may be addressed.

Sophie

When Sophie was in her first program, if her behavior was not interrupted, it would escalate to the point of doing serious harm to others and herself. When that occurred, students and staff were removed from the area, and her grandmother was called to take her home. The school began to talk about the possibility of using physical management procedures when her self-injurious behavior increased. In her new school, the BSP, based on the functions of her behavior, was successful in decreasing the incidents of problem behavior and providing her with ways to initiate peer interactions and appropriately communicate her requests for preferred activities. Consequently, the use of physical management procedures was no longer a topic of conversation.

Roberto

When Roberto's cursing or yelling behavior began to escalate, the nursing staff gave him a verbal warning that he was going to lose all his points. Instead of calming down, the threat seemed to serve as a trigger for him, and his behavior would often further increase. If he did not calm down, staff implemented one of two options: emergency medication or a "code." "Code" meant that all individuals were to be removed from the area of the incident so that Roberto could not hurt anyone; a restraint was likely to follow. The new plan that was developed for Roberto was based on the FBA that the PBS team conducted and focused on eliminating

as much as possible the triggers for the behavior, providing him with increased attention from staff throughout the day, and teaching him how to have appropriate conversations with female staff.

When Positive Behavior Intervention Strategies Fail, Additional Functional Assessment Strategies Are Required to Develop More Effective Intervention Plans

The *analysis* component of *applied behavior analysis* requires the use of data to make timely decisions regarding the effectiveness of an intervention. For example, Farlow and Snell (2005) suggested that if a program has not progressed according to the aim line, program modifications are necessary. It is the type of program modification, however, that may differ across the various behavioral approaches. PBS approaches suggest that when a program is not effective or not progressing in the planned way, it is appropriate to conduct additional functional assessments to determine the intervention elements that might not be effective. This approach differs greatly from the "least restrictive alternative" approach that suggests that less intrusive procedures should be tried and found to be ineffective before more intrusive strategies are implemented (Cooper, Heron, & Heward, 2007). The concern with this type of continuum of interventions is that if an intervention is available for use, it will be used—especially when a behavior is particularly challenging. Regarding the concept of continuum, Taylor (1988) suggests that to conceptualize services in terms of a continuum of restrictiveness is to legitimate those more restrictive components of the continuum. In terms of intrusiveness of interventions, this would translate into accepting the use of aversive interventions for certain people who "need it." Having "permission" to increase the level of aversive consequence (because it is available), even under only certain conditions, is condoning its use and impeding the need to become more innovative and thoughtful about positive interventions.

Sophie

The preventive and instructional procedures that were implemented were effective in reducing Sophie's problem behavior in the classroom. However, Sophie's aggression toward classmates continued on the playground. Instead of focusing on changing consequences for her behavior on the playground (e.g., increasing reinforcement for appropriate behavior or increasing negative consequences for the display of inappropriate behavior), the team conducted further observational assessment and found that she was attempting to initiate interactions. Structured games with a small number of peers were established to teach Sophie turn taking and other social interaction skills. This function-driven revision to her BSP was effective in addressing her playground behavior.

Roberto

One component of Roberto's initial function-based intervention plan developed by the PBS team was to have him receive his medications before the other patients so that he did not have to wait in line. This strategy was designed in response to the hypothesis that the stress of standing for several minutes with his fellow patients triggered behavioral episodes. If Roberto's behavior around the nursing station did not improve with this new strategy, the team would work with Roberto to design another positive function-based intervention to address this component of the plan. It may be that this one component of the intervention is ineffective, although many other components of his multicomponent plan may be effective.

Features of the Environmental Context Affect Behavior

As will be described across all chapters in the book, behavior is a function of the environment. This means that behavior does not occur in a vacuum; it is influenced by and influences an endless variety of environmental variables. An individual may have problem behaviors in one situation or context but not in another; if this occurs consistently, we must assume that

there are specific environmental variables occurring in that situation that are associated with the problem behaviors. As environments are complex, it can be challenging to identify the specific elements of an environment that are associated with the behavior. Collecting data that potentially reveal these associations is critical to analysis of the behavior.

Sophie

Sophie's behavior had been perceived as completely random and unpredictable prior to gathering data for the comprehensive functional assessment. As the data were analyzed, a number of patterns appeared and environmental variables that triggered the problem behavior were identified. Sophie was easily overstimulated by and sensitive to loud noises. Thus, transition times in and out of the classroom, when all the students in the class were moving around and making noise, would often serve as antecedents to a tantrum. When excited about an activity, especially on the playground, Sophie could quickly escalate from playing to screaming and aggression. Her sensory issues included tactile defensiveness that made the almost nonexistent personal space between preschool children difficult for Sophie. It was determined that she could tolerate being with other students if they were at least 8 inches apart. The teachers tried to keep Sophie at a good distance away from one student in particular, as he seemed to enjoy "pushing her buttons" to elicit problem behavior. Other triggers included having to wait for a preferred item or activity and behavioral corrections or reprimands from adults, particularly when these were delivered in a loud, stern voice. Once the contextual variables were analyzed, the team was able to design function-based interventions to help Sophie learn to succeed in the school context.

Roberto

Incident reports are a mainstay of psychiatric settings. These reports typically detail variables such as what time the incident occurred, where the incident occurred, who was involved in the incident, what led up to the incident, how staff reacted, and so forth. An analysis of incident reports for Roberto's unit was conducted in two ways. First, the PBS team conducted an analysis of where and when (i.e., environment and time of day) incidents were occurring with all patients on the unit. This gave the team information that could be used to analyze general practices on the unit (e.g., a high percentage of incidents occurred between 9 and 9:30 and 4:30 and 5:30; a high percentage of incidents occurred near the nursing station). The PBS team now needed to explore what there was about these times of day and locations that could be changed to reduce problem behaviors on the unit. It was assumed that if they could have an impact on the routines occurring during these times, there would be an improved quality of life for everyone on the unit. Second, the contexts in which Roberto displayed aggression to other patients were analyzed. These data revealed that incidents were occurring in two areas of the unit: waiting in line for his medication in the morning and in the day room. The PBS team needed to understand what about these locations might be triggering Roberto's behavior. For example, was it the larger number of patients together in one space that was an issue for Roberto? Or was it that Roberto had no choices about what was on the television in the day room? Once the staff had a better understanding of the environmental variables affecting his behavior, they could begin to work on a BSP.

....

Reduction of Problem Behavior Is an Important but Not the Sole Outcome of Successful Intervention; Effective PBS Results in Improvements in Quality of Life, Acquisition of Valued Skills, and Access to Valued Activities, Settings, and People

Early research in the area of behavior analysis focused predominantly on the reduction of problem behavior. The field of behavior analysis has evolved over time; this evolution is congruent with our changing expectations regarding individuals. PBS has helped behavior analysts see the value of focusing on increasingly socially important responses versus focusing primarily on reducing problem behavior. Where once we were trying to prove that individuals with disabilities could learn (and what they were learning was not necessarily relevant) and that we could reduce interfering behavior, we are now focused on using our behavioral strategies to support

individuals to accomplish a self-determined quality of life. Spooner and Brown (2011) describe four historical benchmarks of change in the way we conceptualize problem behaviors and outcomes. The first benchmark was the demonstration that *behavior can change*. This was a significant paradigm shift, as individuals with significant disabilities were historically considered "untrainable." The second benchmark was that *problem behavior can be reduced*. This benchmark was remarkable in that reducing problem behavior was somewhat more socially valid—at least in terms of decreasing injury to the individual and others. However, there was little concern regarding the methods used to affect behavior change. The third benchmark was that *adaptive behavior can be increased*. The significance of this benchmark is that in addition to our ability to reduce problem behavior, we could increase adaptive behavior. This more educative and constructive approach helped pave the way for teaching useful and functional skills that can contribute positively to an individual's life. The fourth benchmark was that *meaningful behavior change could occur in inclusive environments*. The significance of this shift in perception is that our strategies could not only lead to access to more inclusive environments but be *implemented* in inclusive environments, including school, work, and community settings. The many historical changes in services (see Chapter 1) combined to promote a change in our expectations of what is possible and what visions we could have for individuals with problem behaviors. Meyer and Evans (1989) delineate eight outcomes that demonstrate program success:

1) improvement in target behavior, 2) acquisition of alternative skills and positive behaviors, 3) positive collateral effects and the absence of side effects, 4) reduced need for and use of medical and crisis management services for the individual or others, 5) less restrictive placements and greater participation in integrated community experiences, 6) subjective quality-of-life improvements (happiness, satisfaction, and choices for the individual), 7) perceptions of improvement by the family and significant

others, and 8) extended social relationships and informal support networks.

Sophie

Sophie's problem behaviors decreased dramatically as she acquired the skills to communicate her needs and desires; label her feelings; play independently at school, home, and church; and begin to regulate her behavior by requesting a break when she became overstimulated. Attendance at school- and homelife improved for Sophie and her grandmother as she learned to make choices within her daily routines, such as what she would have for breakfast and which clothes she would wear each day. Her grandmother was able to go back to church services and social activities, taking Sophie with her. The quality of life improved greatly for Sophie and her grandmother, teachers, and classmates.

....

Roberto

Although Roberto did not want to participate in the team meeting, his grandmother and sister met with the hospital staff to talk about transition goals and outcomes. While his family was in agreement that his behavior on the unit was of concern, they were also concerned with his transition to the community, as previous transitions were always problematic. They wanted to talk about volunteer or part-time job placements, living in an apartment with some level of support, and having healthy relationships with male and female peers. Everyone felt that if he had access to typical activities and relationships in the community, his behavior changes would more likely be sustainable.

....

POSITIVE BEHAVIOR SUPPORT ASSUMPTIONS ABOUT INTERVENTIONS

Plans Are Person-Centered, Including the Identification of Outcomes that Enhance Quality of Life and Are Valued by the Individual, His or Her Family, and the Community

Historically, behavior intervention focused predominantly on the goal of reducing problem behavior, whereas the primary goal of PBS interventions is to improve the quality of the lives of target individuals, their families, and those around them (Carr et al., 1999). Person-centered assessment and planning processes, where the individual and his or her team gather to share the individual's history and strengths/talents along with fears and dreams for the future, are the vehicle for identifying valued quality-of-life outcomes (see Chapters 4 and 14). The vision developed by the team, and the identified outcomes and strategies to achieve them, must be reflected in the BSP. These targeted outcomes, which may be referred to as *broad goals* (Positive Behavioral Support Project, 1999), become the driving force behind all interventions and supports.

Sophie

The PBS process began with a team meeting following the McGill Action Planning System (MAPS; Chapter 4) person-centered format, where history, strengths/talents, dreams, nightmares, and needs were shared and an action plan developed to take steps toward improving the quality of Sophie's and her grandmother's lives. The team achieved consensus on broad goals for Sophie. Sophie's grandmother wanted her to be able to stay in school every day; make friends with other children; successfully go to church, Sunday school, and community outings; and be able to stay at home with a babysitter. School staff wanted Sophie to remain in inclusive school programs with needed supports and services, socialize successfully with classmates, acquire self-management skills, and progress in the general education curriculum. Their fears about Sophie's future were also discussed and included concerns about her ending up in a segregated setting or a residential program, not having friends, or not being able to participate in community activities with her grandmother. All interventions and supports were designed as steps toward meeting these broad goals and avoiding any "nightmare" scenarios.

....

Roberto

Roberto's team needed to develop a plan that focused on two levels—the first for his remaining time on the unit and the second for his transition into the community. His family was most concerned with him returning to the community and wanted the plan to focus on whatever it would take to help him maintain a job, live in an apartment, interact appropriately with peers when he returned to the community, and stay on his medications. Their fear was that Roberto might go home and either live an isolated life or end up getting arrested for inappropriate sexual behavior. The professionals on the team agreed with these concerns and identified additional goals to be included in Roberto's plan that were relevant for his stay on the unit, such as getting along with staff and patients and participating in groups, including cross-unit groups with women. The team discussed ways in which the unit staff (i.e., nurses, mental health aides) could support these goals. The social worker on the team was going to contact the local mental health agency to enter Roberto into a day treatment program and continue working with him and his family. The team also discussed how they could facilitate Roberto's participation with the social worker to contribute to his own transition plan.

....

Plans Must Be Based on Functional Behavioral Assessments and Include Functionally Derived Interventions

The process of determining the function of the problem behavior along with the conditions under which the behavior does and does not occur is referred to as *functional behavioral assessment* (FBA; O'Neill et al., 1997). (See Chapters 14 and 15 for further information on FBA.) The key to effective PBS interventions is to determine the purpose (function) the problem behavior serves for the focus individual. Once the function is identified, socially acceptable behavior that achieves the desired outcome can be taught and used by the individual to replace the problem behavior. Instruction and/or reinforcement of desirable behavior that is not function based is unlikely to result in durable change, as the individual will continue to attempt to get the desired outcome. In addition, knowledge of the conditions under which the problem behavior occurs informs us of the "triggers" or antecedents of the behavior. All this information drives the development of a BSP. The effectiveness of function-based interventions has been demonstrated repeatedly (e.g., Carr & Durand, 1985; Ingram, Lewis-Palmer, & Sugai, 2005; Lewis & Newcomer, 2004; Sailor, Dunlap, Sugai, & Horner, 2009).

Sophie

MAPS (person-centered planning) was used to gather information from Sophie's family, friends, teachers, and other staff to determine both the functions of her behavior and goals for intervention. The FBA included the use of a variety of tools and strategies to further understand her behavior. Sophie's grandmother, her teachers, and paraprofessionals each completed the Motivation Assessment Scale (MAS; Durand & Crimmins, 1992). This allowed the team to see differences in Sophie's behavior with certain people and, more important, facilitated conversation regarding the "function" of behavior rather than the problems Sophie was causing. The collection of extensive data at school provided the team with rich information regarding the interaction between Sophie and the environment. Behavior mapping was done on the playground to determine where, when, and with whom problem behavior occurred. Interviews with Sophie's grandmother and speech therapist yielded important information about the messages Sophie's behavior was relaying and about her communication repertoire in general. The communication system that was developed was based on these data, giving her access to a vocabulary that reflected her preferences and provided her with a communicative alternative to her problem behaviors.

....

Roberto

The strategies for meeting the goals identified in Roberto's plan were based on an analysis of incident report forms and observation on the units, as well as the issues identified by his family. The behavior specialists were interested in looking at unit changes that might have an impact on all patients, as well as individual analyses specific to Roberto. Without understanding the function of Roberto's behavior and the environmental variables influencing the behavior, an effective support plan was less likely. For example, Roberto's problem behavior in the day room may have been related to not having control of the television. Data also reveal that other patients have problems in the day room as well. The intervention plan that is designed for Roberto and environmental changes on the unit should include a strategy that allows alternating control of the television among patients. A visual schedule should be posted that indicates who controls the selection. This antecedent function-driven approach is qualitatively different from offering rewards and punishments for appropriate and inappropriate behavior in the day room.

Behavior Support Interventions Promote Self-Determination and Teach Useful and Valued Skills

As noted by Lucyshyn, Dunlap, and Freeman in Chapter 1, PBS emerged from the movements toward normalization (Wolfensberger, 1972), community and school inclusion for individuals with developmental disabilities (Brown et al., 1977; Turnbull & Turnbull, 2000), and self-determination. These movements were based on acknowledgment of the right for every citizen to participate in the same school, home, and community environments as his or her peers and families and to work toward self-defined visions of a good quality of life. This focus dramatically changed the way we looked at interventions. We started to ask, "How do we provide supports that promote participation and are respectful of individuals, their preferences, and their dreams?" This yielded as unacceptable the often aversive and dehumanizing behavior reduction interventions that were designed to control the individual according to preferences of professionals or the "system." In addition, the acceptable outcomes of behavior intervention expanded from a focus on merely reducing

problem behavior to a focus on developing meaningful skills and improving quality of life (Carr et al., 2002). The primary vehicle for achieving the targeted meaningful and valued skills is the instructional component of BSPs. A focus on skills that promote self-determination (Wehmeyer, 2005) supports individuals in building the capacity within themselves to increase control over their lives and advocate for themselves, thus increasing the quality of their lives and often reducing the need for external supports and resources.

Sophie

Sophie's multicomponent BSP included a variety of interventions to teach 4-year-old Sophie initial self-determination skills such as making choices in daily routines, working/playing independently, and beginning to self-regulate her behavior by asking for a break if she needed one. She also learned to evaluate the status of her emotional state via the use of colored cards representing her different moods and had a class job (feeding the rabbit). Learning symbolic communication was a priority, initially with pictures and then moving to speech. Sophie was taught to use her communication strategies for social interaction with her peers and teachers, as well as for self-regulation, requesting, and protesting.

Roberto

The PBS team created a proposal to establish new groups for patients who were interested. These would be in addition to other groups that were already established on the unit (e.g., Alcoholics Anonymous, Narcotics Anonymous, dialectical behavior therapy). Two groups were proposed: the first for self-advocacy and the second for social relationships. Staff would encourage Roberto and other patients to attend these groups but decided not to make any privileges contingent on attendance. One component of the self-advocacy group was to have the patients rotate in leading the discussions. Participation in these groups was intended to give Roberto skills that would be useful not only for his stay on the unit but also when he returned to the community.

....

Behavior Support Interventions Are Acceptable in Inclusive Community Settings and Do Not Use Techniques that Cause Pain or Humiliation or Deprive the Individual of Basic Needs

A critical component of the technology of PBS, evident from the earliest descriptions, is the use of interventions for problem behavior that are consistent with community norms for all people—that is, interventions that are respectful and do not cause pain or tissue damage (Horner et al., 1990; Lavigna & Donnellan, 1986; Meyer & Evans, 1989). (See Chapter 1 for an expanded description of the history of PBS.) Although it is unthinkable that causing pain or tissue damage would be considered in any way acceptable for typical children in public schools or adults in our communities, interventions that do so have been (and in some cases continue to be) used regularly with individuals whose disabilities include problem behavior (Brown, Michaels, Oliva, & Woolf, 2008; Michaels, Brown, & Mirabella, 2005). The U.S. Government Accountability Office (GAO) report titled *Examining the Abusive and Deadly Use of Seclusion and Restraint in Schools* (2009) reveals that the use of these procedures continue nationwide and have led to death and abuse in public and private schools and treatment centers. The GAO also reports that as of 2012, there are no federal regulations restricting or prohibiting these practices but only a wide variety of divergent state regulations (U.S. Government Accountability Office, 2012). Brown and Bambara (2014) suggest that for these types of aversive practices to be banned and for PBS to become the norm will take a four-component approach: 1) a legal ban on the use of aversive interventions, 2) a legal requirement to use PBS, 3) continued growth of evidence-based PBS strategies, and 4) a commitment to the implementation of PBS.

The use of effective positive intervention strategies that do not cause pain or humiliation or deny access to basic needs is a primary assumption for all BSPs. Such positive interventions are, by definition, acceptable in inclusive school and community settings, particularly when age appropriateness is also considered when designing BSPs.

Sophie

In contrast to the reactive strategies implemented in prior school placements, all assessment and interventions for Sophie in her new program were positive, respectful, and conducted in inclusive settings (typical preschool program, home, community, church). Initially, Sophie required an adult to be with her most of the time to prevent harm to herself or others by gently redirecting Sophie and to systematically teach her the steps to participate in new routines such as taking a break (e.g., requesting the break, going to the book area, selecting a book, looking at it, returning it to the shelf, selecting another, and returning to the group when the timer went off), setting up her schedule each day, and feeding the rabbit while other students were returning from recess. The intensive support was gradually faded as Sophie learned to complete the routines independently or with minimal support. It took longer for Sophie to learn to identify her emotional escalation or the potential for this and to request a break. However, this process was also conducted using a systematic and positive process by staff observing her closely and prompting her to request a break at the first sign of potential problem behavior (i.e., at the precursor level). She was also taught to identify how she was feeling using colored pictures of cars. A green car indicated that her engine was running smoothly, a red car indicated her engine was too revved up and she needed an immediate break, and yellow indicated that she was just a little revved up and needed to stop and take a few deep breaths. Reinforcers for Sophie included stickers (especially of cars), enthusiastic praise, hugs (when Sophie initiated this type of contact), and selecting small prizes from the class prize box. Earned reinforcers were never taken away for problem behavior; rather, she did not earn the next available reinforcer. Long-term goals were that she remain in general education classes, make friends, enjoy activities as engaged

in by her same-age peers, and successfully participate in church and community activities. All these
contexts required positive, respectful interventions,
were proactive, and avoided the use of any negative consequences or coercion.

....

Roberto

Roberto's BSP replaced physical and chemical
restraints (i.e., emergency medication) for disruptive behavior on the unit with antecedent-based
strategies (e.g., allowing him to wait in his room for
his turn to get his medications) aimed at reducing
the likelihood that dangerous situations would
occur. Emergency physical restraint was to be used
only if he or others were in imminent physical
danger. The behavior specialists were also going
to work with Roberto to teach him to predict
his problems and proactively ask for prescribed
emergency medication when needed. Meetings
were going to be arranged with his family before
his return home to discuss handling dangerous
situations that might occur there. After using the
planned antecedent and calming approaches, if
Roberto were to become aggressive at home, his
family was to call the police. However, prior to his
return home, his family was urged to go to the
police and discuss Roberto's mental health problems and request that they be as nonconfronta-
tive as possible and try to calm him before they made
any threat of physical restraint or handcuffs.

....

Behavior Support Interventions Are Constructive, Respectful, and Multicomponent, Emphasizing Antecedent Interventions, Instruction in Prosocial Behaviors, and Environmental Modifications

PBS is an educational model with a focus
on constructive efforts to increase the
capacity of the focus individual and those
around him or her to live quality lives. As
noted in descriptions of earlier assumptions, interventions and interactions are
always respectful of the focus individuals
and their families. Over time it has become

increasingly obvious that behavior reduction alone will not result in the achievement of broad goals and improvements in
quality of life that are targeted outcomes of
PBS. Therefore, BSPs are always multicomponent and include a variety of interventions for each individual. BSPs minimally
include antecedent interventions to render
problem behavior unnecessary by removing
triggers and include instructional plans to
teach replacement prosocial and communication skills and provide positive feedback
for desirable behavior (Section V).

Sophie

Two multicomponent intervention plans were developed for Sophie based on functional assessment
data—one for school and one for home and the
community. The school plan was more complex than
the home plan, as the special education teacher had
the training to implement and monitor the plan daily.

School

School interventions included the following:

- A picture schedule that Sophie organized with
  the teacher each morning
- Seating next to the teacher and away from the
  previously mentioned antagonistic student
  during circle and other group/class activities
- A break card and instruction in its use
- A book area designated as her "quiet place"
  where she would go to calm down when getting
  overstimulated (initially with a teacher but with
  the goal of independently requesting a break)
- A class job (e.g., feeding the rabbit) to get her
  back into the classroom and engaged before
  the rest of the class came in from recess
- Systematic instruction in learning to make
  choices and work/play independently
- A picture communication system (Although
  Sophie did have some verbal communication
  skills as demonstrated by her "cussing," she was
  often unable to use it for communication or conversational purposes, especially if she was upset.)
- A timer used to increase Sophie's ability to wait
  (e.g., for her turn on the bike at recess) that began
  with a 2-second delay and was gradually increased

- Enthusiastic praise, stickers, and little "prizes" for desirable behavior (Staff had to be reminded that nothing that Sophie earned would ever be taken away contingent on future problem behavior.)

Home

The home plan, to be implemented by Sophie's grandmother, included the following:

- In the evening, Sophie chose her outfit and breakfast items for the following morning. Sophie was allowed to change her mind using pictures as often as she wanted until it was bedtime, as doing this in the morning had her missing the school bus. The last selection prior to bed was what she would eat and wear in the morning.
- A bag was filled with quiet activities for church. Sophie was to play with one item, put it away, get out the next item, play with it, and so forth. Her break card was also in the bag, and her grandmother would encourage her to use it if Sophie seemed like she was getting restless. She and her grandmother would walk outside for a few minutes and then return to church. The play sequence and use of the break card were both taught at school before these strategies were used by her grandmother.
- A sticker chart and a timer were used in Sunday school, and Sophie received a sticker for participating in activities or sitting quietly along with the other children. This began with an interval of 1 minute and gradually increased as Sophie was successful. Sophie's grandmother went with her to Sunday school to implement the intervention until the interval was 8 minutes and then gradually faded from the room so the teachers could take over Sophie's support.
- Reinforcers were used at home and in church. In addition to stickers, she and her grandmother would go for an ice cream cone on the way home from church after a "good" day. At home, she was rewarded with hugs, praise, her grandmother reading to her, and access to her favorite videos.

Roberto

Two separate but related intervention plans were designed for Roberto—one for the unit and one

for when he made the transition back home. These intervention plans were composed of many elements, including, for example, the following:

Unit

- A visual schedule for control of the television
- New patient-run group sessions on self-advocacy
- A new group on social relationships
- A modified medication dispensing routine
- Teaching Roberto to recognize the need for PRN medication and requesting it

Home

- A continued psychiatric and medication regime
- Participation in individual and group counseling sessions at a day treatment program
- Continued Alcoholics Anonymous and Narcotics Anonymous groups
- Caseworker support to find a job in the community
- Caseworker support to address financial and health insurance complications
- Caseworker support to find an apartment in the community
- Family lessons on calming techniques
- Family meetings with police

Behavior Support Interventions Are Based on Evidence-Based Strategies and Are Socially and Empirically Valid to Achieve Desired Outcomes

PBS as a process for successful behavior intervention is an evidence-based practice for achieving valued and desired outcomes (see Carr et al., 2002; Sailor et al., 2009; Chapters 1, 23, and 29). In addition to PBS as a process, there is an evidence base for a number of intervention categories that are often components of comprehensive BSPs. Some of these include the following:

- Antecedent interventions, such as environmental modifications (Kern & Clemens, 2007; Mace, 1985; Simons & Klein, 2007; Sugai & Horner, 2009), choices (Bambara,

2005; Kern, Bambara, & Fogt, 2002), and curricular modifications (Halvorsen & Neary, 2009; Katz, 2013; Sanford & Horner, 2013)

- Visual support strategies such as story-based interventions (Mirenda, MacGregor, & Kelly-Keough, 2002), visual schedules (Koyama & Wang, 2011; Lequia, Machalicek, & Rispoli, 2012), contingency maps (Brown & Mirenda, 2006; Tobin & Simpson, 2012), and power cards (Campbell & Tincani, 2011; Keeling, Myles, Gagnon, & Simpson, 2003)

- Systematic instruction, including task analysis, chaining procedures, prompt/fading, self-management, and monitoring (Agran & Wehmeyer, 2006; Shogren, Faggella-Luby, Bae, & Wehmeyer, 2004)

- Pivotal Response Training (Koegel, Koegel, Hurley, & Frea, 1992; Koegel, Koegel, & Steibel, 1998; Neft et al., 2010)

- Functional communication training (Durand, 2012; Kurtz, Boelter, Jarmolowicz, Chin, & Hagopian, 2011; Mancil, 2006, for reviews)

- Self-determination training (Algozzone et al., 2001; Sugai & Simonsen, 2012; Wehmeyer, 2005)

Individualized combinations of these types of interventions will comprise components of effective PBS.

Sophie

The intervention strategies used with Sophie were all evidence based and socially valid. The behavior assessment and intervention processes were based on the PBS literature in which her teachers were trained. The effectiveness of visual supports such as the picture schedule, break cards, and picture communication systems are well documented, as are the use of choice-making strategies and reinforcement and systematic instructional strategies. No one strategy alone would meet Sophie's needs; rather, all these strategies worked together to provide Sophie with the necessary supports. Sophie adopted the socially acceptable replacement behaviors as she learned that they were more effective and took less energy on her part than the problem behaviors she had been relying on in the past.

Roberto

Although there is a growing amount of research to support the use of a variety of strategies in school, home, and community settings with participants with varying levels of skills, types of disabilities, and ages, little has been published specifically focused on implementation of PBS strategies for individuals with mental illness and in psychiatric settings. Roberto's PBS team was aware of the literature, and although little was specifically focused on "someone like Roberto," they felt confident that the strategies they read about were likely generalizable across disabilities and settings; they thought that this was at least a promising place to start. Based on their assessment information, they would consider evidence-based strategies such as visual supports and self-monitoring. Frequent evaluation of his behavior would allow the team to determine if these strategies were indeed effective for Roberto.

Intervention Plans Include Ongoing Measurement of Impact on Multiple Measures

Strategies for measuring and evaluating the impact of interventions are critical for the success of PBS implementation. Three characteristics of data must be present in order for measurement to be meaningful: data must reflect important behavior, be contextually appropriate, and be sufficiently accurate and reliable (Brown & Snell, 2011). As PBS is focused on contextually appropriate and collaborative assessment and program development and individually determined visions of quality of life, it naturally meets these standards of measurement. Although hypotheses developed via FBA and person-centered assessments provide direction for interventions that are likely to be effective, there is no way to know whether hypotheses are accurate or interventions will be effective unless the effect of implementation is measured in ways that can provide meaningful and accurate information. Further, the use of an evidence-based strategy does not ensure that any one individual will benefit from it (Brown & Snell, 2011). Because comprehensive BSPs are multielement, multiple measurement strategies are required to evaluate the various components of intervention. Counting problem and replacement behaviors, for example, cannot tell us whether the individual has more friends or is interacting more with family members. (See Chapter 10 for a discussion of measurement strategies.) In addition to the need for information regarding the effectiveness of initial implementation, ongoing evaluation is necessary to identify the need for adjustments or modifications to all or any component of the BSP. There are many factors that, over time, may render previously successful interventions ineffective or unnecessary. Some of these may include changes in the context (e.g., a new teacher or job coach, movement from one school level to the next or a change in residence), fidelity of BSP implementation, changes in the interests of the focus individual without the proper adaptive or communicative skills, and the acquisition of skills that make components of intervention unnecessary (e.g., replacement behavior).

Sophie

The impact of the team-designed interventions on Sophie's behavior was measured in several ways. Data were recorded daily on problem and replacement behaviors. Sophie's attendance and on-time arrival, calls to her grandmother, and the amount of time she spent participating in group/circle activities were also documented. Implementation of the home BSP was also monitored. Sophie's grandmother was taught to use a data sheet developed by the teacher to mark *yes* or *no* to indicate whether Sophie ate or refused the breakfast she had selected just before bed the previous evening and also marked *yes* or *no* regarding whether Sophie did or did not receive a "treat" after church and/or Sunday school. She also wrote a brief weekly summary of church, Sunday school, and other community outings. The team met bi-weekly to review the various data and make adjustments to the plan. As problem behavior decreased and desirable behavior increased, the meetings were extended to one time per month. Data indicated that Sophie's disruptive behavior went from an

average of 14 occurrences per 10-minute intervals during the baseline period to 0 per day after the implementation of the BSP. The only exception to this dramatic progress was when there were interruptions in the implementation of her plan (e.g., when an assembly was not included in her daily schedule). The design of strategies to address the specific events that were the "exceptions" would be the next challenge for the team to address.

Roberto

The PBS team planned to measure Roberto's progress in a variety of ways. First, the number of incidents within the context of the challenging routines (at the nurse's station, in the day room) would be recorded. In this way, progress or problems in each context would be apparent, even if the total number of incidents was not significantly decreased. Second, Roberto's frequency of participation in groups was going to be counted. Third, improvements in his attitude (as indicated in Roberto's self-management reports) were going to be reviewed weekly and discussed with him. Finally, his requests for PRN medications were monitored.

Behavior Support Interventions Are Based on a Collaborative Team Process Throughout Assessment, Intervention, and Evaluation

Collaborative teaming is the process whereby the various members of the focus individual's team come together to agree on common goals and through shared decision making and joint action work to accomplish these goals (Fleming & Monda-Amaya, 2001; Snell & Janney, 2005). PBS teams are composed of individuals representing various disciplines and roles in the individual's life and thus bring differing perspectives and expertise to the process. This variety of perspectives provides incredible richness to the discussions but can also create barriers to achieving consensus on both priority goals and the means with which to accomplish them. Clearly the PBS assumptions described in this chapter and illustrated through Sophie and Roberto's stories could not be accomplished without the collaborative efforts of team members and the focus individual to the greatest degree possible. Sophie had a functional collaborative team, and they successfully worked together throughout assessment, intervention, and evaluation. Roberto's PBS team, due to the culture in the hospital and their unsuccessful efforts at collaboration, worked in isolation, apart from the other staff. Consequently, although the PBS team was competent in their analysis of behavior and their design of intervention and evaluation plans, the plans were never implemented.

The person-centered planning (PCP) processes described in Chapters 4 and 13 provide an excellent vehicle for centering the focus on the individual, their family, and the outcomes that will improve the quality of their lives and the lives of those around them. Action plans directed specifically toward accomplishing these valued goals are developed as a part of the PCP process. Shared decision making is required to conduct FBAs and develop a comprehensive support plan that includes intervention strategies and evaluation measures. Implementation and monitoring of the BSP requires coordinated joint actions and continued shared decision making. In addition to actions for the focus individual, the collaborative process allows team members to support each other in the planning and implementation process. Clearly, participation and "buy-in" are required from *all* team members if the supports are to be successful.

Sophie

Sophie's team includes her grandmother, general education and special education teachers, speech therapist, and a representative from the Vulnerable Children's Project at a local hospital. The program manager also participated in the initial meetings and on occasion over time. Due to the past adversarial experiences between the district and the family, there was a need for the manager to serve as a facilitator and at times a mediator until the team agreed

on ground rules and began to trust one another. The team worked together initially to discuss Sophie's "issues" from each participant's perspective. The initial meeting was structured so all participants were able to share target behavior that they felt should be a priority for intervention, the rationale for this, and their thoughts on why the behavior was occurring. The second meeting focused on preparing for a PCP session. The MAPS process was described; time, location, and people to be invited were determined; and an action plan was developed for preparation for the meeting. The MAPS process resulted in the development of the major goals for Sophie. At school, the goal was for her to remain in the inclusive preschool program and socialize successfully with peers. At home, the major goal was for her to choose clothing and breakfast items for the next day before going to bed and to successfully attend church and Sunday school. The determination of these goals was followed by team meetings to plan and conduct a comprehensive FBA, develop a function-based multielement BSP, and monitor implementation.

Roberto

The PBS team made a variety of attempts to include Roberto, unit staff, nursing staff, and his psychiatrist in all discussions and meetings. For a variety of reasons, participation was minimal. Roberto did not want to sit in a room with so many professionals or with his family. However, recruiting his input was relatively easy, as an individual with whom he had rapport met privately with him to discuss his thoughts concerning living on the unit and making the transition back into the community. The many interpersonal and interdisciplinary challenges that were so ingrained within the hospital culture, however, could not be overcome. In the end, these challenges proved insurmountable, and the PBS team was allowed only to implement changes that focused on individuals—not the unit as a whole. Further, nursing staff were unwilling to make the necessary changes in their daily routines to support the individual strategies that the team developed for Roberto. Although the administration of the hospital was interested in implementing PBS for individuals, their actions prohibited any changes that required cultural shifts in behavior support (e.g., focus on antecedent changes rather than consequence changes, change the method of medication delivery). In the end, change was not supported, and Roberto's BSP was not implemented.

....

CONCLUSION

This chapter describes, through the application to two individuals with diverse needs and characteristics, the foundational assumptions of PBS. With Sophie, a young girl with developmental disabilities and problem behaviors, a collaborative team worked together to develop and successfully implement a plan to maintain and benefit from her attendance in a general education classroom alongside her peers without disabilities, with the goal of helping her live a more satisfying and self-determined life with her grandmother. We are confident that Roberto, a young adult identified as having a psychiatric disorder, could have benefited from the BSP that his team developed. However, due to reluctance of many hospital staff to change the culture of the hospital, Roberto's plan was never implemented. Thus, although his PBS team was competent in the analysis of behavior and design of intervention and evaluation plans, the plans remained unrealized.

We have come a long way with individuals like Sophie. We are only at the first steps with individuals like Roberto. Singh and Strand (2008) point out that individuals with mental illness in hospital settings are rarely consulted about their perspectives on their problems or regarding what, if any, behavior should be targeted for change. Their efforts involved including the individual as a member of the treatment team instead of having a treatment team conceptualize goals and interventions in the absence of the patient. This, however, is only the first step. As Roberto's story teaches us, a person-centered treatment plan cannot be implemented or sustained without the broader systemic support.

The foundational assumptions about behavior and behavior interventions described in this chapter are the cornerstone of PBS. Our vision is that these PBS assumptions will become the standard of practice for all individuals with disabilities.

REFERENCES

Agran, M., & Wehmeyer, M. (2006). Child self-regulation. In M. Hersen (Ed.), *Clinical handbook of behavioral assessment* (pp. 181–199). San Diego, CA: Elsevier Scientific.

Algozzine, B., Browder, D., Karvonen, M., Test. D.W., & Wood, W.M. (2001). Effects of interventions to promote self-determination for individuals with disabilities. *Review of Educational Research, 71,* 219–277.

Association for Positive Behavior Support (APBS). (2007). *Positive behavior support standards of practice: Individual level.* Retrieved from http://www.apbs.org/files/apbs_standards_of_practice_2013_format.pdf

Bambara, L.M. (2005). Overview of the behavior support process. In L.M. Bambara & L. Kern (Eds.), *Individualized supports for students with problem behaviors: Designing positive behavior plans* (pp. 47–70). New York, NY: Guilford Press.

Brown, F., & Bambara, L.M. (2014). Providing respectful behavior supports. In M. Agran, F. Brown, C. Hughes, C. Quirk, & D. Ryndak (Eds.), *Equity & full participation for individuals with severe disabilities: A vision for the future* (pp. 99–121). Baltimore, MD: Paul H. Brookes Publishing Co.

Brown, F., Michaels, C.A., Oliva, C., & Woolf, S. (2008). Personal paradigm shifts in ABA and PBS experts. *Journal of Positive Behavior Interventions, 10,* 212–228.

Brown, F., & Snell, M.E. (2011). Measuring student behavior and learning. In M.E. Snell & F. Brown (Eds.), *Instruction of students with severe disabilities* (7th ed., pp. 186–223). Upper Saddle River, NJ: Pearson.

Brown, K., & Mirenda, P. (2006). Contingency mapping: A novel visual support strategy as an adjunct to functional equivalence training. *Journal of Positive Behavior Interventions, 8,* 155–164.

Brown, L., Wilcox, B., Sontag, E., Vincent, E., Dodd, N., & Gruenewald, L. (1977). Toward the realization of the least restrictive educational environments for severely handicapped students. *The AAESPH Review, 2*(4), 195–204.

Campbell, A., & Tincani, M. (2011). The power card strategy: Strength-based intervention to increase direction following of children with autism spectrum disorder. *Journal of Positive Behavior Interventions, 13,* 240–249.

Carr, E.G., Dunlap, G., Horner, R.H., Koegel, R.L., Turnbull, A.P., Sailor, W. . . . Fox, L. (2002). Positive behavior support: Evolution of an applied science. *Journal of Positive Behavior Interventions, 4,* 4–16.

Carr, E.G., & Durand, V.M. (1985). Reducing behavior problems through functional communication training. *Journal of Applied Behavior Analysis, 18,* 111–126. doi:10.1901/jaba.1985.18-111

Carr, E.G., Horner, R.H., Turnbull, A.P., Marquis, J.G., McLaughlin, D.J., McAtee, M.L., . . . Doolabh, A. (1999). *Positive behavior support for people with developmental disabilities: A research synthesis.* Washington, DC: American Association on Mental Retardation.

Cooper, J.O., Heron, T.E., & Heward, W.L. (2007). *Applied behavior analysis* (2nd ed.). Upper Saddle River, NJ: Pearson.

Durand, V.M. (2012). Functional communication training to reduce challenging behavior. In P. Prelock & R. McCauley (Eds.), *Treatment of autism spectrum disorders: Evidence-based intervention strategies for communication and social interaction* (pp. 107–138). Baltimore, MD: Paul H. Brookes Publishing Co.

Durand, V.M., & Crimmins, D.B. (1992). *The Motivation Assessment Scale (MAS) administration guide.* Topeka, KS: Monaco and Associates.

Farlow, L.J., & Snell, M.E. (2005). Making the most of student performance data. In M.L. Wehmeyer & M. Agran (Eds.), *Evidence-based practices for teaching students with mental retardation and intellectual disabilities* (pp. 27–54). Upper Saddle River, NJ: Pearson.

Fleming, J.L., & Monda-Amaya, L.E. (2001). Process variables critical for team effectiveness. *Remedial and Special Education, 22,* 158–171.

Halle, J., Bambara, L.M., & Reichle, J. (2005). Teaching alternative skills. In L.M. Bambara & L. Kern (Eds.), *Individualized supports for students with problem behaviors: Designing positive behavior plans* (pp. 237–274). New York, NY: Guilford Press.

Halvorsen, A.T., & Neary, T. (2009). *Building inclusive schools: Tools and strategies for success* (2nd ed.). Upper Saddle River, NJ: Pearson.

Horner, R.H., Carr, E.G., Halle, J., McGee, G., Odom, S., & Wolery, M. (2005). The use of single-subject research to identify evidence-based practice in special education. *Exceptional Children, 71,* 165–180.

Horner, R.H., Dunlap, G., Koegel, R.L., Carr, E.G., Sailor, W., Anderson, J., . . . O'Neill, R. (1990). Toward a technology of "nonaversive" behavioral support. *Journal of The Association for Persons with Severe Handicaps, 15,* 125–132.

Ingram, K., Lewis-Palmer, T., & Sugai, G. (2005). Function-based intervention planning: Comparing the effectiveness of FBA indicated and contraindicated interventions plans. *Journal of Positive Behavior Interventions, 7,* 224–236.

Katz, J.N. (2013). The three block model of universal design for learning (UDL): Engaging students in inclusive education. *Canadian Journal of Education/Revue canadienne de l'éducation, 36*(1), 153–194.

Kazdin, A.E. (1977). Assessing the clinical or applied importance of behavior change through social validation. *Behavior Modification, 1,* 427–452.

Keeling, K., Myles, B.S., Gagnon, E., & Simpson, R. (2003). Using the power card strategy to teach sportsmanship skills to a child with autism. *Focus on Autism and Other Developmental Disabilities, 18,* 103–109.

Kern, L., Bambara, L., & Fogt, J. (2002). Class-wide curricular modification to improve the behavior of students with emotional or behavioral disorders. *Behavioral Disorders, 27*(4), 317–326.

Kern, L., & Clemens, N.H. (2007). Antecedent strategies to promote appropriate classroom behavior. *Psychology in the Schools, 44*(1), 65–75. doi:10.1002/pits.20206

Koegel, L.K., Koegel, R.L., Hurley, C., & Frea, W.D. (1992). Improving social skills and disruptive behavior in children with autism through self-management. *Journal of Applied Behavior Analysis, 25*(2), 341–353.

Koegel, L.K., Koegel, R.L., & Steibel, D. (1998). Reducing aggression in children with autism toward infant or toddler siblings. *Journal of The Association for Persons with Severe Handicaps, 23,* 111–118.

Koyama, T., & Wang, H. (2011). Use of activity schedule to promote independent performance of individuals with autism and other intellectual disabilities: A review. *Research in Developmental Disabilities, 32,* 2235–2242.

Kurtz, P.F., Boelter, E.W., Jarmolowicz, D.P., Chin, M.D., & Hagopian, L.P. (2011). An analysis of functional communication training as an empirically supported treatment for problem behavior displayed by individuals with intellectual disabilities. *Research in Developmental Disabilities, 32*(6), 2935–2942. doi:10.1016/j.ridd.2011.05.009

Lavigna, G.W., & Donnellan, A.M. (1986). *Alternatives to punishment: Solving behavior problems with non-aversive strategies.* New York, NY: Irvington Publishers.

Lequia, J., Machalicek, W., & Rispoli, M. (2012). Effects of activity schedules on challenging behavior exhibited by children with autism spectrum disorders: A systematic review. *Research in Autism Spectrum Disorders, 6,* 480–492.

Mace, R. (1985). *Universal design: Barrier-free environments for everyone.* Los Angeles, CA: Designers West.

Mancil, G.R. (2006). Functional communication training: A review of the literature related to children with autism. *Education and Training in Developmental Disabilities, 41*(3), 213–224.

Meyer, L.H., & Evans, I.M. (1989). *Non-aversive intervention for behavior problems: A manual for home and community.* Baltimore, MD: Paul H. Brookes Publishing Co.

Michaels, C.A., Brown, F., & Mirabella, N. (2005). Personal paradigm shifts in PBS experts: Perceptions of treatment acceptability of decelerative consequence-based behavioral procedures. *Journal of Positive Behavior Interventions, 7,* 93–108.

Mirenda, P., MacGregor, T., & Kelly-Keough, S. (2002). Teaching communication skills for behavioral support in the context of family life. *Families and positive behavior support: Addressing problem behavior in family contexts* (pp. 185–207). Baltimore, MD: Paul H. Brookes Publishing Co.

Newcomer, L.L., & Lewis, T. (2004). Functional behavioral assessment: An investigation of assessment reliability and effectiveness of function-based interventions. *Journal of Emotional and Behavioral Disorders, 12,* 168–181.

No Child Left Behind Act of 2001, PL 107-110, 115 Stat. 1425, 20 U.S.C. §§ 6301 *et seq.*

O'Neill, R.E., Horner, R.H., Albin, R.W., Sprague, J.R., Storey, K., & Newton, J.S. (1997). *Functional assessment and program development for problem behavior: A practical handbook* (2nd ed.). Pacific Grove, CA: Brooks/Cole.

Positive Behavioral Support Project. (1999, November). *Facilitator's guide: Positive behavioral support.* Rehabilitation, Research & Training Center on Positive Behavioral Support, University of South Florida. Retrieved from http://www.apbs.org/files/pbswhole.pdf

Sailor, W., Dunlap, G., Sugai, G., & Horner, R. (2009). *Handbook of positive behavior support.* New York, NY: Springer.

Sanford, A.K., & Horner, R.H. (2013). Effects of matching instruction difficulty to reading level for students with escape-maintained problem behavior. *Journal of Positive Behavior Interventions, 15*(2), 79–89. doi:10.1177/1098300712449868

Shogren, K., Faggella-Luby, M., Bae, S.J., & Wehmeyer, M. (2004). The effect of choice making as an intervention for problem behavior: A meta-analysis. *Journal of Positive Behavior Interventions, 6*, 228–237.

Simons, K.D., & Klein, J.D. (2007). The impact of scaffolding and student achievement levels in a problem-based learning environment. *Instructional Science, 35*, 41–72.

Singh, A.N., & Strand, P.S. (2008). A person-centered, strength-based treatment of aggression and sexually inappropriate behavior in mental health. *Clinical Case Studies, 7*, 397–408.

Snell, M.E., & Janney, R.E. (2005). *Teachers' guides to inclusive practices: Collaborative teaming* (2nd ed.). Baltimore, MD: Paul H. Brookes Publishing Co.

Spooner, F., & Brown, F. (2011). Educating students with significant cognitive disabilities: Historical overview and future projections. In J.M. Kauffman &

D.P. Hallahan (Eds.), *Handbook of Special Education* (pp. 503–515). New York, NY: Routledge.

Sugai, G., & Simonsen, B. (2012). *Positive behavioral interventions and supports: History, defining features, and misconceptions.* University of Connecticut: Center for Positive Behavioral Interventions and Supports. Retrieved from http://www.pbis.org/common/pbisresources/publications/PBIS_revisited_June19r_2012.pdf

Taylor, S.J. (1988). Caught in the continuum: A critical analysis of the principle of the least restrictive environment. *Journal of the Association for the Severely Handicapped, 13*, 41–53.

Tobin, C.E., & Simpson, R. (2012). Consequence maps: A novel behavior management tool for educators. *Teaching Exceptional Children, 44*, 68–75.

Turnbull, H.R., & Turnbull, A.P. (2000). *Free appropriate public education: Law and the education of children with disabilities* (6th ed.). Denver, CO: Love.

U.S. Government Accountability Office. *Seclusions and restraints, selected cases of death and abuse at public and private schools and treatment centers.* U.S. GAO Report, May 19, 2009.

Wang, P., & Spillane, A. (2009). Evidence-based social skills interventions for children with autism: A meta-analysis. *Education and Training in Developmental Disabilities, 44*, 318–342.

Wehmeyer, M.L. (2005). Self-determination and individuals with severe disabilities: Reexamining meanings and misinterpretations. *Research and Practice in Severe Disabilities, 30*, 113–120.

Wolf, M.M. (1978). Social validity: The case for subjective measurement or how applied behavior analysis is finding its heart. *Journal of Applied Behavior Analysis, 11*, 203–214.

Wolfensberger, W. (1972). *The principle of normalization in human services.* Toronto, ON: National Institute on Mental Retardation.

Effective Teaming for Positive Behavior Support

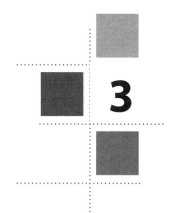

3

Linda M. Bambara and Catherine Kunsch

Emmanuel

Emmanuel, a 6-year-old first grader, recently moved from New York City to a small suburban town in Pennsylvania. When he arrived at his new school, none of his previous school records arrived with him. However, his mother reported that he received special education services for a speech and language delay and provided the school with a copy of his individualized education program (IEP) from kindergarten. Currently, he is enrolled in a regular first-grade classroom and receives speech and language therapy 1 day per week and additional reading instruction through a Title I program at his new school.

When Emmanuel arrived at his new school in late October, his teacher noticed immediately that he had difficulty following the classroom routine and that his reading skills were lower than expected of a first grader. By mid-December, his teacher referred Emmanuel to the school's instructional support team for his inability to follow classroom directions, inability to work independently, and high rates of disruptive behaviors (i.e., lying under his desk or table during independent seat work). On at least several occasions, redirection to sit at his desk resulted in screaming outbursts ("No! I

hate you. I hate this school"). At the first instructional support team meeting, Emmanuel's teacher expressed lots of frustration. She expressed that although Emmanuel is somewhat behind academically, he is more than capable of doing the work she assigns. She stated that he was simply refusing to work and was too disruptive for a regular first-grade classroom. Emmanuel's classroom teacher wants him to be reevaluated for an emotional behavior disorder and removed from her classroom as soon as possible. Other teachers on the instructional support team quickly sided with Emmanuel's teacher. They supported her decision to have Emmanuel reevaluated for placement in a self-contained classroom or school.

Lynn

Lynn is a 38-year-old woman diagnosed with autism and intellectual disabilities. She lives in a private home with two other women with developmental disabilities, where she receives 24-hour staff support for assistance with daily living. With the aid of a job coach, Lynn works part time at a local pharmacy stocking shelves.

Recently, Lynn has been engaging in physically aggressive behavior toward her roommates and support staff who work in her home. Prior to recent bouts of hitting, pushing, and kicking, Lynn has not engaged in any challenging behaviors in about 10 years. Her support staff, some of whom have worked with her for 6 years or more, are very surprised by her behaviors. When interviewed by their supervisor, they reported that Lynn's behaviors occur "out of the blue," and acts of aggression can persist almost all day long. They say on some days it's impossible to redirect Lynn to something she likes, so they let her sit alone in the living room, avoiding interaction with her; but even then, she will leap up and attack whomever is in her path. Lynn's support staff have heard that autism can evolve into serious mental health issues later in adult life. They recommend short-term hospitalization and a psychiatric evaluation for possible bipolar disorder. Regardless, they believe that Lynn needs immediate medication to stop her aggression.

· ·

It is hard to imagine that at one time, in challenging situations like those described in Emmanuel and Lynn's cases, behavior interventions were developed with little team involvement. Not too far in the distant past, behavior support plans (BSP) were primarily expert driven as opposed to team driven, wherein a behavioral consultant or psychologist ("the expert") was called in to assess the situation (typically by taking data on just the frequency of problem behaviors) and then prescribe an intervention plan that teachers, support staff, and/or family members were expected to follow. Not surprising, this approach often resulted in ineffectual outcomes; not necessarily because the intervention plan was poor or that the expert lacked critical know-how but because the plan failed to take into consideration the expertise, knowledge, skills, values, beliefs, and resources of the very people who were required to implement the plan.

Positive behavior support (PBS) proponents have long recognized that the success of any behavior support plan is chiefly dependent on the workings of a collaborative team to design and implement interventions (Snell, Voorhees, & Chen, 2005). A PBS team consists of the focus person (if possible) and relevant people in the focus person's life who are most likely to carry out or be affected by the plan (e.g., family members, teachers, support staff), as well as selected professionals who can inform team decision making and/or support team actions (e.g., behavior support specialist, psychologist, special educator, related services personnel, administrator), as needed. Collaborative teams differ from multidisciplinary teams commonly found in education and human service fields, in that in multidisciplinary teams, team members often set different goals based on their unique disciplines and work independently from one another to address a student's needs. For example, Emmanuel's classroom teacher, speech therapist, and title I reading teacher independently work on goals and objectives that are included in Emmanuel's IEP, while other team members work on different goals and objectives. By contrast, a *collaborative team* is defined as people working together to achieve *common goals through joint action and shared decision making* (Fleming & Monda-Amaya, 2001; Snell & Janney, 2005).

At least five essential characteristics contribute to the makeup of a successful collaborative team (Bambara, Nonnemacher, & Koger, 2005): 1) shared vision and goals, 2) parity or a sense of equity across team members, 3) shared participation and decision making, 4) positive team relationships, and 5) shared accountability. When translated into practice, a PBS collaborative team does the following:

· Is committed to applying person-centered values and PBS standards of practice to establish agreed-on goals and direct team actions and activities

· Uses agreed-on processes that respect the diversity of opinions and each team member's contribution to the team regardless of their role or expertise

- Engages in shared problem solving and consensus building among team members across all phases of the PBS process (i.e., prioritizing and defining problem behavior, conducting a functional assessment, developing hypotheses, designing a BSP, and monitoring and evaluating implementation)

- Employs strategies to foster positive interpersonal relationships among team members such as open communication, listening to understand each other's perspectives, blameless conflict resolution, and support for learning new concepts and skills

- Holds all team members accountable for agreed-on responsibilities and shares both successes and failures as a team, while also working jointly to find solutions to problems

Ultimately, successful collaborative teams produce positive outcomes and engage in processes that are satisfactory to *all* team members, especially the focus individual and his or her family.

CHAPTER PURPOSE AND OVERVIEW

Like designing an effective BSP, successful teaming is a process, not a single event, that requires careful attention to the strategies that enhance its success (Fleming & Monda-Amaya, 2001). The purpose of this chapter is to make these strategies explicit so that school personnel, other professionals, support staff, and families can work together to design effective behavior supports for individuals who engage in challenging behaviors. We begin by discussing first why teaming is important and then some challenges to the teaming process. Understanding challenges to teaming will help to elucidate the necessity for teaming strategies. Next, we outline essential components for structuring successful teaming within the PBS process.

Why Teaming Is Important

Teaming serves two central purposes (Bambara et al., 2005). The first, which is focused on the individual, is to enhance the integrity and effectiveness of a BSP and ensure that the team is responsive to the individual's needs. The second purpose, which is team centered, is to provide ongoing support to team members as they engage in the PBS planning process and carry out behavior supports.

Enhance Integrity and Effectiveness
Teaming can enhance the effectiveness of a support plan in several important ways. First, teaming brings together different ideas and perspectives from various team members that can lead to a comprehensive understanding of the individual, reasons for problem behaviors, and effective strategies that can be applied across multiple settings, such as in school, home, and community. As noted by Dunlap and colleagues (Dunlap, Newton, Fox, Benito, & Vaughn, 2001), no one person holds all the answers to understanding an individual's problem behaviors nor can one person succeed with creating effective supports in all relevant settings. Therefore, a team approach is necessary for all parties, including professionals, family members, and the individual, to exchange vital information for assessment and intervention. Second, teaming fosters consensus building as well as shared responsibility and accountability among team members. Effective behavior support can only happen when all team members are invested in the process, come to a common agreement, and are committed to carrying out behavior supports in cohesive way.

Third, teaming guides team members to select relevant and "doable" interventions and supports that can be realistically carried out in typical classroom, home, or community settings. A support plan is only as effective as its *contextual fit* with resources of a setting and the values, skills, and culture of the team members responsible for implementing the plan (Albin, Lucyshyn, Horner, & Flannery, 1996). Although interventions must be technically adequate (e.g., address the function of behavior), it is a misnomer to assume that interventions applied in all settings and by relevant people must be exactly the same. For example, if Lynn begins to exhibit challenging behaviors in her workplace, it makes little sense to apply the same exact interventions as in the home because work and home are vastly different settings; what is doable at home may not be doable or even appropriate at work. Further, the functions of Lynn's problem behaviors, as well as the antecedents and maintaining consequences, may differ to some degree in these two settings. To ensure that BSPs are feasible and sustainable, teams will need to consider the demands, resources, routines, and expectations of a setting, as well as the skills, preferences, and values of the people who will be affected by the plan, including the focus individual. Consistency is measured not by all team members implementing the same strategies in exactly the same way but with adherence to the integrity of support plans as designed to address the individual's needs across various settings and circumstances.

Provide Ongoing Supports to Team Members Teaming is not just about the focus individual; it is also about team members and, as such, involves a social process of support for team members. Team members bring different and often conflicting views about the reasons for problem behaviors and what constitutes effective behavior management practices. Thus a central goal of teaming is to help individual team members let go of long-standing beliefs and assumptions and, as a team, adopt a like mind-set that is consistent with PBS values and strategies. Quite often this involves shifting perspectives from seeing problem behaviors as being caused by factors that cannot be controlled to seeing problem behaviors as being caused by factors that *can be changed* by the team, and from viewing effective behavior interventions as those consisting of only reactive strategies (e.g., punishment) to viewing these interventions as encompassing a proactive or preventive approach.

The process of changing these perspectives is greatly influenced by team members experiencing success as a result of their efforts (Gersten & Dimino, 2001). Thus

another important purpose of teaming is to help team members build the critical skills and confidence needed to implement interventions and provide the supports needed for team members to try new practices and persist during times of frustration and difficulty. This goal can be accomplished through direct coaching, shared problem solving, and establishing a sense of camaraderie among team members (Janz, Colquitt, & Noe, 1997).

Challenges to Teaming

The following vignettes depict a variety of challenges that often arise in teams:

> I've tried everything—animal stickers when he's good and warnings that he'll miss recess if he doesn't get his work done. Nothing works! He's ADHD and EBD and needs help.
>
> *(Mrs. Rios, first-grade teacher)*

> Even if we can find the time, is it fair to devote so much time and energy to this one kid? Emmanuel will be better served in classroom where teachers are trained to address his needs.
>
> *(Ms. Jackson, lead instructional support teacher)*

> I can't believe Lynn would hit me after all I've done for her.
>
> *(Cyndi, long-term direct support staff)*

> I've worked with others like Lynn. She's bipolar and needs medication.
>
> *(Rick, new direct support staff)*

These vignettes illustrate that perhaps the most challenging aspect of teaming is that not all team members will come together sharing the same perspectives about how to address problem behaviors and best support the individual. The result is varying degrees of team conflict, which is inherent in all teams but problematic when individual team members cannot let go of challenging beliefs that impede the PBS process. Certainly, establishing an organizational culture that is respectful of individual differences and is proactive in its approach to addressing problem behaviors can lay the foundation for team members to share common values and processes for providing behavior support. For example, schoolwide positive behavior support (SWPBS) at the primary prevention level can create schoolwide expectations for teaming, problem solving, data-based decision making, and preventive interventions, laying a solid foundation for school personnel to be receptive to individualized interventions, should they be needed by students (Freeman et al., 2006; Horner, Sugai, & Anderson, 2010). Further, organizations committed to PBS can create time for teams to meet, provide training, and dedicate resources (e.g., extra personnel, materials) to support team activities. Nevertheless, the very nature of intensive problem behaviors is that they are *challenging*, even when supportive organizational systems are in place. Numerous studies have documented that problem behaviors can contribute to high levels of teacher, staff, and parent stress (e.g., Baker, Blacher, Crnic, & Edelbrock, 2002; Klassen, 2010; Mitchell & Hastings, 2001), which in turn can erode team members' feelings of self-efficacy (i.e., beliefs that they can make a difference) and impair their judgment about the individual's behavior and effective practices (Chang, 2009; Hastings & Brown, 2002).

In a series of studies, Bambara and colleagues (Bambara, Goh, Kern, & Caskie, 2012; Bambara, Lohrmann, Nonnemacher, Goh, & Kern, 2014; Bambara, Nonnemacher, & Kern, 2009) assessed the perspectives of school-based personnel and families regarding perceived barriers and supports to implementing and sustaining individualized PBS in school settings. Not surprising, the most challenging and pervasive barriers had to do with team members' beliefs, feelings, or attitudes. Perhaps due a lack of experience with designing PBS plans or the stress associated with challenging behaviors, team members often struggle with accepting and following PBS practices because of competing beliefs and emotions, such as those illustrated in the previous vignettes. Some of the most common challenges, derived from the findings of Bambara and colleagues, are summarized

in Table 3.1, along with potential solutions that will be discussed in the following section on team structure. These challenges are also consistent with our experiences leading teams in nonschool settings (e.g., adult residential, family home) for children and adults.

Time Many teams struggle with beliefs related to time. Team members may perceive PBS as being too time consuming or labor intensive, adding burdensome responsibilities to their already busy routines. This perception may in part reflect realistic, practical concerns about how individual team members will be able to find the time to plan or adjust their routines to implement interventions. Perceptions that PBS is too time consuming may also reflect a "quick-fix" expectation for behavior change and a lack of understanding that developing effective interventions requires a systematic process that takes time. Sometimes, concerns about time, such as expressed by Ms. Jackson in Emmanuel's case, are tied to beliefs of efficacy, such as, "It's not worth investing the time with a particular individual because nothing will work!"

Attribution of Problem Behavior A core challenge to the PBS process well documented by researchers (e.g., Lambrechts, Petry, & Maes, 2008; Westling, 2010; Wilson, Gardner, Burton, & Leung, 2006) is the misattribution of problem behavior. PBS requires that team members acquire a functional understanding of problem behavior so that they can make critical changes to teach new and alternative behaviors and prevent problem behaviors from occurring. Unfortunately, when faced with difficult behaviors, many team members tend to attribute the "cause" of problem behaviors to factors beyond their control, creating a perception that they are powerless to make a difference. This includes external attributions, such as a poor home situation, bad parenting, or a history of ineffective disciplinary practices, as well as attributions internal to the individual. Internal attributions, such as "He's doing

Table 3.1. Teaming challenges and solutions

Challenging beliefs and emotions	Solutions
Time • Process takes too much time. • Process is time consuming. • Effective interventions are quick acting.	• Infuse positive behavior support (PBS) planning into regularly scheduled team meetings. • Make use of alternative means for communication (e.g., e-mail, conference calls, virtual meetings, Skype). • Divide responsibilities among team members. • Break tasks down. • Ensure a contextual fit for both assessment and intervention.
(Mis)attribution of problem behavior • Problem behavior is caused by external factors beyond the team's control (e.g., homelife, parenting, past history). • Problem behavior is inherent to the individual's disability (e.g., autism, bipolar disorder). • Problem behavior is deliberate (i.e., done purposefully to aggravate). • Problem behavior occurs for "no reason" or out of the blue.	• Use a visually explicit process for functional assessment so all team members can see data. • Use data to guide interpretations. • Come to consensus on hypotheses for problem behaviors.
Behavior management/efficacy • Bad behavior should be punished (and punishment is effective). • Individual is better served elsewhere (exclusion). • Proactive strategies are "unfair" to others or "too soft" on the individual. • Nothing works!	• Secure team members' commitment to try PBS strategies. • Make the PBS process explicit every step of the way; revisit frequently to facilitate an understanding. • Use data to evaluate success. • Celebrate all success; big and little.
Uncompromising beliefs • There are conflicting views on best intervention or solutions to problems.	• Use group problem-solving and consensus-building strategies throughout the PBS process. • Ensure that interventions are assessment based and linked to hypotheses of problem behavior. • Stay student focused. • Modify interventions to fit different activities/settings.
Self-efficacy/personalization • Person has a lack of confidence. • Person is afraid to change or try new things. • Person is afraid of being judged for failure. • Person takes problem behavior personally and is feeling hurt.	• Model new strategies and provide coaching. • Reassure team members and praise efforts. • Encourage open and blameless conversation. • Team as a whole (not individual team members) assumes success and failure of the team.

it on purpose" or "She has bipolar disorder," suggest that problem behavior is caused by the individual's disability or personality. Although not tied to a specific cause, statements such as "She did it for no reason" or "Problem behavior occurred out of the blue" also imply that the reasons for problem behaviors are not within the team member's control and certainly not well understood.

Behavior Management/Efficacy Stemming from traditionally held views on behavior management and a lack of understanding of how PBS could work, team members may struggle with viewing preventive

interventions as potentially effective strategies. Instead, when faced with intense behavioral challenges, team members may cling to traditionally held beliefs that difficult behaviors must be met with strong consequences, that the individual may be better served in another setting or program where personnel are specifically trained to address behavioral challenges, and that nonpunitive interventions are equivalent to "spoiling," "giving in," or "being soft" on the individual. Some team members may perceive individualized supports as being unfair to the individual's peers (e.g., classmates, housemates) who do not receive the same accommodations: "Is it fair to the other students to give Emmanuel extra rewards for following directions when he should be doing what is expected?" Unfortunately, as teachers, support staff, or families attempt to apply behavior management practices that have been successful with others but are not individualized to the person's needs, they may quickly conclude that "Nothing works" when their efforts fail. Suffice it to say, many team members enter into the PBS process feeling frustrated and highly skeptical that preventive strategies could work.

Uncompromising Beliefs About Right and Wrong   Similar to strongly held beliefs about behavior management, some team members will stubbornly advocate for what they think is best and fail to consider other intervention options. Typically, competing or problematic beliefs about what is right or wrong are tied to the team member's experiences and not the focus individual's needs, demands of the setting, or needs of other team members. Open discussion about different ideas or sharing potential solutions to problems is healthy; uncompromising beliefs that do not consider the needs of the individual or the goals of the team can prevent the team from moving forward.

Self-Efficacy/Personalization of Problem Behaviors   Challenging situations evoke a range of emotions. Perhaps due to the intensity of problem behavior, previous unsuccessful efforts, or unfamiliarity with positive interventions, some team members may express uncertainty or lack of confidence that they can be personally effective, even when strategies have worked for others. Some may be reluctant to try new approaches, fearful of making a mistake, or fearful of being judged by others for their mistakes or lack of success. Closely related to negative feelings of self-efficacy, some team members may take instances of problem behavior "personally." That is, rather than viewing problem behavior objectively (i.e., asking what might be the trigger or possible function), they respond to problem behavior

as a personal insult. As reflected in Cyndi's statement, "I can't believe she would hit me after all I've done for her," team members may feel hurt and sometimes angry because they believe their efforts or positive relationships alone should have made a difference in preventing problem behavior; unfortunately, this is not often the case. Although good relationships are important and can positively influence intervention effectiveness (e.g., McLaughlin & Carr, 2005), incidents of challenging behavior may have nothing to do with shared experiences or the degree of "likingness" between two people. Rather, these incidents have everything to do with independent events that are problematic to the individual. Similar to misattributions of problem behaviors, hurt feelings can blind team members from seeing real contributions to the problem.

In summary, team members' beliefs and feelings can greatly affect the extent to which they are receptive to new approaches, are willing to try new strategies, and persist during challenging situations. Certainly, not all team members will display all the challenging beliefs and emotions previously described; however, the beliefs are common enough that all teams will encounter one or more of these belief challenges during the course of the team. The key to successful teaming is to help team members become aware of these challenging beliefs and feelings while guiding them to understand and feel confident with implementing PBS practices. The process for making this happen occurs within the structure and strategies of collaborative teaming described next.

ESTABLISHING A STRUCTURE FOR SUCCESSFUL TEAMING

Just as PBS is a process that continually revisits and revises steps and stages, building a collaborative team is also a process. Although we will discuss the structure in a somewhat linear fashion, successful team building does not necessarily occur in a locked sequence. In each PBS phase, there are two categories of actions the team needs to accomplish. First, the team will need to complete the *student or individual-centered* activities, which lead to the development and implementation of the PBS plan. Second, the team should engage in *team-centered* activities, which focus on supporting the team members, encouraging collaboration, and when needed, shifting team members' perspectives from "can't do" to "can do" thinking. Table 3.2 outlines each phase, both individual *and* team-centered activities that need to occur, and guiding questions to promote collaboration as the team engages in the individual-centered activities. Detailed information and descriptions of the individual-centered PBS activities are found elsewhere in this book. This chapter focuses on building collaboration through team-centered activities.

Phase 1: Creating Team Structure and Purpose

The first collaborative phase of the PBS process has two main purposes. First, a team needs to be initiated or created, and, second, the newly formed team will need to prioritize the behaviors of focus. The individual-centered team actions in this phase include identifying team membership, prioritizing the behaviors of concern, defining the behaviors, and agreeing on the student or individual's outcomes. As shown in Table 3.2, there are several collaborative questions that team leaders may ask of team members to help accomplish the individual-centered tasks in a joint manner. In addition to guiding collaboration on individual-centered activities, team leaders need to be concerned with a number of team-centered activities during this first phase, which will lay the foundation for effective collaboration and team decision making throughout the remaining phases of the PBS process.

Determining Team Membership and Roles The first step in building an effective

team may seem obvious, but determining who should serve on the team is an important first step. The team should be constructed around the individual's needs, but members may also serve on other teams for the individual, such as his or her IEP or instructional support team. When determining team membership, consider three questions to guide selection (Thousand & Villa, 2000).

First, who has the necessary expertise and skills to help the team make the best decisions for the individual (e.g., knowledge of the PBS process, knowledge of the individual, knowledge of the setting or context)? Consider the strengths that each person may bring to the team. For example, Lynn's program supervisor has an excellent background in PBS, but does she know Lynn as well as the staff who work in her home? Both the direct care staff and the program supervisor would make equally important contributions to the team and should be considered. In addition to considering who may know the individual the best, consider individuals who will have the authority to assist in the implementation of the plan or provide resources to the team, such as administrators. Being sure to also include someone with PBS experience (besides the team leader or PBS expert) may serve as a solution to some of the teaming challenges likely to occur in the process. Including team members who have had positive experiences with implementing PBS can be useful in establishing a "can do" climate and may aid in securing team members' commitment to PBS. Further, having team members with PBS experience may be helpful, as they can serve as a resource and model for other team members new to PBS.

The second question to consider in determining membership is who will be affected by the team's decisions? Family members, teachers, direct support staff, and the focus individual will most likely emerge when considering this question. Including team members who will likely implement the plan or have a stake in the decision-making process promotes respect for those who will

Table 3.2.   Team actions in the positive behavior support (PBS) process

Collaborative phase 1: Creating the team structure and purpose

PBS steps	Team actions (individual/ student centered)	Questions for collaboration	Team actions (team centered)
Initiate the PBS team.	• Identify team membership.	• Who will be included on the PBS team? • What strengths does each person bring to the team? • What will each team member's responsibilities be? • What is the team's purpose? • What are our ground rules for our team meetings? • How often will we meet? • Where will we meet? • How will we communicate between the meetings?	• Agree on the team purpose and goals. • Set ground rules for collaboration. • Establish meeting times and opportunities for communication between meetings. • Establish a structured meeting agenda. • Solicit team concerns to determine what behaviors should be prioritized for change.
Prioritize and define the behavior.	• Prioritize behaviors for change. • Define behaviors. • Agree on individual outcomes.	• What challenging behaviors are we going to address? • Which challenging behaviors, when modified, will result in the most significant changes in focus individual's quality of life? • Can we count/measure the behavior as defined? • What are the individual's and his or her family's vision for the future? What do we want to happen as a result of our intervention?	

Collaborative phase 2: Assessment and planning

PBS steps	Team actions (individual/ student centered)	Questions for collaboration	Team actions (team centered)
Conduct a functional assessment.	• Decide what information should be gathered. • Determine how and who will gather the information. • Decide who will summarize the information for the team.	• Who is the individual? What are his or her strengths and preferences? • What is the individual's history? • In what activities is problem behavior most likely to occur? • What might be the triggers for problem behavior? • What function does problem behavior serve? What might the individual be communicating? • Are there gaps in our understanding?	• Use a collaborative problem-solving process. • Enhance the team's capacity for understanding. • Reframe challenging beliefs and diffuse team conflict. • Create an atmosphere of openness and honesty. • Ensure that there is a contextual fit. • Divide the responsibilities.
Develop a hypothesis.	• Analyze and interpret the gathered information. • Agree on hypothesis statement(s).	• What patterns have emerged from the data? • Can we all agree with this initial hypothesis? • Do we still have gaps in our understanding? What additional information needs to be collected?	

(continued)

Table 3.2.   *(continued)*

Collaborative phase 2: Assessment and planning

PBS steps	Team actions (individual/ student centered)	Questions for collaboration	Team actions (team centered)
Develop the support plan.	• Develop a mutually agreed-on PBS plan. • Develop action steps for implementing the PBS plan.	• What events can we change to prevent problem behavior and make desired behaviors more likely? • What alternative skills should we teach to replace problem behaviors or produce desirable outcomes? • Are there lifestyle changes that can be made that would prevent the need for the focus person to engage in problem behavior and improve quality of life for the individual? • Does our support plan address our hypotheses and desired outcomes? • Are our interventions doable in targeted settings?	

Collaborative phase 3: Implementing the PBS plan

PBS steps	Team actions (individual/ student centered)	Questions for collaboration	Team actions (team centered)
Implement, monitor, and evaluate the support plan.	• Decide on important outcomes. • Determine how to measure progress and outcomes. • Evaluate whether the plan is working. • Make changes to the plan, as necessary.	• What information do we need to collect? • What's our plan for collecting data (who, how, tools)? • What help do *we need* in order to carry out the plan? • Are the interventions being implemented properly? • Are we seeing progress? Are the changes meaningful to the person and other team members? • How can we change the plan to improve outcomes?	• Support the team. • Celebrate often and problem-solve when needed. • Focus on treatment integrity. • Reflect on the team process. • Evaluate satisfaction with outcomes.

be affected—a good contextual fit when creating a PBS plan.

The final question to aid in determining team membership is asking who wants to participate or who has a vested interest in participating. Perhaps one of the student's teachers has the interest and wants to learn how to conduct a functional behavioral assessment (FBA) but lacks the skills. This teacher's motivation and interest may more than make up for her lack of skills, making her an excellent and highly motivated team member.

After answering these three questions, teams may be faced with a long list of possible team members that may pose a real logistical challenge for active participation (e.g., scheduling a meeting everyone can attend). One suggestion for addressing this issue is to create a core team and an extended team (Snell & Janney, 2005). The core team, or the "working group," is a small group of people who are most involved with the individual (which always includes parents or family), meets regularly, and coordinates the PBS process. The extended team does not meet regularly, but extended team members may be called in as needed for their specific skills or expertise. Creating two subgroups for the overall team may address the time challenges often faced by teams. Creating a core group eliminates the need to accommodate everyone's schedules for meetings and also helps divide responsibilities so team members will not feel overwhelmed or burdened.

Emmanuel

Emmanuel's PBS team consisted of a core group and an extended team, so everyone who was needed or wanted to be involved could be included but each member would not have to attend every meeting. Emmanuel's core group consisted of his mom and dad, his general education teacher, the behavior specialist (a PBS expert), the reading specialist, and the school counselor (who is the PBS team leader). The extended team included Emmanuel's grandmother (who lives with him), the school psychologist (a PBS expert), the school principal, the speech pathologist, and the special education supervisor.

....

Lynn

Lynn's PBS team is also composed of a core (or working) group and an extended group to facilitate meeting schedules of the members. Lynn's core group includes Lynn, the direct care staff members from her home, Lynn's sister, the program supervisor (a PBS team leader and PBS expert), the site supervisor, and a behavior specialist (a PBS expert). The extended team includes the clinical director, Lynn's job coach, a staff psychiatrist, Lynn's primary care physician, and a coworker at Lynn's job who asked if she could help in any way.

....

Once a team is established, it is time to delegate each team member's responsibilities. Not only does this help team members understand their roles and responsibilities, but also it will help identify any missing areas of expertise, and additional team members can be added. There are three major roles on a PBS team: 1) team leader or facilitator, 2) a PBS expert, and 3) a general team member. The team leader, who will coordinate all team activities, must be organized, goal and action oriented, and a skilled communicator and

facilitator. The team leader must be respectful of all team members and the process. In addition to following the team agenda and focusing on outcomes, the team leader will need to encourage, coach, and communicate with all team members. The team leader will need to assess the team's challenging beliefs and feelings as they arise and work toward solutions to keep the team on track. When team members feel overburdened by the process or have disagreements with one another regarding the best course of action, the team leader not only recognizes these challenges but also addresses them through reexamining meeting schedules or assignments, for example, or engaging the team in a problem-solving process rather than arguing differing viewpoints, thus keeping the team focused on the individual. Indeed, the team leader position is important to the team's success. Another critical role is that of the PBS expert. The PBS expert will be called on to ensure the team is adhering to a PBS framework and values, provide or organize training to team members as necessary, serve as a PBS resource to the team, and serve as a general team member. It is possible that the team facilitator will also be the PBS expert or one of the experts, but this is not always the case. In Lynn's example, the program supervisor is the PBS team leader and a PBS expert. However, the behavior specialist is also a member of the team and one of the PBS experts who has specialized knowledge in many PBS areas. Also, one of Lynn's extended team members is the clinical director, who also has generalized PBS expertise and experience to share when needed.

The remaining role of "general team member" is a shared role for all team members. That is, as a general team member, all members assume responsibility for actively participating in team discussions and carrying out specific team activities or responsibilities assigned by the team. Because specific responsibilities may change throughout the PBS process, it is important to define team roles and determine who does what at the beginning of each phase or step of the PBS process.

Agreeing on Team Purpose and Goals During this first collaborative phase, the central individual-centered activity is for the team to prioritize behaviors for change and to agree on individual outcomes (i.e., what the team hopes to achieve for the individual). However, in order to prioritize behaviors for change and agree on individual outcomes, the team must first agree on its purpose—that is, the team must commit to using PBS practices to create change for the individual.

Clearly stated purpose or goal statements such as, "Our goal is to understand what Lynn may be communicating through her problem behavior and develop an intervention that best addresses her needs," will keep the team working together toward a joint purpose. Not infrequently, when members initially come together, they may all have different goals and agendas in mind that may pull a team in different directions and make it nearly impossible to achieve any outcome for the individual. Often, team members may not even be aware they share different visions or goals for the team. In the following example, all team members are in agreement that Emmanuel is experiencing difficulties in school; they all know this as they join together. However, what they do not realize is that some members are hoping he can be moved to another setting or placement, while others are committed to keeping him in his general education classroom. One can only imagine how difficult it will be to move forward if these beliefs are not revealed, addressed, and discussed right away. By explicitly discussing the team purpose and establishing goals early on in the PBS process, team members can come to an agreement and move in one direction as a team. Goal statements should be brief, easily understood, agreed on by all members, and consistent with PBS values.

Emmanuel

Initially, when Emmanuel's PBS team came together, team members had different agendas. Some of the team members believed the team was coming together to have him assessed and removed from the general education classroom. Other team members wanted to explore options to keep him in his first-grade classroom. With the help of the school counselor (PBS team leader) and the behavior specialist (PBS expert), the team agreed to use the PBS process and set a goal of understanding Emmanuel's problem behaviors and where they come from and to generate a plan that would be acceptable to his classroom teacher, his family, and the rest of the team. All the team members ultimately agreed that the overall goal is to help Emmanuel have a positive educational experience and that the first step in reaching this goal would be to focus on why he was misbehaving.

Establishing Ground Rules for Collaboration In addition to agreeing to a team purpose and goals, the PBS team should consider setting rules for how they will collaborate with one another. Establishing ground rules early in the PBS process can help teams articulate how they will operate, stay focused on the PBS process, and interact with fellow team members in respectful ways. In other words, establishing ground rules is a proactive strategy for minimizing team conflict and enhancing team accountability. One way to start the conversation is to ask "trigger questions" (Snell & Janney, 2005), such as the following:

1) "Given our goals, what will it take for us to get our work done?," 2) "What are our responsibilities as team members?," 3) "What PBS assumptions are central to accomplishing our work?," 4) "What processes will we follow?," 5) "How should we behave to ensure our interactions are respectful of one another?," and 6) "What are rules for communicating with one another even though we disagree?"

Once ground rules are established, the team can review them periodically, to keep the team working together: "Remember, we all agreed to use the data to help us make decisions about our success. What is the graph telling us?" Or, "Wait a minute; we agreed to listen to one another's ideas without interruption. After we hear from everyone, let's see how the suggested strategies fit our hypotheses for problem behavior."

Setting a Schedule and Structure for Meetings The next set of team actions includes setting meeting times, creating a structure for the actual meetings, and developing a process for communications in between meeting times. Finding a time to meet may be the most challenging step in the process of initiating a PBS team, but successful completion of this step may help reduce the time challenges a team will face. First, determine how often the team will meet. There is no hard and fast rule for how often a team should meet. The frequency should be determined by the team's purpose, goals, and experience level. The core team may need to meet on a frequent basis if there are many goals, if the behavior intensity is great, or if many of the team members are inexperienced and need more frequent coaching, modeling, and support. Frequent meetings may assist in providing an opportunity to work on solutions to team challenges. Finding a mutual time to meet is never an easy task, but this is an opportunity to think creatively. Whenever possible, the team should try to use an existing meeting time that most members already have "blocked out" in their schedules. For example, are there grade-level meetings, instructional support team meetings, or other previously established meeting times that can be utilized for the PBS team meeting? Utilizing times slots that are normally used for a meeting may improve attendance and help reduce any stress regarding establishing a new schedule. Next, decide on where the team should meet and for how long. If possible, teams should meet in a convenient location with minimal distraction. Meetings of 1 hour or less may be ideal if the team is meeting frequently. Also, the team should attempt to accommodate members with different schedules. For example, how can you include an overnight staff member when all meetings occur during the day? Can the staff member call in to a meeting or attend via Internet video call software (e.g., Skype)? Creating an inclusive team atmosphere requires addressing these issues in this initial phase. Next, a meeting format and a plan for communication should be developed. A 1-hour meeting can quickly become derailed by chatting or complaints. Creating a meeting framework with time allotments (e.g., agenda review—5 minutes, updates on assignments—10 minutes, data review—10 minutes, group discussion—15 minutes) will help keep the team focused and productive. Also, the team should decide how and how often updates will be shared in between meetings (e.g., weekly e-mail updates each Friday afternoon or Monday morning). To enhance communication in between actual meetings, the team leader can designate one person to share updates and information to all team members regularly. Expectations for updates and reports from team members in between meeting dates should be clearly defined and discussed. For example, a staff member implementing an intervention may want to share progress or ask other team members questions but is not sure if it is okay to send multiple e-mails to the team. Discussing this ahead of time and encouraging this level of communication early in the PBS process may aid collaboration during subsequent phases. In addition, team members should be asked what method of communication they prefer for updates. While e-mail is typical and convenient for many, if a parent has only sporadic access to a computer or a printer, e-mailed updates may have a negative impact on the collaborative process. Some staff members may not have access to e-mail during the day and would prefer to send or receive text messages. Communication preferences should be discussed early in the PBS process and revisited as needed.

SOLICITING TEAM CONCERNS REGARDING BEHAVIORS THAT SHOULD BE PRIORITIZED FOR CHANGE

Emmanuel

Emmanuel's team quickly agreed that Emmanuel's disruptive behaviors and refusals to work independently were high priorities for change. However, when the school counselor asked Emmanuel's teacher (Mrs. Rio), "What do you need? What behaviors are most important to you?," she blurted out: "I just need him to be engaged the first 20 minutes of class. I need him to work quietly and independently like the rest of the class so that I can get my class off to a good start. If I could just have 20 minutes without interruption, I feel like I could get my day started in the right direction and I'd be in a better position to address his needs." Although the team's priorities did not change as a result of Mrs. Rios's comments, the team did agree that a focus on Emmanuel's morning routine was also critical. The team decided that they would work quickly with Emmanuel's teacher to find a solution to the problem. For example, perhaps Emmanuel could engage in preferred activity during the first 20 minutes of class time.

....

Because individuals with pervasive behavior challenges often present more than one behavior of concern, teams will need to prioritize which behaviors are important to change first, which can be addressed at a later time, and which are relatively unimportant to address. Decisions for prioritization should first and foremost center on the individual's needs. Certainly, problem behaviors that are harmful to the individual or threaten the safety of others and/or interfere with the individual's learning, participation in inclusive activities, and social relationships are high priority for change. However, prioritization based on individual needs will also need to be balanced with team member concerns. How do problem behaviors affect the daily functioning of families, teachers, and support staff who are committed to the support of the individual? Listening to team members' concerns about how problem behaviors interfere with their routines and ability to provide support can help teams decide relatively quickly which problem behaviors or what situations cause team members the greatest stress or frustration. Prioritizing team activities to address both the individual's and team members' needs can help team members

feel supported, knowing that the team will work to address their concerns as well. Supported team members are less likely to resist and more likely to generate solutions to problems.

Phase 2: Assessment and Planning

The second phase encompasses the core of PBS activities. During this phase, team members center their work on completing individual-focused activities as they conduct the functional behavioral assessment, develop hypotheses based on the assessment data, and develop an intervention plan that addresses the individual's needs. Like the other three PBS phases, the role of the team is to engage in shared decision making throughout each of the core individual-centered activities of this phase. Table 3.2 provides some guiding questions that can facilitate shared decision making for each of the core tasks. Teams will work the hardest during the assessment and planning phase; therefore, team-centered activities are needed to keep the team motivated and directed. The team activities during this second phase focus largely on improving the team's understanding of the PBS process, providing a supportive atmosphere for collaboration, and problem solving as they take on these responsibilities.

Use Collaborative Problem Solving Collaborative problem-solving strategies can be utilized by the team when important decisions need to be made or when there is a conflict or disagreement regarding how to address a situation. During this phase, there are numerous important decisions to be made that could be cast as problems to be solved, such as, "How will we collect data given our busy schedules? What types of interventions are needed, and how can we implement them?" Although collaborative problem solving is presented in this assessment and planning phase, a problem-solving framework can be used during any phase of the PBS process. Numerous team problem-solving strategies exist (Welch, Brownell, & Sheridan, 1999). One framework described by Snell and Janney (2005) can be implemented across a variety of team activities:

- *Step 1—Identify the problem:* What is the single most important issue that needs to be resolved now? (For example, What assessment should we use? The data look bad—what do we do now?)

- *Step 2—Brainstorm potential solutions to the problem:* The team generates as many possible solutions as they can without criticism or evaluative remarks. The PBS team leader will need to ensure everyone is open and nonjudgmental to the ideas shared.

- *Step 3—Evaluate the solutions:* The team narrows down the list created in the previous step to a shorter list of possible solutions (e.g., collect more data, change the data collection procedure, try another intervention). At this point, the team leader may guide the team to consider contextual fit and integrity with PBS processes as the team narrows down solutions. (See other team activities in this phase.)

- *Step 4—Choose a solution:* Together, the team decides on the best solutions.

- *Step 5—Develop an action plan:* A written action plan is created by the team that details who is responsible and when it will be completed.

Enhancing the Team's Capacity for Understanding and Reframing Challenging Beliefs

During the assessment and planning phase, many challenges can surface regarding the beliefs associated with the attribution of problem behaviors and behavior management practices, even when team members initially agree to use PBS practices during the first phase. Therefore, helping team members shift their thinking and keeping them "bought in" to the PBS process becomes critical. Enhancing the team's capacity for understanding not just the "how" but also the "why" of assessment and planning becomes the central focus of the team leader and the PBS experts on the team.

Lynn

During the first collaborative phase, some of Lynn's team members shared a belief that she was experiencing bipolar depression, which was the cause of her problem behaviors. During the FBA, the data revealed that Lynn only exhibited the behaviors on Tuesdays and Thursdays. When it came time to develop hypotheses, several team members felt the behavior was a function of Lynn's possible bipolar disorder. The team leader listened to their ideas but brought out the data summaries and the patterns of behavior Lynn exhibited during the assessment. Everyone agreed the data were sufficient and appeared to be accurate. The team leader then posed a question to the team: "Is it possible for bipolar disorder to cause a predictable data pattern?" She then urged the team to brainstorm and think of what was different on Tuesdays and Thursdays (including issues related to medication) that may trigger Lynn's challenging behaviors. What else might be going on here?

....

One strategy for enhancing the team's understanding is to make the PBS assessment and planning processes explicit (Bambara et al., in press). For example, following the model of the initial line of inquiry (Lohrmann-O'Rourke, Knoster, & Llewellyn, 1999), the team could make wall charts of the setting events, antecedents, and consequences to help the team focus on environmental determinants of the problem behaviors and help reinforce this framework for understanding for team members who are new to PBS or have shifted their thinking. Also, the team should share, visually display, and review the assessment data when developing hypotheses. For example, after collecting several days of antecedent-behavior-consequence (ABC) data, the team member in charge of summarizing data has a stack of ABC cards to summarize. Rather than summarizing the data in words, the team member could visually display these data in a bar graph. Even the least experienced team member could clearly review the data and see what could be possible triggers and nontriggers to problem behavior. The use of data is one of the most effective trans-formative tools for changing beliefs (e.g., Lohrmann, Martin, & Patil, 2012).

Another idea is for the team to use the competing pathways model (O'Neill et al., 1997) to generate interventions. This way, the entire team can see how selected inter-ventions link back to their stated hypotheses for problem behavior. Once a team adopts an explicit process and uses it regularly to guide the understanding of problem behaviors and plan for effective interventions, the same processes can be used to *reframe challenging beliefs as they emerge.* For example, the team facilitator may notice a drift in discussions of data or observations as the team works to formulate a hypothesis. Team members may begin to say things like, "She just knows it drives me crazy!" or "His mother refuses to consider medication for his ADHD," rather than focus on the environmental explana-tions for behavior. Perhaps the team leader needs to ask the members, "What are your beliefs about the reasons for challenging behavior?" in order to assess if team mem-bers are still sticking with "old" ways of thinking about challenging behaviors rather than keeping "new" PBS assumptions in mind. This may help bring team members' apprehension to the surface where it can be discussed. When this begins to happen, it is important for the entire team to reframe challenging beliefs within the PBS context. This entails going back to visual displays of data or the team's intervention plan to rethink and challenge faulty assumptions (e.g., "In what ways will this suggested inter-vention address Emmanuel's need to escape a difficult task? Let's go back to our model to figure this out."). At times, the team may need to be reminded about the goal they developed together, as a team, in the first phase.

Create an Atmosphere of Openness and Honesty   In order for team members to feel comfortable to discuss their beliefs about challenging behavior or their struggles with adopting the PBS process, team leaders should strive to maintain an *open and hon-est atmosphere.* Despite being asked to share their concerns, members will not be able to honestly communicate if they feel they will be judged, dismissed, or put down by fellow team members. Team facilitators will need to display exemplary manners and com-munication skills to create an atmosphere where differing opinions can be shared and discussed. Team leaders should make sure the team is following the ground rules they set when establishing the team structure. Also, the team leader serves as a model in responding and encouraging team member communication. If another team member responds in a noncollaborative manner (e.g., "That will never work!"), it is the team lead-er's role to shape this discussion (e.g., "I'm not sure we understand why you are opposed to this idea. Help us understand why you feel so strongly about this."). The team leader must help show value in everyone's contri-butions, refrain from blaming others for fail-ure, and encourage team members to listen to each other.

Lynn

In the first meeting, Lynn's team established a time limit for each individual team member to speak during the discussion portion of their meetings. However, over time, the site supervisor tended to take twice as much time as the others, often leav-ing one direct care staff member, Margo, without any time to contribute. Over time, Margo felt her role was not valued, and she was reluctant to con-tribute or to complete her tasks on time. She often had interesting insights and stories to share, as she spent the most time with Lynn compared with the other team members, but now she was hesitant to do so. After a meeting, the team leader asked Margo about why she was so quiet in the meet-ings now. Margo mentioned her frustration with the other team member dominating the time. The team leader admitted she did not realize this was happening and resolved to get the team back on track. At the next meeting, the team leader reminded everyone of the ground rules, admitted drifting from the rules, and asked for a volunteer to watch the time during the meeting. When

Margo's turn came, she was able to discuss how she felt betrayed by Lynn, even though she now knew she should not take it personally. She also shared information about the times of day when she noticed Lynn not exhibiting any problem behaviors, which was helpful to the team as they developed hypotheses.

....

Ensure Contextual Fit All the student or individual-focused activities in this phase lead to the development of a BSP. Central to this mission is making certain that each proposed intervention or support developed by the team is assessment based and linked to hypotheses for problem behavior. Thus when considering interventions, teams must come to consensus on the critical questions outlined in Table 3.3 to ensure a fit between the interventions and the assessment information gathered. Teams might ask, for example, "Given our hypotheses for problem behavior, what antecedent events can we change to prevent problem behavior from occurring? What alternative skills can we teach to replace problem behaviors? Will our interventions lead to desired outcomes for the individual?" At the same time, teams must also be concerned with *contextual fit*. A good plan has to have "good fit" with the goals, values, and skills of the team, as well a "good fit" with the typical activities and routines of the individual and plan implementers—at school and at home. No matter how many

plans the team has developed in the past or how successful they have been, each plan will be unique and different because of differences associated with each individual of focus, team membership, and settings in which support plans will be implemented. A support plan with good contextual fit is more likely to have good outcomes, lead to long-term change, and be satisfactory to the individual and the team. Table 3.3 lists some questions teams might ask to evaluate interventions' contextual fit. Answers to these questions can verify the appropriateness of the proposed intervention or lead to modifications or considerations of alternative interventions or supports. In some cases, discussions may lead to additional training or supports for team members.

Divide Responsibilities Each phase consists of a myriad of tasks related to the team actions. In this phase, the team will be faced with tasks such as collecting assessment data, conducting interviews, summarizing data, and reviewing records, just to name a few. Each time the team meets or creates an action item or plan, it is important to clearly assign the task to a team member and that the team member understands his or her responsibility and when the task needs to be completed. Thinking back to Phase 1 and creating a meeting structure, each meeting may end with creating a "to-do" list or "action plan" and assignments for each item. For the team to work collaboratively,

Table 3.3. Questions to evaluate a good contextual fit

- Is the plan doable?
- Is it time efficient?
- Do team members feel they have the skills to carry out the plan?
- Do team members feel confident in carrying out the plan?
- Do team members believe that the plan will result in desired outcomes?
- Are additional resources or supports needed?
- Does the plan address team member priorities and concerns?
- Are the proposed interventions satisfactory to all team members?
- Do the proposed interventions fit routines and settings?
- Are the proposed interventions age appropriate and respectful of the individual?

the work will need to be divided so that everyone feels as though he or he is contributing but not unfairly burdened by his or her responsibilities to the team. By engaging in the previously mentioned team-centered activities such as creating an open and honest atmosphere and collaborative problem solving, responsibilities can be assigned and communicated in a fair manner that takes advantages of each team members' strengths and skills.

Phase 3: Implementing the Positive Behavior Support Plan

During this last phase of the PBS process, the team will implement, monitor, and evaluate the support plan. In this phase, the individual-focused team activities center on implementing interventions, collecting data, and reviewing the data to ensure the plan is indeed working as the team intended. Refer to Table 3.2 for questions to assist the team in their completion of the individual-focused activities. At this time, perhaps more than ever, the team will need to be supported and directed toward team-focused activities as the team begins the very important task of implementing the support plan.

Support the Team The team has created a support plan based on assessment data, which matches the hypotheses, and has identified empirically supported interventions with a good contextual fit. Now what do we do? The attention now shifts back to the team and the importance of the team members. What supports does the *team* need to carry out this plan? What do individual team members need to be successful? How can we build the team's confidence? How can we provide extra support to those implementing interventions or responsible for data collection? What are our fears and concerns about beginning the plan? Supporting the team during implementation helps ensure continuous contextual fit.

One way of supporting the team is to determine the best way to implement the plan. For example, should the team implement several interventions or just focus on prevention strategies first? Asking the team members what makes sense is a way of supporting the team so the process does not overwhelm them. The plan can be implemented all at once, in stages, or in small steps. Another way to support the team is to simply praise and encourage team members who are new or fearful about the process. Providing training and support on specific topics or areas in which the team lacks confidence is yet another means of supporting the team. Training can take the form of formal group training or less formal, more hands-on mentoring and modeling. For example, one of Lynn's direct care staff will be collecting observational data for the first time and is scared she will "screw it all up." Another team member with more experience has volunteered to observe alongside the other team member for the first few days and provide some onsite training and feedback. Team members can also support one another by checking in with each other during the week via phone calls, e-mails, or text messages. Finally, if a team member is particularly stressed after working through some stressful experiences or a crisis with the focus individual, provide a break by having another team member implement the intervention for a brief period of time.

Focus on Treatment Integrity As the interventions begin, the team will need to focus on maintaining a high degree of treatment integrity. An intervention with a high degree of treatment integrity is one that is being implemented exactly as planned. Without treatment integrity, we cannot be certain if the intervention is not working because it is a poor match for the behavior or if the intervention is being implemented incorrectly. Before the interventions even begin, there are several things the team can do to promote treatment integrity. First, they can work on translating the support plan into simple checklists or graphic organizers. User-friendly materials for staff will help everyone understand their role and the procedures. For example, Emmanuel's team created a one-sheet checklist containing the steps of the interventions they decided to put in place in his classroom (see Figure 3.1). The checklist was designed to be used as self-monitoring checklist for the teacher as well as an observation checklist another team member can complete to assess the fidelity of the implementation. Checklists such as these can be easily created and used by the team to ask questions about what is going well and what is not working and why.

Another way of promoting treatment integrity is to translate the plan into a user-friendly format that can be easily and quickly reviewed. Lynn's team created a one-sheet description of each intervention (antecedent, alternative skills, and responses to problem behavior) that shows the hypotheses, the intervention components and purpose, and who is responsible. The interventions were then reviewed with team members and staff, and copies were placed in easily accessible locations. Rather than reviewing a long, detailed support plan, teams can quickly review the

Checklist for Strategies for Emmanuel's Support Plan	
Teacher:	Date:
Increased Use of Praise	
Yes / No	1. Teacher uses praise statements for any positive behavior with a focus on in-seat behavior.
Yes / No	2. Teacher makes four positive statements for every one correction.
Classroom Aide Involvement	
Yes / No	1. Aide is positioned near Emmanuel in classroom.
Yes / No	2. Aide praises Emmanuel when appropriate and/or ignores minor misbehavior.
Rules for Classroom and Other Settings	
Yes / No	1. Teacher reviews expectations.
Yes / No	2. Teacher provides a precorrection (reminder) and/or provides praise to students following rules at least once during observation.
Self-Monitoring of Independent Seat Work	
Yes / No	1. A self-monitoring sheet is on Emmanuel's desk.
Yes / No	2. A cueing device (timer, clock) is utilized to cue intervals for self-monitoring.
Yes / No	3. Emmanuel records his behavior at the end of the interval.
Yes / No	4. Teacher praises Emmanuel for intervals of in-seat behavior.
Yes / No	5. At the end of the specified time, Emmanuel receives feedback for his performance.
Yes / No	6. Teacher checks and records accuracy of Emmanuel's ratings.
Consequence Strategies	
Yes / No	1. Teacher ignores minor misbehavior.
Yes / No	2. Teacher redirects Emmanuel to an alternative task or behavior rather than removal of the work.
Total number of steps completed (tally total number of yeses): _____	
Total number of steps (tally total number of yeses plus nos): _____	
Percentage of plan in place (# of yeses/total # of Steps × 100) = _____	

Figure 3.1. Checklist for strategies for Emmanuel's support plan.

"need to know" information in simple, clear steps. Lynn's summary BSP for antecedent interventions is shown in Figure 3.2.

Despite their best preventive efforts, the team may become concerned because an intervention does not appear to have the desired effect, it was effective but now seems to not work for the individual, or is just progressing too slowly. Although it may be tempting to stop the intervention, declare it unsuccessful, and implement something different, the team needs to resist this temptation and first determine if the intervention is actually being implemented the way it was designed to be implemented or if there has been some change or drift in the procedure. If there is a problem with treatment integrity, the team will need to not only determine

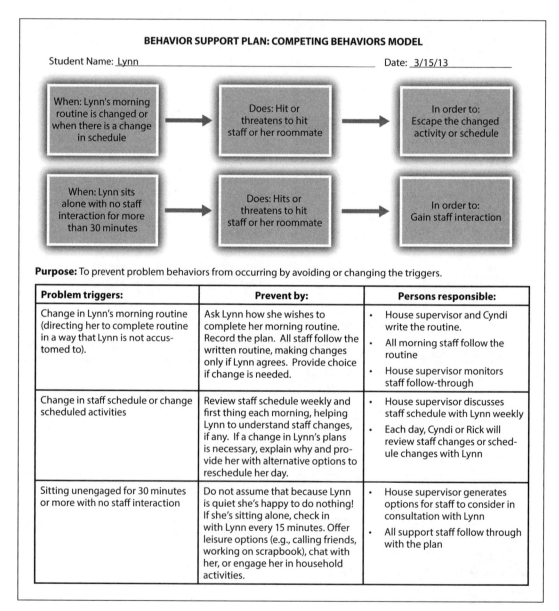

BEHAVIOR SUPPORT PLAN: COMPETING BEHAVIORS MODEL

Student Name: Lynn   Date: 3/15/13

When: Lynn's morning routine is changed or when there is a change in schedule → Does: Hit or threatens to hit staff or her roommate → In order to: Escape the changed activity or schedule

When: Lynn sits alone with no staff interaction for more than 30 minutes → Does: Hits or threatens to hit staff or her roommate → In order to: Gain staff interaction

Purpose: To prevent problem behaviors from occurring by avoiding or changing the triggers.

Problem triggers:	Prevent by:	Persons responsible:
Change in Lynn's morning routine (directing her to complete routine in a way that Lynn is not accustomed to).	Ask Lynn how she wishes to complete her morning routine. Record the plan. All staff follow the written routine, making changes only if Lynn agrees. Provide choice if change is needed.	• House supervisor and Cyndi write the routine. • All morning staff follow the routine • House supervisor monitors staff follow-through
Change in staff schedule or change scheduled activities	Review staff schedule weekly and first thing each morning, helping Lynn to understand staff changes, if any. If a change in Lynn's plans is necessary, explain why and provide her with alternative options to reschedule her day.	• House supervisor discusses staff schedule with Lynn weekly • Each day, Cyndi or Rick will review staff changes or schedule changes with Lynn
Sitting unengaged for 30 minutes or more with no staff interaction	Do not assume that because Lynn is quiet she's happy to do nothing! If she's sitting alone, check in with Lynn every 15 minutes. Offer leisure options (e.g., calling friends, working on scrapbook), chat with her, or engage her in household activities.	• House supervisor generates options for staff to consider in consultation with Lynn • All support staff follow through with the plan

Figure 3.2.   Summary behavior support plan (BSP).

what went wrong (e.g., intervention did not adequately address the hypothesis for behavior) but also ask *why* it went wrong (e.g., the team member was not sure what to do, the team member did not understand when to do the intervention, it was unclear to the team who was responsible for the intervention). The *why* of treatment integrity shifts the focus to the team. For example, Emmanuel's team included several reading interventions in his plan. When the team came together to review his reading probe data, reading grades, and other related data, they were surprised to see very little improvement. The data were increasing, but not as quickly as they hoped. One team member expressed dismay and wanted to add even more reading interventions and boost the intensity. After further discussion, the team realized Emmanuel had missed approximately half of the scheduled sessions with the specialist that month because of assemblies, statewide tests, a field trip, and teacher absences due to illness. Also, when the sessions were missed, the teacher did not realize she should let the specialist know. The reading specialist did not realize Emmanuel's teacher would be able to excuse him for makeup sessions, either. The interventions may not have been working as intended because they were being delivered less frequently than planned. The team found creative ways to ensure that there was time for the reading interventions when other school events interfered with the schedule and also ensure good communication between the teacher and specialist when there are absences and missed sessions. A team member was assigned to monitor missed sessions and schedule makeup sessions.

Review the Data to Celebrate and Problem Solve When Needed An important team function during this phase is regularly reviewing the data. The team leader must ensure the data are being reviewed frequently and ask, "Is sufficient progress being made?" If *yes*, the team should celebrate. Just like an effective teacher who praises each step in the learning process, not just the final product or outcome, a team should find reasons to celebrate its progress along the way. Although this concept is being introduced in this latter phase, celebrations can take place in any step or phase and can be as simple as sharing a checklist of completed tasks by the team, sending a thank-you note or e-mail to a team member, or sharing cookies at the meeting to celebrate some documented changes in behavior or implementation of the plan. The PBS process is a journey, and praise and recognition should not be withheld until the very end. Rather, team leaders and members should look for opportunities to praise and encourage one another throughout the journey. Routine data review provides the team with a ready-made opportunity to see success. Seeing success in the data can motivate team members and transform beliefs about the effectiveness of the PBS process.

Lynn

Margo, a direct care staff member on Lynn's team, was feeling discouraged. Lynn's plan had been in place for 3 weeks, and Margo was still seeing Lynn engage in some challenging behaviors. She came to the team meeting feeling discouraged and tired. But when the team leader displayed Lynn's data, there was a clear downward trend in the frequency of Lynn's challenging behavior. In addition, the behaviors were shorter in duration. Margo was surprised by the data and even more surprised when the team leader thanked and praised her and several other staff for contributing to the change. Margo left the meeting feeling much better about things. Afterward, she thought about the past week or two and realized Lynn did calm down more quickly than she had before. Maybe she was hoping for a "quick fix," but at least the data were moving in the right direction!

In addition to celebration throughout the journey, problem solving also occurs at any point in the process. As in any journey, there will be bumps along the way. If the data show less progress than expected, the team needs to come together, trouble-shoot, and if necessary, revise the plan. For example, a team member discovers that data collection has been happening only sporad-ically for the last 2 weeks, and when data are collected, they may be unreliable. An impromptu meeting is called to deal with this issue, and the necessary training and changes in responsibility are made through collaborative problem-solving steps. Rather than wait for 2 more weeks and cast blame, the team can work together to fix the issue and move forward. If an intervention is not working and treatment integrity is not an issue, maybe the plan should be changed and a different intervention implemented or devised. Teams should anticipate experienc-ing problems somewhere along the way and be prepared to work through them. Even a successful problem-solving episode can be grounds for a celebration.

Evaluate Satisfaction with Outcomes and Reflect on Team Process   By regularly reviewing the individual's data and the team's accomplishments, the team is con-tinually evaluating its progress toward the goals. But what about the team's progress in working as a team? Of equal importance is taking time to reflect on whether or not team members feel as though they are suc-cessful in working together as a team. One way of assessing this is to create a checklist of the important team activities to evaluate team functioning. An example (see Figure 3.3) is provided and can be used during any phases to assess team "health."

CONCLUSION

PBS is an outcome of effective teaming. How the team functions has a direct impact on the planning and delivery of supports and successful outcomes for individuals. Active monitoring of the team process and engaging in team-based activities can lead to improve-ment in team functioning. Effective teaming not only successfully addresses the individu-al's concerns but also has a successful impact

on the team member's understanding and capacity to provide supports for the individ-ual. In this chapter, we provide a number of team-based activities to engage in and mon-itor as a means of improving team function-ing. These activities and strategies provide a starting point for team members to begin to understand and focus on the importance of teaming.

REFERENCES

Albin, R.W., Lucyshyn, J.M., Horner, R.H., & Flannery, K.B. (1996). Contextual fit for behavior support plans: A model for "goodness of fit." In L.K., Koegel, R.L. Koegel, & G. Dunlap (Eds.), *Positive behavioral support: Including people with difficult behaviors in the community* (pp. 81–98). Baltimore, MD: Paul H. Brookes Publishing Co.

Baker, B.L., Blacher, J., Crnic, K.A., & Edelbrock, C. (2002). Behavior problems and parenting stress in families of three-year-old children with and without developmental delays. *American Journal on Mental Retardation, 6,* 433–444.

Bambara, L.M., Goh, A., Kern, L., & Caskie, G. (2012). Perceived barriers and enablers to implementing individualized positive behavior interventions and supports in school settings. *Journal of Positive Behavior Interventions.* Advanced online publica-tion. doi:10.1177/1098300712437219

Bambara, L.M., & Kern, L. (2005). *Individualized sup-ports for students with problem behaviors: Designing positive behavior plans.* New York, NY: Guilford.

Bambara, L.M., Lohrmann, S., Nonnemacher, S., Goh, A., & Kern, L. (2014). *Facilitators' perspectives on fac-tors influencing the implementation of individualized positive behavior supports.* Manuscript submitted for publication.

Bambara, L.M., Nonnemacher, S., & Kern, L. (2009). Sustaining school-based individualized positive behavior support: Perceived barriers and enablers. *Journal of Positive Behavior Interventions, 11,* 161–176. doi:10.1177/1098300708330878

Bambara, L.M., Nonnemacher, S., & Koger, F. (2005). Teaming. In L.M. Bambara & L. Kern, *Individual-ized supports for students with problem behaviors: Designing positive behavior support plans.* New York, NY: Guilford.

Chang, M. (2009). An appraisal perspective of teacher burnout: Examining the emotional work of teach-ers. *Educational Psychology Review, 21,* 193–218. doi:10.1007/s10648-009-9106-y

Dunlap, G., Newton, J.S., Fox, L., Benito, N., & Vaughn, B. (2001). Family involvement in functional assess-ment and positive behavior and support. *Focus on Autism and Other Developmental Disabilities, 16,* 215–222.

Fleming, J.L., & Monda-Amaya, L.E. (2001). Process variables critical for team effectiveness: A Delphi study of wraparound team members. *Remedial and Special Education, 22,* 158–171.

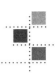

TEAM PROCESS CHECKLIST

Rate each item (Yes/No/Needs Improvement). List barriers and solutions to any issues in each area.

Rating	Evaluation area	Barriers	Solutions
Y/N/NI	We have defined goals, roles, ground rules, and meeting times.		
Y/N/NI	Meetings have an agenda and there is enough time to share ideas and concerns.		
Y/N/NI	The team uses collaborative problem solving to work through issues.		
Y/N/NI	Team members can openly and honestly share information; communication is respectful.		
Y/N/NI	Responsibilities are fairly divided among the team.		
Y/N/NI	The team works to ensure a good contextual fit.		
Y/N/NI	The team consistently uses a positive behavior support (PBS) framework to reframe challenges.		
Y/N/NI	The team supports each other while implementing the plan.		
Y/N/NI	The team is focused on treatment integrity.		
Y/N/NI	The team uses data to celebrate success and problem-solves issues.		
Y/N/NI	The team reflects on "team health" and strives to make changes when needed.		

Figure 3.3. Team process checklist.

Freeman, R., Eber, L., Anderson, C., Irvin, L., Horner, R., Bounds, M., & Dunlap, G. (2006). Building inclusive school cultures using school-wide positive behavior support: Designing effective individual support systems for students with significant disabilities. *Research and Practice for Persons with Severe Disabilities, 31*, 4–17.

Gersten, R., & Dimino, J. (2001). The realities of translating research into classroom practice. *Learning Disabilities Research and Practice, 16*, 120–130. doi:10.1111/0938-8982.00013

Hastings, R.P., & Brown, T. (2002). Coping strategies and the impact of challenging behavior on special educators' burnout. *Mental Retardation, 40*, 148–156. doi:10.1352/0047-6765(2002)040<0148:CSATIO>2.0.CO;2

Horner, R.H., Sugai, G., & Anderson, C.M. (2010). Examining the evidence base for school-wide positive behavior support. *Focus on Exceptional Children, 42*(8), 1–14.

Janz, B.D., Colquitt, J.A., & Noe, R.A. (1997). Knowledge worker team effectiveness: The role of autonomy, interdependence, team development, and contextual support variables. *Personnel Psychology, 50*, 877–904.

Klassen, R.M. (2010). Teacher stress: The mediating role of collective efficacy beliefs. *Journal of Educational Research, 103*, 342–350. doi:10.1080/00220670903383069

Lambrechts, G., Petry, K., & Maes, B. (2008). Staff variables that influence responses to challenging behaviour of clients with an intellectual disability: A review. *Education and Training in Developmental Disabilities, 43*, 454–473. doi:10.1111/j.1365-2788.2009.01162.x

Lohrmann, S., Martin, S.D., & Patil, S. (2012). External and internal coaches' perspectives about overcoming barriers to universal interventions. *Journal of Positive Behavior Interventions.* Advanced online publication. doi:10.1177/1098300712459078

Lohrmann-O'Rourke, S., Knoster, T., & Llewellyn, G. (1999). Screening for understanding: An initial line of inquiry for school-based settings. *Journal of Positive Behavior Interventions, 1*, 35–42. doi:10.1177/109830079900100105

McLaughlin, D.M., & Carr, E.G. (2005). Quality of rapport as a setting event for problem behavior: Assessment and intervention. *Journal of Positive Behavior Interventions, 7*, 68–91.

Mitchell, G., & Hastings, R.P. (2001). Coping, burnout, and emotion in staff working in community services for people with challenging behaviors. *American Journal on Mental Retardation, 106*, 448–459.

O'Neill, R.E., Horner, R.H., Albin, R.W., Sprague, J.R., Storey, K., & Newton, J.S. (1997). *Functional assessment and program development for problem behavior: A practical handbook* (2nd ed.). Pacific Grove, CA: Brooks/Cole.

Snell, M.E., & Janney, R. (2005). *Teachers' guides to inclusive practices: Collaborative teaming.* Baltimore, MD: Paul H. Brookes Publishing Co.

Snell, M.E., Voorhees, M.D., & Chen, L. (2005). Team involvement in assessment-based interventions with problem behavior 1997–2002. *Journal of Positive Behavior Interventions, 7*, 140–152. doi:10.1177/.741932508327466

Thousand, J.S., & Villa, R.A. (2000). Collaborative teaming: A powerful tool in school restructuring. In R.A. & J.S. Thousand (Eds.), *Restructuring for caring and effective education* (pp. 254–291). Baltimore, MD: Paul H. Brookes Publishing Co.

Welch, M., Brownell, K., & Sheridan, S.M. (1999). What's the score and game plan on teaming in schools? A review of the literature on team teaching and school-based problem solving teams. *Remedial and Special Education, 20*, 36–49.

Westling, D.L. (2010). Teachers and challenging behaviors: Knowledge, views and practices. *Remedial and Special Education, 31*, 48–63. doi:10.1177/1098300705 0070030301

Wilson, C., Gardner, F., Burton, J., & Leung, S. (2006). Maternal attributions and young children's conduct problems: A longitudinal study. *Infant and Child Development, 15*, 109–121.

Person-Centered Planning Teams

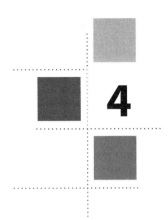

4

Jennifer McFarland-Whisman

Jayelyn

Jayelyn is nearly 3 years old. She is a lively little girl with an adorable smile and bright green eyes. Jayelyn was recently diagnosed with autism—she doesn't speak; has problems with toileting, sleeping, and eating; and has frequent severe tantrums.

Brady

Brady is 9 years old and in the third grade. He has a real talent for drawing, performs academically on grade level, and attends a regular education classroom. Brady has multiple diagnoses, including attention-deficit/hyperactivity disorder (ADHD), oppositional defiant disorder, bipolar disorder, and generalized anxiety disorder. Brady has a reputation at school and is well known by the teachers, administrators, and other students. His behavior can be very disruptive and includes screaming, threatening to hurt others, and throwing and destroying materials. His teachers consider him a real problem, and

some of his peers have expressed being afraid of him. Despite his academic ability, school administrators and his teacher are considering a placement in a special education class.

Stephanie

Stephanie is 21 years old. She recently graduated from high school and lives at home with her parents. She has severe obsessive compulsive disorder. If Stephanie's strict daily routine or obsessive compulsive rituals are disrupted, she can become aggressive (e.g., hitting, pinching, and kicking others). Her parents report that Stephanie has recently become socially avoidant and won't leave the house. She also started to wet her bed, and they are not sure why.

Taken at face value, the behavior challenges faced by these three individuals seem straightforward. In all three cases, behavior problems should be targeted, prioritized, and defined; a functional behavioral assessment conducted; and a plan developed to assist in reducing challenging behavior and increasing adaptive skills. Those most directly involved with the individual—parents, teachers, employers—should be trained to implement the plan, and data collected should be to assist in evaluating and modifying the plan as needed. Now consider some additional information related to these families.

Jayelyn

Jayelyn's parents are stunned by their daughter's diagnosis and not sure where to turn. They recently immigrated to a large city and have no extended family nearby. For both parents, English is their second language. Given that they just moved to this city, they have few friends to rely on for support. Jayelyn's family was recently referred to early intervention services, but they are now being told that their daughter will need to make the transition to school-age services by age 3. They've hardly gotten to know their early intervention providers and now will be interacting with a whole new set of professionals. The learning curve is steep, as they are bombarded with information about Jayelyn's diagnosis, treatment options, and available services all in a language that they are still struggling to learn. Jayelyn's mother works at a local grocery store and is considering quitting her job but wonders how they will make it financially; as the family also just found out they are expecting their second child.

Brady

Brady's parents are divorced and don't communicate well with each other. Brady's mother is an alcoholic, so much of the parenting is left up to his father, who has full custody. Brady has been in and out of inpatient psychiatric hospitals over the past year, and he is on multiple medications. The family has limited financial resources. The family does have some close friends they can rely on for support. The school system is pressuring the family to "discipline" Brady at home, seek another

inpatient admission, or change his medication regime. Brady's behavior is difficult at home too, and his father is at a loss as to what to do.

Stephanie

Stephanie's family lives in a very rural community. They have a large extended family, and they all live on the same family-owned property. Stephanie's father is a coal miner with a disability; he is at home full time but finds it difficult to care for Stephanie due to his disability. Stephanie's mother works full time to make ends meet. There are very few services for Stephanie in the area, transportation is an issue because there is no public transit system, and employment options are very limited for anyone living in the area. While they usually enjoy being with extended family, the fact that Stephanie has a hard time leaving the house has made it difficult for them to leave as well.

These stories help us recognize the context in which we all live, providing us with a better understanding about how to develop behavior support plans (BSPs) that are more closely aligned with the individual and his or her family's lifestyle. This chapter will discuss how the broader context of a person's life can and should drive the development of BSPs. The chapter will focus on person-centered planning (PCP), a process commonly employed by practitioners of positive behavior support (PBS). With PCP, a team is assembled to gather information about the individual and the broader context of his or her life and, armed with that information, develop a more comprehensive support plan that considers and is responsive to those variables.

MODELS OF SERVICE DELIVERY AND HISTORY OF PERSON-CENTERED PLANNING

There exist two broad, mutually exclusive approaches to service delivery. The first, an *expert-driven approach*, typically involves an expert in a particular field (e.g., behavioral consultant, special educator, speech therapist) who is the sole designer of intervention plans (Becker-Cottrill, McFarland, & Anderson, 2003). The expert plays a directive role in assessment, educational and behavior plan development, evaluation, and plan modification. While information from others may be taken into consideration, the expert commonly is seen as having the background and experience in his or her field to address and answer questions or problems as they arise. The expert may provide some combination of direct services to the individual and training for others (e.g., teachers, parents) to implement the intervention plan. Services may take place in clinical and/or natural settings. The focus is on improving skills and reducing the challenging behavior of the individual. There is, however, no formal focus on the context of an individual and his or her family's life or overall quality of life.

The other service delivery model, an *ecological approach,* takes a broader view of the individual and his or her life (see Becker-Cottrill, McFarland, & Anderson, 2003; Greene & McGuire, 1998). Factors such as the individual and his or her family's history, resources, living situation, financial status, strengths, and goals are taken into consideration when developing plans. PBS is a service delivery model that uses an ecological approach (Albin, Lucyshyn, Horner, & Flannery, 1996; Clark & Hieneman, 1999; Horner et al., 1990). Within a PBS approach, a team of invested stakeholders, including the individual, his or her family, and other caregivers, friends, and service providers, meet to develop, implement, and evaluate intervention plans. As with an expert-driven approach, skill development and decreasing challenging behavior is still a focus; however, a PBS approach addresses broader issues such as variables related to quality of life and contextual fit (Albin et al., 1996). Ideally, addressing broader lifestyle issues will improve skills and decrease challenging behavior. For example, through PCP and a functional behavioral assessment, the team for an individual who is engaging in

severe challenging behavior and lives with a roommate at a group home with six other residents may come to understand that the individual needs more personal space. The team's focus would then be on providing the individual with more personal space within the group home or, ideally, to advocate for a different living arrangement. If the team was correct in their hypothesis that the individual's behavior was due, in part, to a nonpreferred living arrangement, the team may find that his challenging behavior naturally decreases without an intrusive or complicated intervention plan. In other words, changing the living environment in this case would be the intervention—decreasing problem behavior by improving quality of life.

One way for PBS teams to structure their assessment of broader issues in an individual and/or family's life is through PCP. PCP emerged in the mid-1970s—the outcome of a group of individuals interested in exploring how the quality of life of people with disabilities could be enhanced by applying the principles of normalization (O'Brien & O'Brien, 2002). PCP became a commonly used term by the mid-1980s and was used in part to address the needs of individuals with intellectual and developmental disabilities who were moved from large institutions to smaller community-based settings during the large-scale deinstitutionalization movement (O'Brien, 1987; O'Brien & O'Brien, 2002). Many of those making this transition had lived most of their lives in large institutions, and the change to smaller community settings, while believed to be in their long-term best interest, was potentially disruptive and frightening. PCP provided an avenue for individualizing support needs and providing a smoother transition for these individuals. At about the same time PCP was beginning to be more widely used, PBS was in its infancy (Carr et al., 2002). Because of PBS's emphasis on the principles of normalization, inclusion, and self-determination, dovetailing PCP with PBS seemed a natural fit. PBS provided the structure and strategies to assist in meaningful behavior change and skill development.

PCP provided an avenue to develop cohesive teams, address broader quality-of-life changes, assist in finding natural and systemic supports for the individual in the community, and create a better fit between BSPs and the context of the individual's life (Albin et al., 1996; Horner et al., 1990). While initially developed to address the needs of individuals with severe disabilities, PCP has been expanded to more diverse populations and settings, including mental health and addiction (Adams & Grieder, 2005; Curtis et al., 2010), human services (Freeman et al., 2005; Reid et al., 2003), health care (Briggs, 2004; Thompson & Cobb, 2004), and dementia care (Ryan & Carey, 2009).

WHAT IS PERSON-CENTERED PLANNING?

PCP is a process through which the strengths, wishes, future goals, and support needs of an individual are identified (Holburn, 2002; Mount, 2000; O'Brien, 1987; O'Brien & O'Brien, 2002). The common goals of PCP are to assist the focus person to become a valued and respected part of his or her community, help the individual develop and maintain satisfying relationships with others, provide important choices related to his or her life, and support the development of new skills (Kincaid, 1995; Kincaid & Dunlap, 2003). A team of individual stakeholders, including the focus person and his or her family, friends, important supporters, and service providers, gather to complete one or more tools with preestablished topics to lead their discussion. The views and opinions of the focus person and those close to him or her take priority and are recorded by a neutral facilitator.

PCP differs from traditional interview or client-centered assessments in several ways. First, the views or perceived wishes of the focus person or his or her caregiver, depending on the individual's age and ability to participate, are given precedence in a PCP process. This avoids placing an emphasis on a person's impairments and deviates from viewing the expert as the authority (Holburn,

2002). Rather than fitting the person to the needs of the service system, the system is shaped to fit the needs of the person. For example, a traditional model might provide a list of standard services that all individuals receive, even if one person has different needs from the standard services provided by that agency. A person-centered approach first looks at the individual's expressed needs and goals; then a unique and tailored plan for services and supports is developed. To address the full range of needs, this plan may blend agency and natural supports (e.g., parents, friends, individuals in the community) to fit the person's expressed goals, lifestyle, and support needs. Even if the individual is unable to fully participate in his or her PCP process, steps are taken to identify and understand the interests and desires of the individual by observing him or her in his or her home and community and gathering information from caregivers and other stakeholders. Care is taken by the facilitator to ensure the PCP process reflects the goals of the focus person rather than those of caregivers, agency representatives, or other team members. If safety, health, or legal issues might be compromised or some goals are clearly unattainable, the team works to find a satisfactory alternative. For example, an underage individual might express a desire to learn to roll and smoke his own cigarettes—something that is both a health and legal concern. The team might explore what he is really interested in doing and problem-solve to find a possible alternative. If the motivation to engage in the behavior was, for example, rolling things up, perhaps the individual would enjoy helping a local paper delivery person roll newspapers for a paper route. However, if the motivation was to socially connect with others, the team might further analyze the individual's interests and leisure skills and assist him in connecting with others who have similar interests. For example, if the individual had a passion for trains, he could be introduced to a local group of miniature train collectors and taught the social skills needed to effectively participate in the group.

The second difference between PCP and traditional assessment is that information is typically recorded on large sheets of paper posted in view of all team members, rather than team members taking notes on a pad of paper or computer individually. The rationale behind using large sheets of paper is to enhance the team's ability to work together and focus their attention on the same information. Usually, information is recorded in writing, using the focus person and teams' wording rather than professional jargon, and graphically to facilitate understanding for all team members, including those who might have literacy, second language, or other cognitive challenges. Finally, several PCP tools are used not only for assessment purposes but also lead directly to an action plan where goals, responsible parties, and due dates are recorded and acted on. Thus PCP may have a dual role of both assessing a person's individual desires and needs and providing a way for teams to begin putting the plan into action to move toward those goals.

Commonly used PCP tools include Planning Alternative Tomorrows with Hope (PATH; Falvey, Forest, Pearpoint, & Rosenberg, 1997; O'Brien & Pearpoint, 2003; Pearpoint, O'Brien, & Forest, 1993), personal profiles (O'Brien, Mount, & O'Brien, 1990), the McGill Action Planning System (MAPS; Falvey et al., 1997; Vandercook, York, & Forest, 1989), essential lifestyle planning (Smull, 1997), personal futures planning (Mount, 2000; Mount & Zwernick, 1988), circle of friends (Falvey et al., 1997), solution circles (O'Brien & Pearpoint, 2003), and the PICTURE method (Holburn, Gordon, & Vietze, 2007). Ecomaps, culturagrams, and genograms, originally developed by social workers, share many of the same characteristics as PCP tools and may also be useful for gathering information specific to the family and/or focus person within the context of PCP (Green & Barnes, 1998).

All the PCP tools include the focus person and his or her team of invested stakeholders (family, friends, school personnel, and service providers) and a neutral facilitator who records information and decisions in writing and graphically for the whole team PCP tools differ in the types of information gathered, whether or not an action plan is developed, and the length of time it takes to complete each. This chapter will concentrate on how to develop a PCP team and then focus on the first three PCP tools mentioned previously, the PATH, MAPS, and personal profiles, providing descriptions and examples of each. The chapter will conclude by illustrating how PCP can be used to enhance the BSP by promoting stakeholder commitment, addressing quality of life, and raising sensitivity to cultural diversity issues.

Building a Collaborative Person-Centered Planning Team

While some systems have adopted PCP agencywide, for others, the need for a PCP team emerges when a problem develops or is anticipated. For example, a PCP team might be developed to address issues related to an individual engaging in severe challenging behavior, an individual making the transition between service delivery systems or settings (e.g., early intervention to preschool, preschool to kindergarten, high school to adulthood, moving to a new home), or discord among service providers and the individual or his or her caregivers. Invitations to participate on the team are usually made to individuals who have a direct connection to the focus person, including family members, friends, teachers, direct services providers, and outside agency personnel. Others, with specific expertise who might provide useful information and resources to the team, may be invited and include an individual with behavioral expertise, administrators, or others with knowledge or experiences specific to the needs of the focus person (e.g., a speech therapist with specific training in the Picture Exchange Communication System [PES] or a vocational rehabilitation counselor).

Determining *who* should be on the team may be less difficult than helping teams function in a truly collaborative manner.

PCP and subsequent team meetings may be called to address a particularly difficult issue for a focus person; however, the team may or may not work collaboratively to approach the issue(s). Six key components of effective collaboration have been identified (Blue-Banning, Summers, Frankland, Nelson, & Beegle, 2004; Blue-Banning, Turnbull, & Pereira, 2000): communication, equality, commitment, skills, trust, and respect.

Communication Collaborative teams that function well together have a mechanism for communicating with each other, often through regularly scheduled meetings. Effective communication among team members may occur formally during PCP meetings and less formally outside of meetings. Communication is respectful, honest, and open and serves to convey information necessary to move the process forward (Blue-Banning et al., 2004). Communication occurs not only between professionals on the team but most important with the focus person and his or her family.

Equality All members of collaborative PCP teams are treated respectfully and seen as equal partners, and the information they provide is given as much consideration as everyone else's input. Within PCP, equality among individuals on the team is especially important when considering the role of the focus person and his or her family. Parents and caregivers who participated in a study by Blue-Banning et al. (2004) indicated their trust and collaboration with professionals was strengthened when they felt their opinions and views were valued. Professionals reported better collaboration when "turfism" was avoided by team members. PCP is limited in effectiveness if a team fails to share power and control with each other, especially with the focus person and their family (Holburn, 2002).

Commitment Better collaboration and relationships with professionals occur when focus people and families see professionals as committed beyond their job description,

working with or around the system to help the focus person realize their goals. Blue-Banning et al. (2004) found these professionals tended to view the focus person and his or her family as individuals rather than "clients," "cases," or "numbers."

Skills Valuing the skills of everyone on the team, making a commitment to continue learning new skills, and keeping up-to-date on research are also important aspects of collaboration. For a professional, being able to admit he or she does not know everything but is willing to learn appears to be highly valued by parents and focus people (Blue-Banning et al., 2004). Team members recognize the value of learning new skills and are open to sharing materials and resources so all team members learn new information.

Trust Working within the context of a PCP team means having the ability to trust that others will follow through on their promised actions—that is, once an individual on the team makes a commitment to do something, the rest of the team is relying on them to follow through. Parents and professionals agreed that reliability is an important factor related to strong parent–professional relationships (Blue-Banning et al., 2004). Other key aspects of trust reported by parents involved safety and confidentiality—they needed to know that their child was safe and that professionals respected their privacy by keeping information confidential.

Respect Respect is an important aspect of PCP teams. While team members may not agree on every point, PCP team members are asked to consider the views of all other team members and come to a consensus on issues. This requires not only listening to others but also being able to compromise and come to a joint decision. Other aspects of respect involve treating others with courtesy; understanding and empathizing with others' circumstances; and acknowledging the hard work of all team members (Blue-Banning et al., 2004).

The role of the team facilitator is critical to the team's success or failure. Typically, the facilitator is someone who takes a neutral role providing support and guidance to the team. Effective facilitators assist the PCP team by setting firm ground rules, moderating conflict, maintaining communication, and helping the team follow through on actions. The facilitator also plays a key role in helping the team problem-solve as barriers arise.

Jayelyn

Because of an impending transition to preschool, Jayelyn's early intervention team decides it would be beneficial to expand its membership to include the preschool's receiving staff. Jayelyn's parents and her early intervention developmental specialist, speech therapist, occupational therapist, and new preschool teacher and speech therapist meet to begin developing a transition plan. While Jayelyn's parents see the value in involving the members from the preschool, they are nervous, as they have come to trust their early intervention team, especially their developmental specialist who is open to their concerns, shares information easily, and has worked hard to understand their unique cultural perspective. They are concerned about what their relationship with the new staff will be like and worried about cultural and linguistic barriers that might be problematic. Given the family's concern, the early intervention specialist works with the family to find a local college student who would be interested in serving as an interpreter for the family to increase their ability to understand the information they are receiving regarding Jayelyn.

Brady

Due to Brady's severe and persistent challenging behavior, a team is developed to discuss a behavior plan and the possibility that Brady would be better served in a special education setting. Brady's mother, father, and his stepmother meet with the school principal and assistant principal, psychologist, Brady's third-grade teacher, a district administrator, school district lawyer, and a behavior specialist. The family sits on one side of the table while the school team, many with their arms crossed, sits on the other. While the family is familiar with some of the school staff, they have never met the district administrator, lawyer, or behavior specialist. Many of their interactions with the staff they do know have been negative, as the principals and teacher have talked with the family numerous times about Brady's behavior and have implied the family needs to discipline him better at home, have him hospitalized, or have his medication changed. The family is nervous and speaks very little during the meeting. Many of the terms used by the district personnel are new to the family, but there are few opportunities for questions and the family leaves the meeting confused, worried, and unsure about what they've agreed to.

Stephanie

Stephanie's parents are increasingly concerned about her behavior. They had previously been involved with a statewide program that provides PCP and PBS services and are still in contact with their support person. They make a call to the support person to ask for advice and additional help. The support person suggests a small team meeting with Stephanie and her family. The family feels relieved and begins thinking about how they can best address Stephanie's current issues.

These scenarios reveal apparent discrepancies between the functioning of the three teams. It is obvious that some interactions among team members have the potential to be more effective than others. For example, Jayelyn and Stephanie's teams will most likely benefit from the positive relationships that have been established by professionals on their teams. Jayelyn's early intervention specialist recognizes the family's concerns regarding meeting new team members and the potential for cultural and language barriers to impede progress. She is working with the family to address these probable barriers and has obviously gained their trust and respect. In Stephanie's case, they have ready access to a trusted professional they worked well with previously. The approach of Brady's team, however, is likely to put the family on edge even more and exacerbate an already tense situation. Their body language and interaction with the family is unlikely to encourage any of the important aspects of parent–professional working relationships discussed previously.

PERSON-CENTERED PLANNING TOOLS

A variety of PCP tools are available that may be used to gather information about a family and/or focus person. The tools differ from each other in a variety of dimensions (see Meaden, Shelden, Appel, & DeGrazia, 2010, for a comparison of the tools). In this section, three tools will be discussed in more detail: PATH, MAPS, and personal profile.

A PATH usually takes about 2.5 to 3 hours to complete and is used in more complex, challenging situations where there may be a long history of problems, disagreement, and/or strong emotion (Falvey et al., 1997; O'Brien & Pearpoint, 2003; Pearpoint, O'Brien, & Forest, 1993). The PATH involves gathering in-depth information about a focus person's dream or vision for the future. This vision becomes the "North Star" that guides the future actions of the individual and their team. The focus person is encouraged to dream about his or her future without constraints or barriers. No limits are placed on the person's dream, with the facilitator ensuring that no one on the team questions how realistic the dream is. Usually, the focus person or a designated representative who knows the individual well is the only one allowed to speak during this initial step of articulating the dream. The PATH begins by looking into the future then proceeds by working backward from the near future to the present. The team determines an appropriate time line to work toward the personalized goals, usually between 1 and 2 years. These goals must meet the criteria of being both "positive" and "possible." The team is then asked to reflect on what is happening currently by providing

single words or short phrases that represent "now." Teams often find there are both negative and positive aspects to what is happening now, and there should be enough tension between the dream and the current situation to propel and motivate them to move forward together. Last, the facilitator assists the team in looking at whether other stakeholders should be at the table, what resources/actions will help the team become stronger, and setting goals to be met in the next few days, in a month, and in 6 months to 1 year. The more immediate goals are written as an action plan, detailing specific action steps to be taken, who is responsible for completing the actions, and due dates.

Brady

Not sure where to turn, Brady's father contacts a local advocacy agency. After hearing his concerns, the advocate suggests contacting an individual she knows who has experience with PCP. The PCP facilitator meets individually with Brady, Brady's family, and the school team to assess the situation and determine a course of action. Given the complexity of Brady's needs, family dynamics, and the tension that exists between the school personnel and family, she determines it might be best to use a PATH to assist the team in uniting and moving forward to address the situation. A copy of Brady's PATH can be found in Figure 4.1.

The MAPS process is shorter in length, taking approximately 1.5 to 2 hours to complete, and is usually chosen for less complex situations where the focus person or team is stuck and needs help moving forward—in other words, a situation exists that impedes the progress toward accomplishing the focus person's dream. The MAPS process begins by asking the focus person or his or her trusted representative to tell his or her story and dream (Falvey et al., 1997; O'Brien & Pearpoint, 2003; Vandercook, York, & Forest, 1989). The team is then facilitated through questions related to the individual's "nightmare" while reiterating who the focus person

Brady's dream

Take art classes

Get a dog

Be a mechanic

Participate in first communion

Go to the pool more often

Graduate and move to my own house

Have a sleepover Birthday party

Now	Enroll	Teamwork	First steps	1-month goals	Positive and possible (6-month goals)
• Good with his hands • Smart • Tension • Doesn't like school • Frustration • Behavior problems • Loves art • Having more problems during math and writing activities	• Art teacher • School-based therapist • Behavior consultant	• Work together • Better communication • Meet regularly	Determine who is collecting data	Functional assessment results reviewed by team and strategies developed	Behavior support plan in place and working
			Change school schedule so he can be in art every day	Identified a place to take art classes and potential funding	Attending art class outside of school
				Dad has identified new hands-on activities at home	Working with Dad on other hands-on activities (build a bird house, help fix things at home)
			Principal to make referral to school psychologist for an assessment	Learning assessment completed by school psychologist	Curriculum changed to include more hands-on activities
				Dad and stepmother discuss problems at church with behavior consultant	A plan in place at home and Brady is attending church activities more often

Figure 4.1. Sample Planning Alternative Tomorrows with Hope (PATH) for Brady.

79

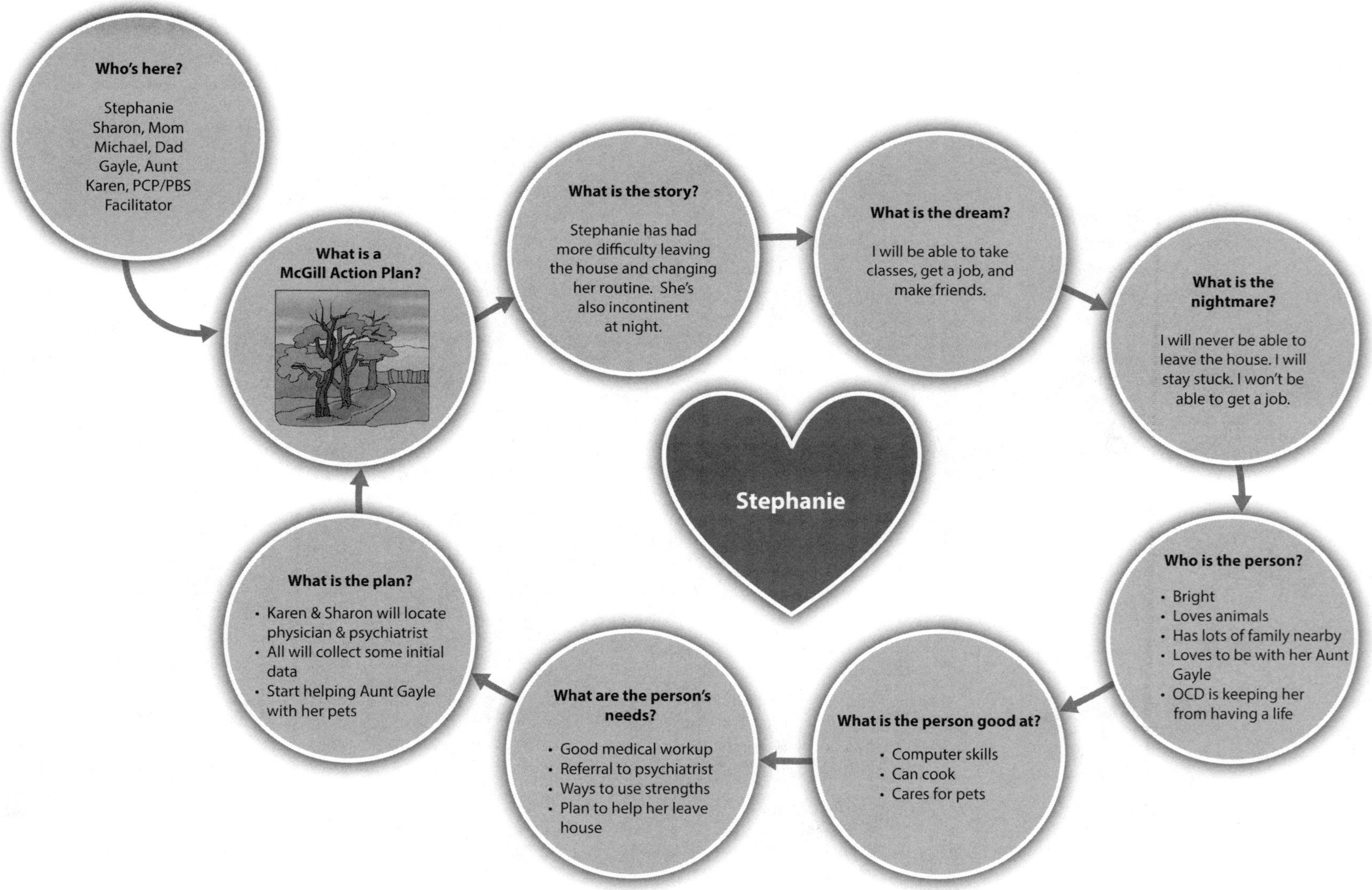

What is the nightmare?

I will never be able to leave the house. I will stay stuck. I won't be able to get a job.

Who is the person?

- Bright
- Loves animals
- Has lots of family nearby
- Loves to be with her Aunt Gayle
- OCD is keeping her from having a life

What is the dream?

I will be able to take classes, get a job, and make friends.

Stephanie

What is the person good at?

- Computer skills
- Can cook
- Cares for pets

What is the story?

Stephanie has had more difficulty leaving the house and changing her routine. She's also incontinent at night.

What are the person's needs?

- Good medical workup
- Referral to psychiatrist
- Ways to use strengths
- Plan to help her leave house

What is a McGill Action Plan?

What is the plan?

- Karen & Sharon will locate physician & psychiatrist
- All will collect some initial data
- Start helping Aunt Gayle with her pets

Who's here?

Stephanie
Sharon, Mom
Michael, Dad
Gayle, Aunt
Karen, PCP/PBS
Facilitator

Figure 4.2. Sample McGill Action Planning System (MAPS) for Stephanie.

is, his or her dreams, what he or she is good at, and what needs he or she has. In MAPS, the nightmare serves a similar function as reflecting on the "now" in the PATH. The team is forced to face what could or has happened and thus propelled to make changes in course to help the focus person avoid the "nightmare." Similar to the PATH, MAPS concludes with a specific action plan to assist the team in implementing the plan.

Stephanie

While Stephanie's situation is fairly complex, the current issues have evolved more recently, her family situation is stable, the PCP facilitator knows Stephanie and her family very well, and her family generally has a good relationship with service providers. The PCP facilitator decides the best PCP tool to use would be MAPS. MAPS will allow the team to focus on the present situation and move forward with an action plan. See Figure 4.2 for more information about Stephanie's MAPS.

....

A useful tool for gathering in-depth information about a focus person's or family's story is the personal profile (O'Brien, Mount, & O'Brien, 1990). The personal profile usually takes about 3 hours and is composed of several distinct pages or "frames" that detail specific aspects of a person's life. Some of the topics that may be addressed in compiling the personal profile and about which additional information may be gathered include the person's history, their choices, routines, fears and hopes, and the places they go. In some applications of the personal profile, teams expand their focus to gather additional information such as stressors and resources (Becker-Cottrill, McFarland, & Anderson, 2003). Many of the frames include color coding and/or graphics to indicate emotion attached to the topic. For example, in the history frame, neutral events are coded blue or black, stressful ones are coded red, and good times are coded green. Stressful events also may be noted by lightning bolts and good times by happy faces or other icons representing positive and

negative emotions. The personal profile does not lead directly to an action plan, although it may be combined with the development of a futures plan, noting the common themes across frames and developing goals or a vision for the future (Mount, 2000; Mount & Zwernick, 1988; O'Brien & Lovett, 1992).

Jayelyn

Jayelyn's early interventionist has previous training and experience using several PCP tools. Just after meeting Jayelyn and her family, she conducts a personal profile to better learn about the family's circumstances and assess their priorities for Jayelyn. (See Figure 4.3 for some of Jayelyn's personal profile.) Before meeting with Jayelyn's new preschool team, the early interventionist updates the personal profile and reviews the information with the family and their new interpreter to determine if there is information they would be willing to share with the new team members. She feels it will provide the future preschool staff with a richer understanding of the family in addition to traditional skills assessment information. The early interventionist, family, and interpreter share this information with the preschool staff as a part of their first meeting. Because they now have a better understanding of the family, the preschool staff leaves with a better appreciation and more respect for the family. At the end of the meeting, having learned more through the personal profile, the full team agrees that MAPS would be a useful additional tool in helping them plan steps for Jayelyn's impending transition.

....

While many individuals will be able to fully participate in the PCP process, some will have limitations that inhibit their ability to express their vision, strengths, and needs. In those situations, people close to the focus person such as family members and/or friends may take the role of spokesperson. The spokesperson does not replace the focus person but serves to facilitate the communication of his or her wishes. One difficulty faced by PCP facilitators in these situations is to ensure the PCP actually represents the desires of the focus person and not his or her spokesperson. For example, parents

History

Jayelyn born (2/12/2009)

Easy baby at first; content to be in crib or playpen

Had some feeding problems (reflux and didn't breastfeed well); started on formula

Held head up and sat early; loved toys but didn't enjoy playing patty-cake

Walking at age 1; had a fun birthday party

Worried at 18 months, as she isn't saying any words and isn't responding to her name; hearing test normal and doctor says not to worry

Moved to the city when Jayelyn was 2 years old; love the city but miss family and friends

Still not saying words; diagnosed as having autism at 2.5 years

Started early intervention services; trying to figure out best preschool program and services

Places

Home

Live in apartment downtown

Medical/other services

Dr. Smith, pediatrician

Dr. Kasey, gastroenterologist

Stacy Jones, speech therapist

Early intervention team

Walk or use city bus/subway

School/child care

Will attend preschool and child care

Has nanny right now

Community

Park

Fast food restaurants (only go through drive-through)

Choices

Child's

- What time we get up
- When we go to bed
- What she eats
- If we can go out
- Which restaurants we go to
- What she will wear
- If we have company over or not

Family's

- What we watch on television
- Where we live
- Where Jayelyn will go to school
- What we eat
- Where we work

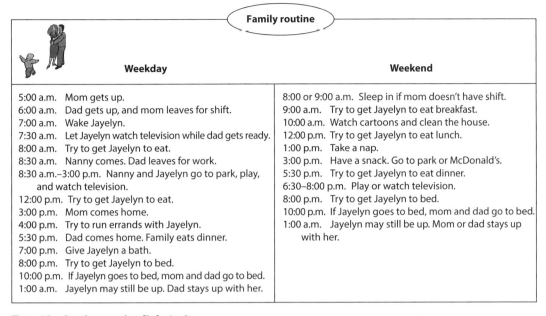

Figure 4.3. Sample personal profile for Jayelyn.

of a teenager with a severe disability who is nonverbal may indicate their child's dream is to continue to live at home with them and learn independent living skills such as cooking, cleaning, and laundry. However, the focus person's dream may be to live away from home with support and to employ someone to do household chores for him or her. In order to be sure this is the focus person's "dream," the facilitator will need to take time prior to beginning the PCP to get to know and interact with the focus person and his or her family or other spokesperson. The facilitator will also need to explain the process, fully making sure the spokespeople understand their role is to convey *what the focus person would want*, not *what they want for the focus person*.

MAINTAINING MOMENTUM AND ACCOUNTABILITY

Many times teams leave the PCP meeting energized, motivated, and feeling more positive about the focus person. However, if follow-up meetings are not scheduled and specific plans and time lines are not formalized, PCP action plans are less likely to be carried out. If teams

are not provided with some continued support by the facilitator (e.g., organize meetings, assist with problem solving, and ensure actions are being implemented), they may encounter barriers, be unable or unsure about problem-solving techniques, and may abandon the PCP plan, falling back to their previous methods for providing service delivery, declaring that "PCP doesn't work" (Holburn, 2002). Often, the systems that adopt PCP may themselves prove to be barriers to its implementation. PCP has been adopted systemwide by numerous state agencies with good intentions; however, while the language of PCP may be embedded in the system, PCP may not be implemented with fidelity (Holburn, 2002). Systems may not change the nature of their service structure and working policies to accommodate the PCP philosophy and principles; thus PCP becomes another form of paperwork with little meaning to focus people.

When adopting PCP, systems need to analyze their own structure and determine how PCP does or does not fit into current team practices and flexible support arrangements. Systems need to ensure that facilitators have appropriate knowledge, skills, resources, and a philosophical base to successfully implement PCP tools and assist teams in problem solving and continued action planning (Holburn, 2002). PCP should be implemented in a responsible and well-thought-out manner. The facilitator will not only need to understand how to effectively gather information using PCP tools but also need the skills to help teams make a commitment to continue meeting, implement action plans, evaluate where things stand with the plan, problem-solve, and make modifications to the course of the action plan as needed (see Figure 4.4).

THE RELATIONSHIP BETWEEN PERSON-CENTERED PLANNING AND THE BEHAVIOR SUPPORT PLAN

PCP informs and contributes to the BSP in several ways. PCP allows teams to focus on the broader context of a focus person's life, placing an emphasis on improving quality of life for the focus person and assisting the focus person and/or his or her family in pursuing a desired lifestyle. Such self-determined changes in quality of life may naturally lead to reduction of problem behavior (Beadle-Brown, Hutchinson, & Whelton, 2012; Carr et al., 2002; McClean & Grey, 2012). PCP assists teams in subscribing to the process, coming to consensus, and working together toward the same goals. Finally, PCP contributes to a better understanding of how a focus person's culture has an impact on the behavioral norms and expectations within their community, helping teams develop culturally responsive BSPs.

Quality-of-Life Outcomes

Traditionally, the evaluation of BSPs has focused on reducing problem behaviors, with less emphasis placed on broader changes within a person's life and the life of their family. Improvement in skill development (e.g., communication, social skills, self-help skills) and decreases in challenging behavior are the hallmarks of an effective BSP. Within the field of PBS, however, there also is an emphasis on measuring the impact of positive BSPs on quality of life (Carr et al., 2002; Kincaid, Knoster, Harrower, Shannon, & Bustamante, 2002; Smith-Bird & Turnbull, 2005). Measures of quality of life generally focus on several different dimensions, including emotional, social, personal, physical, and material satisfaction, as well as self-determination, inclusion, and rights (Kincaid et al., 2002).

The definition of quality of life is individualized. What one person views as important to their life will naturally be different from another person's views on quality of life. For example, one person may express a desire to have a large group of friends and be socially active, and another might express the desire to have a smaller group of friends and have opportunities for more time alone. Both may report being equally happy, despite differences in the size

Strategies to Assist Teams in Maintaining Momentum and Accountability
- Adopting a regular schedule for meetings and keeping to an agenda and time frame.
- Developing a "to do" list documenting individual team members who have volunteered to oversee specific actions and commit to a specific deadline.
- Asking team members to report on progress toward implementing specific actions during each team meeting.
- Providing assistance to team members if they have difficulty implementing specific actions.
- Using a variety of communication strategies between meetings (e.g., e-mail listserv, texts, private Facebook page, GoTo meetings, private Google page).
- Helping teams problem-solve barriers to implementation.
- Making meetings fun by bringing food or beverages.
- Celebrating and pointing out accomplishments of the team and consumer.

Figure 4.4. Strategies to assist teams in maintaining momentum and accountability.

of their social networks and how much time they spend with others or alone.

PCP tools gather information useful to assisting teams in personalizing behavior supports to fit lifestyle needs, person by person, without imposing external expectations or definitions of what a quality life should look like. PCP's focus on gathering information directly from the focus person and/or those most invested in them provides an opportunity for teams to use the focus person's input to develop responsive BSPs that assist the individual in developing necessary skills to attain a lifestyle suited to their own desires. In turn, the effectiveness of a BSP may be enhanced because the focus person's interests, strengths, and desired outcomes become the focus.

Team and Administrative Commitment

In a traditional expert approach to service delivery, the focus person and those closest to him or her (e.g., family, friends, coworkers, service providers, and educators) may not be included in the development of the BSP, yet they may be expected to fully implement the plan. While some may willingly implement plans developed by others, there may also be active or passive resistance to implementation if the plan does not take into account the context in which the focus person lives or the system under which service providers work. (See Delprato, 2002, for a discussion of "countercontrol.") Such resistance to implementing plans may include directly questioning the plan, outright refusal to implement the plan, complaints about the plan "not working," lackluster data collection, unreliable data, or implementing the plan inconsistently.

Part of the job of those facilitating the BSP is to actively recruit commitment, not only from those implementing the plan but also from system administrators, who will have access to resources that may assist the team in plan implementation. One way to generate commitment and avoid or temper the potential for others to undermine the BSP is to include the focus person and important stakeholders from the beginning.

PCP offers one method for allowing the focus person and stakeholders to contribute their expertise and express which strategies will best fit the context that they live and work in (Kincaid & Dunlap, 2003).

Cultural Diversity Issues

With the advent of modern technology, the world has truly become a "global" community. People are more mobile than their counterparts a generation ago, with the advent of the Internet, cell phones, television, high-speed rails, an interconnected highway system, and more efficient and available airplane services. Within the United States alone, the diversity of the population has changed drastically in the last 10 years. According to the 2010 U.S. Census, the Asian population, the fastest growing population in the United States, grew 43%, while those describing themselves as white alone grew the slowest (6%), with most of the growth in this population due to increases in the Hispanic population (U.S. Census Bureau, 2011). The makeup of individual households has changed drastically as well. Nearly half (40%) of all households were reported as headed by unmarried couples, with a 52% increase in same-sex couples and a 40% increase in opposite-sex couples. There was also a 31% increase in the number of single men as head of the household (U.S. Census Bureau, 2012).

Clearly, it is imperative for individuals facilitating the PCP and PBS processes to be sensitive to a variety of cultural impacts that influence how individuals and families view child rearing, disabilities, service providers, education, religion, and so forth (Chen, Downing, & Peckham-Hardin, 2002; Wang, McCart, & Turnbull, 2007). In addition, facilitators come to the table with their own set of cultural influences and norms, which have the potential to bias their view of others' perspectives. To be sensitive to cultural differences, facilitators need to first recognize and understand the influences of their own culture and then be open to the views and traditions of others. Cultural competence requires being able to individualize supports, identify the contextual variables influencing problems, and listen and communicate effectively (Green, Watkins, McNutt, & Lopez, 1998).

Implemented well, PCP can address these requirements of culturally competent practice. Within PCP, the focus people and those closest to him or her provide the greater part of the information guiding the PCP process. The facilitator's role is to listen and assist the team in communicating successfully. Contextual variables, such as living situation, job constraints, service limitations, and relationships with others, are identified. Variables that are supportive are strengthened, and barriers are addressed. Taking into account the focus person's wishes and needs and the context of his or her life, the facilitator helps the team develop a BSP that is unique and individualized to the focus person.

Jayelyn

Jayelyn's parents come from a family that values education. Jayelyn's father and both of her grandfathers are highly educated. Jayelyn's mother is interested in pursuing her education further, perhaps eventually entering a nursing school. Jayelyn's father is the CEO of a large business. He takes advantage of educational opportunities in his field and encourages his employees to do the same. Since her birth, both parents have had high expectations for Jayelyn's education, which continue despite her diagnosis. Jayelyn's mother, with the help of her interpreter, also has taken it upon herself to read as much as she can about autism and treatment. She plans to become as much of an expert on issues Jayelyn might face as she can. Given this information, Jayelyn's team will need to be sensitive about how they provide and receive information, and they will need to respect the family's desire to be highly involved in Jayelyn's education. Including Jayelyn's family in all aspects of BSP development will take into account contextual factors in addition to helping the family feel competent to implement plans.

Brady

Brady's parents are very interested in Brady acquiring skills to obtain a job in the future and live independently. Brady's father comes from a long line of blue-collar workers. He has worked most of his life at a local aluminum factory. He enjoys the camaraderie with fellow workers and hopes Brady will find an interest in something similar. Brady and his father enjoy working on old cars at home, and Brady's father is proud that his son has such a knack for mechanics. Both of Brady's parents and extended family attend church regularly. Their hope is that Brady's behavior will improve enough for him to attend church and participate in the various church rites as he grows older. Brady's team will need to be sensitive to the family's religious beliefs, assist the family in finding strategies to help Brady participate more in the church community, and continue to support Brady in developing his strength in manual/hands-on activities.

Stephanie

For Stephanie's family, being a part of their extended family and local community is very important. While increasingly open to other service providers, Stephanie and her family would rather rely on other family members for support. They have expressed that they are uncomfortable having "strangers" in their home. The family enjoys many outdoor activities, including camping, fishing, four-wheeling, and hunting. Stephanie used to enjoy these activities with her family but due to increasing social isolation has not done so for several years. Stephanie's PCP and PBS team will need to help the family educate other family members about Stephanie's situation, use extended family as support, and assist Stephanie and her family in developing strategies to help them enjoy outdoor and family activities again.

CONCLUSION

Jayelyn, Brady, and Stephanie all come from unique and varied situations. Jayelyn is young, her parents value education, and they have access to many resources in their urban community. However, they lack social support from friends and family, may face language barriers, and have different cultural values regarding child rearing than others in their community. Brady has many strengths, which may initially be disregarded or unrecognized by his school team because of his behavior challenges. While struggling with several issues, Brady's family, given the right support, has the potential to be able to advocate for a plan that incorporates Brady's strengths and interests. Unlike Jayelyn and Brady, Stephanie lives in a rural community with few formal services and resources but has a strong, close-knit extended family nearby. Stephanie and her family have very different interests from the other individuals. Certainly, a technically sound plan could be developed for each of the three focus people to address his or her challenging behavior, but implementation of the plan may be compromised and less effective if information about the focus person and his or her life circumstances is not taken into account. PCP does not supplant the need for a functional assessment and a technically sound plan grounded in evidence-based practices. Rather, PCP enhances the BSP by providing a philosophy and tools to assist those developing and implementing BSPs in addressing the needs, strengths, resources, and unique lives of those they serve.

REFERENCES

Adams, N., & Grieder, D.M. (2005). *Treatment planning for person-centered care: The road to mental health and addiction recovery.* Burlington, MA: Elsevier Academic Press.

Albin, R.M., Lucyshyn, J.M., Horner, R.H., & Flannery, K.B. (1996). Contextual fit for behavioral support plans: A model for "goodness of fit." In L.K. Koegel, R.L. Koegel, & G. Dunlap (Eds.), *Positive behavioral support: Including people with difficult behavior in the community* (pp. 81–98). Baltimore, MD: Paul H. Brookes Publishing Co.

Beadle-Brown, J., Hutchinson, A., & Whelton, B. (2012). Person-centered active support—increasing choice, promoting independence, and reducing challenging behavior. *Journal of Applied Research in Intellectual Disabilities, 25*(4), 291–307.

Becker-Cottrill, B., McFarland, J., & Anderson, V. (2003). A model of positive behavioral support for individuals with autism and their families: The family focus process. *Focus on Autism and Other Developmental Disabilities, 18,* 110–120.

Blue-Banning, M.J., Summers, J.A., Frankland, H.C., Nelson, L.L., & Beegle, G. (2004). Dimensions of family and professional partnerships: Constructive guidelines for collaboration. *Exceptional Children, 70,* 167–184.

Blue-Banning, M.J., Turnbull, A.P., & Pereira, L. (2000). Group action planning as a support strategy for Hispanic families: Parent and professional perspectives. *Mental Retardation, 38,* 262–275.

Briggs, L. (2004). Shifting the focus of advance care planning: Using an in-depth interview to build and strengthen relationships. *Journal of Palliative Medicine, 7,* 341–349.

Carr, E.G., Dunlap, G., Horner, R.H., Koegel, R.L., Turnbull, A., Sailor, W., . . . Fox, L. (2002). Positive behavior support: Evolution of an applied science. *Journal of Positive Behavior Interventions, 4*(1), 4–16.

Chen, D., Downing, J.E., & Peckham-Hardin, K.D. (2002). Working with families of diverse cultural and linguistic backgrounds: Considerations for culturally responsive positive behavior support. In J.M. Lucyshyn, G. Dunlap, & R.W. Albin (Eds.), *Family and positive behavioral support: Addressing problem behavior in family contexts* (pp. 133–152). Baltimore, MD: Paul H. Brookes Publishing Co.

Clark, H.B., & Hieneman, M. (1999). Comparing the wraparound process to positive behavioral support: What can we learn? *Journal of Positive Behavior Interventions, 1*(3), 183–186.

Curtis, L.C., Wells, S.M., Penney, D.J., Ghose, S.S., Mistler, L.A., Mahone, I.H., . . . Lesko, S. (2010). Pushing the envelope: Shared decision making in mental health. *Psychiatric Rehabilitation Journal, 34* (1), 14–22.

Delprato, D.J. (2002). Countercontrol in behavior analysis. *Behavior Analyst, 25*(2), 191–200.

Falvey, M.A., Forest, M., Pearpoint, J., & Rosenberg, R. (1997). *All my life's a circle. Using the tools: Circles, MAP's and PATH.* Toronto, ON: Inclusion Press.

Freeman, R., Smith, C., Zarcone, J., Kimbrough, P., Tieghi-Benet, M., Wickham, D., . . . Hine, K. (2005). Building a statewide plan for embedding positive behavior support in human service organizations. *Journal of Positive Behavior Interventions, 7*(2), 109–119.

Green, R.R., & Barnes, G. (1998). The ecological perspective, diversity, and culturally competent social work practice. In R.R. Greene & M. Watkins (Eds.), *Service diverse constituencies: Applying the ecological perspective* (pp. 63–96). New York, NY: Aldine De Gruyer.

Green, R.R., Watkins, M., McNutt, J., & Lopez, L. (1998). Diversity defined. In R.R. Greene & M. Watkins (Eds.), *Service diverse constituencies: Applying the ecological perspective* (pp. 63–96). New York, NY: Aldine De Gruyer.

Holburn, S. (2002). How science can evaluate and enhance person-centered planning. *Research and Practice for Persons with Severe Disabilities, 27,* 250–260.

Holburn, S., Gordon, A., & Vietze, P.M. (2007). *Person-centered planning made easy: The PICTURE method.* Baltimore, MD: Paul H. Brookes Publishing Co.

Horner, R.L., Dunlap, G., Koegel, R.L., Carr, E.G., Sailor, W., Anderson, J., . . . O'Neill, R.E. (1990).

Toward a technology of "nonaversive" behavioral support. *Journal of The Association for People with Severe Handicaps, 15*(3), 125–132.

Kincaid, D. (1995). Person-centered planning. In L.K. Koegel, R.L. Koegel, & G. Dunlap (Eds.), *Positive behavioral support: Including people with difficult behaviors in the community* (pp. 439–465). Baltimore, MD: Paul H. Brookes Publishing Co.

Kincaid, D., & Dunlap, G. (2003). Laying the foundation for positive behavior support through person-centered planning. *Positive Behavioral Interventions and Support Newsletter, 2*(1). Retrieved June 18, 2012, from http://www.pbis.org/pbis_newsletter/volume_2/issue1.aspx

Kincaid, D., Knoster, T., Harrower, J.K., Shannon, P., & Bustamante, S. (2002). Measuring the impact of positive behavior support. *Journal of Positive Behavior Interventions, 4*(2), 109–117.

McClean, B., & Grey, I. (2012). A component analysis of positive behavior support plans. *Journal of Intellectual and Developmental Disability, 37*(3), 221–231.

Meaden, H., Shelden, D.L., Appel, K., & DeGrazia, R.L. (2010). Developing a long-term vision: A road map for students' futures. *Teaching Exceptional Children, 43*(2), 8–15.

Mount, B. (2000). *Person-centered planning.* New York, NY: Graphic Futures.

Mount, B., & Zwernick, K. (1988). *It's never too early, it's never too late: An overview on personal futures planning.* St. Paul, MN: Governor's Council on Developmental Disabilities.

O'Brien, C., & O'Brien, J. (2002). The origins of person-centered planning. In S. Holburn & P.M. Vietze (Eds.), *Person-centered planning: Research, practice and future directions* (pp. 3–27). Baltimore, MD: Paul H. Brookes Publishing Co.

O'Brien, J. (1987). A guide to life-style planning: Using the activities catalogue to integrate services and natural support systems. In G.T. Bellamy & B.A. Wilcox (Eds.), *Comprehensive guide to the activities catalogue: An alternative curriculum for youth and adults with severe disabilities* (pp. 175–189). Baltimore, MD: Paul H. Brookes Publishing Co.

O'Brien, J., & Lovett, H. (1992). *Finding a way toward everyday lives: The contribution of Person-Centered Planning.* Harrisburg, PA: Pennsylvania Office of Mental Retardation.

O'Brien, J., Mount, B., & O'Brien, C. (1990). *The personal profile.* Lithonia, GA: Responsive Systems Associates.

O'Brien, J., & Pearpoint, J. (2003). *Person-centered planning with MAPS and PATH: A workbook for facilitators.* Toronto, ON: Inclusion Press.

Pearpoint, J., O'Brien, J., & Forest, M. (1993). *Planning alternative tomorrows with hope: A workbook for planning possible and positive futures.* Toronto, ON: Inclusion Press.

Reid, D.H., Rotholz, D.A., Parsons, M.B., Morris, L., Braswell, B.A., Green, C.W., & Schell, R.M. (2003). Training human service supervisors in aspects of PBS: Evaluation of a statewide, performance-based program. *Journal of Positive Behavior Interventions, 5*(1), 35–46.

Ryan, J., & Carey, E. (2009). Developing person-centered planning in dementia care. *Learning Disability Practice, 12*(5), 24–28.

Smith-Bird, E., & Turnbull, A.P. (2005). Linking positive behavior support to family quality-of-life outcomes. *Journal of Positive Behavior Interventions, 7*(3), 174–180.

Smull, M. (1997). *A blueprint for essential lifestyle planning.* Napa, CA: Allen, Shea & Associates.

Thompson, J., & Cobb, J. (2004). Person-centered health action planning. *Learning Disability Practice, 7*(5), 12–15.

U.S. Census Bureau. (2011). *Overview of race and Hispanic origin: 2010 (C2010BR-02).* Washington, DC: Government Printing Office. Retrieved August 22, 2012, from http://www.census.gov/prod/cen2010/briefs/c2010br-02.pdf

U.S. Census Bureau. (2012). *Households and families: 2010 (C2010BR-14).* Washington, DC: Government Printing Office. Retrieved August 22, 2012, from http://www.census.gov/prod/cen2010/briefs/c2010br-14.pdf

Vandercook, T., York, J., & Forest, M. (1989). The McGill Action Planning System (MAPS): A strategy for building the vision. *Journal of The Association for Persons with Severe Handicaps, 14,* 205–215.

Wang, M., McCart, A., & Turnbull, A.P. (2007). Implementing positive behavior support with Chinese American families: Enhancing cultural competence. *Journal of Positive Behavior Interventions, 9*(1), 38–51.

Supporting Individuals with Challenging Behavior Through Systemic Change

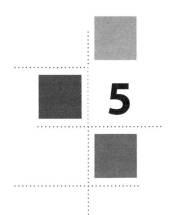

5

Randall L. De Pry, Kavita V. Kamat, and Richard Stock

Increasing our understanding of human behavior is central to understanding how positive behavior support (PBS) practitioners provide comprehensive behavior support for individuals within and across systems. PBS practitioners rely on an extensive literature that is founded on three broad categories of understanding: applied behavior analysis, normalization and inclusion, and person-centered values (Carr et al., 2002). Each of these categories informs our understanding of human behavior across a wide variety of contexts and systems and has come to be known as PBS.

Central to understanding systemic change is defining how and why we respond in various settings or contexts. Our responses involve a complex interplay among the environment, the individual, and the consequences that maintain, increase, or decrease future responding within identified settings, contexts, or systems (Baer & Pinkston, 1997; Cooper, Heron, & Heward, 2007).

Using a wide variety of assessment methods, PBS practitioners gather information to understand the function(s) or purpose that a problem behavior serves for an individual within identified settings or as part of a typical routine. Following data collection, information that was gathered is reviewed by critical stakeholders as a means for designing a plan of support that seeks to *prevent* future problem behavior from occurring; *teach* new responses that are more efficient, effective, and relevant for the person of concern than engaging in the identified problem behavior(s) (O'Neill et al., 1997); and provide ongoing support and *reinforcement* for the use of these new strategies in a manner that increases the likelihood that these strategies will be implemented in the future (Dunlap et al., 2010).

The Association for Positive Behavior Support's (APBS; 2007) Standards of Practice: Individual Level (SOP-I) provide research-based guidelines for the development of multielement plans of behavior support. The standards emphasize collaboration, assessment, self-determination, contextual fit, and evaluation related to the development and implementation of plans of support. Each of these is briefly discussed in the following section.

As an applied science, PBS actively promotes collaboration over consultation. In other words, expertise extends to all critical stakeholders, and plans of support are developed in collaboration with the person of concern and his or her team, family, and friends. Plans are predicated on the collection of data from multiple sources, including person-centered and functional behavioral assessments (FBAs; Carr et al., 2002). Multiple methods are used to understand the problem behavior across contexts or systems to provide a clearer picture of what is actually occurring and to serve as a method of triangulating data to better inform decision making. Multielement plans of support are designed to affirm the individual's dreams, preferences, and choices as a means to a higher quality of life (Martin, Marshall, & De Pry, 2008; Schalock & Alonso, 2002). Contextual fit, which is defined as "the congruence or compatibility that exists between specific features and components of a behavioral support plan and a variety of relevant variables relating to individuals and environments" (Albin, Lucyshyn, Horner, & Flannery, 1996, p. 82), is a guiding principle for PBS practitioners. Contextual fit is achieved when critical stakeholders agree on the need, vision, process, and resources that are necessary to implement PBS plans with fidelity. Finally, multielement plans of support include methods for evaluating and adjusting implementation over time and across settings.

SYSTEMS AND NATURAL COMMUNITIES OF SUPPORT

The purpose of this chapter is to discuss systemic change from the perspective of multicomponent behavior support planning and implementation. Case studies illustrate key points and provide practical examples of systemic change in a workplace system, family system, and school-based system. Systems, for purposes of this chapter, are defined as *the environmental contexts that we encounter in our daily lives.* Examples can include home, school, community, work, and social systems. Systems have specific people, practices, and policies that are unique to that context (Scott, 2007). For example, within a workplace system, colleagues work together to achieve a common goal. The workplace has specific practices that are established through education, training, and professional development. Implementation of these practices is guided by defined procedures and policies. The workplace system, in other words, has specific people who are engaged in specific practices that lead to valued outcomes. Natural communities of support, on the other hand, are *systems that are preferred by the individual and result in an increased quality of life.* Natural communities of support are identified by the person of concern (e.g., person-centered planning, or PCP) and include relevant stakeholders, resources, and other supports that are necessary to fully and successfully implement the behavior support plan (BSP). The following example by Schall (2010) illustrates the development and implementation of a plan of support for an individual within a defined workplace system. The example includes critical stakeholders that are working together to support a young man who demonstrated challenging behavior while at work.

Systemic Change in the Workplace

Schall (2010) described a young man named "DJ" in his mid-20s with autism. He was employed at a sandwich shop and was successful in most aspects of his job, including food preparation and cleanup tasks. However, his problem behavior became a barrier to working independently since he made loud noises and pushed others out of his way when he was upset. To understand and ultimately address this issue, an FBA was conducted that included interviews and direct observation of DJ in his work setting. According to Schall, "After observation and data collection, the team met to analyze the data and proposed the hypothesis that DJ's noises and pushing others was an attempt to avoid correction. They observed that DJ became most noisy and pushed others away when he made a mistake and required verbal correction and redirection" (p. 111). The team focused on the development of antecedent strategies, which were intended to prevent the behavior from occurring; teaching DJ a new skill that replaced the old responses (yelling and pushing); and reinforcing the new skill when DJ used it successfully. The team identified two replacement responses for DJ to learn: One focused on teaching DJ to take a break instead of making noises or pushing (i.e., functionally equivalent replacement response), and the second was focused on problem-solving skills that DJ could learn that helped him accept work-related corrections. The author noted that DJ had considerable support at work, including a job coach and an employer who were able to work with DJ around communication needs, routines, work tasks, and implementation of the behavior intervention plan. The author used a single-case research design where tallies for targeted behaviors were collected for a month by the job coach then graphed as a single data point. The baseline phase included cumulative data per month for a total of 2 months (2 data points), and the intervention phase had 5 months of data (5 data points). Data from this study provide support for the methods used. For example, pushing decreased to "0" and yelling decreased from a high of "30" incidents during the baseline phase to a low of "4" incidents for the last month of the intervention. The authors noted that DJ was able to become more independent and improve the quality of his work life by learning his new skills and receiving support from his colleagues and coach within his workplace system.

An analysis of Schall (2010) suggests that collaboration, assessment, self-determination, contextual fit, and evaluation were all evident in the planning and implementation of the BSP for DJ. His plan took into account his 1) personal preferences, 2) workplace setting considerations, 3) implementation of strategies by critical stakeholders that prevented the problem behavior from recurring, 4) teaching and learning new skills and strategies that replaced the problem behavior, and 5) reinforcement of plan components that supported DJ's work goals. This example illustrates that DJ was not fully independent at his workplace prior to plan implementation due to his yelling and pushing following corrections related to his work performance. In fact, his ability to be fully included and maintain employment may have been in jeopardy if these issues were not resolved at the individual and systems level. The multielement plan that was designed and implemented first sought to improve the quality of DJ's work life (Carr, 2007) and only secondarily focused on the reduction of the problem behavior (Carr et al., 2002) within this workplace system.

DEFINING SYSTEMIC CHANGE

Our tendency to want to "fix problem behavior" can result in a misplaced focus on behavior reduction as our primary intervention method. Unfortunately, the daily news is replete with examples of how frequently aversive strategies are used in our society and the negative and dehumanizing effects they can have on the person of concern, their families, and friends. This includes testimonies about the use of seclusion and restraint for people with disabilities in school-based settings (Government Accountability Office [GAO], 2009). Carr et al. suggest an alternative that serves as one of the guiding principles of PBS:

> In providing support, we should focus our efforts on fixing problem contexts, not problem behavior. Behavior change is not simply the result of applying specific techniques to specific challenges. The best technology will fail if it is applied in an uncooperative or disorganized context. This principle has made efforts at systems

Table 5.1. Definitions

Systems	The environmental contexts that we encounter in our daily lives.
Natural communities of support	Systems that are preferred by the individual and result in an increased quality of life.
Systemic change	The adoption and sustained use of evidence-based practices by relevant stakeholders in natural communities of support.

change one of the defining features of PBS. (2002, pp. 8–9)

Therefore, systemic change is defined as *the adoption and sustained use of evidence-based practices by relevant stakeholders in natural communities of support* (see Table 5.1). This definition is built on our understanding of systems and natural communities of support discussed previously.

The following scenario provides a tangible example of definition components and illustrates positive outcomes that resulted from the development and implementation of a family-centered multielement BSP. Pay close attention to the family system (a natural community of support), relevant stakeholders (the focus individual, parents, siblings, interventionist, school personnel), and the adoption and sustained use of behavior support strategies that were incorporated into the individual's multielement BSP. This example shows that by focusing on the family system, as opposed to "fixing the individual," positive changes were accrued within the family system, including dramatic improvements in the individual's behavior.

Systemic Change in a Home

Zane, who was 10 years old at the time of this intervention, lived with his parents and two younger siblings, ages 4 and 7. He was diagnosed as having autism and a developmental coordination disorder. His mother was the primary caregiver in the family, as the father worked long hours and was often not home. Zane attended a public elementary school and received support from a full-time special education assistant (SEA). Zane was referred

for behavior consultation services due to significant challenging behavior directed toward his parents and siblings. These behaviors included 1) use of inappropriate language such as calling a family member stupid, telling them to shut up, or swearing at a family member; 2) engaging in inappropriate gestures such as pointing to his or other's private parts; and 3) leaving his chair during meals at home. Over the past year, these behaviors had increased at home and were a significant source of stress for Zane's parents. In addition, his younger brothers had begun to imitate Zane's problem behaviors during their interactions with each other. Given these problems, the parents requested referral for behavior consultation services offered by a nonprofit agency. An interventionist from the agency was assigned to the family and initiated a process of family-centered PBS. The steps in the process included a comprehensive ecological assessment and FBA, the collaborative development of a PBS plan in the home, and ongoing evaluation of outcomes. Two assessments guided the development of the PBS for Zane and his family: the family ecology assessment (Albin et al., 1996) and FBA (O'Neill et al., 1997), which are described in the following sections.

Family Ecology Assessment

During this assessment, the interventionist gathered information relevant to the design of a contextually appropriate BSP. First, semistructured questions were posed in an informal, conversational style to assess broad aspects of the family's ecology, including Zane's strengths and positive contributions to the family, family strengths and resources, and family stressors (Albin et al., 1996). Zane's parents spoke passionately about his strengths. He was very talented in music, enjoyed playing the drums, was an avid reader of science and other fact-based books, and enjoyed Legos and robotics. He also was well informed about marine life and had expressed an interest in becoming a marine biologist. He often checked out books from the library and shared interesting facts with his parents. His younger brothers looked up to him and sought his attention. Zane also had a good sense of humor and enjoyed telling jokes and making family members laugh. Zane's parents were highly motivated to support him. His mother was very knowledgeable about autism and an effective advocate for her son. However, when faced with stressors, Zane's parents were very troubled by his problem behavior and felt helpless in regard to supporting him. In addition, their second son was recently referred for autism assessment due to social problem behaviors at school. This was a new cause for worry and concern for the family.

The interventionist and family completed a focused informal assessment of family activities or routines in the home and community to identify priority routines for intervention. Zane's parents informed the interventionist that he engaged in two to three community-based activities, all of which reflected his interests. The rest of his nonschool hours were spent at home with his mother and siblings. Zane's mother was very busy in the early morning, afternoon, and evening, managing three boys in addition to cooking and other household chores. On most days, his father joined the family later in the evening, close to dinnertime. Zane's parents identified four problematic routines that they wanted to improve: 1) breakfast time routines, 2) transitions from car to school and school to car, 3) free time with siblings in the afternoon, and 4) homework routines. Both parents chose the breakfast routine as their first priority. Zane's parents were then asked to describe their vision of a successful breakfast routine. They envisioned a routine that began at about 7:45 a.m. and lasted 25–30 minutes: enough time for the boys to eat and get to school on time. Due to the father's work hours, he would not be present. Breakfast would consist of cereal, sometimes eggs, and juice or milk. The routine would be calm and not chaotic—one in which the boys stayed seated while eating, took turns talking and listening to each other, and used polite language with each other and with their mother. The routine also would help Zane get off to a good start for his day at school.

Functional Assessment

A functional assessment interview (FAI; O'Neill et al., 1997) was completed with both parents and a preliminary hypothesis about the function of Zane's problem behaviors was developed with the family. Functional assessment observations (FAO) were conducted to confirm the hypothesis by observing a video of the breakfast routine that Zane's mother had created (O'Neill et al., 1997). Functional assessment results indicated that Zane's problem behaviors were maintained by family member attention. The interventionist and mother collaboratively developed a summary hypothesis statement about Zane's problem behaviors during the breakfast routine, they wrote:

> At breakfast time when mom is busy getting items to the table and is focused on his younger siblings, Zane engages in inappropriate language and gestures to get attention from his mother and siblings. These behaviors are more likely when he has had a poor night's sleep and when his younger brother whines at the table.

Completing the family ecology and functional assessment together in a collaborative manner proved to be an important step for Zane's mother. It brought her to the realization that in order to change Zane's behavior, she would have to make changes in the way she set up the breakfast routine and how she responded to Zane and his brothers during breakfast. Changes in breakfast routines are a practical example of systemic change within this family system.

Based on the results of the comprehensive assessment, the interventionist and family worked together to develop a technically sound and contextually appropriate multicomponent PBS plan for the breakfast routine (see Figures 5.1 and 5.2). Strategies in the plan were logically linked to each feature of the problem identified in the competing behavior pathway diagram (O'Neill et al., 1997) and were based on the principles of PBS. Setting event support strategies included 1) setting up a predictable bedtime routine to ensure sufficient sleep and 2) Zane's mother deciding to use a communication book to inform Zane's teacher about his progress in the morning routine. Antecedent strategies included 1) using a visual sequence that predicted the steps in the routine and a reward he would receive for successfully completing the routine, 2) providing Zane with a choice of breakfast items, and 3) encouraging him to

share a joke or fact with mother and brothers as a positive and fun way to access attention. Consequence strategies included 1) providing a high-level praise and access to a preferred item when Zane engaged in desired behavior at the table (i.e., sitting at the table, eating his breakfast, taking turns, and using polite language), 2) providing him with immediate attention when he requested it appropriately, and 3) actively ignoring (i.e., extinction) and/or redirecting minor problem behavior.

During the plan design process, Zane's mother and the interventionist also worked together to ensure that the BSP was a good contextual fit with the ecology of the breakfast routine. An important contextual fit consideration, particularly because Zane's mother had to manage the routine by herself, was ensuring that the plan supported all three boys at the breakfast table. Zane's mother emphasized the need for strategies that taught and encouraged the three boys to engage in appropriate behavior. She also wanted the plan to be designed in a way

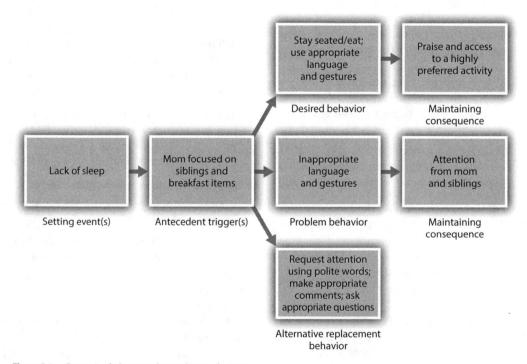

Figure 5.1. Competing behavior pathways diagram for Zane.

Setting event strategies	Preventive strategies	Teaching strategies	Consequence strategies
Set up a regular bedtime routine. Have a home–school communication book to inform teachers of Zane's sleep and morning routines.	Inform Zane of behavior expectations and the positive contingency. Offer choices of breakfast, place to sit, and juice. Ask him to share a fun fact of the day with his brothers.	Teach Zane to use the behavior expectation card to self-manage his behavior at the table. Teach him to use polite words to request attention from mom and brothers.	Praise Zane and provide him a preferred item/activity when he uses appropriate language and gestures at the table. Give attention when he asks for it using polite words. Ignore inappropriate language and gestures.

Figure 5.2. Positive behavior support (PBS) plan for Zane's morning routine.

that was appealing to the boys. Given this, the plan was augmented with additional strategies and supports. These included 1) reviewing the plan with the boys prior to implementation, 2) identifying and using rewards that all three boys found reinforcing (i.e., a surprise bag with a variety of small toys and treats), 3) modeling appropriate behavior by sitting and eating breakfast with the boys, 4) the boys using personalized self-monitoring cards that showed the steps and expectations of the routine, and 5) using an interdependent group contingency (Cooper et al., 2007) presented in an appealing game format. In addition, Zane helped to create a set of "bonus" cards that represented fun activities that the family could do together if the child whose turn it was to select a bonus card had behaved well during the routine. The opportunity to contribute to the plan's development appeared to help Zane buy into the plan and accept his mother's use of plan strategies (Martin, Marshall, & De Pry, 2008).

Implementation support included the provision of an implementation checklist that the mother used to self-monitor her use of plan strategies, a review of plan procedures, role play of strategies and supports, problem-solving meetings, and video-based feedback. Prior to initiating the plan in the breakfast routine, Zane's mother decided to first implement the plan in a simpler routine—a brief afterschool snack time. Doing so provided Zane's mother with an opportunity to practice the use of plan strategies

without the added stress of getting the children ready for school and also allowed the children to come into contact with the positive contingency and reinforcement. The mother quickly mastered implementation of the plan in the snack routine, and all three boys' behavior improved markedly. As a result, they became excited about receiving positive reinforcement at breakfast time. Implementation support to the family occurred over a period of 3 months. During the first 3 weeks, Zane's mother recorded the routine one to two times per week, and these data were used to evaluate initial progress.

Video observations taken during the first 3 weeks of implementation support showed an immediate decrease in problem behavior to near zero levels for Zane and his two brothers. Following five consecutive days of zero levels of problem behavior, the delivery of tangible reinforcement (i.e., small toys and treats) was faded to an intermittent schedule (Cooper et al., 2007). By the fourth week of intervention, the delivery of tangible reinforcement was completely faded except for the bonus activity (i.e., family activity), which the family decided to continue. During the subsequent months, the family reported that improvements in Zane and his brothers' behavior maintained and that it was a pleasure to sit together with the boys at the breakfast table. In addition, Zane's father reported collateral effects during dinnertime. During dinner, Zane waited for his turn to talk and used appropriate language during interactions with his parents and siblings. Similar effects were observed in his younger brothers as well. In follow-up conversations with the interventionist, the parents expressed a strong sense of pride in their achievement.

In summary, focusing on the family system placed Zane's parents in the role of collaborative partners during each step of the assessment and intervention process, with the interventionist remaining responsive to the goals, values, preferences, and input of family members. Doing so allowed Zane's mother to quickly take ownership of the plan and implement plan strategies with growing confidence and skill. Systemic change within the home environment was evident given the adoption and sustained use of evidence-based strategies by relevant stakeholders (e.g., members of the Zane's family), including modifications of routines and practices within their family system (e.g., a natural community of support for Zane and his family). Ensuring that the plan worked for all three boys also helped gain their "buy-in" such that they responded with not only cooperation but also enthusiasm. By collaborating with Zane's family to develop a function-based BSP that was a good contextual fit within the family system, the family was able to achieve outcomes that were meaningful, durable, and sustainable.

TOWARD A FRAMEWORK OF SYSTEMIC CHANGE

Fixsen, Blase, Horner, and Sugai (2009) delineate stages of program implementation that provide a framework for understanding change within systems. This framework includes the following stages: exploration, installation, initial implementation, full implementation, innovation, and sustainability. The authors note that, in some systems (e.g., schools), a team may move in or out of a particular stage depending on their need at any given time. It is notable that individual learning follows a similar structure (Wolery, Bailey, & Sugai, 1988) where

a learner (system) moves from initial acquisition of content to fluent responding that is maintained and demonstrated across settings (sustainability). Given that systems represent groups of individuals learning together and working toward valued outcomes, considering systemic change as analogous to learning theory may be useful as you consider the following content. Each stage will be described and briefly discussed, followed by a school-based example that illustrates a successful PBS implementation over an extended period of time.

Exploration

The exploration stage is where teams establish a need and readiness to provide behavior support. The word *readiness* suggests interest, preparation, or capacity. Readiness can be established in a variety of ways and includes a focus on collaboration, teaming, and delineation of need (see APBS, 2007, Section 11). For example, relevant stakeholders and other interested people are identified and agree to meet. Stakeholders meet in support of the person of concern and establish that a need exists for comprehensive PBS. The need may be documented by data that demonstrate chronic or persistent problem behavior across settings and how it is diminishing the quality of life for the person of concern, family, and friends. A vision for support is typically articulated during this stage.

Installation

The installation stage focuses on preparation and resource attainment. Building on our example, once the vision for support has been established by the team, additional work is still needed. For example, the vision for support might serve as the framework for agreements about processes, team roles, and other systems-level considerations that are necessary to support the person of concern. During the installation stage, discussions about resources (e.g., time, personnel, training, and system considerations) are reviewed and established prior to implementation.

Initial to Full Implementation

For our purposes, these stages are combined to show that a continuum exists from initial implementation to full implementation. Fixsen et al. (2009) suggest that this continuum can follow a pattern of first attempts at implementation, with some initial awkwardness, to skillful implementation that is well integrated into the system. Nersesian, Todd, Lehmann, and Watson (2000) illustrate this continuum in their description of a district implementation of schoolwide positive behavior interventions and supports over a period of 4 years. Initially, five school-based teams began to implement behavior support during the first year. After reviewing outcome data, district-level implementation extended to other schools in subsequent years. Nersesian et al. write, "A satisfying result of the process has been the durability of change. Schools require 2 to 3 years of district-level support to establish schoolwide discipline systems" (p. 245). The 2 to 3 years highlighted here demonstrate how schools moved along the continuum from initial to full implementation with systems-level support at the school and district levels. The authors go on to substantiate this continuum by showing growth over time as measured by the School-Wide Evaluation Tool (Sugai, Lewis-Palmer, Todd, & Horner, 2005).

Innovation

The innovation stage is represented by data-based changes to implementation processes and practices. During full implementation, behavior support strategies are often implemented in multiple contexts, with evaluation data being collected to gauge effectiveness. These data can result in new knowledge, skills, and the use of new (innovative) implementation strategies by the team. Sugai et al. (2010) summarize this approach in the context of schoolwide positive behavior support (SWPBS):

> A hallmark of the School-wide Positive Behavior Support (SWPBS) process is the emphasis on *data* to guide decision making about what *practices* should be put in place to support student learning and social behavior. The third essential component of effective SWPBS is *an equal emphasis on the system supports that will be needed to build fluency with new or revised practices among all teachers and staff within the school* . . . The basic problem solving process of data, practices and systems is then applied across the continuum of supports students will need to increase the likelihood of their academic and social behavior success. (p. 3, emphasis added)

Sustainability

The final stage, sustainability, suggests that a high level of support must exist within the identified system for continued implementation over time. McIntosh, Horner, and Sugai (2009) define sustainability as "durable, long-term implementation of a practice at a level of fidelity that continues to produce valued outcomes" (p. 328). To illustrate this point, a school-based example of a student named Freddy is provided in the following section. Pay close attention to how systemic changes resulted in positive academic and social outcomes for Freddy over an extended period of time and across systems. This example also provides a practical demonstration of the stages of implementation that the school and family system went through as they worked to support Freddy, including an exploration stage (kindergarten), installation stage (Grade 1), initial to full implementation stages (Grades 2–7), innovation stage (Grades 6–7), and sustainability stage (Grades K–7).

Systemic Change in a School Setting

In preschool, Freddy was significantly affected by his autism with significant delays in language, communication, social skills,

and high rates of self-stimulatory and problem behaviors. He was unable to participate
in the regular classroom setting throughout kindergarten and most of first grade.
Now in seventh grade, with the support of
his parents and school-based PBS teams, he
has made remarkable progress to the point
that he is independently meeting grade-level
outcomes, has meaningful friendships with
his peers, enjoys recreational and extracurricular activities, independently uses
public transit to go home from school each
day, and is excited to make the transition
to high school. Freddy lived at home with
his mother, father, and maternal grandmother. Both of his parents work in professional fields outside of the home; thus his
grandmother has been actively involved as
a primary caregiver. Despite their busy professional careers, his parents have both been
actively involved in his home and school-
based educational programs.

Freddy's transition from preschool to
public school, his kindergarten year, presented a number of challenges for the school
system. The first months of kindergarten for
Freddy were characterized by high levels of
escape and attention-maintained problem
behavior, as well as delays in language, communication, and social skills and high rates
of self-stimulatory behavior. The school was
often in crisis mode responding to his escalating problem behaviors. Given the need to
focus on Freddy's behavior needs, including
instances of property destruction, the school
principal eventually secured extra funds to
provide some help to "put out fires"—a typical approach of *reacting* to problem behavior.

First grade began with the same high
rates of problem behavior experienced in
kindergarten. However, the school-based
team agreed to participate in an FBA process (O'Neill et al., 1997), which began in
early October. While the first-grade general education classroom teacher was not
actively involved in the development of the
PBS plan, his teachers in subsequent grades
(grades 2–7) were increasingly involved in
supporting Freddy. The school principal was

in her second year at the school and did not
have an extensive background in autism but
knew Freddy well from the previous year and
was very motivated and active in providing
administrative, systems-level support to
Freddy's school-based team.

The outcome of the FBA process was
the identification of two high-value routines.
The first involved making the transition from
recess back to the classroom each morning.
The expectation was that Freddy would listen
for the bell and independently make the transition with his peers back to the classroom.
However, he would suddenly and without
permission "bolt" by turning and running
back outside to the rear of the school, where
he could observe a neighboring construction
site. He would typically remain there until
an adult came to find him. The hypothesis
obtained from the FAI and FAO was that this
behavior was maintained by escape from
nonpreferred activities and access to the
construction site (see Figure 5.3). This was
a high-value routine for the PBS team, due
to the safety risks it posed (e.g., staff did not
know where Freddy was, the construction site
posed dangers to an unsupervised child).

The second routine also involved "bolting" problem behavior but occurred in
physical education classes during activities
that were too difficult or boring for him. He
would suddenly and without permission bolt
to one of the two emergency exit doors and
run outside where he would either wait for an
adult to give chase or run around to the front
of the school and come back to the gym via
the main hallway. The hypothesis obtained
from the FAI was a multifunctional problem
behavior of escape and attention. This was
supported by the FAO. The problem behavior was originally triggered by a difficult or
unengaging activity but then morphed into
an attention maintained problem behavior,
as evidenced by his desire to be "chased." This
routine is depicted in a competing behavior
pathways diagram (see Figure 5.4). Two plans
were developed around these high-priority
routines. The strategies are indicated in Figure 5.5.

Setting event strategies	Preventative strategies	Teaching strategies	Consequence strategies
Change the location of recess activities so they are far away from the construction site. Increase reinforcement for appropriate transitioning if Freddy does see the construction site.	Use a visual schedule that shows what activities follow recess and specifically include preferred activities following recess. Precorrect transitions and redesign the actual transition to include a peer buddy and/or a motivating activity that is potentially incompatible with bolting, such as putting equipment away.	Teach Freddy how to self-monitor and how to ask for access to the construction site. Develop a Social Story about making transitions.	Give praise/reinforcement contingent on appropriate transitions (no bolting). Add access to construction site into visual schedule contingent on asking for it. Redirect back to transition or redesigned transition activity (e.g., putting balls away) Enforce a loss of recess time if behavior continues.

Figure 5.3. Behavior support strategies for Freddy: transition from recess to classroom.

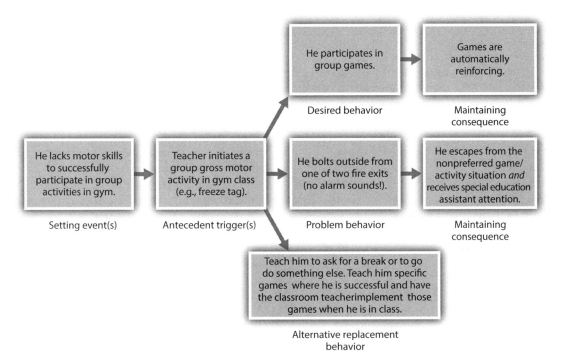

Figure 5.4. Competing behavior pathway diagram for Freddy.

"Bolting" behavior in both routines decreased to zero levels before the end of first grade. Having experienced the success and empowerment of a multicomponent PBS process, the school-based team was able to apply the process and behavior strategies to subsequent challenging behaviors with similar effectiveness for the remainder of the school year. By second grade, Freddy was spending more time in the classroom with lower levels of problem behavior. This was also the first year that the general education classroom teacher was actively involved in the development of plans and strategies, which certainly contributed to his overall success. In addition, both the classroom teacher and LST attended many of the monthly home-team meetings throughout the year, which greatly

Setting event strategies	Preventative strategies	Teaching strategies	Consequence strategies
Enroll him in related/ relevant community activities such as gymnastics and so forth. Preteach specific games/ skills at home.	Precorrect him concerning how to ask for help, and allow him to watch. Use natural, positive, contingency statements (e.g., "After the game, we get free time"). Modify the games to include choices, and intersperse easy and difficult tasks.	Teach him how to ask for a break or help. Teach him a specific skill set that can be incorporated in to the majority of the class games.	Give attention/praise contingent on desired behavior of participating in group games. Give break or help contingent on request. If minor problem behavior (PB), prompt to ask for help or a break. If major PB, spend more time in gym immediately or during recess/lunch.

Figure 5.5. Behavior support strategies for Freddy: bolting behavior in physical education.

enhanced home-school communication and collaboration. The educators' systems-level responsiveness contributed to the success that Freddy had to this point.

The same trend continued into third, fourth, and fifth grade, where the classroom teachers attended the home-team meetings and were active participants in developing support plans and strategies and the collaborative system that, developed over the course of several school years, ensured that plans were ecologically sensitive and contextually appropriate each year, with different teachers and classroom expectations. Correspondingly, during this time, the intensity of home-based intervention was reduced and extracurricular activities took its place. Similarly, behavioral consultation to the school was scaled back, as there was less need for consultation due to his excellent progress and the school-based team was able to develop PBS plans, as needed, with less external consultation and support.

In sixth grade, a new principal entered the school and Freddy entered an experimental model of a combined sixth- and seventh-grade classroom that was cotaught by two teachers and was structurally similar to the high school schedule/model. However, his SEA remained the same. Although he required less support, both coteachers were actively involved in Freddy's regular and special education programming, with one of them having taught him in a previous year. In addition, his sixth-grade individualized

education program (IEP) meeting included a PCP component where Freddy actively participated in selecting some of his own social and academic goals.

Freddy is now in seventh grade, and data suggest that problem behaviors appear to be a thing of the past. Indeed, new staff can hardly believe it when his early elementary school problem behaviors are described to them. Freddy is primarily independent at school but still needs some help with language arts, creative writing, and the occasional social skills issue. He has learned to be responsible for his own personal and academic materials; to manage his own work load, deadlines, and assignments; and to set his own academic goals. He has true friendships and enjoys watching and playing sports. During the second half of elementary school, as problem behaviors decreased and language/communication/social-skills improved, he began to participate in leisure and extracurricular activities including piano lessons; French and Farsi lessons; baseball; going to movies; joining the school band in sixth grade (percussion); family vacations; community outings, including NHL hockey games; and developing social relationships with peers, including use of phone and Skype.

The significant reduction of problem behaviors that began with the use of PBS in first grade and the concurrent improvements in his communication, language, and social skills over the course of his elementary school career have permitted him to access curricular and extracurricular activities and demonstrate a significant improvement in Freddy's overall quality of life at school and home.

Freddy's case provides an example of a school sustaining practices and supports that lead to a variety of positive outcomes for a student. At the school system level, providing support for teacher and administrative participation, team-based assessment, and plan implementation and innovation was a critical factor that sustained the work of supporting Freddy. This, combined with collaboration between the school and home, produced increased communication and aligned support strategies that were sustainable. In other words, the school and family engaged in a number of systemic change strategies to fully support Freddy.

McIntosh, Horner, and Sugai (2009) and McIntosh et al. (2013) describe four factors that support sustainability within systems. They include 1) priority, 2) effectiveness, 3) efficiency, and 4) continuous regeneration. Table 5.2 provides definitions of these concepts, and each are briefly discussed in light of Freddy's multicomponent plan of support.

PBS was a *priority* for the team and remained so as Freddy moved through his grades. Implementation efforts were long term and focused on valued outcomes and systems-level changes that improved the quality of Freddy's school life and homelife. Priority was demonstrated by systems supports such as general education teacher participation in meetings, ongoing administrative support, full participation in the collection of assessment data, collaborative plan development, and resource allocation. *Effectiveness* was demonstrated by the focus on the identification of evidence-based strategies around high-value routines and ongoing review of data to inform team decisions. *Effectiveness* and *efficiency* are illustrated by the team's significant changes to how support was allocated, as illustrated by the following statement:

> Correspondingly, during this time, the intensity of home-based intervention was reduced and extracurricular activities took its place. Similarly, behavioral consultation to the school was scaled back as there was less need for consultation due to his excellent progress and the school-based team was able to develop PBS plans, as needed, with less external consultation and support.

Finally, *continuous regeneration* was evident since data were used regularly and served as a guide for informing team decision making and practices as Freddy's plan was updated based on his need (Baer, Wolf, & Risley, 1968). This was illustrated by the team's decision to add PCP to Freddy's IEP teaming processes in sixth grade.

CONCLUSION

Systems change is foundational to understanding PBS. O'Neill et al. (1997) writes, "If we consider problem behaviors as occurring in contexts, it becomes logical to change the context" (p. 5). Multi-element plans of support

Table 5.2. Factors related to sustained implementation

Priority	Effectiveness	Efficiency	Continuous regeneration
• "The relative importance of the practice in comparison to other practices." (McIntosh, Horner, et al., 2009) • "It includes general, often intangible support for the specific practice, amidst competing initiatives." (McIntosh et al., 2013, p. 294)	• "The extent to which the practice results in valued outcomes. . . . effectiveness depends on both the quality of the practices itself and the quality of implementation." (McIntosh et al., 2013, p. 295)	• "Consideration of the resources needed to implement the practice. When practices are perceived as more efficient, they are judged to be more worthwhile and, therefore, more sustainable." (McIntosh et al., 2013, p. 296)	• "Continuous regeneration includes collecting fidelity and outcome data regularly and using data to adapt practices to make them more relevant, efficient, and effective." (McIntosh et al., 2013, p. 296)

include antecedent- and consequence-based strategies as well as environmental modifications that support systemic change. When successful, systemic change is evidenced by *the adoption and sustained use of evidence-based practices by relevant stakeholders in natural communities of support.* Systemic change involves an exploration phase where relevant stakeholders establish their readiness to engage in PBS; an installation phase where preparation and resource attainment occurs; implementation phases (initial and full) where plans of support are implemented within and across systems; an innovation phase, where new knowledge, skills, and implementation strategies based on data are incorporated into implementation efforts; and a sustainability phase that is predicated on the prioritization, effectiveness, efficiency, and continuous regeneration of regeneration of PBS systems.

REFERENCES

Albin, R.W., Lucyshyn, J.M., Horner, R.H., & Flannery, K.B. (1996). Contextual fit for behavioral support plans: A model for "Goodness of Fit." In L.K. Koegel, R.L. Koegel, & G. Dunlap (Eds.), *Positive behavioral support: Including people with difficult behavior in the community* (pp. 81–98). Baltimore, MD: Paul H. Brookes Publishing Co.

Association for Positive Behavior Support (APBS). (2007). *Positive behavior support standards of practice: Individual level.* Retrieved from http://www.apbs.org/files/apbs_standards_of_practice_2013_format.pdf

Baer, D.M., & Pinkston, E.M. (1997). *Environment and behavior.* Boulder, CO: Westview.

Baer, D.M., Wolf, M.M., & Risley, T.R. (1968). Some current dimensions of applied behavior analysis. *Journal of Applied Behavior Analysis, 1,* 91–97.

Carr, E.G. (2007). The expanding vision of positive behavior support: Research perspectives on happiness, helpfulness, and hopefulness. *Journal of Positive Behavior Interventions, 9,* 3–14.

Carr, E.G., Dunlap, G., Horner, R.H., Koegel, R.L., Turnbull, A.P., Sailor, W., . . . Fox, L. (2002). Positive behavior support: Evolution of an applied science. *Journal of Positive Behavior Interventions, 4,* 4–16, 20.

Cooper, J.O., Heron, T.E., & Heward, W.L. (2007). *Applied behavior analysis* (2nd ed.). Upper Saddle River, NJ: Pearson.

Dunlap, G., Iovannone, R., Wilson, K.J., Kincaid, D.K., & Strain, P. (2010). Prevent-teach-reinforce: A standardized model of school-based behavioral intervention. *Journal of Positive Behavior Interventions, 12,* 9–22.

Fixsen, D.L., Blase, K.A., Horner, R., & Sugai, G. (2009). *Readiness for change: Scaling up brief 3.* Chapel Hill: University of North Carolina.

Government Accountability Office. (2009). *Seclusion and restraints: Selected cases of death and abuse at public and private schools and treatment centers (GAO-09-719T).* Washington, DC: Government Printing Office.

Martin, J.E., Marshall, L.H., & De Pry, R.L. (2008). Participatory decision-making: Innovative practices that increase student self-determination. In R.W. Flexer, T.J. Simmons, P. Luft, & R. Baer (Eds.), *Transition planning for secondary students with disabilities* (3rd ed., pp. 340–366). Columbus, OH: Merrill.

McIntosh, K., Horner, R.H., & Sugai, G. (2009). Sustainability of systems-level evidence-based practices in schools: Current knowledge and future directions. In W. Sailor, G. Dunlap, G. Sugai, & R. Horner (Eds.), *Handbook of positive behavior support* (pp. 327–352). New York, NY: Springer.

McIntosh, K., Mercer, S.H., Hume, A.E., Frank, J.L., Turri, M.G., & Mathews, S. (2013). Factors related to sustained implementation of schoolwide positive behavior support. *Exceptional Children, 79,* 293–311.

Nersesian, M., Todd, A.W., Lehmann, J., & Watson, J. (2000). School-wide behavior support through district-level system change. *Journal of Positive Behavior Support, 2,* 244–247.

O'Neill, R.E., Horner, R.H., Albin, R.W., Sprague, J.R., Storey, K., & Newton, J.S. (1997). *Functional assessment and program development for problem behavior: A practical handbook* (2nd ed.). Pacific Grove, CA: Brooks/Cole.

Schall, C.M. (2010). Positive behavior support: Supporting adults with autism spectrum disorders in the workplace. *Journal of Vocational Rehabilitation, 32,* 109–115.

Schalock, R.L., & Alonso, M.A.V. (2002). *Handbook on quality of life for human service practitioners.* Washington, DC: American Association on Mental Retardation.

Scott, T.M. (2007). Issues of personal dignity and social validity in schoolwide systems of positive behavior support. *Journal of Positive Behavior Interventions, 9,* 102–112.

Sugai, G., Horner, R.H., Algozzine, R., Barrett, S., Lewis, T., Anderson, C., . . . Simonsen, B. (2010). School-wide positive behavior support: Implementers' blueprint and self-assessment. Eugene, OR: University of Oregon. Retrieved from http://www.pbis.org

Sugai, G., Horner, R.H., Dunlap, G., Hieneman, M., Lewis, T.J., Nelson, C.M., . . . Ruef, M. (2000). Applying positive behavior support and functional behavioral assessment in schools. *Journal of Positive Behavior Interventions, 2,* 131–143.

Sugai, G., Lewis-Palmer, T., Todd, A., & Horner, R.H. (2005). *School-Wide Evaluation Tool* (v. 2.1). Eugene: Educational and Community Supports, University of Oregon.

Wolery, M.R., Bailey, D.B., Jr., & Sugai, G.M. (1988). *Effective teaching: Principles and procedures of applied behavior analysis with exceptional children.* Boston, MA: Allyn & Bacon.

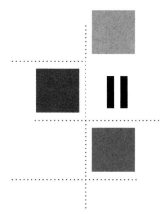

Basic Principles of Behavior

 STANDARDS ADDRESSED IN THIS SECTION

I. A. Practitioners of positive behavior support (PBS) have the following historical perspectives on the evolution of PBS and its relationship to applied behavior analysis (ABA) and movements in the disability field:
1. History of applied behavior analysis and the relationship to PBS
2. Similarities and unique features of PBS and ABA

III. A. Practitioners of PBS utilize the following behavior assessment and support methods that are based on operant learning:
1. The antecedent behavior consequence model as the basis for all voluntary behavior
2. Operational definitions of behavior
3. Stimulus control, including discriminative stimuli and S-deltas
4. The influence of setting events (or establishing operations) on behavior
5. Antecedent influences on behavior
6. Precursor behaviors
7. Consequences to increase or decrease behavior

III. B. Practitioners of PBS understand and use antecedent manipulations to influence behavior, such as the following:
1. Curricular modifications
2. Instructional modifications
3. Behavioral precursors as signals
4. Modification of routines

(continued)

5. Opportunities for choice/control throughout the day
6. Clear expectations
7. Precorrection
8. Errorless learning

III. C. Practitioners of PBS understand and use the following consequence manipulations to increase behavior:
   1. Primary reinforcers and conditions under which primary reinforcers are used
   2. Types of secondary reinforcers and their use
   3. Approaches to identify effective reinforcers, including the following:
      a. Functional assessment data
      b. Observation
      c. Reinforcer surveys
      d. Reinforcer sampling
   4. Premack principle
   5. Positive reinforcement
   6. Negative reinforcement
   7. Ratio, interval, and natural schedules of reinforcement
   8. Pairing of reinforcers

III. D. Practitioners of PBS understand the following consequence manipulations to decrease behavior:
   1. The use of punishment, including characteristics, ethical use of punishment, and potential side effects of punishment procedures.

      Any use of punishment, including strategies that are found within integrated natural settings, must be within the parameters of the 11 key elements identified in IC, with particular attention to IC9, "Techniques that do not cause pain or humiliation or deprive the individual of basic needs."

   2. Differential reinforcement, including the following:
      a. Differential reinforcement of alternative behavior
      b. Differential reinforcement of incompatible behavior
      c. Differential reinforcement of zero rates of behavior
      d. Differential reinforcement of lower rates of behavior
   3. Extinction, including the following:
      a. Characteristics of extinction interventions
      b. How to use extinction
      c. Using extinction in combination with interventions to develop replacement behaviors
   4. Response cost, including the following:
      a. Cautions associated with use of response cost
      b. Using response cost with interventions to develop replacement behaviors
   5. Time-out, including the following:
      a. Types of time-out applications
      b. How to implement time-out
      c. Cautions associated with use of time-out
      d. Using time-out with interventions to develop replacement behaviors

III. E. Practitioners of PBS understand and use the following methods for facilitating generalization and maintenance of skills:
   1. Forms of generalization, including the following:
      a. Stimulus generalization
      b. Response generalization
      c. Generalization across subjects
   2. Maintenance of behaviors across time

IV. A. Practitioners of PBS understand that data-based decision making is a fundamental element of PBS and that behavioral assessment and support planning begins with the following techniques for defining behavior:

1. Using operational definitions to describe target behaviors
2. Writing behavioral objectives that include the following:
   a. Conditions under which the behavior should occur
   b. Operational definition of behavior
   c. Criteria for achieving the objective

IV. B. Practitioners of PBS understand that data-based decision making is a fundamental element of PBS and that the following techniques for measuring behavior are critical components of behavioral assessment and support:

1. Using data systems that are appropriate for target behaviors, including the following:
   a. Frequency
   b. Duration
   c. Latency
   d. Interval recording
   e. Time sampling
   f. Permanent product recording
2. Developing data collection plans that include the following:
   a. The measurement system to be used
   b. Schedule for measuring behavior during relevant times and contexts, including baseline data
   c. Manageable strategies for sampling behavior for measurement purposes
   d. How, when, and if the interobserver agreement checks will be conducted
   e. How and when procedural integrity checks will be conducted
   f. Data collection recording forms
   g. How raw data will be converted to a standardized format (e.g., rate, percentage)
   h. Use of criterion to determine when to make changes in the instructional phase

IV. C. Practitioners of PBS use the following graphic displays of data to support decision making during the assessment, program development, and evaluation stages of behavior support:

1. Converting raw data in standardized format
2. Following graphing conventions, including the following:
   a. Clearly labeled axes
   b. Increment scales that allow for meaningful and accurate
3. Representing the data in the following ways:
   a. Phase change lines
   b. Clearly labeled phase change descriptions
   c. Criterion lines

IV. D. Practitioners of PBS use the following data-based strategies to monitor progress:

1. Using graphed data to identify trends and intervention effects
2. Evaluating data regularly and frequently
3. Sharing data with team members for team-based, person-centered decision making
4. Using data to make decisions regarding program revisions to maintain or improve behavioral progress, including decisions relating to maintaining, modifying, or terminating interventions
5. Using data to determine if additional collaborations, support, and/or assistance is needed to achieve intended outcomes

The seven chapters that make up Section II provide a comprehensive introduction to a science of human behavior commonly referred to as applied behavior analysis (ABA). ABA is a systematic approach to understanding human behavior that is based on an extensive and replicable research literature (Baer, Wolf, & Risley, 1968). ABA has played a critical role in the evolution and current practice of positive behavior support (PBS). Carr et al. (2002) write, "Applied behavior analysis has made two major contributions to PBS. First, it has provided one element of a conceptual framework relevant to behavior change. Second, and equally important, it has provided a number of assessment and intervention strategies" (p. 5). The chapters that follow will provide the reader with a strong grounding in ABA, including outlining the basics of behavior, behavioral assessment, and research-based interventions that support the practice of PBS. Finally, each of these chapters provide case examples that help illustrate major points.

Chapter 6, "Applied Behavior Analysis as a Conceptual Framework for Understanding Positive Behavior Support," provides a historical overview of ABA and introduces key concepts that are used throughout the book. The chapter illustrates how ABA provides a rich literature that informs PBS practices for improving the quality of life of those receiving positive behavior interventions and supports. Chapter 7, "Antecedent Strategies to Change Behavior," focuses on strategies that are instituted prior to a response. The authors discuss a number of research-based strategies that can be used in both school and community-based settings by PBS practitioners, such as curricular modifications, modification of routines, opportunities for choice, and precorrection. Chapter 8, "Consequence Strategies to Change Behavior," examines the role that consequences play

for increasing, decreasing, or maintaining responding. Pay close attention to the discussion on the use of aversive strategies and how a PBS framework differs from a more traditional behavior analytic perspective when it comes to behavior reduction strategies. Chapter 9, "Facilitating Generalization and Maintenance of Behavior Change," examines evidence-based strategies for facilitating the generalization and maintenance of responses. The chapter provides an overview of the research basis for generalization and maintenance and covers critical topics such as stimulus and response generalization and schedules of reinforcements. Chapter 10, "Defining, Measuring, and Graphing Behavior," provides a comprehensive overview of key concepts such as data, operational definitions, behavioral objectives, stages of learning, measuring and recording behavior, reliability, and graphing basics. Chapter 11, "Single-Case Designs and Data-Based Decision Making," extends content presented in the previous chapters and examines how practitioners make data-based decisions based on graphic displays of data. Specific single-case designs are discussed, including assumptions and guidelines for their use. Chapter 12, "Systematic Instruction," serves as a capstone for this section and illustrates an approach—systematic instruction—that incorporates principles of applied behavior analysis in a structured format for teaching new skills for people who experience challenging behavior.

Randall L. De Pry

REFERENCES

Baer, D.M., Wolf, M.M., & Risley, T.R. (1968). Some current dimensions of applied behavior analysis. *Journal of Applied Behavior Analysis, 1,* 91–97.
Carr, E.G., Dunlap, G., Horner, R.H., Koegel, R.L., Turnbull, A.P. Sailor, W., . . . Fox, L. (2002). Positive behavior support: Evolution of an applied science. *Journal of Positive Behavior Interventions, 4,* 4–16, 20.

Applied Behavior Analysis as a Conceptual Framework for Understanding Positive Behavior Support

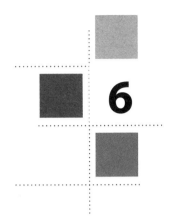

6

Teri Lewis

A student stops what she is doing to hold the door for a classmate entering the same building. A person is startled and moves away from a dog when walking through his neighborhood. While one person enjoys camping by a lake, another person delights in listening to a symphony orchestra. A song comes on the radio and the person listening begins to tear up and thinks of her grandmother whom she hasn't thought of for months. How do we develop habits (e.g., always put your keys in the same place)? Why do we choose what to do when (e.g., decide whether you would like to try bowling)? And why is it that something in your day suddenly sparks a memory of friend you haven't thought of for years?

Behavior analysis is a systematic approach to understanding behavior within an environmental context. Based on the principles of both classical and operant conditioning, behavior analysis is aimed at understanding and improving behavior (e.g.,

Alberto & Troutman, 2008; Cooper, Heron, & Heward, 2007). Critical to this scientific approach is a focus on determinism, empiricism, and philosophical doubt. Determinism is the belief that events are lawful and orderly and, as such, understandable (Cooper, Heron, & Heward, 2007). However, the understanding of phenomena must be based on empirical methods, including objective assessment, repeated measurement, and quantitative analysis. Philosophical doubt requires the scientist to continually question assumptions and rely on objective measurement over subjective beliefs. These guiding principles continue to influence both the science and practice of behavior analysis today. Research in behavior analysis covers a wide range of phenomena, populations, environments, and behaviors and includes both a basic and applied focus. An "experimental analysis of behavior" (EAB) concentrates on basic research with the intent of understanding behavior principles in their simplest and purest forms, whereas "applied behavior analysis" (ABA) developed with the purpose of applying this technology to improve behavior in real-world settings by focusing on socially important behaviors (Baer, Wolf, & Risely, 1968; Wolf, 1978).

In addition to providing a basis for understanding behavior, ABA is the foundation for the development of a variety of interventions and programs. Positive behavior interventions and supports (PBIS) is a systems-level approach to developing proactive school discipline systems (e.g., Horner, Sugai, Todd, & Lewis-Palmer, 2005; Sugai & Horner, 2002). PBIS involves establishing a three-tier model of behavior support for all staff, students, and settings within a school. Within each level, particularly at the secondary and tertiary levels, the focus of PBIS is on individuals with or at risk of developing behavior challenges. Given the proactive and preventive philosophy of PBIS, support goes beyond the school to include the individual's family and the community (e.g., employment, afterschool programs, counseling, medical). In other words, PBIS can be viewed as a framework for supporting and improving the use of positive behavior support (PBS) with individuals, with groups, and within systems (Sugai & Horner, 2002).

The focus of PBS is to enhance the quality of individual's lives by reducing problem behavior and increasing quality of life using methods from ABA, focusing on inclusion and normalization, and emphasizing person-centered approaches (Carr et al., 2002). PBS achieves this goal by blending 1) comprehensive lifestyle change, 2) a life-span perspective, 3) ecological focus, 4) stakeholder participation, 5) social validity, 6) systems-level and comprehensive interventions, 7) emphasis on prevention, 8) flexibility in practices, and 9) multiple perspectives. This chapter will focus on how ABA provides an empirical basis for PBS and its goal of improving the lives of individuals.

At each level, ABA provides the foundation for assessment and intervention. PBIS provides an example of how the principles of ABA, specifically direct observation and data-based decision making, stimulus control, reinforcement and punishment, and function-based assessment, are integrated into a comprehensive effective program. Sean and Maria, described here, illustrate a need for comprehensive and effective programs of support.

Sean

Sean is in third grade but only reads at the first-grade level. Sean and his brother spent much of their early life homeless and living with their father. Both boys were recently adopted. Sean's teachers have noticed that he is withdrawn, rarely interacts with the other children in his class, and doesn't appear to have much interest in his teacher or the teaching assistant. Because of Sean's low reading level, he receives special education support. Sean's teachers are concerned that his limited engagement in both the academic and social aspects of his classroom will put Sean even further behind in school.

....

Maria

Maria is a young adult with Down syndrome who is working on her high school equivalency and spends part of her day working in the community. Maria has a job in an office delivering mail, managing the recycling, and doing some basic cleaning and hopes to find a similar full-time position that will allow her to move out of her parents' home and live in a group home with other young adults.

....

Originally, the focus of ABA was on improving the lives of individuals (Baer, Wolf, & Risley, 1968; Wolf, 1978). As the field developed, so has the application of ABA principles. Early applications focused on responding to behavior primarily using consequent interventions, but current applications emphasize the prevention of problem behavior by focusing on antecedent interventions. Present-day ABA involves both antecedent (prevention, teaching) and consequent (feedback, reinforcement and punishment) interventions as well environments designed to increase the capacity of the individual and the key stakeholders. The remaining chapters in this section each focus on different aspects of a comprehensive ABA approach to PBS. The purpose of this chapter is to provide an overview of the conceptual foundation of ABA for understanding PBS.

HISTORICAL DEVELOPMENT

Classical Conditioning

While studying canine digestive systems, Ivan Pavlov (1927) observed that the dogs anticipated food before being fed. Classical conditioning provides an understanding of respondent or reflexive behaviors. We are born with reflexive (involuntary) behaviors such as blinking when a puff of air hits our eye or being startled when we hear a loud noise. These behaviors are unlearned, biological, and predictable. An unconditioned stimulus results in the emission of an unconditioned response. For Pavlov, this would have been food in mouth resulting in the canine's salivation. However, Pavlov noticed that the canines began salivating before they were given food again, as if they anticipated the food. From this observation, Pavlov investigated what is now known as classical conditioning—one of the two ways we learn behavior from our experiences. Pavlov's canine's learned that when the feeders approached, food was soon to follow. Therefore, the feeders became a

conditioned stimulus, and the salivation before eating was a conditioned response (see Figure 6.1).

Pavlov's research explains how events in the environment provide predictability and consistency to our day. Whether we are aware of it or not, we respond to environmental stimuli throughout our day. While we are born with reflexive (unlearned) responses, we also learn how the environment guides or shapes our behavior. When driving a car we know to stop at a red light and drive at a green light. What happens at a yellow light depends on complex information from the environment. Are you running late to work? Is your mother sitting in the car with you? How many other cars or pedestrians are around the intersection? We use information, often complex, from the world around us to decide what behavior or response is appropriate for the situation and what will likely happen as a result of our choices. If you run a light, you run the risk of getting a ticket or getting into an accident. If you stop, then you won't get a ticket or be in an accident.

Building from the work of Pavlov, John B. Watson demonstrated that phobias and many other behaviors are often established as a result of classical conditioning. In the famous Little Albert experiment, Watson and Raynor (1920) examined the development of a fear response using the principles of classical conditioning. While often criticized, the

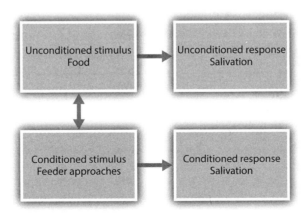

Figure 6.1. Model of classical conditioning.

importance of this study is twofold. First, it clearly illustrated the ease with which we learn behavioral and emotional responses from environmental stimuli and how important the early environment is for the development of young children. Second, this line of research helped us understand how phobias are developed and, more important, how to help individuals overcome those phobias.

Operant Conditioning

Pavlov's and Watson's contributions to the science of ABA provided a model for how we are influenced by our antecedent events. However, classical conditioning only explains part of people's behavior. Sometimes individuals behave in ways we wouldn't expect or don't seem to be influenced by things in their immediate environment. While classical conditioning focused on reflexive (unlearned) behaviors, operant conditioning expanded to focus on learned or voluntary behaviors. Operant conditioning, most associated with the work of B.F. Skinner, expands learning to those behaviors or responses that are not reflexive but are instead learned, elicited, and influenced by antecedent and consequent stimuli (before and after a behavior). Operant conditioning provides a model for understanding when and why a behavior occurs and why some behaviors stop occurring.

In addition to Skinner, Edward Thorndike's (1911) law of effect states that if the result of our behavior is pleasing, we are likely to repeat the behavior, and if it is unpleasant, we are unlikely to repeat the behavior. Reinforcement then refers to a consequence that increases the likelihood of a behavior occurring again, and punishment then refers to a consequence that decreases the likelihood of a behavior occurring again. Sean and Maria help illustrate these points.

Sean

Over time, Sean has learned that becoming withdrawn at school allows him to escape academic

and social demands. Because teachers and peers leave Sean alone when he puts his head down or walks away from class activities, he has learned that withdrawing and not participating allow him to escape academic demands and the likelihood of struggling or not being able to complete the academic demand. This is an example of how consequences increase the continued use of a response, such as withdrawing from academic demands.

....

Maria

While Maria's supervisor is generally pleased with her work ethic, she doesn't always get all her tasks done and occasionally needs reminders to return from her breaks. Other employees have commented that Maria occasionally interrupts them while they are working. Maria has learned that being in the break room allows her to interact with the other employees and gets her attention.

....

While the law of effect describes the influence of consequence events (those that happen after a response), to understand the larger environmental context requires a model of what was going on before as well as what happened after. The four-term operant includes events that occur before, to prompt or occasion a response, and those that occur after to increase, decrease, or maintain a response. The four-term operant is composed of the behavior of interest (response), the immediate antecedent (discriminative stimuli), the maintaining consequence (reinforcement), and distal antecedent events (setting events). Figure 6.2 illustrates the four-term operant from earliest event (setting events) to last event (maintaining consequence). Together, the components of the four-term contingency allow us to think about behavior from an environmental perspective that focuses on the individual's need, not just the behavior. In other words, it tells us the what (response), when (discriminative stimuli), why (reinforcement), and distal events that make it more likely

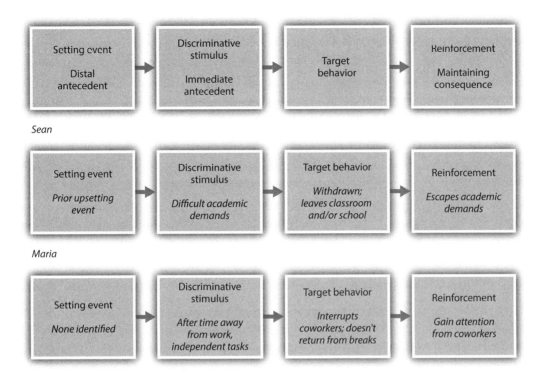

Figure 6.2.   Four-term contingency.

that the behavior will occur (setting events; Alberto & Troutman, 2008; Cooper, Heron, & Heward, 2007; Woolery, Bailey, & Sugai, 1988). Sean and Maria help illustrate the four-term operant.

Sean

For Sean, his target behavior was becoming withdrawn, which sometimes included leaving the classroom or the school. His triggering antecedent was any difficult academic demand, particularly any that involved reading, and his maintaining consequence was escaping the difficult demand. During conversations with his teachers and mother, it became clear that while school was difficult, it was more so on days when there had been an upsetting event. Upsetting events then acted as a setting event for Sean—that is, they increased the likelihood of his withdrawing from activities or leaving school grounds.

Maria

When considering Maria's not returning from scheduled breaks on time and interrupting other employees while they are working, her supervisor noticed that this occurred more often on Mondays or after other breaks (e.g., holidays, vacations, sick days). Thus days away from work appear to be the triggering antecedent, which makes sense because she didn't have many opportunities to socialize outside of work. Therefore, the maintaining consequence was gaining her co-worker's attention. For Maria, there didn't appear to be specific setting events that increased the likelihood she would interrupt coworkers or stay in the break room beyond her scheduled break time.

Combined, classical, and operant conditionings offer an understanding of how responses are influenced by the environment and develop into patterns of responding for an individual. For example, if a child is startled by a loud noise while playing at a friend's house (unconditioned stimulus), they may pair their fear of the noise (unconditioned response) with their friend's house and become afraid (conditioned response) of going to other children's homes (conditioned stimuli) to play. However, over time, that same child might learn that by saying they are afraid, they get out of doing many unpleasant activities (e.g., going to school, the store, the dentist). So a response, being afraid, that began as an unlearned startle response has now been reinforced by being able to avoid many other activities and has become a learned behavior. See Table 6.1 for a comparison of operant and classical conditioning.

Reinforcement and Punishment The terms *reinforcement* and *punishment* are often misunderstood, but from a behavior analysis perspective they are words that describe the likelihood of future behavior—that is, reinforcement *increases* the likelihood of a response occurring in the future, and punishment *decreases* the likelihood of a response occurring in the future. ABA examines environmental events that influence increases or decreases in responding. When something is presented, it is called *positive*, and when something is removed, it is called *negative*. Again, confusion often arises with the terms *positive* and *negative*. In this context, thinking of these terms "mathematically," where positive (+) equals addition and negative (–) equals subtraction, may help keep the definition clear. To begin to understand consequences, these elements are combined.

Positive reinforcement is when a behavior has an increased likelihood of occurring in the future following the presentation (positive) of reinforcing stimuli. For example, when teachers praise Miranda privately, she continues to turn her work in on time. When friends laugh, Jacob tells jokes at lunch more often, or when Heather talks to customers while bagging their groceries, they ask her about her day and engage in casual conversation (Alberto & Troutman, 2008; Cooper, Heron, & Heward, 2007; Woolery, Bailey, & Sugai, 1988). Negative reinforcement, then, is the increased likelihood of behavior occurring in the future following the removal (negative) of aversive stimuli (Alberto & Troutman, 2008; Cooper, Heron, & Heward, 2007; Woolery, Bailey, & Sugai, 1988). For example, when Bradley is sent to the office for talking out in class, he is talks out more often in class. In this example, being in the classroom is aversive to Sean, and he has learned that by talking out he can avoid being in class. When Lolita is asked to sort the mail, she complains that she gets paper cuts from the mail and that it isn't fair that she always get asked to do this task. Over time, Lolita's supervisor has stopped asking her to sort the mail, and Lolita has learned that complaining gets her out of undesirable tasks.

Both positive and negative reinforcement result in increases in future behavior occurrence. However, one involves presenting a reinforcing stimulus (positive) and one involves removing an aversive stimulus (negative).

Punishment, as well, is classified as either positive or negative. Positive punishment is the decreased likelihood of behavior occurring in the future following the presentation of aversive stimuli (Alberto & Troutman, 2008; Cooper, Heron, & Heward, 2007; Woolery, Bailey, & Sugai, 1988). For example,

Table 6.1.   Two models of learning: Comparison of classical and operant conditioning

Classical conditioning	Operant conditioning
• Elicited	• Emitted
• Involuntary	• Voluntary
• Unlearned	• Learned
• Occasioned by antecedents (before)	• Occasioned by antecedents (before)
	• Influenced by consequences (after)

when Kyle and Kristen have to clean the cafeteria after pushing in the lunch line, their pushing of other students decreases. Negative punishment is the decreased likelihood of behavior occurring in the future following the removal of reinforcing stimuli (Alberto & Troutman, 2008; Cooper, Heron, & Heward, 2007; Woolery, Bailey, & Sugai, 1988). When Michael has to sit on the side of the building during recess because he called Tim names, Michael's name calling decreases. Both positive and negative punishment decrease future occurrence of behavior. Positive punishment does this by presenting an aversive event and negative punishment by removing reinforcing stimuli. Figure 6.3 summarizes the relationship between the action (presentation or removal) and the effect (increase or decrease). For additional discussion on the role of consequences, including guidelines for decreasing the use of aversive or punishment-oriented consequences in school and community settings, see Chapter 8. Sean and Maria illustrate the role of reinforcement as follows.

Sean

Because Sean's low reading ability made participating in academic activities difficult for him, his feelings about school and his teachers had changed so that he no longer wanted to go to school. His withdrawing from classroom activities and the school allowed him to escape this aversive situation. His behavior is explained using negative reinforcement—that is, withdrawing continues to occur because it removes the academic demand.

Maria

Maria's behavior is explained using positive reinforcement. Maria is very social and easy to talk with. She brings up interesting topics and often asks people about how they are doing or if they had a good weekend. Because of her social skills, Maria has learned how to start and keep conversations going. She has also learned that staying in the break room allows her more opportunities to talk to her coworkers.

Stimulus Control The relationship between behaviors and consequences provides a model for understanding how behaviors are learned and why they either continue or do not continue to happen. However, we use information from the environment to help us decide when to choose one behavior or response over another. Again, antecedent stimuli provide environmental information about the expected consequences to our behavior—in short, whether engaging in a behavior will result in something pleasant or unpleasant.

Most of us have cell phones. We have learned that when our phone rings, we should answer to be able to talk the person. Few, if any of us, pick up our phone when it isn't ringing to see if someone might be on the line waiting to speak to us. While this may sound obvious, it is an example of stimulus control. We answer our phones when they ring (antecedent stimuli present) and do not answer when they are quiet (no antecedent stimuli present). As with Pavlov's research, the ringing of the phone is a conditioned stimulus that

		Action	
		Present	Remove
Effect	Increase	Positive reinforcement	Negative reinforcement
	Decrease	Positive punishment	Negative punishment

Figure 6.3.   Summary of positive and negative reinforcement and punishment. (*Source:* Sulzer & Mayer, 1972.)

Stimulus "What shape is this?"	Response	Consequence
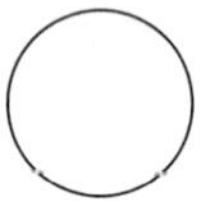 ◯	"Circle"	Praise (reinforcement)
▢	"Square"	Correction procedure (no reinforcement; punishment)
▢	"Square"	Praise (reinforcement)

Figure 6.4. Example of stimulus control influencing learning shapes.

results in a conditioned response (answering the phone). Yet understanding our behavior is more complicated than simple stimulus–response relationships. We are able to predict whether talking on the phone will be pleasant or unpleasant. We consider what else is happening at the time (e.g., sitting at home, in a meeting at work) and whom it is we will get to talk with. So antecedent stimuli both increase and decrease our behavior by providing us with information about likely consequences—that is, will the behavior result in reinforcement or punishment? Stimulus control, or using the environment to predict outcomes, also serves as the basis for learning. For example, when asking a child to identify shapes, the child learns to pair the correct response by receiving praise and by receiving correction/redirection for an incorrect response (see Figure 6.4). More information about how antecedent influences may be used to build interventions are presented in the Chapter 7, which focuses on the role of antecedents in teaching and arranging environment, and in Chapter 12, which provides an understanding of systematic instruction. Stimulus control is further illustrated using our examples of Sean and Maria.

Sean

While teachers making academic demands on Sean increased the likelihood of his withdrawing,

this was not true for all classroom activities. When the class would engage in an art project, Sean would participate and often choose art activities when he had free time during his day. Sean also joined Boy Scouts and looked forward to meetings. When Sean would earn a badge, he would immediately want his mother to sew the new badge onto his uniform when he got home from the meeting. Therefore, Sean's withdrawing occurred in the presence of academic demands but not in the presence of other requests (e.g., art).

Maria

Maria's supervisor noticed that when Maria gets to work in tasks in the front office where she could talk and work at the same time, she rarely had to be reminded to stay focused on her task or to return from her breaks. On days when Maria hasn't seen her coworkers for a while and on tasks where she works alone, she is more likely to take long breaks and interrupt coworkers. However, when she gets to work with others, she stays on task and returns promptly from her breaks.

THE BEGINNING OF APPLIED BEHAVIOR ANALYSIS
Some Current Dimensions

Baer, Wolf, and Risley's article is still used as the standard description of ABA (Baer,

Wolf, & Risley, 1968). The seven dimensions of ABA provide the field with both a scientific and an ethical base. First and foremost, ABA is applied, behavioral, and analytic. *Applied* refers to focusing on societal interests and not on advancing basic science. Because of this, ABA is concerned with environments, not just behavioral response. *Behavioral* means the emphasis is on what individuals do, not what they say they are going to do. However, thoughts and feelings are behaviors, just private instead of public. Because thoughts and feelings are difficult to "see," ABA has been cautious to make judgments about how someone might be feeling. Therefore, while these private events are important, they are more difficult to measure directly. (See Chapter 10 for more information on defining, measuring, and graphing behavior to improve decision making.) While we know that people feel insecure, we cannot look at a child and know that is what they are feeling unless they tell us. We can however, describe that they sit alone with their head down and rarely play when peers ask them to. Beyond precise measurement, ABA is also *analytic*—that is, the researcher can provide "a believable demonstration of the events that can be responsible for the occurrence or nonoccurrence of that behavior" (Baer, Wolf, & Risley, 1968, pp. 93–94). In addition, ABA is *technological*, which means that procedures and practices are completely described to facilitate accurate use within applied settings. Baer, Wolf, and Risley's *conceptual systems* refer to the practices and procedures being embedded within a theoretical basis. Where technological aspects of ABA explore "how" the procedure works, conceptual systems explore "why" a procedure works. It is key to ABA that the application of procedures and practices is *effective*. From an ABA perspective, effectiveness is not based on statistical change alone but is heavily based on whether the outcomes have practical value. Finally, ABA has *generality*. While requests to provide support for an individual with behavior challenges often focus on one particular setting (e.g., recess, during math, dinnertime at home), ABA is interested with increasing the person's success across all aspects of their life. Providing individuals with more socially acceptable behaviors will not only improve their ability to meet their current needs but also give them the skills to be successful in other environments in the future. Immediate changes in the person's behavior are important, but long-term change and success are the ultimate goal of PBS.

Expansion of Values

Heward et al. (2005) added their belief that five characteristics should be added to those presented by Baer, Wolf, and Risley (1968, 1987). They suggest that ABA should be *accountable*. In essence, this means that ABA relies on direct and frequent measurement to evaluate the effectiveness of procedures and practices and that we should use the data to improve, change, or discontinue the practice. In addition, they propose the addition of *public* and *doable* to the tenets of ABA. *Public* indicates that the entire process (assessment, results, theoretical explanation) should be public and therefore open to evaluation by anyone. Related to this is the concept of being *doable*. *Doable* involves extending the definition of *applied* beyond the setting and population to include the ability of practitioners and families to implement and benefit from procedures and practices. Finally, Heward et al. assert that ABA should be both *empowering* and *optimistic*. By being both *applied* and *doable*, ABA should empower practitioners, participants, families, and so forth as a means to effectively change behavior. Optimistic then incorporates the previous tenets and concludes that if we have done the others well, we will have established a knowledge base that has validated effective practices to address real-world issues that emphasize ongoing evaluation and revision to increase learning and eventually increase the independence of individuals.

Social Validity

Soon after the original definition of ABA as a field unique and complimentary to EAB, Montrose Wolf (1978) proposed the concept of social validity. Social validity brings to the forefront the importance of subjectivity when addressing applied settings and issues. Specifically, social validity is threefold: the social significance of the goals, the social appropriateness of the procedures, and the social importance of the effects. Echoing the premise of Baer, Wolf, and Risley (1968, 1987), Wolf (1978) states that intervention effectiveness must result in important, not simply statistical, outcomes. Strain, Barton, and Dunlap (2012) found that addressing social validity as part of an ABA intervention 1) improves the design of service delivery systems, 2) informs implementers when to fade support, 3) increases clients and implementers' willingness to employ complex strategies, 4) allows implementers to identify important and unanticipated effects, and 5) provides focus for future research efforts, all of which relate to the values of ABA (Baer, Wolf, & Risley, 1968, 1987; Heward et al., 2005).

A core tenet of PBS is the focus on the individual and involves assessing both strengths and needs as well as preferences and life goals. Functional behavior assessments (FBAs) have guided the development of individualized behavior intervention plans (BIPs) for decades (see Chapters 14 and 15). In general, an FBA provides a framework for understanding the environment from the perspective of the individual in need of behavior support—that is, it provides information about the 1) target behavior so that a complete and accurate description can be developed, 2) antecedent events that influence the occurrence of problem behavior, 3) consequence events that maintain the problem behavior, and 4) setting events that may increase the intensity of likelihood of the target behavior occurring. The point of an FBA goes beyond understanding behavior within an environmental context. Having a comprehensive understanding of what

is currently happening provides interventionists (e.g., teachers, employers, parents, behavior specialists) with a framework for designing support. When traditional FBA information is combined with the individual's preferences, strengths, and life goals, the interventionist has an understanding of where to begin, where the individual wants to be, and what practices would be appropriate to include in the BIP.

However, the FBA-BIP involves both empirically supported practice and contextual fit to the individual of concern. Benazzi, Horner, and Good (2006) assessed the usability and acceptability of FBA, resulting in a BIP. FBA-BIPs developed by those with strong behavioral expertise were rated as being technically adequate but with low usability and acceptability. FBA-BIPs developed by key stakeholders (e.g., teachers, parents) were seen as usable and acceptable but lacking technical adequacy. However, when the behavior experts and key stakeholders collaborated on the FBA-BIP process, plans were considered both acceptable and technically adequate. Focusing on key stakeholders and setting features, also known as the contextual fit (Albin, Lucyshyn, Horner, & Flannery, 1996), increases the immediate acceptability and effectiveness of interventions and provides a foundation for the sustainability of efforts. Ensuring a contextual fit means including multiple stakeholder perspectives and considering the local capacity of implementers, availability of resources of implementation settings, as well as preferences and values of the stakeholders (Albin et al., 1996). Sean and Maria's case study illustrates the importance of collecting contextualized information from key stakeholders.

Sean

Identifying individual strengths and preferences is a key part of the FBA process. Learning that Sean enjoyed art and Boy Scouts, in particular earning badges, allows us to tailor an intervention to his needs (i.e., maintaining consequence) and not have a standard intervention for not participating/withdrawing. In an interview, Sean's teacher stated that she often sent notes home to his mother when he had a great day at school. However, Sean's mother stated that she never got these notes. Knowing that Sean had limited reading ability, the teacher would even read the note to Sean before sending it home. Sean's behavior here indicates that he did not trust what the adults were telling him and had learned that notes home usually meant he had done something wrong and would get in trouble at home. Again, this information was critical to developing an intervention that relied on empirically supported practices but also incorporated Sean's strengths, needs, and perspective.

. . . .

Maria

Maria's supervisor understood that Maria's need for socialization is both a concern and a strength for Maria. In addition to alternating Maria's activities to include more time working with colleagues and reinforcing her hard work with longer break time, her supervisor worked with Maria's family to help Mara identify a hobby, learning to paint, so she could take group classes and meet other people who also enjoy painting and go out for lunch with them at the end of their Saturday painting class.

. . . .

EXPANDED LEVEL OF ANALYSIS

Early ABA focused on understanding the behavior of individuals. However, as the field has grown, so has the focus of analysis. Currently ABA addresses a wide range of settings and populations. It is common for interventionists to work with individuals, groups (e.g., classroom, family, individuals with similar needs), organizations (e.g., school, agency, company), and large-scale systems (e.g., regional organizations, school districts, state departments of education).

PBIS is an example of an ABA-based program that addresses multiple levels of analyses. Based on a three-tiered model of prevention, PBIS addresses the needs of large organizations, with Tier-1 primary interventions of groups, Tier-2 secondary interventions of individuals, and Tier-3 tertiary interventions. *Primary interventions* consist of school- or organizationwide discipline and management systems and practices that prevent the development of nonadaptive social behavior and promote the development of prosocial skills. *Secondary interventions* address the educational needs of individuals who are at risk of academic and/or social behavior failure. *Tertiary interventions* provide specific behavior supports to individuals with emotional and behavioral challenges and their families.

PBIS emphasizes the use of systems, data, evidenced-based practices, and outcomes, which are continually monitored by a school-based leadership team of representative staff. By ensuring that research-based practices are employed in a systematic fashion and that data are collected to monitor results, schools can increase the likelihood that they will achieve positive outcomes. Early on, the focus of ABA was on interventions at the individual level. With the expansion to systems-level approaches, such as PBIS, the focus moved to establishing environments that support all students, staff, and family across all environments. Schools report that relying on a strong preventive schoolwide foundation increased their ability to successfully support individuals with intense needs. In addition, PBIS establishes a culture of individuals who rely on data-based decision making and focus on arranging environments for success. Because of this, the move to adopt PBS as a means to enhance the quality of life for individuals with intense behavioral needs is a natural next step.

The ultimate goal for practitioners is that effective practices and programs sustain. Fixsen and colleagues (2005) have suggested that sustainability is a function of how well adoption and implementation has been handled. Similarly, Elliott and Mihalic (2004) have suggested that sustainability is related to how well programs provide technical assistance, train staff, prepare sites for a new program, and have the program supported by organizational resources.

Traditionally, organizations implement programs that rely solely on training using what is sometimes referred to as a "train and hope" approach (Stokes & Baer, 1977). However, the "train and hope" approach results in little sustainable change. Literature shows that simply telling teachers or other practitioners what to do or providing written instructions is not sufficient for obtaining high integrity of implementation. Coaching improves implementation and sustained use of effective interventions (e.g., Fuchs & Fuchs, 1996; Wickstrom, Jones, LaFleur, & Witt, 1998). Training provides the technical skills and coaching support necessary for implementation fidelity. When training and coaching are combined, the best outcomes are achieved (see Figure 6.5).

In 2002, Carr et al. worked the seven tenets of ABA from Baer, Wolf, and Risley (1968) into a PBIS framework. While the original tenets of ABA remain important to PBS, Carr et al. (2002) expanded the philosophy to a broader systems-level perspective. This expansion is similar to the one presented in the Heward et al. (2005) article discussed earlier. Carr et al. (2002) focus the expanded perspective on the inclusion movement and the subsequent belief that person-centered planning represents the blending of empirically supported treatments and thoughtful, ethical implementation. In person-centered planning (e.g., Kincaid, 1996), the short- and long-term goals of the individual guide the development of the intervention. In this regard, behavior change includes not just what behavior but why and how the change will occur.

Given the change in culture as well as advancement in science, Carr et al. (2002) frame PBIS as concerned with 1) change in quality of life, 2) taking a comprehensive life-span perspective, 3) stakeholder participation, 4) inclusion of both ecological and social validity, and 5) supporting efforts via systems-level interventions. By expanding the level of intervention from individual intervention to systems and by including multicomponent interventions, the likelihood of practitioners and settings engaging in prevention efforts—and thereby reducing the need for more intensive reactive interventions—is increased.

Table 6.2 compares the original seven tenets from Baer, Wolf, and Risley (1968) to the expanded and evolved views of both Heward et al. (2005) and Carr et al. (2002).

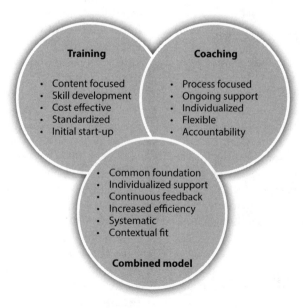

Figure 6.5. Benefit of providing a combined model of training and coaching.

Table 6.2. Comparison of applied behavior analysis (ABA) critical features across Baer, Wolf, and Risley (1968); Heward et al. (2005); and Carr et al. (2002)

	Baer, Wolf, and Risley (1968)	Heward et al. (2005)	Carr et al. (2002)
Theoretical basis	Behavioral ──────────────▶		
	Analytic ──────────────▶		
	Technological ──────────────▶		
	Conceptual systems ──────▶		Respect for scientific practice(s)
			Multiple theoretical perspectives
Setting and participant role	Applied ──────────────▶		Ecological validity
	Effective ───────▶	Accountable	
	Generality ──────────────▶		Systems change
		Public	
		Doable	Stakeholder participation
Subjective assessment		Empowering	Lifestyle change
		Optimistic	
			Lifespan perspective
			Social validity
			Emphasis on prevention

Over time, ABA has grown to use evidence-based practices in broader application of environments, stakeholders, and populations:

> The extension of PBS represents part of a larger movement in the social sciences and education away from traditional models that have emphasized pathology toward a new positive model . . . with a view to improving quality of life and preventing behavior problems. (Carr et al., 2002, p. 14)

Promoting New Responses: Prevention, Teaching, and Reinforcement

The focus of this chapter was to provide an introduction to how ABA provides a conceptual framework for PBIS. Key concepts such as reinforcement, punishment, and stimulus control combine to guide both assessment and intervention (i.e., FBA-BIP). Furthermore, ABA provides key stakeholders with guidelines and values for choosing and implementing behavior strategies whether the focus is on universal, secondary, or tertiary levels of support and across contexts (i.e., school, home, work, community). As indicated by Benazzi, Horner, & Good (2006), the FBA-BIP process requires a balance between empirically supported practices and social validity. While there are many empirically supported practices, there are a few that are effective, efficient, and commonly utilized.

Increasing Existing Behaviors

The ultimate goal of a BIP is to increase the individual's independence. Self-management (e.g., Cooper, Heron, & Heward, 2007) is a strategy that may be used with a variety of behaviors and places the individual in a central role for implementation of the strategy. Most of us use self-management strategies daily (e.g., alarm clocks, day planners, to-do lists). When working with an individual to increase the consistency of an existing behavior, self-management may be useful and effective. Self-management involves having the individual monitor his or her behavior and track how often or how well he or she has completed the behavior that day. Maria could be given a chart so that she could track when she went on break and when she returned and then determine if she returned on time. If she successfully returned on time for break, then she would receive some type of reinforcement. For Maria, it could be earning an extra 5 minutes of break on her next scheduled break since being able to socialize is so reinforcing for her. Because Sean wanted to avoid school but was close to his mother, he could keep track of his successful day (i.e., participation, use of his stress management system) and then go over this at the end of the school day with his mom. Having Sean monitor his behavior in one environment (school) and receive reinforcement in another (home) highlights an advantage of having the individual increase his or her independent management of his or her behavior—that is, individuals rely on themselves to assess, record, and report their successes.

Another strategy, differential reinforcement, involves four variations of interventions that combine both positive reinforcement and negative punishment (extinction) (e.g., Cooper, Heron, & Heward, 2007). Because this set of interventions combine both strategies to increase and decrease behavior in one intervention, they offer easy-to-implement yet effective options. In addition, the four variations make them applicable to a broad range of behaviors. All four variations include extinction (or not attending to problem behavior), with differences concerning how reinforcement is incorporated. Differential reinforcement of other behavior (DRO) provides reinforcement for the nonoccurrence of the target behavior, or behavior other than the target behavior. Differential reinforcement of low-rate behavior (DRL) provides

reinforcement for reduced rates or levels of the target behavior. The intent of DRL is to maintain behaviors at lower, more appropriate rates. For example, if an individual raises their hand to ask questions several times an hour, a DRL intervention would result in the individual continuing to ask questions but at a reduced rate (e.g., once per hour). Differential reinforcement of incompatible behavior (DRI) and differential reinforcement of alternative behavior (DRA) both strengthen a replacement behavior. With DRI, the replacement and target behavior cannot be performed at the same time (e.g., in seat and out of seat), and with DRA, the replacement meets the same maintaining consequence or need of the target behavior (e.g., teaching someone to shake hands or say hello instead of hitting someone to get their attention). Together the differential reinforcement procedures provide varied, efficient, and effective options for BIP.

Preventing Target Behaviors

While some interventions are aimed at responding to problem behaviors, others are aimed at preventing them before they occur. Precorrection (Colvin, Sugai, Good, & Lee, 1997) involves providing reminders or prompts to the individual before they are going to be in an environment likely to trigger the target behavior. For Maria, this would include reminding her of the length of her break, asking her when she needed to be back to work, or asking her what her plan for the break is. For Sean, his teachers could teach him how to identify when he is becoming upset/anxious and provide him with strategies to reduce his stress. Then when they notice him becoming upset, they could remind him of his three cool-down options (i.e., art basket at desk, back of the classroom, or main office). The goal of providing the precorrections is to compete with and reduce the reliance on the problem behavior. That is, Sean could cool down when he is just beginning to becoming stressed instead of waiting until he becomes so upset that he feels the need to leave the school grounds.

Teaching New Behaviors

Finally, an ABA approach involves teaching new skills to increase the individual's competence and ultimately their independence. Task analysis is an effective strategy to teach new skills. With a task analysis, complex skills such as getting dressed or cooking a meal are broken down into smaller steps. Then each individual step is modeled and practiced with prompts until the person is successful at completing the step, and the next step is modeled and practiced. Finally, the person can complete each smaller step in the correct order so that they are able to be successful and independent with the entire complex skill. For example, if Maria was responsible for office mail, she could begin by going to get the mail from the mailbox. Once she was able to complete this step independently, she would learn to sort and alphabetize the mail. Then she would learn to put the sorted mail in the correct boxes, and then she could learn to collect outgoing mail and take this to the mailbox, and so forth.

CONCLUSION

ABA began as an application of EAB to demonstrate how a scientifically based theory can increase the success of individuals and improve the structure and predictability of environments. While originally focused on responding to behavior challenges of individuals, the field has grown to focus on prevention and larger systems-level application. PBIS is an example of how the science of ABA can be applied to environments to build a comprehensive model that begins with prevention and continues to specialized interventions.

The focus on environmental influences to describe both behavior deficits and excesses has allowed the field to address diverse populations while focusing on individualized interventions aimed at increasing the success of individuals. Returning to our case studies, we can see the benefits of implementing comprehensive, multicomponent plans of support.

Sean

For Sean, adopting an ABA perspective allowed us to develop a plan that reflects both the science and the art of behavior interventions. A key component of Sean's intervention was increased academic instruction. However, given that increasing his reading skills is a long-term goal, we wanted Sean to let adults know when work was too difficult and he was becoming stressed. Since Sean was unlikely to tell his teachers directly, we taught him to move a paper clip up a stress thermometer that was placed on his desk. We also taught Sean that he could take a break. Also, because we knew some days were harder for Sean than others, we wanted him to have a choice of the type of break he could earn. Sean could work on art projects at his desk. In fact, we had him create "good day" badges that he could take home to his parents at the end of the day. If that wasn't enough of a break, we set up a cooldown area at the back of the classroom that he could go to. Sean could also participate in class circle activities from his desk. Initially, he was actively involved, but by being allowed to stay at his desk, he did remain in the area and listened to the instruction and other students' responses. Finally, if Sean was a having a particularly difficult day, he could place a card on the classroom door and go to the principal's office (an area he identified as being one he enjoyed). In addition, teachers and parents would alert each other if anything out of the ordinary happened so that they would know Sean might have a harder time than usual with academic demands.

....

Maria

While Sean's plan focused on increasing his communication and addressed his limited academic engagement and growth, Maria did not have difficulty verbally communicating with peers and coworkers; her focus was knowing under what conditions to socialize while at work. Again, applying ABA and a function-based support increases the focus on individual strengths and needs. The goal for Maria's intervention plan was not to stop her from talking with colleagues while at work but to teach her when and where it is appropriate to talk with colleagues and when she needs to work independently and quietly on tasks. As with

Sean's plan, Maria's plan went beyond her workday to look for ways to improve her independence and quality of life during her weekends, with the hope of opening more social opportunities for her. Furthermore, Maria's supervisor understood that for Maria to be successful, she would need more than a self-management program, and she involved both Maria's family (to help with evening and weekend activities) and her colleagues. While Maria's initiating conversations in the break room and around the office disrupted some coworkers, others looked forward to the minibreaks and were inadvertently reinforcing Maria's off-task talking by engaging Maria in conversation. For Maria to be successful, all coworkers were asked to redirect Maria to the task at hand when it was not an appropriate time to talk and continue to have conversations with Maria when they were working together on a task or on break.

By focusing the assessment of Sean's target behavior (withdrawing from activities and school) and Maria's behavior (talking with colleagues too much and when she was supposed to be working independently) in an ABA framework, we were able to understand the respective situations through Sean's and Maria's perspectives and develop an intervention that focused on both their needs and their strengths.

REFERENCES

Alberto, P.A., & Troutman, A.C. (2008). *Applied behavior analysis for teachers* (8th ed.). Upper Saddle River, NJ: Pearson.

Albin, R.W., Lucyshyn, J.M., Horner, R.H., & Flannery, K.B. (1996). Contextual fit for behavior support plans. In L.K. Koegel, R.L. Koegel, & G. Dunlap (Eds.), *Positive behavioral support: Including people with difficult behaviors in the community* (pp. 81–92). Baltimore, MD: Paul H. Brookes Publishing Co.

Baer, D.M., Wolf, M.M., & Risley, T.R. (1968). Some current dimensions of applied behavior analysis. *Journal of Applied Behavior Analysis, 1*, 91–97.

Baer, D.M., Wolf, M.M., & Risley, T.R. (1987). Some still-current dimensions of applied behavior analysis. *Journal of Applied Behavior Analysis, 20*, 313–327.

Benazzi, L., Horner, R.H., & Good, R.H. (2006). Effects of behavior support team composition on the technical adequacy and contextual-fit of behavior support plans. *Journal of Special Education, 40*(3), 160–170.

Carr, E.G., Dunlap, G., Horner, R.H., Koegel, R.L., Turnbull, A.P., Sailor, W., . . . Fox, L. (2002). Positive behavior support: Evolution of an applied science. *Journal of Positive Behavior Interventions, 4*, 4–16.

Colvin, G., Sugai, G., Good, R.H., & Lee, Y. (1997). Using active supervision and precorrection to improve transition behaviors in an elementary school. *School Psychology Quarterly, 12*(4), 344–363.

Cooper, J.O., Heron, T.E., & Heward, W.L. (2007). *Applied behavior analysis* (2nd ed.). Upper Saddle River, NJ: Pearson.

Elliott, D., & Mihalic, S. (2004). Issues in disseminating and replicating effective prevention programs. *Prevention Science, 4*, 83–105.

Fixsen, D.L., Naoom, S.F., Blase, K.A., Friedman, R.M., & Wallace, F. (2005). *Implementation research: A synthesis of the literature.* Tampa, FL: University of South Florida, Louis de la Parte Florida Mental Health Institute, The National Implementation Research Network.

Fuchs, D., & Fuchs, L. (1996). Consultation as a technology and the politics of school reform: Reactions to the issue. *Remedial and Special Education, 17*, 386–392.

Heward, W.L. Heron, T.E., Neef, N.A., Peterson, S.M., Sainato, D.M., Cartledge, G., . . . Dardig, J.C. (Eds.). (2005). *Focus on behavior analysis in education: Achievements, challenges, and opportunities.* Upper Saddle River, NJ: Pearson.

Horner, R.H., Sugai, G., Todd, A.W., & Lewis-Palmer, T. (2005). School-wide positive behavior support. In L. Bambara & L. Kern (Eds.), *Individualized supports for students with problem behaviors: Designing positive behavior plans* (pp. 359–390). New York, NY: Guilford Press.

Stokes, T.F., & Baer, D.M. (1977). An implicit technology of generalization. *Journal of Applied Behavior Analysis, 10*, 349–367.

Strain, P.S., Barton, E.E., & Dunlap, G. (2012). Lessons learned about the utility of social validity. *Education and Treatment of Children, 35*(2), 183–200.

Sulzer, B., & Mayer, G.R. (1972). *Behavior modification procedures for school personnel.* Hinsdale, IL: Dryden Press.

Sugai, G., & Horner, R.H. (2002). The evolution of discipline practices: School-wide positive behavior supports. In J.K. Luiselli & C. Diament (Eds.), *Behavior psychology in the schools: Innovations in evaluation, support, and consultation* (pp. 23–50). New York, NY: Haworth.

Thorndike, E. (1911). *Animal intelligence.* New York, NY: Macmillan.

Watson, J.B., & Raynor, R. (1920). Conditioned emotional reactions. *Journal of Experimental Psychology, 3*, 1–14.

Wickstrom, K.F., Jones, K.M., LaFleur, L.H., & Witt, J.C. (1998). An analysis of treatment integrity in school-based behavioral consultation. *School Psychology Quarterly, 13*, 141–154.

Woolery, M.R., Bailey, D.B., Jr., & Sugai, G.M. (1988). *Effective teaching: Principles and procedures of applied behavior analysis with exceptional children.* Boston, MA: Allyn & Bacon.

Wolf, M.M. (1978). Social validity: The case of subjective measurement of how applied behavior analysis is finding its heart. *Journal of Applied Behavior Analysis, 11*, 203–214.

Antecedent Strategies to Change Behavior

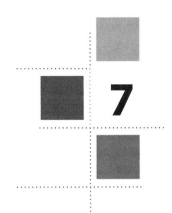

Sheldon L. Loman and Amanda K. Sanford

Preventing challenging behaviors while simultaneously actively promoting appropriate behaviors is a hallmark of positive behavior support (PBS; Carr et al., 2002). Research has adjusted the lens of behavior management from its historic focus on reactive strategies to include a more comprehensive, proactive vision that seeks to modify antecedent events that precede problematic behavior (e.g., Kern, Choutka, & Sokol, 2002). Antecedent strategies play an integral role in deeming problem behavior irrelevant, inefficient, and ineffective (Horner, 2000), while concurrently making replacement responses more likely (Wolery & Gast, 1984). Strategies based on the manipulation and arrangement of antecedents have tremendous implications in the design of comprehensive behavior supports for individuals in home, school, and community settings.

This chapter addresses the basic principles of behavior so practitioners of PBS can understand and use antecedent manipulations to influence behavior (APBS, 2007, section III-B, 1–8). The antecedent strategies that will be discussed include 1) curricular modifications, 2) instructional modifications, 3) modification of routines, 4) opportunities for choice/control throughout the day, 5) clear expectations, 6) precorrection, and 7) errorless learning. Guiding principles for designing antecedent strategies based on PBS values and technology will be presented along with examples of the application of these principles with three individuals of differing ages and abilities within school and community settings.

ANTECEDENT AND SETTING EVENT STRATEGIES DEFINED

The framework and principles behind the four-term contingency (see Figure 7.1) are central to the design of individual behavior supports. Interventions can be designed to address any or all levels of the four-term contingency; however this chapter focuses on antecedent interventions that address

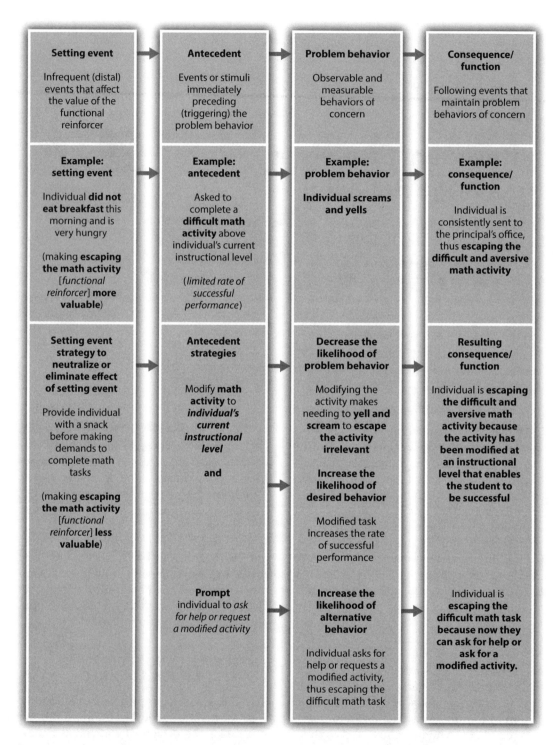

Figure 7.1. Four-term contingency with definitions of terms and examples. (From Borgmeier, C., & Loman, S. [2011]. *Training school personnel to facilitate brief FBA/BIP through problem-solving teams.* Paper presented at the 2011 National PBIS Leadership Forum, Rosemont, IL. Adapted by permission of OSEP Technical Assistance Center on Positive Behavioral Interventions and Supports.)

behavior occurrences. Two classes of antecedent strategies will be addressed in this chapter: 1) distal antecedents and 2) proximal antecedents. Distal antecedents, or "setting events" (Horner, Vaughn, Day, & Ard, 1996), are events that "change the likelihood of a targeted behavior at a later point in time by momentarily altering the value of consequences" (p. 382). Setting events may also be considered "distal" in proximity to the problem behavior, as they usually occur in environments other than where a problem behavior occurs. Examples of setting events include missed medications, sleep deprivation, and hunger. Strategies that address distal antecedents in this chapter will hereafter be termed *setting event strategies*. Setting event strategies seek to minimize the likelihood or neutralize the effect of setting events (e.g., Horner, Albin, Todd, Newton, & Sprague, 2011).

Proximal antecedents (also referred to as *discriminative stimuli*, or S^d) are those events or stimuli that immediately precede (or signal) the occurrence of a targeted behavior. A targeted behavior following a proximal antecedent that is reinforced is likely to continue to occur (Cooper, Heron, & Heward, 2007). For example, a teacher may present a difficult task (proximal antecedent event) to a student. Immediately, the student screams and throws materials (problem behavior), which results in the student being sent to the principal's office. The difficult task immediately preceded the problem behavior that was reinforced by being sent to the principal's office; if this pattern continued, the difficult task may be considered a proximal antecedent. From this point forward in this chapter, strategies that address proximal antecedents (or discriminative stimuli) will be referred to simply as *antecedent strategies*. Antecedent strategies have been defined as interventions that alter events prior to the occurrence of problem behavior that result in a decrease in the likelihood of problem behavior and/or an increase in the likelihood of desired behavior (Carr, Reeve, & Magito-McLaughlin, 1996; Carr et al., 2002).

Antecedent strategies hold several advantages in reducing problem behavior as compared with consequence-based, reactive strategies (Bambara & Kern, 2005). Kern and Clemens (2007) reported that antecedent strategies 1) "prevent problematic behavior from occurring" (p. 66) by removing events that precede the problem behavior; 2) tend to be "quick acting" (p. 66) because removing triggering events usually results in an immediate reduction of problem behavior (Kern, Bambara, & Fogt, 2002); 3) correct a mismatch between the environment and an individual's skills, strengths, and preferences (Kern, Gallagher, Starosta, Hickman, & George, 2006); and 4) enhance the environment by eliminating aversive events while increasing events that promote desirable behavior. Despite the strengths of antecedent-based strategies, antecedent events are strongly influenced by the context of consequences (Miltenberger, 2006). Consequently, interventions based solely on antecedent strategies without addressing consequence strategies may not be sufficient to change problem behavior or teach new appropriate behaviors (Walker, Shea, & Bauer, 2004). Therefore, this chapter will frame antecedent strategies as one component of a comprehensive behavior support plan (BSP) in which all components of the four-term contingency should be addressed.

POSITIVE BEHAVIOR SUPPORT TECHNOLOGY AND VALUES GUIDING PRINCIPLES OF ANTECEDENT STRATEGIES

PBS has emerged as a field because of its strong commitment to both values and technology focused on improving an individual's overall quality of life (Dunlap, Sailor, Horner, & Sugai, 2009). The values and technology of PBS have emphasized the use of the empirically supported principles of applied behavior analysis (ABA; Baer, Wolf, & Risley, 1968) guided by a person-centered (Holburn & Vietze, 2002; see Chapters 4 and 13), team-based approach that promotes an individual's self-determination (e.g., decision making, control over environment; Wehmeyer, 2005; see Chapters 17 and 18) and inclusion in natural settings, such as general education classrooms and community settings (Carr et al., 2002; Fox, Vaughn, Dunlap, & Bucy, 1997). These values critically inform the design and implementation of antecedent strategies based on ABA principles that appropriately fit the individual and context where strategies are implemented.

Though there has not been a consensus as to the features that are essential to the design of antecedent strategies, several guidelines have been recommended that epitomize PBS values and practices (Chandler & Dahlquist, 2010; Crone & Horner, 2003; Horner et al., 2011; Kern & Clarke, 2005; O'Neill et al., 1997). This chapter will present a number of specific research-based practices but will place an emphasis on designing antecedent strategies based on the five guiding principles that are consistent with PBS values and technology, presented in Table 7.1.

Guiding Principle 1: Antecedent Strategies Should Be Person Centered and Individualized

This feature is consistent with PBS values of person-centered approaches to increase self-determination (Dunlap et al., 2009). In addition, the incorporation of preferences and

respect for an individual's choice are important aspects of an intervention that seeks to prevent the occurrence of problem behavior (Bambara, Ager, & Roger, 1994; Carlson et al., 2008). Including the individual in the assessment and design of their behavior interventions may increase their personal investment in the plan, increasing the likelihood of success (Kincaid, 1996). Furthermore, presenting materials and content that are functional, interesting, and stimulating may decrease the likelihood of problem behavior (Ferro, Foster-Johnson, & Dunlap, 1996).

Guiding Principle 2: Antecedent Strategies Must Directly Address the Function that Problem Behavior Serves

A central assumption of PBS is that problem behavior serves a function for the individual engaging in the behavior (Kern & Clarke, 2005). Interventions that address the function of problem behavior are more successful than those that are not function based (e.g., Ingram, Lewis-Palmer, & Sugai, 2005; Newcomer & Lewis, 2004). Furthermore, functional communication training (Carr & Durand, 1985) has been established as an effective practice for teaching individuals appropriate, alternative means to express their desires or request a functional reinforcer. Therefore, once it is determined that an individual is engaging in challenging

Table 7.1. Positive behavior support (PBS) values and guiding principles for designing antecedent strategies

Guiding principle	PBS values/technology
1. Antecedent strategies should be person centered and individualized.	• Person-centered planning (Holburn & Vietze, 2002) • Self-determination strategies (Wehmeyer, 2005) • Wraparound services (Eber, Sugai, Smith, & Scott, 2002)
2. Antecedent strategies must directly address the function that problem behavior serves.	• Function-based support (O'Neill et al., 1997)
3. Antecedent strategies should directly address the antecedents that trigger the problem behavior and seek to neutralize setting events when possible.	• Applied behavior analysis (ABA; Baer, Wolf, & Risley, 1968) • Social and ecological validity (Wolf, 1978)
4. Antecedent strategies should be practical and fit the context, values, and resources of implementers.	• Contextual fit (Albin et al., 1996) • Multicomponent planning (Crone & Horner, 2003)
5. Antecedent strategies should reflect the types of procedures that occur within typical settings.	• Inclusion (Sailor, 1996) • Normalization (Wolfensberger, 1983)

behaviors in order to obtain or avoid something, alternative communication methods that serve the same function as the challenging behavior should be taught and prompted using antecedent strategies. (See Chapter 21 for more information on functional communication training.)

Antecedent interventions should be based on assessment results that present a hypothesis of the maintaining function (e.g., obtaining/escaping attention, obtaining/escaping stimuli, obtaining/escaping tangibles; Horner & Day, 1991) of an individual's problem behavior. For example, if gaining attention is hypothesized as the function of an individual's behavior, antecedent interventions should be outlined that ensure that attention is available or that those events that triggered the behavior are adjusted. The individual should be taught to elicit attention in appropriate ways. If avoiding or escaping an aversive stimuli or event is the hypothesized function of an individual's behavior, preventive steps should be taken to eliminate or modify those stimuli or the events affecting the problem behavior. The individual should be taught to escape nonpreferred stimuli by using more appropriate forms of communication. In cases where sensation or automatic reinforcement is a hypothesized function, antecedent strategies might involve enriching the individual's environment so that sensory stimuli that serve the same function as the problem behavior are accessible. Antecedent strategies organized by behavior function are summarized in Table 7.3, later in the chapter.

Guiding Principle 3: Antecedent Strategies Should Directly Address Immediate Antecedents that Trigger the Problem Behavior and Seek to Neutralize Setting Events When Possible

Strategies should be outlined that seek to remove or modify the hypothesized antecedent events to eliminate the occurrence of problem behavior. For example, if a student is engaging in problem behaviors in order

to escape a difficult math task (e.g., double-digit multiplication), an antecedent strategy may involve simplifying the task (e.g., single-digit multiplication) or removing the task entirely. Antecedent strategies may also seek to associate stimuli (or prompts) with desirable behavior (Kern, Sokol, & Dunlap, 2006). For example, a teacher may 1) verbally prompt a student to use his augmentative communication device to make a request (desired behavior) and 2) remind him that he may receive a reinforcing item or activity when using his device to make this request. Other examples of antecedent prompts include gesturing, modeling, pictures, written directions, and physical guidance. Furthermore, when it is known that a setting event has occurred, setting event strategies may 1) remove or modify triggering antecedents that increase the likelihood of problem behavior or 2) add events that increase appropriate behavior (e.g., attention from a positive adult figure).

Guiding Principle 4: Antecedent Strategies Should Be Practical and Fit the Context, Values, and Resources of Implementers

The development of interventions by a collaborative team consisting of staff and parents that will implement the plan will help ensure that interventions fit the skills, resources, and values of the implementers (Albin et al., 1996; Benazzi, Horner, & Good, 2006; Kern & Dunlap, 1998). This collaborative team should ensure they outline interventions that are 1) consistent with the philosophy and practices of staff or family and 2) realistic for staff or family members to implement with fidelity.

Guiding Principle 5: Antecedent Strategies Should Reflect the Types of Procedures that Occur within Typical Settings with Other Individuals

Based on the principles of normalization and inclusion that are central to the values of PBS (Carr et al., 2002), antecedent strategies for individuals that display problem behavior should resemble strategies for students who do not display problem behaviors. Natural stimuli (or artificial stimuli paired with natural stimuli) used within situations that already exist in natural settings will increase the likelihood that new appropriate behaviors will be maintained and generalized (Chandler, Lubek, & Fowler, 1992; Falvey, 1995). In addition, normative interventions (i.e., interventions that would typically be used with other individuals within the same setting) have been described by Chandler and Dahlquist (2010) as more acceptable to staff, students, and families. They surmised that normative strategies might be easier to implement due to the staff's familiarity with ongoing procedures or their natural occurrence within typical routines. For example, a normative intervention may involve a student carrying a point card (with his or her daily expectations listed for the teacher to rate), much like the point cards carried by his or her peers. The similarity in the point cards makes the intervention easier for the teacher to implement and less stigmatizing for the student.

ESTABLISHING EFFECTIVE HOST ENVIRONMENTS

PBS researchers recognize that the effective implementation of behavior supports for individuals is highly dependent on the context in which they are delivered. Even a well-designed individualized BSP that is technically sound and contextually consistent will fail when implemented in chaotic environments (Dunlap et al., 2009). Therefore, it is critical to establish home, school, and community environments that can host effective practices. Antecedent strategies applied within a broader context (i.e., classrooms, community settings) strive to establish environments that are safe, positive, predictable, and motivating (Sugai, Horner, & Gresham, 2002). The application of antecedent strategies within these larger contexts based on PBS values and

technology holds promise for preventing the need for intensive individualized supports, while also setting the foundation for effectively supporting individuals that require them (Bradshaw, Koth, Thornton, & Leaf, 2009; Horner et al., 2009).

Addressing challenging behaviors involves first focusing on establishing effective host environments whereby the occurrence of problem behavior is reduced and problem behaviors are dealt with more efficiently and effectively when they occur (Sugai & Horner, 2009; Sugai, Horner, & Gresham, 2002; Kern & Clemens, 2007). Literature suggests that we can prevent the occurrence of problem behavior by 1) creating positive classroom, school, and community climates (e.g., Epstein, Atkins, Cullinan, Kutash, & Weaver, 2008; Greenberg et al., 2003); 2) providing opportunities for choice throughout the day (e.g., Carlson, Luiselli, Slyman, & Markowski, 2008; Kern, Bambara, & Fogt, 2002); 3) establishing effective community (Lucyshyn, Dunlap, & Albin, 2002), schoolwide (Horner & Sugai, 2000), and classroom behavior management systems (Colvin & Lazar, 1995; Kern & Clemens, 2007); and 4) ensuring high rates of success (e.g., Preciado, Horner, & Baker, 2009; Sanford & Horner, 2013).

ASSESSMENTS TO DEFINE ANTECEDENT VARIABLES

When broader preventive strategies are implemented with high fidelity but chronic problem behaviors continue to occur for an individual, further assessments need to identify the variables that are triggering and maintaining problem behaviors. Person-centered planning approaches (Holburn & Vietze, 2002), preference assessments (Lohrmann, O'Rourke, & Browder, 1998), functional behavioral assessments (FBA; O'Neill et al., 1997; see Chapter 15), structural analysis procedures (Gage & Lewis, 2010), curriculum-based assessments (Payne, Marks, & Bogan, 2007), and ecological inventories (Browder & Spooner, 2011) have all been used to identify antecedent variables that affect an individual's behavior. Table 7.2 summarizes these assessments, their outcomes, their procedures, and measures available. All the assessment methods presented in Table 7.2 are not necessarily used in the development of every individual BSP; however, these methods are used to essentially outline a hypothesis statement (e.g., the four-term contingency displayed in Figure 7.1) that clearly identifies the setting events, antecedents to the problem behavior, and the functions that the problem behavior serves for the student (Horner et al., 2006). Consistent with the person-centered values of PBS, it is emphasized that, to every extent possible, individuals are included throughout the assessment process.

COMPETING BEHAVIOR PATHWAY: LINKING ASSESSMENTS TO INTERVENTIONS

A competing behavior pathway (see Figure 7.2) visually frames the FBA hypothesis statement, forming the center of the pathway, to guide the BSP (Crone & Horner, 2003; Horner, Albin, Todd, Newton, & Sprague, 2011; see Chapters 14 and 15). An FBA summary statement within the competing behavior pathway should read, "When 'A' (antecedent events immediately preceding problem behavior), the individual will 'B' (observable behavior of concern), which typically results in 'C' (following events occurring directly after the problem behavior). It

Table 7.2. Assessments for identifying antecedent strategies

Assessment	Outcomes in identifying antecedent strategies	Procedures	References
Person-centered planning approaches	Identification of learning history, cultural values, and motivating influences of behavior	Meetings held where the focus participant (and their family) is involved and offers perspectives on their values, goals, and concerns	• Planning Alternative Tomorrows with Hope (PATH; Pearpoint, O'Brien, & Forest, 1993) • Personal futures planning (Mount, 1984)
Preference assessments	Identification of preferred items or activities for individuals with limited verbal skills	Systematically provide access to perceived desired items or activities to determine actual preferences of the individual	• Systematic preference assessments (Lohrmann-O'Rourke & Browder, 1998) • Free access or constrained choice assessments (Johnston, Reichle, Feeley, & Jones, 2012)
Functional behavioral assessment (FBA)	Identification of variables triggering and maintaining functions of problem behaviors	Records review, interviews, checklists, rating scales, and surveys of participant and family, direct observations of individual in problematic routines/situations	• (Chandler & Dahlquist, 2010; Crone & Horner, 2003; O'Neill et al., 1997)
Structural analysis	Systematically testing hypotheses developed from FBA by examining the frequency of problem behavior in the presence and absence of specific antecedent variables	Reversal or alternating treatment designs where typical conditions are contrasted with conditions in which the instructional or environmental antecedents are modified or eliminated	• (Gage & Lewis, 2010; Kern, Sokol, & Dunlap, 2006; Stichter, Randolph, Kay, & Gage, 2009)
Curriculum-based assessments and ecological inventories	Identification of instruction-level materials so that demands of instruction match student skill levels	Survey-level assessment and direct observations within instructional environments	• (Browder & Spooner, 2011; Payne, Marks, & Bogan, 2007)

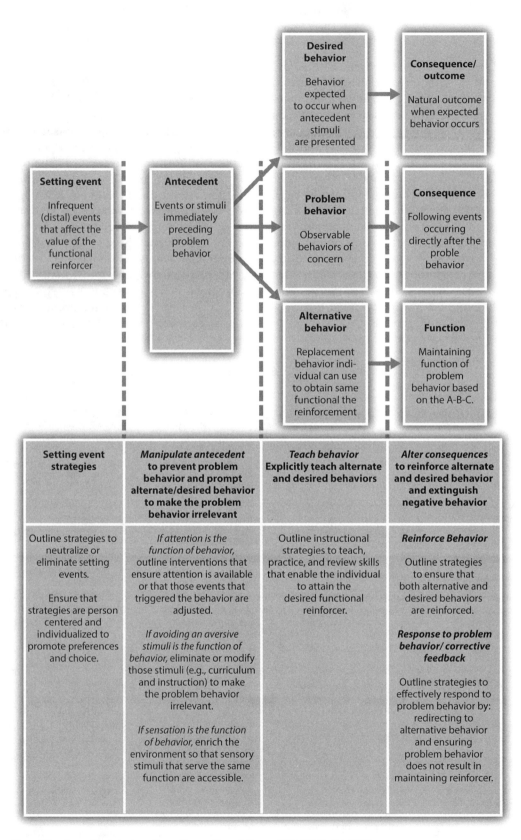

Figure 7.2. Competing behavior pathway. (*Sources:* Crone & Horner, 2003; O'Neill et al., 1997.)

is hypothesized the individual's behavior is maintained by 'X' (maintaining function of problem behavior based on the FBA). These behaviors are more likely to occur when 'Y' (setting event occurs)."

The competing behavior pathway in Figure 7.2 also identifies the desired behavior (box above the problem behavior) and common responses for engaging in those behaviors as well as an alternative behavior that serves the same function (box below problem behavior) but has increased social acceptability when compared with the problem behavior. This model provides a framework to logically link the multiple intervention procedures and support strategies of a comprehensive BSP to information collected in the FBA. The competing behavior pathway framework seeks to ensure that all elements of a BSP are technically sound.

A technically sound BSP should include antecedent interventions based on the five guiding features presented earlier in this chapter (see Table 7.1) that seek to neutralize or eliminate possible setting events and antecedents that occasion problem behaviors. In addition, a technically sound BSP should include instructional strategies to prompt and teach replacement behaviors that will enable the student to achieve desired consequences in more socially acceptable ways (e.g., functional communication training; see Chapter 21). Finally, a BSP should outline strategies to provide the student with corrective feedback and reactive strategy procedures that directly address the function of the problem behavior when the problem behavior occurs (specifically addressed in Chapter 8).

FUNCTION-BASED ANTECEDENT STRATEGIES

The goal of antecedent strategies is to structure the environment to prevent problem behaviors, prompt desired behaviors, and enhance motivation (Kern & Clemens, 2007). Because antecedent interventions must address the function of behavior, the following descriptions of antecedent interventions are organized as addressing either negative or positive reinforcement. As a reminder from Chapter 6, negative reinforcement occurs when a behavior increases due to the removal of stimuli. Behavior that results in negative reinforcement is commonly considered escape-maintained behavior that seeks to avoid aversive instructional, physical, sensory, or social experiences. Behavior that is maintained by positive reinforcement can be considered behavior that seeks to obtain desired social attention, sensory experiences, activities, or tangible items. Positive reinforcement occurs when a behavior increases due to the addition of stimuli. Behavior that results in positive reinforcement may be considered behavior that seeks to obtain desired social attention (i.e., attention-maintained behavior), tangibles (e.g., toys, foods), or physical and sensory experiences. (See Chapter 8 for additional discussion of positive and negative reinforcement.)

Examples of function-based antecedent strategies supported by research are presented in Table 7.3. As several antecedent strategies have been shown to be effective across multiple behavior functions, Table 7.3 is organized in such a way to indicate those functions for which a specific strategy is typically applied. Also, within the review of function-based antecedent strategies, in the next sections of this chapter, case study examples with completed competing behavior pathways (see Figures 7.3, 7.4, and 7.5) are provided.

Antecedent Strategies to Address Escaping Instructional and/or Physical Tasks

There are several reasons an individual's problem behavior may be maintained by escaping an instructional or physical task. The individual may find the task too difficult, in which case they may be trying to avoid the frustration of failing repeatedly at the task or avoid embarrassment of failing in front of peers or adults. The individual also may find the task too easy, in which case they may be trying to escape the task because they are bored. The individual also may be disinterested in the task and engaging in problem behavior

Table 7.3. Function-based antecedent strategies

Function						
Negative/escape			Positive/obtain			
Instructional/ physical	Sensory	Social	Social	Sensory	Tangible/activities	Antecedent strategy
X						Precorrect/preteach (or prime) desired behavior (Wilde, Koegel, & Koegel, 1992).
X						Clarify/simplify instructions to the task or activity (Dunlap, Kern-Dunlap, Clarke, & Robbins, 1991; Munk & Repp, 1994).
X	X	X				Provide choices/preference in activity (Dunlap & Kern, 1993; Dyer, Dunlap, & Winterling, 1990; Munk & Karsh, 1999; Reichle et al., 1996).
X	X	X				Provide frequent noncontingent breaks from aversive activity/people (Carr et al., 2000).
	X	X				Allow individual to work independently (Kern & Clarke, 2005).
X						Match task demands to student skill level and interest (Kennedy & Meyer, 1998).
X	X					Modify duration of tasks (Dunlap & Kern, 1993; Smith, Iwata, Goh, & Shore, 1995).
X						Intersperse easy tasks with difficult tasks (Horner, Day, Sprague, O'Brien, & Heathfield, 1991).
X						Reduce the number/frequency of demands (Smith et al., 1995).
X	X					Change the features (e.g., medium, materials, intensity) of task demands (Kern & Dunlap, 1998; Pace, Iwata, Cowdery, Andree, & McIntyre, 1993; Touchette, MacDonald, & Langer, 1985).
X	X	X				Prompt to ask for a break when needed (Carr & Durand, 1985; Wacker et al., 1990).
X			X			Provide assistance with difficult tasks (Ebanks & Fisher, 2003).
X	X	X		X	X	Remove specific stimuli (e.g., people, objects) that set the occasion for the problem behavior (Rapp & Vollmer, 2005).
X	X	X	X	X	X	Prompt self-management strategies (monitor and record own behavior; Koegel & Koegel, 1990).
X			X			Utilize behavior momentum strategies (Mace et al., 1988).
X		X	X	X	X	Embed task demands in reinforcing activities (Carr et al., 1994).
X	X	X	X	X	X	Use visual activity schedules/social stories (Gray & Garand, 1993) to increase predictability of demands (Lalli, Casey, Goh, & Merlino., 1994) or to cue upcoming tasks.
X	X	X	X	X	X	Provide picture symbols, augmentative communication devices, and/or prompts that enable the student to request alternative activities, tasks, materials, people, locations, or break from an activity (Durand, 1999).
			X		X	Precorrect for the transition from a desired item/activity (Kern & Clarke, 2005).
			X	X	X	Introduce stimuli identified by a preference assessment that can compete with triggering antecedent (Morrison & Rosales-Ruiz, 1997).
			X	X	X	Enrich the environment (provide noncontingent access to reinforcers; Carr & LeBlanc, 2006).
			X			Provide peer-mediated instruction/tutoring (Carter, Cushing, Clark, & Kennedy, 2005).

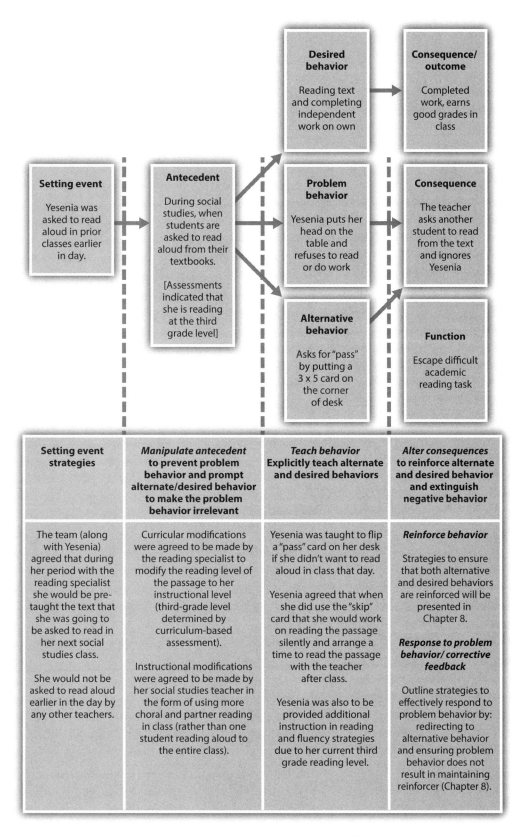

Figure 7.3. Competing behavior pathway for Yesenia. (*Sources:* Crone & Horner, 2003; O'Neill et al., 1997.)

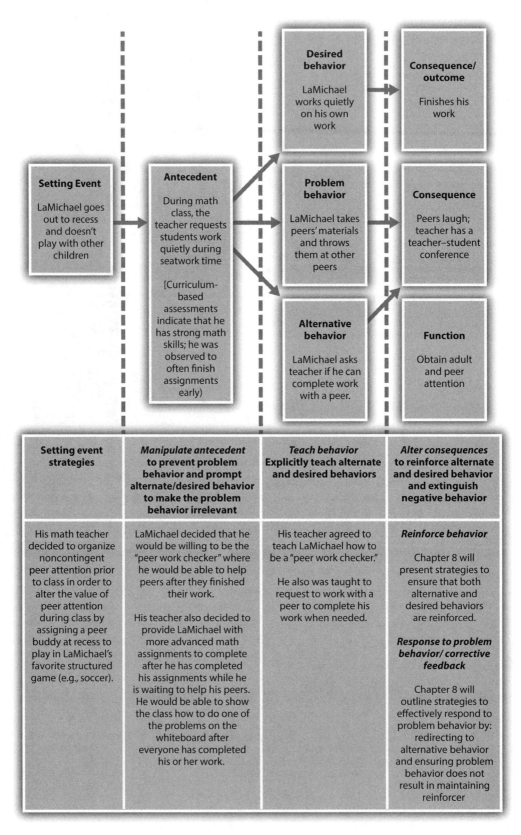

Figure 7.4. Competing behavior pathway for LaMichael. (*Sources:* Crone & Horner, 2003; O'Neill et al., 1997.)

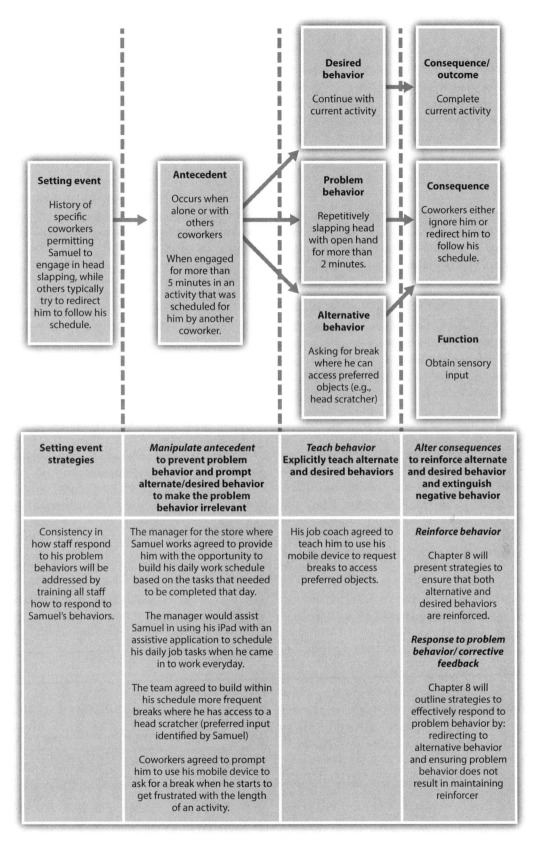

Figure 7.5. Competing behavior pathway for Samuel. (*Sources:* Crone & Horner, 2003; O'Neill et al., 1997.)

to avoid the task. The key feature of interventions designed for individuals escaping such nonpreferred tasks is that the tasks must be perceived as less aversive so that the student is less likely to want to escape the task. Interventions should also teach an appropriate form of behavior that can be used to obtain the same function—that is, escaping or avoiding the task.

Curricular modifications, such as matching task demands to student skill level and interest, may reduce the averseness of tasks. Several studies have shown that problem behavior can be reduced for students engaged in escape-maintained problem behavior if the task demands are adjusted to match the student's skill level (e.g., Preciado et al., 2009; Sanford & Horner, 2013). In reading, for example, this can be accomplished by completing a survey-level assessment to identify the student's instructional level (see Table 7.2; Shapiro, 2004; Tremptow, Burns, & McComas, 2007) and matching the student's reading materials to their instructional level (e.g., Sanford & Horner, 2013). This could involve increasing or decreasing task difficulty depending on the results of the assessment. The difficulty of the task can also be altered by preteaching the academic task as illustrated in Preciado et al. (2009), which pretaught academic content in Spanish and decreased problem behavior and increased students' performance of academic tasks in English reading.

Another curricular modification that may be helpful in preventing problem behaviors involves the reduction in the length of difficulty of a task demand (e.g., Sanford & Horner, 2013) by interspersing easy tasks with more difficult tasks (e.g., Cates & Skinner, 2000), both of which may reduce the aversiveness of the tasks, thereby decreasing the likelihood of the occurrence of problem behavior. Similarly, the use of behavior momentum strategies (also referred to as pretask requesting or interspersed requests; Horner, Day, Sprague, O'Brien, & Heathfield, 1991) can reduce unsafe behaviors (e.g., self-injury, aggression, tantrums) that can be frustrating to parents and teachers (Mace

et al., 1988). Behavior momentum involves the presentation of a series of requests for behaviors that are both easy for a student to perform (i.e., high-probability requests) and commonly associated with a high rate of reinforcement. This is quickly followed by the presentation of a request for a behavior that has a low probability of occurrence (Romano & Roll, 2000). Distributing the difficulty of tasks to ensure high rates of success plays a key role in preventing problematic behaviors while promoting new appropriate skills.

Instructional modifications that include explicit teaching of academic content also reduce the likelihood of problem behavior. When content concepts are taught explicitly, it increases students' likelihood of correctly completing the instructional task, thereby increasing the likelihood of being reinforced for the task. Explicit teaching may involve presenting tasks to students at their instructional level through curricular modifications and guided practice that may involve more significant levels of prompting that are eventually faded. The key is to ensure a high likelihood of success. This kind of teaching is framed as errorless learning (Terrace, 1963), which provides enough prompting that students produce the correct behavior and gradually fades the prompting as students are able to complete the task more independently. This level of support increases the rates for correct completion of the task and also increases the reinforcement students receive for appropriate behavior, thereby decreasing the likelihood they will engage in problem behavior.

Escape Academic Task Example (see Figure 7.3)

Meet Yesenia, an eighth grader who was referred for behavior support strategies to address behavior and academic difficulties. An FBA was conducted for her that involved interviewing 1) Yesenia, 2) her parents, and 3) her teachers and directly observing Yesenia during identified problematic routines. After holding a meeting to discuss the results of the assessments, Yesenia and a team consisting of her mother, the reading specialist, her social studies teacher, and the school's behavior specialist outlined a BSP using a competing behavior pathway. The plan was based on the following summary statement: "When students are asked to read aloud in social studies text, Yesenia puts her head on the table and refuses to read or do work in order to escape the reading and academic tasks. This behavior is more likely to occur when Yesenia has been asked to read aloud in classes earlier in the day." Before the team determined a helpful intervention strategy, they first identified the function of Yesenia's behavior—to escape the academic reading task.

Based on the guiding principles presented in Table 7.1, they identified setting event strategies that might alter the value of the reinforcement. They considered removing the requirement to read in prior classes and in her social studies class, which would have reduced her problem behavior but probably wouldn't have helped with her below-average course work. Since being asked to read in prior classes increased the likelihood that Yesenia would engage in problem behavior, the team considered why Yesenia might find the reading tasks aversive. They wanted to know if the reading was too easy, too difficult, or not interesting to Yesenia. A survey-level assessment (Shapiro, 2004) was conducted by the reading specialist and determined that Yesenia was reading at the third-grade level but was being asked to read an eighth-grade-level text. In order to make the reading task less aversive, the team decided that curricular modifications would be made by the reading specialist that included modifying the content of the social studies text to her instructional reading level. In addition, Yesenia would benefit from participating in the school's extra reading-help period before her social studies class. In this class, Yesenia was taught multisyllabic-word reading and fluency strategies that would help her read more effectively. The reading specialist also pretaught the text Yesenia was being asked to read in social studies, which directly decreased the difficulty of the passage reading she was asked to do in class since she could practice it beforehand. To alter the antecedent, her social studies teacher agreed to highlight the part of the text Yesenia would be asked to read in class so she could practice it with her reading teacher beforehand. The social studies teacher also agreed to use more choral and partner reading in social studies class. Yesenia and her peers were also taught how to be a good reading partner (reading and correcting

their partner's errors). This reduced the aversiveness of reading aloud since Yesenia could get help from a partner if she didn't know a word. Finally, Yesenia was taught to flip a "skip" card on her desk if she didn't want to read in class. Her social studies teacher told her she could use the skip card if she didn't want to be asked to read individually, in which case he would call on another student.

Antecedent Strategies to Address Escaping Sensory Stimulation

Individuals may engage in problem behavior to escape what they may perceive as overstimulating situations, such as excessively loud or bright environments. Antecedent strategies to address this function of behavior might include making environmental accommodations to limit the amount of stimuli that may trigger problem behavior. For example, for a student who seeks to escape from a loud classroom, the use of carpets and soundproofing materials may be an environmental accommodation that reduces the level of noise, thus reducing the likelihood of problem behavior. In addition, individuals may use self-monitoring strategies to identify when they are overstimulated and select to use earplugs or headphones to reduce noise levels. Alternative communication systems may also be used for an individual to appropriately communicate the need to leave a situation. To ultimately eliminate the occurrence of problem behavior due to overstimulating situations, one can modify an individual's schedule to help them avoid aversive settings (Rapp & Vollmer, 2005) or limit the duration of activities by building in regular breaks (Carr et al., 2000).

Antecedent Strategies to Address Escaping Social Attention

In those cases where escaping social attention is the maintaining function of problem behavior, it is important to arrange the environment in such a way that social interaction is not aversive. One way of doing this is arranging the environment so that individuals have enough personal space. In addition, using visual schedules and other visual strategies such as Social Stories (Gray & Garand, 1993) can provide individuals with advanced notice of when social situations will occur. Social Stories may be useful for visually prompting a number of behaviors, including 1) following directions and using a quiet voice (Brownell, 2002), 2) social-communication skills (Norris & Datitilo, 1999; Theimann & Goldstein, 2001), 3) greetings and sharing materials (Swaggert et al., 1995), 4) self-help skills (Smith, 2001; Hagiwara & Myles, 1999), and 5) on-task or compliance behaviors (Brownell, 2002; Smith, 2001). However, in the case of avoiding social attention from a specific person, Social Stories can be used to remind the target individual and others to keep a comfortable proximity (according to the target individual). Finally, a Social Story, when used in conjunction with functional communication training in an alternative behavior, may teach and prompt the individual to appropriately terminate the interaction or request that others give him or her personal space.

Antecedent Strategies to Address Obtaining Social Attention

When a problem behavior is maintained by obtaining peer and/or adult attention, antecedent strategies may rely on providing both contingent and noncontingent reinforcement. Noncontingent reinforcement is a function-based strategy in which the reinforcer for a problem behavior is provided to the individual irrespective of his or her behavior performance (Carr & LeBlanc, 2006). Basically, when noncontingent reinforcement is applied, an individual receives reinforcement on a schedule that is not dependent (i.e., not contingent) on their responses or behaviors. Examples of noncontingent attention may be to schedule peer or adult attention, especially preceding times when the problem behavior is most likely to occur. This could be achieved through pairing students with a peer to complete tasks,

assigning a lunch buddy, ensuring an adult checks in with the student at the beginning and throughout the school day, or using peer-mediated instruction and peer tutoring (Carter et al., 2005) or individualized or small group instruction provided by an adult.

Individuals can also be taught to recruit attention in a prosocial manner in order to gain access to the reinforcing attention without engaging in problem behavior. An example of this may be giving a student a self-monitoring system, in which the student raises her hand to ask the teacher to check her work after a specified number of problems are completed on a worksheet. Students may also be taught to use a communication system that allows them to ask to participate in a game or interact with peers or adults in another prosocial manner.

Obtain Attention from Peers and/or Adults Example (see Figure 7.4)

LaMichael is a third grader who has been referred to the behavior support team at his school for repeatedly throwing materials during math class. LaMichael has strong math skills and often finishes his work early, but his disruptive behavior is creating a problem for other students and the teacher. The behavior specialist conducted an FBA by interviewing LaMichael's teacher and observing LaMichael in routines the teacher identified as problematic. LaMichael's mother and his individualized support team met to outline a BSP using a competing behavior pathway (see Figure 7.4). Review Figure 7.4 and Table 7.1 to see how his team used the guiding principles to identify antecedent strategies to prevent problem behaviors while promoting alternative behaviors that resulted in obtaining adult and peer attention.

Antecedent Strategies to Address Obtaining Tangibles

Individuals may engage in problem behaviors in order to obtain or retain possession of a preferred object (e.g., toys, cell phones). Kern and Clarke (2005) provide a number of antecedent interventions to address this behavior function, including 1) providing a warning before terminating an activity, 2) scheduling a transitional activity, and 3) increasing the accessibility of items (for those individuals with limited communication skills). When it is essential that a preferred object be requested of someone with a history of utilizing problem behavior in order to retain objects, it may be useful to offer a less desirable substitute item in compensation (Morrison & Rosales-Ruiz, 1997). For example, if a student with a history of self-injurious behaviors is playing with a preferred toy that is property of the classroom and the student must make the transition to the bus to return home, classroom staff (after a number of attempts to request the toy from the student) may offer the student his or her own personal (less preferred) toy as a substitute in order to prevent the occurrence of a self-injurious tantrum.

Antecedent Strategies to Address Obtaining Sensory Stimulation

Obtaining sensory input (i.e., sensations of touch, temperature, sound, and movement) may be a reason individuals engage in behaviors such as head banging and hand flapping. When it is determined that an individual's behavior is sensory based (sometimes referred to as *automatic reinforcement*; Lermann & Rapp, 2006), an individual's team must work with him or her to determine whether the behavior is acceptable within the contexts where they are occurring. If the team decides that these behaviors are acceptable (e.g., behaviors that are not dangerous to the student or others like hand flapping or repetitive rocking), activities or times where these behaviors can occur without stigmatization could be offered within their schedule. If the behaviors are deemed harmful or stigmatizing within the environment (e.g., head banging, cutting oneself), an alternative sensory activity should be offered to the individual that meets the same sensory needs. Some examples of such

alternatives may include providing access to equipment such as head/back scratchers or brushes for individuals seeking stimulation of the head or body parts; safe, chewable objects for people seeking oral sensation; and squeezable objects for individuals desiring tactile input. Creating an enriched environment that provides noncontingent access to reinforcing sensory stimuli and activities has been considered an effective strategy for reducing problematic behaviors in individuals seeking to obtain sensory-based reinforcement (Carr & LeBlanc, 2006). Furthermore, sensory-based strategies should be employed with great caution, and the individual, their family, and support teams should determine protocols for use.

Obtaining Sensory Reinforcement Example (see Figure 7.5)

Samuel is a 20-year-old male who was assessed by a behavior specialist for repetitively slapping his head with the palm of his hand while working at the local grocery store. The competing behavior pathway (see Figure 7.5) displays the summary statement derived from a person-centered plan and FBA that included a structural analysis (Gage & Lewis, 2010). Samuel's team included Samuel, his parents, his supervisor at the grocery store, and another coworker that hangs out with Samuel when they are not working. They hypothesized that "during the performance of an activity that Samuel has not selected for more than 5 minutes, whether he is alone or with co-workers, he slaps his head with the palm of his hand in order to gain sensory input (as sometimes he is redirected and sometimes he is ignored by co-workers)." The team decided that the setting event of inconsistent responses from coworkers was something that they would address by training all staff how to respond to Samuel's behaviors. Specific antecedent strategies that the team identified for Samuel involved first providing him with the opportunity to build his daily work schedule based on the tasks that needed to be completed that day. The store supervisor of the grocery store agreed to assist Samuel to use his mobile device to do this when he came in to work every day. Next, Samuel was given more frequent breaks in his schedule, where he had access to a head scratcher (since this was the preferred sensory input identified by Samuel within the person-centered plan and preference assessment). Finally, a coworker agreed to train other coworkers to prompt Samuel to use his mobile device to ask for a break to use his head scratcher when he is frustrated with the length of an activity. Samuel's team agreed to monitor data on the number of "head-slapping" behaviors that occurred daily and present these data at his next team meeting in 2 weeks.

all components of a four-term contingency (setting events, antecedents, behaviors, and consequences) are addressed. The visual framework of a competing behavior pathway presented in this chapter can guide the development of a plan where intervention strategies coherently address the function of an individual's behavior. The case examples of Yesenia, LaMichael, and Samuel show the need for antecedent strategies that work in concert with the consequence strategies presented in Chapter 8.

CONCLUSION

A hallmark of PBS is emphasizing the prevention of problem behaviors while positively promoting appropriate behaviors. Antecedent strategies play an integral role in creating a context where all individuals experience safe, predictable, and consistent environments in which they learn, live, and work. Through enriching environments that provide choice and access to reinforcing events, curricular and instructional modifications, preteaching or prompting of alternative behaviors, or simply removing events that are known to precede the occurrence of problem behavior, antecedent strategies seek to quickly prevent an individual's problem behaviors and enhance their motivation. Five principles consistent with PBS research, values, and technology were presented in this chapter. These principles outlined that antecedent strategies should 1) be person centered and individualized; 2) directly address the function that problem behavior serves; 3) directly address the antecedents that trigger the problem behavior and seek to neutralize known setting events; 4) be practical and fit the context, values, and resources of implementers; and (5) reflect the types of procedures that occur within typical settings.

Despite their strengths, antecedent strategies should be considered necessary but not sufficient for changing problem behaviors or teaching new appropriate behaviors for all individuals. It is important that a comprehensive BSP be developed where

REFERENCES

Albin, R.W., Lucyshyn, J.M., Horner, R.H., & Flannery, K.B. (1996). Contextual fit for behavior support plans. In L.K. Koegel, R.L. Koegel, & G. Dunlap (Eds.), *Positive behavioral support* (pp. 81–98). Baltimore, MD: Paul H. Brookes Publishing Co.

Association for Positive Behavior Support (APBS). (2007). *Positive behavior support standards of practice: Individual level.* Retrieved from http://www.apbs.org/files/apbs_standards_of_practice_2013_format.pdf

Baer, D.M., Wolf, M.M., & Risley, T.R. (1968). Some current dimensions of applied behavior analysis. *Journal of Applied Behavior Analysis, 1*(1), 91–97. doi:10.1901/jaba.1987.20-313

Bambara, L.M., Ager, C., & Roger, F. (1994). The effects of choice and task preference on the work performance of adults with severe disabilities. *Journal of Applied Behavior Analysis, 27*(3), 555–556. doi:10.1901/jaba.1994.27-555

Benazzi, L., Horner, R.H., & Good, R.H. (2006). Effects of behavior support team composition on the technical adequacy and contextual fit of behavior support plans. *Journal of Special Education, 40*(3), 160–170. doi:10.1177/00224669060400030401

Borgmeier, C., & Loman, S. (2011). *Training school personnel to facilitate brief FBA/BIP through problem-solving teams.* Paper presented at the 2011 National PBIS Leadership Forum, Rosemont, IL. Retrieved from http://www.pbis.org/common/cms/files/Forum11_Presentations/B12_Borgmeier%20_Loman.pd

Bradshaw, C., Koth, C., Thornton, L., & Leaf, P. (2009). Altering school climate through school-wide positive behavioral interventions and supports: Findings from a group-randomized effectiveness trial. *Prevention Science, 10*(2), 100–115. doi:10.1007/s11121-008-0114-9

Browder, D.M., & Spooner, F. (2011). *Teaching students with moderate and severe disabilities.* New York, NY: Guilford Press.

Brownell, M.D. (2002). Musically adapted social stories to modify behaviors in students with autism: Four case studies. *Journal of Music Therapy, 39,* 117–144.

Carlson, J.I., Luiselli, J.K., Slyman, A.K., & Markowski, A. (2008). Choice-making as intervention for public disrobing in children with developmental disabilities. *Journal of Positive Behavior Interventions, 10,* 86–90. doi:10.1177/1098300707312511

Carr, E.G., & Durand, V.M. (1985). Reducing problem behaviors through functional communication training. *Journal of Applied Behavior Analysis, 18*(2), 111–126. doi:10.1901/jaba.1985.18-111

Carr, E.G., Dunlap, G., Horner, R.H., Koegel, R.L., Turnbull, A.P., Sailor, W., . . . Fox, L. (2002). Positive behavior support: Evolution of an applied science. *Journal of Positive Behavior Interventions, 4*(1), 4–16. doi:10.1177/10983007020040010

Carr, E.G., Levin, L., McConnachie, G., Carlson, J.I., Kemp, D.C., & Smith, C.E. (1994). *Communication-based intervention for problem behavior: A user's guide for producing positive change.* Baltimore, MD: Paul H. Brookes Publishing Co.

Carr, E.G., Reeve, C.E., & Magito-McLaughlin, D. (1996). Contextual influences on problem behavior in people with developmental disabilities. In L.K. Koegel, R.L. Koegel, & G. Dunlap (Eds.), *Positive behavioral support: Including people with difficult behaviors in the community* (pp.403–423). Baltimore, MD: Paul H. Brookes Publishing Co.

Carr, J.E., Coriaty, S., Wilder, D.A., Gaunt, B.T., Dozier, C.L., Britton, L.N., . . . Reed, C.L. (2000). A review of "noncontingent" reinforcement as treatment for the aberrant behavior of individuals with developmental disabilities. *Research in Developmental Disabilities, 21,* 377–391. doi:10.1016/S0891-4222(00)00050-0

Carr, J.E., & LeBlanc, L.A. (2006). Noncontingent reinforcement as antecedent behavior support. In J.K. Luiselli (Ed.), *Antecedent assessment and intervention: Supporting children and adults with developmental disabilities in community settings* (pp. 147–164). Baltimore, MD: Paul H. Brookes Publishing Co.

Carter, E.W., Cushing, L.S., Clark, H.M., & Kennedy, C.H. (2005). Effects of peer support interventions on students' access to the general curriculum and social interactions. *Research and Practice for Persons with Severe Disabilities, 30,* 15–25.

Cates, G.L., & Skinner, C.H. (2000). Getting remedial mathematics students to prefer homework with 20% and 40% more problems: An investigation of the strength of interspersing procedure. *Psychology in the Schools, 37,* 339–347. doi:10.1002/1520-6807(200007)37:4<349::AID-PITS5>3.0.CO;2-7

Chandler, L.K., & Dahlquist, C.M. (2010). *Functional assessment: Strategies to prevent and remediate challenging behavior in school settings* (3rd ed.). Upper Saddle River, NJ: Merrill Prentice Hall.

Chandler, L.K., Lubek, R.C., & Fowler, S.A. (1992). Generalization and maintenance of preschool children's social skills: A critical review and analysis. *Journal of Applied Behavior Analysis, 25*(2), 415–428. doi:10.1901/jaba.1992.25-415

Colvin, G., & Lazar, M. (1995). Establishing classroom routines. In A. Deffenbaugh, G. Sugai, & G. Tindal (Eds.), *The Oregon Conference Monograph 1995* (vol. 7, pp. 209–212). Eugene: University of Oregon.

Cooper, J.O., Heron, T.E., & Heward, W.L. (2007). *Applied behavior analysis* (2nd ed.). Upper Saddle River, NJ: Pearson.

Crone, D.A., & Horner, R.H. (2003). *Building positive behavior support systems in schools.* New York, NY: Guilford Press.

Dunlap, G., & Kern, L. (1993). Assessment and intervention for children within the instructional curriculum. In J. Reichle & D. Wacker (Eds.), *Communicative approaches to the management of challenging behavior problems* (pp.177–203). Baltimore, MD: Paul H. Brookes Publishing Co.

Dunlap, G., Kern-Dunlap, L., Clarke, S., & Robbins, F.R. (1991). Functional assessment, curricular revision, and severe problems. *Journal of Applied Behavior Analysis, 24*(2), 387–397. doi:10.1901/jaba.1991.24-387

Dunlap, G., Sailor, W., Horner, R.H., & Sugai, G. (2009). Overview and history of positive behavior support. In W. Sailor, G. Dunlap, G. Sugai, & R.H. Horner (Eds.), *Handbook of positive behavior support* (pp. 3–16). New York, NY: Springer.

Durand, V.M. (1999). Functional communication training using assistive devices: Recruiting natural communities of reinforcement. *Journal of Applied Behavior Analysis, 32*(3), 247–267. doi:10.1901/jaba.1999.32-247

Dyer, K., Dunlap, G., & Winterling, V. (1990). The effects of choice-making on the problem behaviors of students with severe handicaps. *Journal of Applied Behavior Analysis, 23*(4), 515–524.doi:10.1901/jaba.1990.23-515

Ebanks, M.E., & Fisher, W.W. (2003). Altering the timing of academic prompts to treat destructive behavior maintained by escape. *Journal of Applied Behavior Analysis, 6*(3), 355–359. doi:10.1901/jaba.2003.36-355

Eber, L., Sugai, G., Smith, C.R., & Scott, T.M. (2002). Wraparound and positive behavioral interventions and supports in the schools. *Journal of Emotional and Behavioral Disorders, 10*(3), 171–180. doi:10.1177/1063426 6602010003050 1

Epstein, M., Atkins, M., Cullinan, D., Kutash, K., & Weaver, R. (2008). *Reducing behavior problems in the elementary school classroom. A practice guide (NCEE 2008–012).* Washington, DC: National Center for Education Evaluation and Regional Assistance, Institute of Education Sciences, U.S. Department of Education. Retrieved from http://www.principals.in/uploads/pdf/Classroom_Management/Reducing_Behavior.pdf

Ferro, J., Foster-Johnson, L., & Dunlap, G. (1996). Relation between curricular activities and problem behaviors of students with mental retardation. *American Journal on Mental Retardation, 101*(2), 184–194.

Falvey, M.A. (1995). *Inclusive and heterogeneous schooling: Assessment, curriculum, and instruction.* Baltimore, MD: Paul H. Brookes Publishing Co.

Fox, F., Vaughn, B.J., Dunlap, G., & Bucy, M. (1997). Parent-professional partnership in behavioral support: A qualitative analysis of one family's experience. *Journal of The Association for Persons with Severe Handicaps, 22*(4), 198–207.

Gage, N.A., & Lewis, T.J. (2010). Structural analysis in the classroom. *Beyond Behavior, 19*(3), 3–11.

Gray, C.A., & Garand, J.D. (1993). Social Stories: Improving responses of students with autism with accurate social information. *Focus on Autistic Behavior, 8*(1), 1–10. doi:10.1177/108835769300800101

Greenberg, M., Wessberg, R., O'Brien, M., Zins, J., Fredericks, L., Resknik, H., & Elias, M. (2003). Enhancing school-based prevention and youth development through coordinated social, emotional, and academic learning. *American Psychologist, 58,* 466–474. doi:10.1037/0003-066X.58.6-7.466

Hagiwara, T., & Myles, B.S. (1999). A multimedia social story intervention: Teaching skills to children with autism. *Focus on Autism and Other Developmental Disabilities, 14,* 82–95.

Holburn, S., & Vietze, P.M. (2002). *Person-centered planning: Research, practice, and future directions.* Baltimore, MD: Paul H. Brookes Publishing Co.

Horner, R.H. (2000). Positive behavior support. *Focus on Autism and Other Developmental Disabilities, 15*(2), 97–105. doi:10.1177/10883576001500205

Horner, R.H., Albin, R.W., Todd, A.W., Newton, J.S., & Sprague, J.R. (2011). Designing and implementing individualized positive behavior support. In M.E. Snell & F. Brown (Eds.), *Instruction of Students with Severe Disabilities* (pp. 257–303). Upper Saddle River, NJ: Pearson.

Horner, R.H., & Day, H.M. (1991). The effects of response efficiency on functionally equivalent competing behaviors. *Journal of Applied Behavior Analysis, 24*(4), 719–732.

Horner, R.H., Day, H.M., Sprague, J.R., O'Brien, M., & Heathfield, L.T. (1991). Interspersed requests: A nonaversive procedure for reducing aggression and self-injury during instruction. *Journal of Applied Behavior Analysis, 24*(2), 265–278. doi:10.1901/jaba.1991.24-265

Horner, R.H., & Sugai, G. (2000). School-wide behavior support: An emerging initiative. *Journal of Positive Behavior Interventions, 2,* 231–232. doi:10.1177/109830070000200407

Horner, R.H., Sugai, G., Smolkowski, K., Eber, L., Nakasato, J., Todd, A.W., & Esparanza, J. (2009). A randomized, wait-list controlled effectiveness trial assessing school-wide positive behavior support in elementary schools. *Journal of Positive Behavior Interventions, 11*(3), 133–144. doi:10.1177/1098300709332067

Horner, R.H., Vaughn, B., Day, H.M., & Ard, B. (1996). The relationship between setting events and problem behavior. In L.K. Koegel, R.L. Koegel, & G. Dunlap (Eds.), *Positive behavioral support: Including people with difficult behavior in the community* (pp. 381–402). Baltimore, MD: Paul H. Brookes Publishing Co.

Ingram, K., Lewis-Palmer, T., & Sugai, G. (2005). Function-based intervention planning: Comparing the effectiveness of FBA function-based and non-function-based intervention plans. *Journal of Positive Behavior Interventions, 7*(4), 224–236.doi:10.1177/1098300705007004401

Johnston, S.S., Reichle, J., Feeley, K.M., & Jones, E.A. (2012). *AAC strategies for individuals with moderate to severe disabilities.* Baltimore, MD: Paul H. Brookes Publishing Co.

Kennedy, C.H., & Meyer, K.A. (1998). Establishing operations and the motivation of problem behavior. In J.K. Luiselli & M.J. Cameron (Eds.), *Antecedent control: Innovative approaches to behavioral support* (pp. 329–346). Baltimore, MD: Paul H. Brookes Publishing Co.

Kern, L., Bambara, L., & Fogt, J. (2002). Class-wide curricular modification to improve the behavior of students with emotional or behavioral disorders. *Behavioral Disorders, 27*(4), 317–326.

Kern, L., Choutka, C.M., & Sokol, N.G. (2002). Assessment-based antecedent interventions used in natural settings to reduce challenging behavior: An analysis of the literature. *Education and Treatment of Children, 25,* 113–130.

Kern, L., & Clarke, S. (2005). Antecedent and setting event interventions. In L.M. Bambara & L. Kern (Eds.), *Individualized supports for students with problem behaviors* (pp. 201–236). New York, NY: Guilford.

Kern, L., & Clemens, N.H. (2007). Antecedent strategies to promote appropriate classroom behavior. *Psychology in the Schools, 44*(1), 65–75. doi:10.1002/pits.20206

Kern, L., & Dunlap, G. (1998). Curriculum modifications to promote desirable classroom behavior. In J.K. Luiselli & M.J. Cameron (Eds.), *Antecedent control: Innovative approaches to behavioral support* (pp. 289–308). Baltimore, MD: Paul H. Brookes Publishing Co.

Kern, L., Gallagher, P., Starosta, K., Hickman, W., & George, M.L. (2006). Longitudinal outcomes of functional behavioral assessment-based interventions. *Journal of Positive Behavior Interventions, 8,* 67–78. doi:10.1177/10983007060080020501

Kern, L., Sokol, N.G., & Dunlap, G. (2006). Assessment of antecedent influences on challenging behavior. In J.K. Luiselli (Ed.), *Antecedent intervention: Recent developments in community focused behavior support* (pp. 53–71). Baltimore, MD: Paul H. Brookes Publishing Co.

Lalli, J.S., Casey, S., Goh, H., & Merlino, J. (1994). Treatment of escape-maintained aberrant behavior with escape extinction and predictable routines. *Journal of Applied Behavior Analysis, 27*(4), 705–714. doi:10.1901/jaba.1994.27-705

Lohrmann-O'Rourke, S., & Browder, D. (1998). Empirically based methods to assess the preferences of individuals with severe disabilities. *American Journal on Mental Retardation, 103*(2), 146–161.

Lucyshyn, J.M., Dunlap, G., & Albin, R.W. (2002). *Families and positive behavior support.* Baltimore, MD: Paul H. Brookes Publishing Co.

Mace, F.C., Hock, M.L., Lalli, J.S., West, B.J., Belfiore, P., Pinter, E., & Brown, D.K. (1988). Behavioral momentum in the treatment of noncompliance. *Journal of Applied Behavior Analysis, 21*(2), 123–141. doi:10.1901/jaba.1988.21-123

Miltenberger, R.G. (2006). Antecedent intervention for challenging behavior maintained by escape from instructional activities. In J.K. Luiselli (Ed.), *Antecedent assessment and intervention: Supporting children and adults with developmental disabilities in community settings* (pp. 101–124). Baltimore, MD: Paul H. Brookes Publishing Co.

Mount, B. (1984). *Creating futures together: A workbook for people interested in creating desirable futures for people with handicaps.* Atlanta: Georgia Advocacy Office.

Morrison, K., & Rosales-Ruiz, J. (1997). The effect of object preferences on task performance and stereotypy in a child with autism. *Research in Developmental Disabilities, 18,* 127–137. doi:10.1016/S0891-4222(96)00046-7

Munk, D.D., & Karsh, K.G. (1999). Antecedent curriculum and instructional variables as classwide interventions for preventing or reducing problem behaviors. In A.C. Repp & R.H. Horner (Eds.), *Functional analysis of problem behavior: From effective assessment to effective support* (pp. 259–276). Belmont, CA: Wadsworth.

Munk, D.D., & Repp, A.C. (1994). The relationship between instructional variables and problem behavior: A review. *Exceptional Children, 60*(5), 390–401.

Newcomer, L.L., & Lewis, T.J. (2004). Functional behavioral assessment an investigation of assessment reliability and effectiveness of function-based interventions. *Journal of Emotional and Behavioral Disorders, 12*(3), 168–181.

Norris, C., & Dattilo, J. (1999). Evaluating effects of a social story intervention on a young girl with autism. *Focus on Autism and Other Developmental Disabilities, 14*, 180–186.

O'Neill, R., Horner, R., Albin, R., Sprague, J., Storey, K., & Newton, J. (1997). *Functional assessment and program development for problem behavior: A practical handbook.* Pacific Grove, CA. Brooks/Cole Publishing Company.

Pace, G.M., Iwata, B.A., Cowdery, G.E., Andree, P.J., & McIntyre, T. (1993). Stimulus (instructional) fading during extinction of self-injurious escape behavior. *Journal of Applied Behavior Analysis, 26*(2), 205–212. doi:10.1901/jaba.1993.26-205

Payne, L.D., Marks, L.J., & Bogan, B.L. (2007). Using curriculum-based assessment to address the academic and behavioral deficits of students with emotional and behavioral disorders. *Beyond Behavior, 16*(3), 3–6.

Pearpoint, J., O'Brien, J., & Forest, M. (1993). *PATH: A workbook for planning positive possible futures.* Toronto, Canada: Inclusion Press.

Preciado, J.A., Horner, R.H., & Baker, S.K. (2009). Using a function-based approach to decrease problem behaviors and increase academic engagement for Latino English language learners. *The Journal of Special Education, 42*, 227–240. doi:10.1177/0022466907313350

Rapp, J.T., & Vollmer, T.R. (2005). Stereotypy I: A review of behavioral assessment and treatment. *Research in Developmental Disabilities, 26*(6), 527–547. doi:10.1016/j.ridd.2004.11.005

Romano, J.P., & Roll, D. (2000). Expanding the utility of behavioral momentum for youth with developmental disabilities. *Behavioral Interventions, 15*(2), 99–111.

Sailor, W. (1996). New structures and systems change for comprehensive positive behavioral support. In L.K. Koegel, R.L. Koegel, & G. Dunlap (Eds.), *Positive behavioral support* (pp.163–206). Baltimore, MD: Paul H. Brookes Publishing Co.

Sanford, A.K., & Horner, R.H. (2013). Effects of matching instruction difficulty to reading level for students with escape-maintained problem behavior. *Journal of Positive Behavior Interventions, 15*(2), 79–89. doi:10.1177/1098300712449868

Shapiro. E.S. (2004). *Academic skills problems: Direct assessment and intervention* (3rd ed.). New York, NY: Guilford Press.

Smith, C. (2001). Using Social Stories to enhance behaviour in children with autistic spectrum difficulties. *Educational Psychology in Practice, 17*, 337–345.

Smith, R.G., Iwata, B.A., Goh, H., & Shore, B.A. (1995). Analysis of establishing operations for self-injury maintained by escape. *Journal of Applied Behavior Analysis, 28*(4), 515–535. doi:10.1901/jaba.1995.28-515

Stichter, J.P., Randolph, J.K., Kay, D., & Gage, N. (2009). The use of structural analysis to develop antecedent-based interventions for students with autism. *Journal of Autism and Developmental Disorders, 39*(6), 883–896. doi:10.1007/s10803-009-0693-8

Sugai, G., & Horner, R. (2009). Responsiveness-to-intervention and school-wide positive behavior supports: Integration of multi-tiered system approaches. *Exceptionality, 17*(4), 223–237. doi:10.1080/0936283090323537

Sugai, G., Horner, R.H., & Gresham, F.M. (2002). Behaviorally effective school environments. In Shinn, M., Walker, H., & Stoner, G. (Eds.), *Interventions for achievement and behavior problems* (Vol. 2, pp. 315–350). Bethesda, MD: National Association of School Psychologists.

Swaggart, B.L., Gagnon, E., Bock, S.J., Earles, T.L., Quinn, C., Myles, B.S., & Simpson, R.L. (1995). Using social stories to teach social and behavioral skills to children with autism. *Focus on Autistic Behavior, 10*(1), 1–15.

Terrace, H.S. (1963). Discrimination learning with and without "error." *Journal of the Experimental Analysis of Behavior, 6*, 1–27.

Thiemann, K.S., & Goldstein, H. (2001). Social stories, written text cues, and video feedback: Effects on social communication of children with autism. *Journal of Applied Behavior Analysis, 34*, 425–446.

Touchette, P.E., MacDonald, R.F., & Langer, S.N. (1985). A scatter plot for identifying stimulus control of problem behavior. *Journal of Applied Behavior Analysis, 18*(4), 343–351. doi:10.1901/jaba.1985.18-343

Treptow, M.A., Burns, M.K., & McComas, J.J. (2007). Reading at the frustrational, instructional, and independent levels: The effects on students' reading comprehension and time off task. *School Psychology Review, 36*, 159–166.

Wacker, D.P., Steege, M.W., Northup, J., Sasso, G., Berg, W., Reimers, T., . . . Donn, L. (1990). A component analysis of functional communication training across three topographies of severe behavior problems. *Journal of Applied Behavior Analysis, 23*(4), 417–429. doi:10.1901/jaba.1990.23-417

Walker, H.M., Shea, T.M., & Bauer, A.M. (2004). *Behavior management: A practical approach for education.* Columbus, OH: Merrill/Prentice Hall.

Wehmeyer, M.L. (2005). Self-determination and individuals with severe disabilities: Re-examining meanings and misinterpretations. *Research and Practice for Persons with Severe Disabilities, 30*(3), 113–120. doi:10.2511/rpsd.30.3.113

Wilde, L.D., Koegel, L.K., & Koegel, R.L. (1992). *Increasing success in school through priming: A training manual.* Santa Barbara, CA: University of California.

Wolery, M., & Gast, D.L. (1984). Effective and efficient procedures for the transfer of stimulus control. *Topics in Early Childhood Special Education, 4*, 57–77. doi:10.1177/027112148400400305

Wolf, M.M. (1978). Social validity: The case for subjective measurement or how applied behavior analysis is finding its heart. *Journal of Applied Behavior Analysis, 11*(2), 203–214. doi:10.1901/jaba.1978.11-203

Wolfensberger, W. (1983). Social role valorization: A proposed new term for the principle of normalization. *Mental Retardation, 21*, 234–239.

Consequence Strategies to Change Behavior

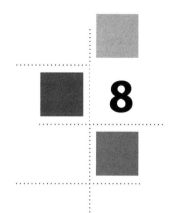

8

Chris Borgmeier and Billie Jo Rodriguez

Though most dictionary definitions of the word *consequence* maintain a neutral status, in everyday use *consequence* often takes on negative connotations. This tendency toward negative connotation is particularly true when *consequence* is mentioned in school or community care settings. For example, when you hear someone say, "If you do that, there will be consequences," it is unlikely you envision the speaker referring to positive consequences. Consequence interventions are an important component of behavior support, yet concern regarding the overreliance on consequence interventions (particularly aversive or punitive interventions) is among the primary influences in the evolution of positive behavior support (PBS; Horner et al., 1990). A second important influence on the PBS movement involves changes in how consequence interventions are used, with a clear emphasis on actively integrating consequences within more comprehensive plans that include proactive, preventive, and teaching strategies. Guided by the Association for Positive Behavior Support (APBS) standards of practice, this chapter provides a framework for understanding and considering the range of consequence interventions.

BEHAVIORAL DEFINITIONS

Given the competing interpretations of the term *consequence*, it is important to begin by defining key terminology. PBS is rooted in the science of applied behavior analysis (ABA; Carr et al., 2002); the following definition is used to guide discussion of consequence interventions throughout this chapter. A *consequence* is a stimulus or event presented contingent on a particular behavior response (Alberto & Troutman, 2013). Within a context of behavior support for individuals with challenging behavior, our focus is on how to apply consequences to behaviors to increase the use of desired behaviors and reduce problematic behaviors.

There are two primary classes of consequence interventions: those that increase behavior (reinforcers) and those that reduce behavior (punishers).

Punishment is another word that often has different meanings in everyday versus a behavioral or PBS framework. In everyday conversation, punishment often focuses on a category of responses to problematic behavior intended to stop the behavior or keep the person from doing it again. Examples of responses commonly considered "punishments," according to the colloquial definition, include scolding, spanking, time-outs, suspension, traffic fines, or prison time. In colloquial use, negative or aversive consequences are often considered punishment whether or not there is an impact on reducing future behavior. For example, many drivers continue to speed even after they have received a speeding ticket (a perceived punisher).

According to a behavioral definition, punishment specifically refers to a consequence response to a behavior that decreases the future occurrence of the behavior (Alberto & Troutman, 2013). What is most meaningful from a behavioral perspective is the effect of the consequence on the future occurrence of the behavior rather than the intent or topography of the consequence. According to a behavioral definition, if the consequence does not reduce future occurrences of the behavior, it is not a punishment. Given the prominent role aversive consequences have traditionally played in the understanding of punishment, some authors (e.g., Alberto &

Troutman, 2013; Scheuermann & Hall, 2012) have begun using the term *behavior reduction intervention* to provide an expanded understanding of punishment. *Behavior reduction intervention* is a broader term for describing consequence manipulations that allow for a distinction between aversive and nonaversive intervention (e.g., differential reinforcement and extinction) to reduce recurring problem behavior. This is a meaningful distinction because the values of PBS require that careful attention is paid to the use of behavior reduction interventions and avoid the use of aversive behavior interventions (APBS, 2007).

Conversely, reinforcement is defined as a consequence response that increases or maintains the future occurrence of a behavior (Alberto & Troutman, 2013). Throughout the remainder of this chapter, the terms *reinforcement* and *punishment* refer to the behavioral definitions provided—that is, the effect of the consequence stimulus on future occurrence of the behavior. Last, it is important to clarify the use of the terms *positive* and *negative* as pertaining to discussions of reinforcement and punishment. When discussing reinforcement and punishment within a behavioral framework, the terms *positive* and *negative* take on very specific meanings. *Positive* means *to give or present* and *negative* means *to remove or avoid*. Figure 8.1 provides a visual for framing these terms.

An example of positive reinforcement is giving a child a sticker contingent on completion of her chores (assuming this maintains

What is done; impact on behavior ⟶	Behavior increases	Behavior decreases
Add something	**Positive** reinforcement	**Positive** punishment
Take away something	*Negative* reinforcement	*Negative* punishment

Figure 8.1. Behavioral terminology for consequence responses.

or increases chore completion in the future), while negative reinforcement involves allowing the child to earn a pass out of chores on Saturday contingent on completion of her chores all week (assuming removal of the chores maintains or increases chore completion behavior in subsequent weeks). An example of positive punishment would be to give Susan extra chores (nondesired stimulus) contingent on the use of disrespectful language (assuming the presentation of extra chores reduces disrespectful language in the future). An example of negative punishment might be to remove access to a privilege, such as going to a regularly scheduled movie contingent on Susan's use of disrespectful language (assuming removal of the privilege reduces use of disrespectful language in the future). Distinguishing between these terms can be confusing because positive and negative are so often used to describe the virtue of the target behavior. In fact, both positive reinforcement and negative reinforcement can be (and are) applied routinely to desired and nondesired behaviors, as are positive or negative punishment. In an effort to avoid confusion throughout this chapter, the terms *positive* and *negative* will be used solely to describe the class of reinforcement or punishment. Meanwhile, the virtue or valence of behaviors or consequences will be described using such terms as *desired* or *nondesired*, *problematic* or *aversive*.

CONSEQUENCES WITHIN A POSITIVE BEHAVIOR SUPPORT FRAMEWORK

Concern with Aversive Consequences

Historically, PBS grew out of the "nonaversive" behavior support movement, a response to widespread use of aversive, dehumanizing interventions with individuals with severe disabilities (Horner et al., 1990). A major emphasis in PBS is the dignity, safety, and well-being of the people receiving intervention or support (Carr et al., 2002). The greatest concern regarding aversive consequences involves the use of positive punishment that causes physical pain, discomfort,

or humiliation (APBS, 2007), such as electric shock, spanking, or intimidation. Supporting the ethical tenets of PBS, 31 states have placed bans on the use of corporal punishment in schools (Center for Effective Discipline, 2010). Although consequences causing physical pain and discomfort often represent examples of the most aversive form of punitive consequences, these represent only one end of the continuum of stimuli that can be presented to reduce behavior. Within a continuum of behavior reduction strategies (presented by Alberto & Troutman, 2013; Scheuermann & Hall, 2012), positive punishment is framed as the delivery of aversive stimuli. The challenge when using aversive stimuli to change behavior is determining how painful, uncomfortable, or humiliating a particular consequence is for an individual. Individual differences make it difficult to differentiate levels of aversion; for example, for one person, being humiliated in front of peers may be as painful as an electric shock is to another person. On the other hand, negative punishment is the removal of a desired stimulus, which in some cases can result in similar feelings of discomfort. For instance, a child can appear to experience a great deal of emotional discomfort when removed from recess for hitting a peer. The challenge in such situations involves determining the personal level of discomfort or anxiety an individual is feeling and then weighing the appropriateness of the intervention. Given this challenge, a PBS framework encourages the use of alternative interventions instead of potentially aversive consequences intended to reduce behavior.

Beyond the potential to compromise the safety, dignity, and well-being of the individual receiving aversive consequences, research suggests a number of potential negative side effects that commonly coincide with the use of aversive consequences, even when they effectively reduce behavior. First, the administration of aversive punishments may elicit aggressive behavior and emotional responses in the individual receiving the punishment (Sobsey, 1990). In addition, the recipient of punishment and observing bystanders learn to use aversive consequences through modeling, increasing the likelihood they will use aversive actions as a strategy in the future (Simons & Wurtele, 2010). Next, aversive consequences often cause the person being punished to avoid the individual who administers the consequences (Alberto & Troutman, 2013). Finally, if the use of aversive consequences is effective in reducing a problem behavior, it can lead to continued use and overreliance on aversive consequences (i.e., negative reinforcement for the person who delivers the punishment). Based on these potential side effects, even when behavior can be changed using aversive consequences, the standards of practice (APBS, 2007; see Standard I-C 9) emphasize the use of "techniques that do not cause pain or humiliation or deprive the individual of basic needs."

Though aversive consequences using physical pain, intimidation, and humiliation to influence behavior change are the most blatant concerns within a PBS framework, there are also important considerations when using consequence interventions that most people would not classify as physically or emotionally aversive. One concern is the unintended effects of many commonly used responses to problem behavior, such as overreliance on the repeated use of negative consequences. For example, schools commonly use a range of consequences for student problem behavior that remove the student from the instructional environment (e.g., sending students to the hall, office, detention, seclusion room) or school (e.g., suspension, expulsion) and limit access to instruction and normalized, inclusive school experiences. In community settings, the consequences may be even direr when people with disabilities engage in behaviors leading to an encounter with a punishment-based legal system, which can result in significant restrictions (e.g., prison, institutionalization) to normalized, inclusive participation in society.

While consequence interventions can be effective in changing behavior in many circumstances, there are many situations and people for whom consequence interventions

(reinforcing or punishing) alone are insufficient. (The intention of the previous statement is not to encourage the use of punitive consequences, but rather to encourage increased use of more positive, proactive and teaching interventions.) Schools and other community entities (e.g., legal system) often rely solely on the use of negative consequences in interventions, failing to teach the appropriate replacement behaviors or skills the individual may need to be successful. In such cases, without teaching and support, the individual is likely to continue to engage in problem behavior and experience a recurring cycle of negative interactions, escalating behavior, and increasingly aversive consequences. This cycle of escalating interactions, problem behavior, and increasingly aversive consequences often leads to interventions and decisions (i.e., seclusion, restraint, specialized placements, institutionalization) presented under the pretext of safety that often increasingly restrict access to normalized, inclusive experiences.

PBS emphasizes a shift from the immediate, short-term amelioration of problem behavior through consequence interventions to comprehensive interventions with a broader focus on quality of life and comprehensive lifestyle change (Carr et al., 2002). In PBS, the only regular use of positive punishment should be the provision of corrective responses (verbal or visual) intended to stop and redirect the nondesired behavior by prompting an alternate, more socially appropriate behavior. When designing behavior support plans for individuals with challenging behavior, the implementation of multicomponent interventions is recommended to integrate consequences with strategies focused on prevention, teaching, and reinforcing functional replacement responses.

Increased Use of Positive and Integrated Interventions

As implied by the name *positive* behavior support, a defining characteristic of PBS is the use of positive, prevention-oriented, reinforcement-based intervention. PBS emphasizes a shift away from a predominant reliance on consequence interventions (reinforcing or punishing) for behavior change, promoting instead the increased use of interventions focused on prevention and teaching (Carr et al., 2002). While consequence strategies remain a vital component of behavior intervention plans, a goal of PBS is to move away from interventions focusing primarily on trying to overpower problem behavior through punishment or reinforcement. In order to do this, more comprehensive plans must be implemented that integrate the use of consequences with prevention and teaching and use reinforcement strategies more effectively. In a PBS approach, consequences are relegated to the role of "equal partner" with strategies focused on teaching and prevention.

A school-based example of using a consequence to "overpower" problem behavior could include the recurring use of detention with a threat of suspension for a student who chronically refuses to work and engages in disruptive behaviors. At home, the child's parents might promise a trip to Disneyland as a reward if the student completes his work and is not disruptive for the rest of the year. Both efforts are attempts to "overpower" the student's problem behavior with high-powered consequences (both punitive and reinforcing). The problem is without a more comprehensive, regimented plan based on a functional assessment of the behavior, consequences are not likely to be successful in reducing behavior. A comprehensive plan would address student skill deficits and build in supports for student success by 1) modifying the schoolwork to be more commensurate with the student's skills and instructional level and 2) teaching the student the academic skills to do the work or the social skills to more appropriately request teacher help, alternate assignments, or breaks from difficult work.

By actively integrating consequence strategies with prevention (antecedent) and teaching interventions, practitioners can reduce the magnitude of consequences (reinforcement and punishment). Greater reliance on consequences in interventions often requires bigger and bigger consequences, which are often dramatically different from naturally occurring consequences. The greater the discrepancy between consequences used in the intervention and naturally occurring consequences, the more challenging it is to fade the use of consequences, maintain the intervention over time, and generalize across settings where such significant consequences may not be readily available (Horner, 2005). Reducing the magnitude of consequences also creates an intervention that is more consistent with what typical members of society are experiencing, thereby creating a more normalized and inclusive experience for the individual. Effectively implementing and fading interventions often requires understanding and recognizing the dynamic and symbiotic relationship among several complementary components of the intervention (antecedent, teaching, and consequence interventions). Integrating each of these three aspects of intervention into a behavior plan is key to the successful implementation of PBS. This integration occurs through an understanding of the function of behavior and can be guided by the competing behavior pathway model (O'Neill et al., 1997) described in the next sections.

Role of Function When a behavior occurs repeatedly, it is *functional,* or serves a purpose by achieving desired outcomes for the individual in a given context. A significant barrier inhibiting many behavior change efforts is a disconnect between the *intentions* of the person delivering the consequence and actual *outcome* of the consequence on recurrence of the targeted behavior. For example, a teacher may send a student to the hall (consequence) for engaging in a tantrum (behavior) when asked to complete an assignment (antecedent) with the "intention" of punishing the child. Instead, the student experiences the problem behavior as an effective,

or functional, means to avoiding an undesired task, and as an added bonus, she gets to
read her favorite book in the hallway. Despite
the teacher's intentions, the child experiences the consequence as a reward. When
the student quickly engages in a tantrum
the next time she is asked to do her assignment, it is clear that being sent to the hall
serves as a reinforcing, rather than punishing, consequence.

To avoid this mistake, a PBS framework
encourages the use of a functional understanding of behavior to guide the selection,
use, and evaluation of consequence interventions, particularly with persons requiring
individualized behavior support. To understand the role of the consequence in the
previous example, we must understand the
"function" of the problem behavior from the
student's perspective. The purpose or function of the student's tantrum was to avoid the
task; by being sent to the hallway, the student
learned a tantrum was a functional means
to achieve the desired outcome. The effective use of consequence interventions can be
maximized when matched to the function of
an individual's behavior. It is equally important to pair consequence interventions with
antecedent and teaching strategies to form
an integrated and comprehensive behavior
intervention. Once we understand why a person is engaging in a particular behavior, we
can begin to develop interventions that align
the person's needs (or wants) with socially
acceptable behaviors.

***Competing Behavior Pathway Frame-
work*** When punishment or reinforcement
are used in an intervention, the value of
reinforcement received for problem behavior is competing with the value of the potential reward for the desired behavior and/or
the value of punishment for the nondesired
behavior. The competing behavior pathway
framework (O'Neill et al., 1997; see Chapter 7, Figure 7.2, and Chapter 14) provides
an efficient organizational framework for
demonstrating the competing consequences
and identifying and integrating the multiple

components (e.g., setting event, antecedent, teaching, consequence, function) of
an intervention. Though the competing
pathway logic emphasizes comprehensive,
integrated interventions, the focus in this
chapter is on the effective use of consequences within this model.

The goal of the competing pathway
model is to devise interventions that ensure
problem behavior is no longer functional
or effective for the individual (extinction)
and to replace the problem behavior with a
more appropriate replacement, or alternative, behavior (differential reinforcement).
The differential reinforcement of alternative
behavior (DRA) is a strategy that involves
reinforcing a more appropriate form of
behavior than the targeted behavior of concern (Alberto & Troutman, 2013). The goal
is that when the individual engages in the
problem behavior, the consequence should
not provide a functional outcome for the
individual (e.g., a tantrum to successfully
escape from a task). Instead, the intervention should encourage a more appropriate
response by prompting use of the replacement or alternative behavior at the earliest
signs of problem behavior; this appropriate
behavior should then be reinforced. A strong
understanding of how to effectively design
and implement consequence interventions is
integral to the competing behavior pathways
model and PBS.

REINFORCEMENT: CONSEQUENCE MANIPULATIONS TO INCREASE BEHAVIOR

As discussed earlier in the chapter and
presented visually in Figure 8.1, positive
reinforcement is the contingent presentation of a stimulus following a behavior that
increases or maintains future occurrence of
the behavior; negative reinforcement is the
contingent removal of a stimulus following a
behavior that increases or maintains future
occurrence of the behavior (Alberto & Troutman, 2013). It is important to understand
that reinforcing consequences can increase

the future occurrence of both desired and undesired behaviors. To demonstrate positive and negative reinforcement, consider Sofia, who enjoys talking with her friends on the phone during free time in the afternoon. Within her residential program, Sofia, who normally resists brushing her teeth, can now earn 5 minutes to talk on the phone each day if she brushes her teeth after each meal. This is an example of positive reinforcement (assuming that earning minutes to talk on the phone each day maintains or increases the likelihood Sofia will brush her teeth after each meal). To illustrate negative reinforcement with a similar example, Sofia can avoid doing a daily chore she doesn't enjoy (e.g., cleaning the bathroom) if she brushes her teeth after each meal.

Effective Use of Reinforcement

There are several principles to understand when planning and implementing consequence interventions for individuals with challenging behavior. The delivery of reinforcing and punishing consequences can be varied in several ways to increase or decrease the salience (or strength) of the consequence, and there are circumstances in which more and less salient applications of consequences are appropriate. As a rule, it is beneficial to apply the least salient example of a consequence that is likely to be effective for the individual. For example, there are many options for how to set up an opportunity to take a break from working. If it will be effective to allow the student a quick break to walk to the water fountain, get a drink of water, and come back to class, that would be less salient than allowing the student take a 20-minute break on the computer. The 20-minute computer break, however, is less salient than giving a student the rest of the afternoon off. The three most common ways to vary the salience of consequence interventions are to vary the consequences' 1) value, 2) contingency, and 3) schedule. Each of these three aspects of consequence interventions should be tailored to best match the needs of each individual case and varied over time based on the efficacy of the intervention.

Value By definition, a *reinforcer* must result in an increase in the future occurrence of the behavior. For this to occur, the individual must value the reinforcer. A common mistake in attempts to use reinforcement strategies is the selection of "reinforcers" that are not meaningful to the individual. If the individual does not value the consequence, there is not likely to be an impact on behavior. Conversely, it is also possible to choose reinforcers that are highly valued, which may bring a separate set of concerns. For example, the use of money, say $100, as an incentive might be effective in increasing an individual's behavior in the short term; however, it may be very challenging to maintain this incentive or to generalize this incentive across settings. It is important to identify valued incentives that provide the least salient example to increase the likelihood of sustained behavior change. The value of a reinforcer may also be affected by satiation and deprivation. *Deprivation* occurs when an individual does not have regular or easy access to a particular reinforcer, which often increases the value of the reinforcer for the individual. However, *satiation* occurs when the individual has easy or recent access to the potential reinforcer, resulting in less value. These principles often have an impact on the success of interventions over time. For example, if Tom loves ice cream, this may typically be a valued reinforcer. If Tom has not had ice cream recently (deprivation), ice cream may be especially motivating. However, if Tom just ate a huge bowl of ice cream (satiation), the typically valued reinforcer (ice cream) may hold less value. Similarly, a child who really likes superheroes may initially be very motivated to work for superhero stickers (due to novelty and deprivation or previous limited access); however, after earning superhero stickers for several weeks, the child may lose interest in working for the stickers (due to the satiation or having lots of stickers). Therefore, it is important to consider the impact of deprivation and satiation regularly during the behavior support process.

There are several strategies for identifying valued reinforcers. The first strategy is to conduct a functional behavioral assessment (FBA). Understanding the function (or purpose) of a person's problem behavior can help determine reinforcers for prosocial behavior. For example, if FBA data suggest a child is talking out to obtain peer attention, we could provide opportunities for the child to earn a special activity with peers (e.g., social activity, free recess) for appropriate behavior. While understanding the function of behavior can be helpful in determining valued reinforcers, it is important to note that reinforcers unrelated to the function of behavior can also be selected (and potentially effective).

Reinforcer sampling is another means for determining effective reinforcers. In reinforcer sampling, the target individual is directly involved in selecting reinforcers. Reinforcer sampling can be done in a variety of ways but typically involves presenting a variety of potential reinforcers and having the individual pick those that are most desirable. Selection can happen in a variety of ways—for example, an individual with physical disabilities may reach for or gaze at a selection. Research demonstrates the value of asking the individual to identify preferred reinforcers (Fisher, Thompson, Piazza, Crosland, & Gotjen, 1997; Lerman et al., 1997). The actual choices can then be used as reinforcers, or if a categorical preference appears (e.g., the person typically chooses reinforcers that involve attention from adults), these types of reinforcers may be presented.

Contingency To maximize the salience of a reinforcer, it is important to ensure the reinforcer is delivered contingent on the occurrence of the desired behavior. This means the delivery of the reinforcer depends on the occurrence of desired behavior, and the individual only has access to the reinforcer if he or she engages in the target behavior. For example, if a teacher identifies a child who has a hard time making a transition from snack time to a math activity, the teacher could offer the child tokens to indicate time earned for playing with puzzles (a high-preference activity) when the child makes transitions appropriately. If the puzzle activity is freely available to all students in the classroom, whether or not they make the transition appropriately, puzzle time has *not* been made contingent on the student's transition. On the other hand, if puzzles are not freely available unless the student makes the transition well, the puzzles are now contingent on appropriate transitions.

Reinforcement can also be delivered noncontingently; noncontingent reinforcement means that reinforcers are delivered at regular intervals regardless of the individual's behavior (Alberto & Troutman, 2013). For example, adult attention may be a valued reinforcer that can be delivered regularly in a classroom regardless of contingencies around productivity. Regular, noncontingent access to adult attention enriches the classroom environment and may reduce off-task or problematic behavior and increase student productivity in the meantime. When targeting specific behaviors, it may be important to be purposeful in choosing which reinforcers will be used and when they will be delivered to balance the benefits of contingent and noncontingent reinforcement. Using the example of puzzles from the previous paragraph, if puzzles were always accessible to the child (as regular noncontingent reinforcement), the value of puzzles as a contingent reinforcement would be diminished. It would be important to select different reinforcers for noncontingent and contingent reinforcement, if used simultaneously.

Closely related to the contingent nature of the relationship between behavior and response is the immediacy or passage of time between a behavior and a consequence. Typically, the immediate delivery of reinforcement is more strongly associated with behavior change (often even more so for younger children or individuals with developmental disabilities). One advantage of providing consequences immediately is that the individual receiving consequences is more likely to associate the behavior and the consequences. For example, Amanda meets her goal of engaging in on-task behavior during math instruction and earns 5 minutes of computer time. If Mr. Jones does not plan to give her the earned computer time until the end of the school day, there is a possibility Amanda may engage in problematic behavior during the last period of the day and then have difficulty attributing her computer time (earned during math instruction) to the appropriate behavior during math instruction. Amanda is much more likely to understand the relationship between on-task behavior in math class and the reinforcement (computer time) if it is provided immediately following her on-task behavior in math. It is also helpful to verbally label the specific behavior being reinforced. In the previous example, Mr. Jones could say, "You did such a great job of staying on task during math time that you've earned computer time."

Schedule Another way to adjust the salience of the reinforcer is to consider the schedule of reinforcement—that is, *when* and *how often* the reinforcer is delivered. It is important to consider whether the reinforcer will be delivered each time the target behavior occurs (continuous) or only following some instances of behavior (intermittent). When initiating a behavior intervention, whether teaching a new skill or breaking an old habit, it is often important to begin with a continuous reinforcement schedule in which reinforcement is delivered each time (or nearly each time) the target behavior occurs. High rates of consistent positive feedback or reinforcement help build the individual's learning history more quickly; in the previous example, the child learned "when I transition appropriately, I receive access to puzzles." Once the behavior has been clearly established, it may be appropriate to switch to an intermittent schedule (providing puzzles every few days for appropriate

transitions, instead of daily). An intermittent schedule is considered more natural (i.e., most people do not receive reinforcement for every instance of appropriate behavior) and is also more likely to maintain behavior over time (Alberto & Troutman, 2013).

When determining schedules of reinforcement, it is important to ensure the time frames and expectations set for the individual are reasonable and achievable, given current levels of performance. Reinforcers that are offered but not achieved (or not perceived as achievable) are not likely to influence behavior and may escalate problem behavior. Initially, it is best to make access to the reinforcer easily achievable; setting the criterion for reinforcement just slightly above the current level of behavior can increase achievability. Once the individual is consistently achieving the initial criterion for success, or receiving reinforcement, it may be time to develop an incremental plan for increasing the criterion to access the reinforcement.

As patterns of appropriate behavior begin to develop, the schedule of reinforcement can be *faded* to decrease the consistency and frequency of reinforcement (see Figure 8.2). For example, if reinforcement initially is administered every 15 minutes based on the individual's behavior, over time the schedule of reinforcement may be progressively and strategically increased to longer and more variable (or less predictable) intervals (e.g., 20 minutes and then 30 minutes). Data should be collected and used to monitor the effectiveness of attempts to fade intervention and determine revisions to the reinforcement schedule as needed. For example, if data suggest that a shift in the reinforcement schedule from accessing a reinforcer every hour to once per day results in increases in challenging behavior, it will be important to revise the schedule of reinforcement to one that will maintain success and lead to a successful transition as the intervention is faded. Shifting to a schedule that reinforces behavior every 90 minutes, up from every 60 minutes, may be a more reasonable progression in fading the reinforcement schedule. (For an

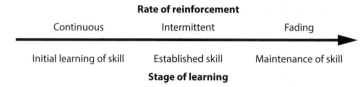

Figure 8.2.   Varying rates of reinforcement.

additional discussion related to schedules of reinforcement, see Chapter 9.)

Applications of Reinforcement

When considering reinforcement in practice, it is often helpful to begin by focusing on the desired behavior. Begin by developing a clear understanding and definition of what you want the person to do. Identifying the target behavior is a critical first step in the successful application of reinforcement. As the person engages in the desired behavior, it is important to provide verbal feedback that is clearly focused on acknowledging the behavior (e.g., "Thank you for completing your chores. As a result you have earned time to play with friends before dinner," is better than, "Wow, I'm so proud of you for earning time with your friends before dinner."). If the person is unable to perform the desired (goal) behavior right away, you should consider an approximation of the behavior the person might be able to perform. As the person gains mastery with the approximation of the behavior, you can gradually adjust the targeted behavior expectation. The process of reinforcing approximations of a behavior is called *shaping* (Alberto & Troutman, 2013).

Once you've identified the target behavior(s), the next step is to select appropriate reinforcers. Natural reinforcers are those that are logical, naturally occurring responses connected to the behavior. For example, natural reinforcers for reading commonly include comprehending and learning new information, being entertained, or knowing what you can order for lunch. As individuals begin engaging in desired behavior, it can be important to make explicit connections between the behavior and natural reinforcers.

For example when the student begins reading, help the student recognize the utility of reading for comprehending one's environment (e.g., "Since you can read the signs, you know which way to go"). Accessing natural reinforcers of behavior in natural contexts is a key to sustaining behavior.

Although many behaviors are maintained by naturally occurring reinforcers, often individuals with challenging behavior do not have the skills to readily access the natural reinforcers. For example, reading for pleasure is a natural reinforcer associated with reading. This is not possible, however, if one cannot read accurately or fluently. Similarly, a person may not access the natural reinforcers often or easily enough for behavior to be maintained (e.g., a struggling reader may take three times longer than is typical to read the paragraph, answer the questions, and complete the homework assignment requirements necessary to get a good grade). When skill impairments (i.e., the student does not know how or cannot perform the behavior) appear to restrict access to naturally occurring reinforcers for a behavior, short-term substitute reinforcers can be used temporarily while the individual develops the skills necessary to access natural reinforcers for the behavior.

The term *substitute reinforcers* is used here to describe reinforcers that are effective in increasing or maintaining behavior but are not naturally tied to the behavior required to obtain them. Substitute reinforcers might include tangible items (e.g., stickers, food, toys), social attention (e.g., time with a preferred peer or adult), activities (e.g., games, computer time), privileges (e.g., team captain, homework pass, star student, free choice time), or token reinforcers to be exchanged for other types of reinforcers (e.g., points, credits, money). For example, if a child is not a fluent reader and is unable to access the natural reinforcer of reading for pleasure or information, a parent might provide a special reward, such as computer time, for time spent practicing reading each day. However, as the child becomes more fluent, the special reward can be faded (e.g., the time required to earn a reward might be increased, the types of rewards can slowly shift to ones more related to reading such as a trip to the library or watching a movie after reading the book) so that the natural reinforcer, reading for meaning or pleasure, begins to maintain and sustain reading. Explicit planning involves a careful bridging of tangible/token or other substitute reinforcers to natural reinforcers. Though initially it may be necessary to provide a substitute reinforcer to motivate learning, it is important to be thoughtful about how this substitute reinforcer can eventually be connected to natural reinforcers as the person develops fluency with a skill.

Sometimes the problem with the application of reinforcement has less to do with the person's ability to access the reinforcer and more to do with limited interest in the natural reinforcers (i.e., they aren't meaningful to the individual) or *competing reinforcers* that may be more powerful. For example, a student named Keith may be capable of doing assigned math problems; however, telling jokes that gets his peers laughing may be a more powerful reinforcer than sitting and working quietly on the math task to access such natural reinforcers as personal satisfaction, a good grade, and/or occasional praise from the teacher. In this case, the natural reinforcers of personal satisfaction from work completion, good grades, or occasional teacher praise are not very meaningful to Keith and cannot compete with the more highly valued attention from peers. In such cases, intervention may require using richer substitute reinforcers that are highly valued by Keith to increase the payoff for work completion, while also trying to diminish access to peer attention for inappropriate behavior during work time.

Another common challenge is that natural reinforcers may not be available contingent on engaging in the desired behavior. Consider Yolanda, a third grader with cognitive impairment, who has a history of engaging in aggressive behavior on the playground. Yolanda is taught to ask politely to join an activity and give compliments to access peer attention at recess. However, when Yolanda uses her new social skills, the students do not allow her to join the activity and do not respond to her compliments because their history with Yolanda has taught them it is safer not to engage with her. In this case, not only do we have to work on Yolanda's skills, but we also have to strategically incorporate access to natural reinforcers (e.g., peer response and entry into the activity) to make Yolanda's new social skills functional and meaningful to her. In this case, we may have to explicitly teach and encourage peers to respond to Yolanda appropriately and to let her join the group activity.

The goal of any behavior change intervention is ultimately for the person to self-manage his or her own behavior and, to the extent possible, fade substitute reinforcers and replace them with natural reinforcers. When delivering reinforcement, it is important that the focus be on the behavior(s) being increased and not on the reinforcer. In addition, it is important to maximize success by ensuring that reinforcement is appropriately paired with antecedent and teaching interventions to increase access to reinforcers, especially natural reinforcers. For example, a student who is struggling to complete reading tasks is likely to be more successful and more quickly access the natural joys of reading when placed in reading instruction that is close to his or her own reading level. This antecedent modification (i.e., adjusting reading instructional level) combined with specific teaching (i.e., literacy skills needed to increase success with reading) may make the natural reinforcement of reading for pleasure more accessible and is likely to reduce the magnitude of the external reinforcers needed.

BEHAVIOR REDUCTION INTERVENTIONS

When working with individuals with behavior challenges, it is important to start by clearly defining and prioritizing the behaviors of concern, as well as the routines in which problem behaviors are most prevalent. In this section, the range of behavior reduction interventions, including differential reinforcement, extinction, negative punishment, and positive punishment, are described with considerations for application within a PBS framework.

Common concerns when responding to problem behavior or the use of behavior reduction interventions include the risk of escalating behavior or extinction burst (i.e., problem behavior increases and/or intensifies before showing reductions when reinforcement is withheld). Escalating behaviors and extinction bursts are often a result of an increased attempt to get a payoff for a previously reinforced behavior. For example, when Maria's mother ignores Maria's negative comments intended to get her mother's attention, Maria escalates to a tantrum. An understanding of behavioral function and the competing behavior pathway (see Chapter 7, Figure 7.2) offer a framework for limiting escalation and guiding the effective use of behavior reduction interventions. Reducing the chances of escalation and extinction burst can occur through the use of "nonaversive" behavior reduction strategies by pairing *extinction* with teaching and DRA. By providing an alternative, more socially appropriate way for an individual to access the desired outcome usually received through problem behavior, it is possible to replace the problem behavior with an alternative behavior in a way that reduces the chance for escalation that occurs when using extinction strategies in isolation. With Maria, the strategy for extinction is to withhold attention for negative comments; however, this is likely to lead to escalation. To prevent escalation at the earliest signs of problem behavior, her mom should redirect Maria to respectfully request her attention,

which would give Maria a more appropriate way to access her mother's attention without the need to escalate behavior. The following section describes in greater detail the nonaversive behavior reduction interventions of differential reinforcement and extinction.

Nonaversive Behavior Reduction Interventions

A PBS framework encourages the use of nonaversive behavior reduction strategies. Nonaversive strategies include differential reinforcement, extinction, and gentle correction or redirection. These strategies are considered not only more acceptable but also an integral component of PBS intervention and the competing behavior pathway logic. Though these interventions can be used independently, the coordinated use of the interventions makes it possible to avoid the use of more aversive interventions and the potential side effects that often undermine sustained implementation of these interventions in isolation.

Differential Reinforcement Differential reinforcement is considered the least aversive form of behavior reduction (Alberto & Troutman, 2013). It is a procedure in which the absence or reduction of the target behavior or the use of a replacement behavior is contingently reinforced. Differential reinforcement can be applied in a variety of ways. Common examples include the differential delivery of reinforcement based on the occurrence of 1) incompatible behavior (DRI), 2) alternative behavior (DRA), 3) lower levels of behavior (DRL), or 4) other behavior (DRO). Research has demonstrated that differential reinforcement of alternative behaviors or the absence or reduction of a target behavior can reduce that behavior (e.g., Anderson & Long, 2002; Dietz & Repp, 1983; Wilder, Harris, Regan, & Ramsey, 2007). An example of DRA is when a teacher provides attention (reinforcer) for requesting appropriately (e.g., asking for teacher attention or teacher help) rather than providing attention when the student speaks out in class and interrupts others. DRA is a hallmark of the competing behavior pathway model, particularly when coordinated with extinction strategies.

Extinction   *Extinction* is actively withholding reinforcement for a targeted problem behavior to reduce the behavior (Alberto & Troutman, 2013). The effective use of extinction depends on understanding the function of the target behavior to be reduced. For example, ignoring a student is an effective extinction strategy to reduce or eliminate minor disruptive behavior *if* the function of disruptive behavior is to gain social attention. If the function of the student's behavior is to avoid a task, rather than seeking attention, then ignoring him or her is not an effective response to extinguish behavior; instead, the response of ignoring the student will reinforce the problem behavior. Extinction strategies for problem behavior aimed at avoiding a task would involve eliminating or limiting opportunities for the student to avoid the task in response to problem behavior. For example, if the student is sent to the office or to another room in response to problem behavior, the student must remain accountable for completing the work. The teacher may send the work with the student to complete or have the student stay in during recess or after school until the work is completed. This assumes that the student is capable of completing the work or that the teacher will provide help with completing the task.

There are challenges and side effects that often impede the successful use of extinction. One challenge is the initial escalation of the behavior that may occur. For instance, Bo, a child with limited verbal communication, frequently moans and screams to request a snack; to extinguish moaning and screaming, it is important to withhold snack in response to those target behaviors. Unfortunately, without a more appropriate or effective way to request a snack, Bo's remaining option is to escalate his behavior by moaning or screaming more loudly or by perhaps becoming more aggressive. This is where it

becomes important to pair extinction with DRA. The goal in this situation is not to withhold a snack from Bo but to teach and reinforce more effective communication skills for requesting a snack than moaning and screaming. So before putting screaming and moaning on extinction, it is critical to teach appropriate alternative behaviors for requesting a snack (e.g., using sign language or a picture communication system). So the next time Bo begins to moan and scream to get a snack, it is important to withhold the snack for those behaviors. Instead, at the earliest signs of moaning, provide a gentle correction or prompt to Bo to use either sign language or his picture communication system to request a snack. As soon as he engages in the alternate behavior of making a more appropriate request, quickly provide him with a snack.

Since problem behavior in most cases serves an important purpose or function for meeting an individual's needs, it is important to offer a more socially acceptable behavior as an alternate means to attain the desired outcome previously achieved by engaging in the problem behavior. Research suggests that if reinforcement for problem behavior is not minimized or eliminated, the problem behavior may continue even if new behaviors have been taught and reinforced (e.g., Fisher et al., 1993; Stahr, Cushing, Lane, & Fox, 2006). By pairing extinction with DRA, it is possible to reduce the escalating behavior that is problematic for implementers of the plan and the person of concern.

Punitive Behavior Reduction Interventions

Punitive interventions are divided into two categories. The first is the removal of desired stimuli that reduces a target behavior, known as negative punishment (e.g., response cost, time-out), and the second is the presentation of aversive stimuli to reduce a target behavior, known as positive punishment (e.g., corrections and redirection, overcorrection; Alberto & Troutman, 2013). These strategies are considered progressively more aversive with the understanding that the level of aversion can vary within each category, depending on specific stimuli being removed or presented. When considering the use of punishment, PBS emphasizes the use of "techniques that do not cause pain or humiliation or deprive the individual of basic needs" (APBS, 2007). Though not encouraged, if used, punitive behavior reduction strategies should be those that "do not cause pain or humiliation or deprive the individual of basic needs," are only used in coordination with PBS strategies (e.g., prevention, teaching, reinforcement), and use data to make decisions about the initial use of punitive interventions and closely monitor outcomes focusing on fading punitive interventions as quickly as possible.

Within a PBS framework, acceptable applications of positive punishment are the use of correction and redirection as responses to problem behavior. Corrections are responses to problem behavior intended to arrest the problem behavior and encourage the use of a more appropriate alternative behavior. For example, if a student is engaging in disruptive and off-task behaviors, it is important to consistently correct or redirect the student disruption to the appropriate alternative (e.g., asking for a break or asking for help) or desired behavior (e.g., to get back on task). One reason it is important to consistently correct or redirect to an appropriate behavior is to minimize opportunities for individuals, particularly individuals with disabilities, to practice inappropriate or incorrect behaviors. Instead, they should receive corrective feedback followed by opportunities to engage in the desired behavior (Berliner, 1980).

Even verbal redirection may be applied in more or less acceptable ways. Therefore, we recommend clear correction or redirection that occurs in an unobtrusive, nonaversive manner, respecting the dignity of the individual. For example, a private, gentle verbal correction is usually considered less humiliating and more respectful to the individual than a harsh, public scolding that includes demeaning language. The use

of redirection or correction at the earliest signs of problem behavior are an important applications of positive punishment within a competing behavior pathway framework but should be combined with proactive interventions setting up the individual for success and limiting the need for correction. The discussion of positive punishment in the following sections primarily focuses on the effective use of correction and redirection and in no way encourages the use of aversive consequences that cause pain, humiliation, or loss of dignity.

Effective Use of Punishment

Similar to reinforcement, there are some clear ways to vary the salience and use of punishment strategies that can have a substantial impact on the strength of the intervention and effectiveness in reducing behavior. The principles for planning and implementing punitive responses to behavior can be understood using the same categories described previously for reinforcement: 1) value, 2) contingency, and 3) schedule. When using punishment strategies, consequences that are specifically relevant to the individual are likely to have a larger, more immediate impact in reducing behavior; however, as described previously, PBS takes a strong position against the use of aversive punishers for behavior change or any strategy that causes pain or humiliation or loss of dignity. Even the use of what might be considered mildly aversive punitive interventions is not recommended in individual intervention. The only forms of positive punishment that are recommended within a PBS framework are gentle correction and redirection as responses to problem behavior.

When committed to reducing a behavior, *corrective* responses to problem behavior are most effective when administered contingent on the problem behavior, consistently, and immediately. It is also beneficial, when possible, to clearly label the specific behavior being corrected. Consistency is extremely important when trying to reduce or extinguish behavior. For behaviors targeted for extinction or correction, nearly every occurrence of problem behavior should receive a corrective response, prompting a more appropriate alternative behavior. At the very least, it is important to try to ensure the problem behavior does not result in the desired reinforcement (extinction). Research on intermittent schedules of reinforcement has demonstrated that inconsistency in responding to problem behavior can actually maintain a problem behavior and make it more resistant to extinction (Bijou, 1957). A significant difference in the application of correction and redirection, when compared to reinforcement, is that the frequency of corrective and extinction responses will not be faded over time. The frequency of corrective and extinction responses should remain consistent and contingent (i.e., a fixed ratio schedule) to be most effective in long-term behavior reduction.

Within PBS, a comprehensive approach to intervention that focuses on prevention, teaching, reinforcement, and corrective behavior reduction interventions (pairing DRA with extinction) is recommended; the use of aversive consequences that cause, pain, harm, or humiliation is never allowed, and punitive intervention is generally not recommended. The competing behavior pathway provides a helpful framework for coordinating reinforcement and "nonaversive" behavior reduction interventions to eliminate the use of aversive interventions. The following case studies provide examples of such coordinated interventions.

CASE STUDY EXAMPLES

The following are case studies that offer an opportunity to apply the consequence strategies learned in this chapter to intervention planning and checking understanding by comparing responses to those of the authors. For each case study, use the competing behavior pathway framework to identify consequence interventions specific to each case that will answer the following questions:

1. How can the team reinforce the use of an appropriate alternative behavior?

2. How can the team reinforce use of the desired behavior(s) or approximations to shape the desired behavior(s)?

3. How can the team provide a corrective prompt or redirection to encourage the use of the alternative or desired behavior at the earliest signs of problem behavior?

4. How can the team use extinction on the problem behavior?

Yesenia

Please see Chapter 7 to review the case and competing behavior pathway (see Chapter 7, Figure 7.3) for Yesenia. Yesenia, an eighth grader, has been referred to the behavior support team for academic difficulties, putting her head down, and refusing to do work in order to escape reading tasks that are beyond her third-grade reading level. In Chapter 7, Yesenia's team determined she would receive additional reading instruction. An instructor would preteach and highlight Yesenia's selected reading text and provide her with a reading partner for extra help. In addition, Yesenia was provided a "pass" card as an appropriate alternative to problem behavior to identify that she wanted to skip her turn reading aloud. After reviewing the case, *answer the focus questions and compare your responses to the following author responses:*

1. How can the team reinforce the use of an appropriate alternative behavior?

   By using the "pass card," Yesenia's teacher was encouraging her to ask for a break in a more acceptable, more mature way when she did not want to read. When Yesenia used her "pass card," the teacher was to reinforce the alternative behavior by simply choosing another student to read so Yesenia could avoid reading.

2. How can the team reinforce use of the desired behavior(s) or approximations to shape the desired behavior(s)?

   In an effort to encourage Yesenia to read aloud in class (desired behavior), she was reinforced with a tally mark on her "pass card." Once Yesenia earned three tallies on her card, she would earn an additional incentive of her choice. (Yesenia's team planned to interview her to identify valued incentives.)

3. How can the team provide a corrective prompt or redirection to encourage the use of the

alternative or desired behavior at the earliest signs of problem behavior?

If problem behavior does occur, it's important to prompt and encourage Yesenia to make a better choice by using the alternative behavior instead of continuing to engage in or escalate problem behavior. At the first sign of work refusal or frustration, the teacher is to redirect Yesenia by prompting her to use her "pass card" if she wants a break.

4. How can the team use extinction on the problem behavior?

   Extinction can be challenging when the function of problem behavior is to escape or avoid. In this case, Yesenia is seeking to escape reading tasks, so the goal of extinction is to eliminate or limit the opportunity to escape or avoid reading, contingent on engaging in problem behavior. The challenge is that, at the moment, if Yesenia wants to avoid the reading task, she will be able. This is largely out of the control of the teacher. In cases of escape, the best plan is to proactively limit the need to escape through antecedent intervention, teach and reinforce the use of an alternative behavior, and finally to try to limit the extent that responses to problem behavior provide access to escape. The antecedent, teaching, and reinforcement interventions are in place to limit Yesenia's need for escape. In order to limit the extent that Yesenia can avoid reading in response to problem behavior, the team has decided she will make up time spent avoiding reading during class by reading aloud with the teacher before going to recess. The team will meet regularly to review data and make decisions about revisions to the plan, which might include increasing or fading supports, depending on Yesenia's progress.

....

LaMichael

Please see Chapter 7 to review the case and competing behavior pathway (see Chapter 7, Figure 7.4) for LaMichael, a third grader who has been referred to the behavior support team at his school for repeatedly throwing materials during math class. To summarize, the team identified *obtaining peer attention* as the function of LaMichael's behavior and identified the following antecedent and teaching interventions: LaMichael would be assigned a peer

buddy at recess, provided with structured activities in which to participate with peers at recess, and taught to ask to play with peers. LaMichael was also taught, upon completion of his work, to be the "peer work checker" in math. After reviewing the case, *answer the focus questions and compare your responses to the following author responses:*

1. How can the team reinforce the use of an appropriate alternative behavior?

   The initial focus on consequence intervention will be to reinforce the alternative behavior as a replacement for problem behavior. In this case, when LaMichael requests to work with a peer, it is important to quickly provide access to working with a peer.

2. How can the team reinforce use of the desired behavior(s) or approximations to shape the desired behavior(s)?

   LaMichael's peers were taught to give positive attention to LaMichael when he was on task and handling materials appropriately, his teacher was told to do the same, especially if he was working independently. This was paired with a more formal reinforcement system during which LaMichael could receive a "caught being good" card each day if he handled materials safely, respected his peers' work without disrupting them, and responded quickly to the teacher's redirection to the alternate behavior. When he earned two cards, he could exchange the cards for the opportunity for the entire class to spend the last 5 minutes of math playing a game, such as "heads up, seven up." Because LaMichael really likes peer attention, the class could celebrate and reinforce his positive behavior through the game. Following LaMichael's first successful week, a goal would be to adjust requirements for earning cards to include increasing independent work (desired behavior).

3. How can the team provide a corrective prompt or redirection to encourage the use of the alternative or desired behavior at the earliest signs of problem behavior?

   The team anticipates that the antecedent intervention of working with a peer from the start of the task should reduce the likelihood of LaMichael's problem behavior and increase opportunities and access to positive peer attention. However, if the behavior does occur, the intervention will include a plan for redirecting problem behavior to the alternate behavior as guided by the competing behavior pathway. At the earliest signs of LaMichael's off-task behavior, the teacher should redirect LaMichael by visually prompting him (limiting social attention) to use the alternative behavior of asking, "Can I work with a peer?" When asking appropriately, LaMichael should quickly be allowed to work with a peer to reinforce the alternative behavior.

4. How can the team use extinction on the problem behavior?

Extinction, or withholding reinforcement, for the problem behavior (throwing materials) can be challenging when the function of behavior is to obtain peer attention since it involves peer behavior. This is a particularly challenging behavior to ignore because it is so disruptive to his peers' work. To put LaMichael's problem behavior (taking and throwing peers' materials) on extinction, peers were taught to ignore his problem behavior or provide a minimal, nonemotional response and instead walk to the teacher's desk if they needed to move away from LaMichael. It's important to remind LaMichael's peers to make sure to provide positive attention to reinforce when he is on task and safe. LaMichael's team planned to meet regularly to review data and make decisions about revisions to the plan, which included increasing or reducing supports, depending on his progress.

....

Samuel

Please see Chapter 7 to review the case and competing behavior pathway (see Chapter 7, Figure 7.5) for Samuel. Samuel is a 20-year-old male who repetitively slaps his head with the palm of his hand to obtain sensory input. Head slapping is most likely to occur when Samuel is anxious because he was not allowed to organize his own schedule for the day and when tasks someone else scheduled are longer than 5 minutes without a break. Samuel's team decided to provide him with the opportunity to build his own work schedule with frequent breaks and give him access to a head scratcher as an alternative means to gain sensory stimulation. After reviewing the case, *answer the focus questions and compare your responses to the following author responses:*

1. How can the team reinforce the use of an appropriate alternative behavior?

Samuel's boss agreed with plans to reinforce the alternative behavior in the short term. When Samuel asked for a break, he would be allowed a 2-minute break with his head scratcher.

2. How can the team reinforce use of the desired behavior(s) or approximations to shape the desired behavior(s)?

Samuel's team decided that if Samuel followed his schedule all day without engaging in any head slapping (desired behavior), Samuel would be reinforced for the desired behavior with the opportunity to wash his hair that evening with a special soap (that made his scalp tingle and was highly preferred) and head scratcher.

3. How can the team provide a corrective prompt or redirection to encourage the use of the alternative or desired behavior at the earliest signs of problem behavior?

Although Samuel's team believed that allowing him to build his schedule with frequent breaks and access to a head scratcher would reduce Samuel's head slapping, they still wanted to identify specific ways to respond when Samuel engaged in head slapping. Fortunately, Samuel's team has been providing support to Samuel regarding his head slapping for years, so he is pretty responsive to redirection unless he is extremely anxious or upset. If Samuel's supervisor or coworkers see that he is beginning to look anxious or engage in head slapping, they are to quickly prompt him to request a break with the head scratcher (alternative behavior).

4. How can the team use extinction on the problem behavior?

If Samuel does not respond to redirection and continues to slap his head, his supervisor is supposed to gently put his arm around Samuel's shoulders to prevent him from continued slapping (extinction) and escort him to the supervisor's office so Samuel can talk to his case manager on the phone. The team will meet regularly to review data and make decisions about plan revisions, which includes increasing or fading supports depending on his progress.

....

CONCLUSION

PBS has reframed the use of consequences in behavior intervention. Most importantly, the use of aversive consequences that cause, pain, harm, or humiliation are never allowed (APBS, 2007), and due to the challenge of predicting individual experiences of aversion to punitive interventions, these other types of punitive consequences are generally not recommended. PBS also suggests strategic and moderate use of consequences for both desired and nondesired behavior, emphasizing the challenges to fading and generalization that can result from interventions relying predominantly on the use of reinforcement and punishment to overpower problem behavior.

PBS suggests a more comprehensive approach to intervention that focuses on prevention, teaching, reinforcement, and corrective behavior reduction interventions with a focus on improving quality of life, not merely reducing problem behavior (Carr et al., 2002). The goal is to implement comprehensive interventions using an understanding of the function of problem behavior to actively integrate antecedent, teaching, and consequence strategies. The competing behavior pathway framework was demonstrated as a useful guide for informing the development of integrated interventions that can reduce reliance on big consequences (rewards or punishments) and maximize meaningful, long-term, positive outcomes.

REFERENCES

Alberto, P.A., & Troutman, A.C. (2013). *Applied behavior analysis for teachers* (9th ed.). New York, NY: Pearson.

Anderson, C.M., & Long, E.S. (2002). Use of a structured descriptive assessment methodology to identify variables affecting problem behavior. *Journal of Applied Behavior Analysis, 35,* 137–154.

Association for Positive Behavior Support (APBS). (2007). *Positive behavior support standards of practice: Individual level.* Retrieved from http://www.apbs.org/files/apbs_standards_of_practice_2013_format.pdf

Berliner, D.C. (1980). Using research on teaching for the improvement of classroom practice. *Theory into Practice, 19*(4).

Bijou, S.W. (1957). Patterns of reinforcement and resistance to extinction in young children. *Child Development, 28*(1), 47–54.

Carr, E.G., Dunlap, G., Horner, R.H., Koegel, R.L., Turnbull, A.P., & Sailor, W., . . . Fox, L. (2002). Positive behavior support: Evolution of an applied science. *Journal of Positive Behavior Interventions, 4,* 4–16.

Center for Effective Discipline. (2010). *U.S. corporal punishment and paddling statistics by state and race.* Retrieved from http://www.stophitting.com/index.php?page=statesbanning

Dietz, D.D., & Repp, A.C. (1983). Reducing behavior through reinforcement. *Exceptional Education Quarterly, 3,* 34–46.

Fisher, W., Piazza, C., Cataldo, M., Harrell, R., Jefferson, G., & Conner, R. (1993). Functional communication training with and without extinction and punishment. *Journal of Applied Behavior Analysis, 26,* 23–36.

Fisher, W., Thompson, R., Piazza, C., Crosland, K., & Gotjen, D. (1997). On the relative reinforcing effects of choice and differential consequences. *Journal of Applied Behavior Analysis, 30,* 423–438.

Horner, R. (2005). General case programming. In M. Hersen, J. Rosqvist, A. Gross, R. Drabman, G. Sugai, & R. Horner (Eds.), *Encyclopedia of behavior modification and cognitive behavior therapy* (Vol. 3, pp. 1343–1348). Thousand Oaks, CA: Sage Publications. doi:10.4135/9781412950534.n3071

Horner, R.H., Dunlap, G., Koegel, R.L., Carr, E.G., Sailor, W., Anderson, J., . . . O'Neill, R.E. (1990). Toward a technology of nonaversive behavioral support. *Journal of The Association for Persons with Severe Handicaps, 15*(3), 125–132.

Lerman, D., Iwata, B., Rainville, B., Adelinis, J., Crosland, K., & Kogan, J. (1997). Effects of reinforcement choice on task responding in individuals with developmental disabilities. *Journal of Applied Behavior Analysis, 30,* 411–422.

O'Neill, R., Horner, R., Albin, R., Sprague, J., Storey, K., & Newton, J. (1997). *Functional assessment and program development for problem behavior: A practical handbook.* Pacific Grove, CA: Brooks/Cole.

Scheuermann, B.K., & Hall, J.A. (2012). *Positive behavioral supports for the classroom* (2nd ed.). New York, NY: Pearson.

Simons, D.A., & Wurtele, S.K. (2010). Relationships between parents' use of corporal punishment and their children's endorsement of spanking and hitting other children. *Child Abuse & Neglect: The International Journal, 34*(9), 639–646.

Sobsey, D. (1990). Modifying the behavior of behavior modifiers. In A. Repp & N. Singh (Eds.), *Perspectives on the use of nonaversive and aversive interventions for persons with developmental disabilities* (pp. 421–433). Sycamore, IL: Sycamore Publishing.

Stahr, B., Cushing, D., Lane, K., & Fox, J. (2006). Efficacy of a function-based intervention in decreasing off-task behavior exhibited by a student with ADHD. *Journal of Positive Behavior Interventions, 8,* 201–211.

Wilder, D.A., Harris, C., Reagan, R., & Rasey, A. (2007). Functional analysis and treatment of noncompliance by preschool children. *Journal of Applied Behavior Analysis, 40,* 173–177.

Facilitating Generalization and Maintenance of Behavior Change

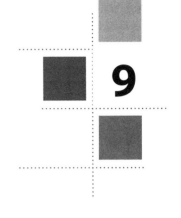

9

Jeffrey Sprague

This chapter provides key terms, concepts, and strategies for promoting generalization and maintenance of responding, which were briefly introduced in the introduction to Chapter 6. The aim of this chapter is to allow the reader to understand and use methods for facilitating the generalization and maintenance of skills (an Association for Positive Behavior Support [APBS] standard of practice). A background and rationale for the importance of promoting generalization and maintenance follows, along with operational definitions of both concepts. A discussion of the essential differences between generalization and maintenance of responding is provided. Response maintenance will also be discussed in the context of schedules of reinforcement (Ferster & Skinner, 1957). A brief review of the research literature on generalization and maintenance precede the closing section on methods for programming and monitoring generalization and maintenance. The closing section includes sample case studies to illustrate the technical content.

BACKGROUND/PROBLEM STATEMENT

Programming for and achieving generalization and maintenance of learned behavior has been a primary goal of behavior change for researchers and practitioners since the inception of applied behavior analysis (ABA). "A therapeutic behavioral change, to be effective, often (not always) must occur over time, persons, and settings, and the effects of the change sometimes should spread to a variety of related behaviors" (Stokes & Baer, 1977, p. 350). However, what we know about life outcomes for individuals with disabilities and/or challenging behavior indicates that they characteristically fail to generalize or maintain learned behavior without careful design of instruction and supports (Horner, Bellamy, & Colvin, 1984). Ideally, instruction is designed and delivered to result in behavior change beyond the context and materials used during teaching. However, the methods for assessing and achieving this outcome are not universally adopted (Harvey, Lewis-Palmer, Horner, & Sugai, 2003). The goal of an instructional or behavior support strategy should be to achieve accurate performance in all settings (stimulus contexts) where the target response is desirable and functional and does not occur in those stimulus contexts where the target response is inappropriate or not functional. The focus individual is taught to discriminate between correct and incorrect performances of a skill or behavior. For example, a student may be able to demonstrate money counting in the classroom, but if she cannot use the skill to purchase valued items in the community, it would be a generalization failure. This example would also apply to a student with behavior challenges who might perform a complex social skill such as conflict resolution in a classroom group but fails to use that skill when confronted with a bully in the school cafeteria. Once the behaviors have been acquired and applied in targeted contexts, the focus should shift to achieving durability or maintenance of behavior change over time (Horner, Dunlap, & Koegel, 1998). The rules and procedures for achieving maintenance are different from those used to achieve generalized responding, as reviewed in the following discussion.

Generalization and maintenance concepts are sometimes defined insufficiently or even incorrectly, and as a result, consistent, technically correct methods for promoting these two outcomes are often misunderstood, misapplied, or simply hoped for and not often achieved. For the purposes of this chapter, there are two types of generalization and one type of maintenance. Stimulus generalization is observed when as a function of training with one set of stimuli, a different (but similar) set of stimuli control the conditioned response. For example, if a student sees .50 cents on a vending machine and adds two quarters to get the item, she should see .50 cents on a different machine and still know to put in two quarters. Response generalization is observed when after training a response to one stimulus, the same or a similar response is observed for another stimulus. For example, if a student learns to button one shirt, she should be able to adjust the buttoning movements to get another shirt buttoned. The response is similar but has to be varied to match the requirements of the new shirt. Maintenance is defined as durability of performance over time. Once a student learns a new skill, we can observe her performing the skill over time.

Trevor Stokes and Donald Baer (1977), in their seminal paper on this topic, noted that in traditional operant research, generalization was considered the natural outcome of failing to learn discrimination (e.g., discriminating "b" from "d"). The authors argued that a "technology of generalization" was needed to advance theory and practice. Their landmark paper set the standard for the field and much of the writing and research regarding generalization and maintenance still uses the typology laid out by these two pioneers in the field of ABA. This paper continues to influence how behavioral researchers and practitioners discuss generalization and maintenance successes and failures. Unfortunately, the typology does not discriminate clearly between generalization and maintenance as defined here (Horner et al., 1984). Each strategy is defined as follows with some simple examples:

1. *Train and hope:* After a behavior change is achieved, generalization may be noted but not actively pursued. For example, we teach a young student to ask for help during math instruction and hope that he or she will use the skill elsewhere without providing any explicit support. We may not even conduct any probes to see if the skill is performed in novel contexts (Redd & Birnbrauer, 1969). Stokes and Baer (1977) addressed maintenance of generalized responding over time under this strategy by suggesting that, like generalization, we often don't directly program for it.

2. *Sequential modification:* In this strategy, a skill is taught and probes for generalization are conducted. Based on the success or failure of the teaching strategy, a revised teaching plan might modify responses, settings, or trainers. For example, if a student learns to give a greeting during 1:1 instruction but does not use the skill elsewhere, teaching examples may be expanded (addressing specific examples, setting, or trainer characteristics) to achieve generalized performance. In this example, the student may simply be prompted to use the greeting response in other settings, with other people, and so forth.

3. *Introduction to natural maintaining contingencies:* Stokes and Baer (1977) described this as a strategy for generalization programming, when it is actually aimed at maintenance of behavior change (Horner et al., 1984). The goal of this strategy is to teach behaviors that might be maintained by naturally occurring contingencies in the environment. For example, we might provide frequent reinforcement for a new skill such as asking for help with a difficult task and then fade that reinforcement until it "matches" the natural need to use that skill in the classroom (Baer & Wolf, 1970).

4. *Training sufficient exemplars:* In this strategy, one example of a skill is taught and a probe for generalization is conducted. If the desired generalization of responding does not occur, then new teaching examples would be introduced. This would continue until "sufficient" examples were presented. For example, if a student was taught to use a problem-solving algorithm (Rooney, Poe, Drescher, & Frantz, 1993) when faced with teasing from peers, he or she might next be taught to use the skill to work through a conflict with a friend. Examples would be added until generalization is observed.

5. *Training loosely:* In this strategy, Stokes and Baer (1977) suggested that teaching be conducted with relatively little control or attention to teaching examples. The goal is to "maximize sampling of relevant dimensions for transfer to other situations and other forms of behavior" (p. 357). For example, if we want a student to ask for help in a variety of situations, we might provide prompts or direct teaching of the skill, without consideration of the range and type of examples. While the goal of sampling a range of examples is of primary importance, this method would certainly not be indicated, given the propensity of support for carefully designed instruction, including example selection and sequencing to achieve maximum efficiency and effectiveness of instruction and support (Horner, Sprague, & Wilcox, 1982).

6. *Indiscriminable contingencies:* Stokes and Baer (1977) suggested that "resistance to extinction may be regarded as a form of generalization" (p. 358) and yet using schedules of intermittent reinforcement (see the next section) is clearly a method for achieving maintenance of behavior change over time (Horner, Dunlap, & Koegel, 1998). For example, if a student is taught to raise his or her hand to gain adult attention (a functionally equivalent replacement behavior), a teaching plan might aim to make the schedule or frequency of actually gaining attention unpredictable or inconsistent to promote maintenance of that behavior.

7. *Programming common stimuli:* In this strategy, teaching examples are specifically chosen to match up the stimulus characteristics found in the targeted generalization setting(s) (Rincover & Koegel, 1977). For example, if using a skill with multiple people is desired, then the selection of teaching examples should include a range of adults and students (Mesmer, Duhon, & Dodson, 2007).

8. *Mediating generalization:* This refers to the idea that a learned skill or behavior would likely be used in other contexts or problem settings as well and that there is sufficient similarity between the original teaching context and the generalization context to result in "generalization" (Stokes & Baer, 1977). For example, teaching a student to self-manage his or her behavior using

the popular "check in–check out" (CICO) system (Crone, Horner, & Hawken, 2004) may result in generalized use of the CICO point card across settings.

9. *Training "to generalize":* In this final strategy, it is suggested that a reinforcement contingency be placed on "generalized responding," as it would with any other behavior or skill. For example, if a student is taught to ask for help when attempting a difficult task, reinforcement may be applied (along with instructions) to use the newly acquired skill when attempting other difficult tasks (Harvey et al., 2003).

Robert Horner and colleagues (1984) published a paper proposing a conceptual model of generalization programming that clearly discriminates the concepts and operational features of generalization and maintenance as originally presented in the Stokes and Baer (1977) paper. Horner et al. argued that generalization and maintenance represented functionally different concepts that are controlled by different behavior mechanisms. They also argued that the Stokes and Baer typology did not lead to an effective and efficient methodology for teaching generalized responding. This paper outlined a methodology for "general case programming" that guided a generation of important research. Before proceeding to the details of general case programming, it is necessary to understand the key vocabulary and concepts of generalization and maintenance. This next section provides definitions and rules of use.

KEY VOCABULARY AND CONCEPTS

Generalization

Horner et al. (1984) used a seminal paper on stimulus control written by H.S. Terrace (1966) as the conceptual and technical basis of their approach. They argued the critical importance of discriminating generalization from transfer of stimulus control as the basis for building a conceptual logic for a technology of generalization. For each of the following definitions, S refers to an antecedent stimulus, and R refers to the response of the individual. Thus S_1 is "Stimulus 1" and R_2 is "Response 2."

Stimulus and Response Classes

One of the most important concepts to understand is that different stimuli can occasion the same response, and different responses can be performed to achieve the same functional effect. Figure 9.1 illustrates this concept. For example, a "difficult task" may take many forms (e.g., making a sandwich, cleaning, completing a math worksheet) and "difficult task" might be considered a stimulus class, meaning that each of these tasks share enough features to occasion a similar response from an individual. In the same logic, an individual might use different responses (typically referred to as *topography*) to achieve the same functional effect. For example, an individual might verbally refuse, hit others, or destroy property in an attempt to avoid a difficult task.

Stimulus Generalization

Stimulus generalization is observed when, after training with one set of stimuli, a different (but similar) set of stimuli control the conditioned response:

- *Prior to instruction:* $S_1 \neq R_1$ and $S_2 \neq R_1$
- *During instruction:* $S_1 \rightarrow R_1$
- *After instruction:* $S_1 \rightarrow R_1$ and $S_2 \rightarrow R_1$

For example, a mother is successful in teaching her son to "take a drink" (S_1), and the father also gives the direction "take a drink" (S_2). If their son complies with both requests, then we can suggest stimulus generalization across the people.

Response Generalization

Response generalization is observed when, after training an $S_1 \rightarrow R_1$ relation and then placing R_1 on extinction (or blocking R_1), a new response R_2 is likely:

- *Prior to instruction:* $S_1 \neq R_1$ and $S_1 \neq R_2$
- *During instruction:* $S_1 \rightarrow R_1$

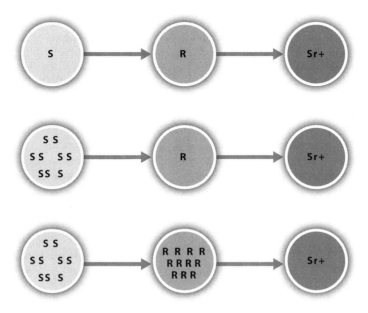

Figure 9.1. Model of stimulus and response classes.

- *After instruction R1 is placed on extinction or blocked:* S1 → R1 and S1 → R2

For example, if a student is asked to complete a task (S1) and uses hitting in an effort to avoid the task, we can continue to present S1 (also known as *escape extinction*) until a novel response is produced. Unfortunately, without directly teaching the student, this will likely produce a new problem behavior (R2). In practical application, we would always teach and prompt the functionally equivalent replacement behavior.

Transfer of Stimulus Control

Transfer of stimulus control is observed when stimulus control exerted by one stimulus *transfers* to a second previously non-controlling stimulus as a function of pairing:

- *Given:* S1 → R1 and S2 ≠ R1
- *Teach:* S1 + S2 → R1
- *Result:* S2 → R1

For example, we can return to the mother who successfully teaches her son to "take a drink" (S1) and the father who also gives the direction "take a drink" (S2). In this case, when the father gives the direction, the son does *not* comply. If the parents take turns (a form of pairing, S1 + S2 → R1) giving the direction "take a drink," over many trials the son begins to take a drink in response to the father's direction (S2 → R1).

Stimulus Control Transfer Strategies

There are three main methods for achieving transfer of stimulus control. These include pairing, fading, and time delay:

- *Simple pairing:* S1 + S2
- *Pair S1 and S2 then fade S1 across trials:*
    - Fade within a prompt
    - Fade across prompts
- *Time delay (given S1 → R1):*
    - S1 + S2 → R1
    - S2 . . . S1 → R1
    - S2 . . . → R1
    - S2 → R1

Simple pairing is illustrated by the son who learned to respond to "take a drink" from the mother and then the father (S1 + S2). *Fading* would simply involve the mother reducing her presence over time, until the child responded to the father's direction. *Time delay* is a special instance of fading (Charlop & Walsh, 1986; Schuster, Gast, Wolery, & Guiltinan, 1988), where an initial prompt (S1) or direction is established (stimulus control) and paired with a second type of prompt (S2). After pairing is successful, then S2 is delivered first, while S1 is "delayed" (either a constant delay or an increasing interval over time [S2 . . . . . . S1 → R1]) until S2 works the same as S1. For example, if a teacher prompts a student to "say apple" (S1) when presented with a picture of an apple (S2), he or she would delay the prompt "say apple" for a few moments to test if the student says "apple" in response to the picture alone. Time delay is a highly successful and well-researched teaching method.

MAINTENANCE

Maintenance refers to the durability of performance over time (Ferster & Skinner, 1957). It also refers to the durability of stimulus control over time and as continued performance of behavior(s) when consequences are removed (extinction; Terrace, 1966). For example, once a student learns to use a skill such as asking for help, he or she continues to use that skill as targeted over time. Maintenance of a behavior is affected by schedules of reinforcement during acquisition (also known as the learning phase) and fluency building (performing the skill "automatically"). A schedule of reinforcement refers to the rate, frequency, or probability that reinforcement will occur. Schedules of reinforcement are reviewed briefly in the next section.

Schedules of Reinforcement: Essential for Facilitating Maintenance and Treating Maintenance Failures

Understanding the rules governing types and schedules of reinforcement is essential to maximize effectiveness in promoting behaviors in all phases of learning (acquisition, fluency building, generalization, maintenance). In this section, a definition of *reinforcement* is provided, followed by a presentation of the types of different *schedules of reinforcement* (see Chapter 8). The *schedule* of reinforcement simply refers to ways to break down how frequently or likely a response or skill will result in a reinforcing consequence.

Reinforcement refers to an increase in the probability of a behavior over time as a function of the contingent delivery (or removal) of a consequence event/object/ stimulus. A *reinforcer* is a stimulus, which when presented contingent on a response, increases the future occurrence of the response. It is critical to understand that reinforcement (and punishment) is a process and cannot be inferred by observing a single event, a common mistake in practice. This may lead practitioners or parents to believe that if they could just deliver a sufficiently powerful consequence one time, they will be effective. This is simply not the case because reinforcement can only be inferred after observing several instances of the behavior.

Continuous versus Intermittent Reinforcement

We can break down how schedules of reinforcement work by illustrating key features. First, continuous reinforcement (CRF) requires that a reinforcer is presented after *every* occurrence of the response. CRF is rarely practical in applied settings, except during early acquisition of a skill or behavior, because it takes a lot of effort and diligence on the part of a teacher or practitioner. In addition, CRF does not result in the maintenance of behavior unless it is sustained. Intermittent schedules are more practical and more desired in the long term. Intermittent reinforcement is in place when the reinforcer is *not* presented after every occurrence of a response but at some fixed or variable ratio or interval. Types of reinforcement schedules are presented next, with practical examples.

Simple Schedules of Reinforcement

Schedule Dimensions We can break sched
ules of reinforcement in to four dimensions
that include the following:

1. *Fixed:* Predictable (the ratio or interval of
   reinforcement is the same)

2. *Variable:* Less predictable (the ratio or
   interval varies)

3. *Ratio:* Based on the number of responses

4. *Interval:* Delivered on the first response
   after a period of time

Table 9.1 illustrates the range of combinations for these four dimensions, along with
examples. A related type of reinforcement is
called *noncontingent* and is also presented.
It is important to remember that reinforcement schedules rarely function alone in
applied settings. Concurrent schedules of
reinforcement will be discussed later.

Effects of Simple Schedules It is critical to understand the predicted effects of
simple reinforcement schedules on the individual. First, we can more effectively support
maintenance of behavior if we understand
the predicted effects. We may also be able to
observe the naturally occurring schedules that
maintain problem (and desired) behavior and
either change that schedule or present a competing schedule to promote the use of adaptive
behavior over time. This will be discussed in a
later section. Table 9.2 provides a summary of
the predicted effects of simple schedules.

Extinction: A Critical Process

Extinction represents a critical process in
teaching and behavior support. Extinction
is a reduction in responding over time as a
function of withholding a previously delivered reinforcer. The classic example of
extinction is withholding attention from a

Table 9.1. Schedules of reinforcement

Schedule type	Definition	Example
Fixed ratio (FR)	A reinforcer is presented contingent on a response occurring a specific number of times (e.g., FR 3, FR 10, FR 100). Note that FR 1 indicates continuous reinforcement (CRF).	Students get a "point" for each correct math problem (CRF).
Fixed interval (FI)	A reinforcer is presented contingent on the first response following a fixed time interval (e.g., FI 10 minutes, FI 30 minutes, FI 3 years).	Students get to go to recess after a correct group response at the end of a 90-minute period (FI 90 minutes). Going to the mailbox is only rewarded the first time after the mail arrives (which is about the same time every day; FI 1 day).
Variable ratio (VR)	A reinforcer is presented after a specific num-ber of responses, "on average." The range and mean need to be defined (e.g., VR 10, 5–12; VR 20, 15–25).	Student receives praise on average every 50 responses (range 2–150, VR 50).
Variable interval (VI)	A reinforcer is presented on the first response after a time interval with a specified range and mean (e.g., VI 20 minutes, 15–25 minutes).	Student receives peer attention for talking out about every 5 minutes (range 3–8 minutes, VI 5 minutes). Student receives praise for remaining seated in accordance with a "time card" (1 minute, 5 minutes, 8 minutes, VI 4 minutes).
Noncontingent reinforcement (NCR; unrelated to student/child behavior)	The reinforcer is delivered at a specific time regardless of the response. Rewards are de-livered based on events and general positive praise is given.	The teacher greets and welcomes students at the door each morning at the beginning of school.

Table 9.2. Predicted effects of simple reinforcement schedules

Schedule type	Predicted effect	When and why to use
Fixed ratio (including continuous reinforcement [CRF])	• High rate of responding • Postreinforcement pause (increased length of pause as ratio increases; go, go, Sr+ [positive reinforcement], pause, pause, go go, Sr+, pause . . .)	• CRF is especially useful when the student is learning new skills to ensure they get a lot of feedback. It is important to "fade" to intermittent so the student does not come to depend on CRF.
Fixed interval	• Moderate rate of responding • Longer post-reinforcement pause (also known as a scallop function; go, go, Sr+, pause, go a little, go more, go, go, Sr+)	• A fixed schedule is predictable, and the student may slow down after receiving reinforcement because they know that it will be coming again soon. Use when a consistent rate of responding is not critical.
Variable interval	• Moderate rate of responding • No post-reinforcement pause	• Variable interval schedules are useful if a student can perform the behavior and you want to keep it going.
Variable ratio	• High rate of responding • No post-reinforcement pause	• Variable interval schedules are useful if a student can perform the behavior and you want to keep it going. You also need to be able to count the number of behaviors, so this may be challenging.
Noncontingent rewards (NCR)	• NCR signals availability of rewards • May be contingent on participation in setting • May establish conditional reinforcers • Proximity to teacher becomes a reinforcer. • Noncontingent rewards do *not* affect levels of specific target behaviors.	• Noncontingent rewards are useful when you want to establish a positive environment and signal to students that rewards are available.

student who is seeking it by using inappropriate behavior, such as not responding to a student who is calling out in class. Extinction is also a critical process that operates when teaching functionally equivalent alternative behaviors as part of a behavior support plan (BSP; Kuhn, Lerman, Vorndran, & Addison, 2006; O'Neill et al., 1997). When we teach a new, functionally equivalent replacement behavior, the "problem" behavior is put on extinction either because we give more reinforcement for the new replacement behavior or because we prevent reinforcement for that problem behavior.

There are three typical effects of extinction: extinction burst, response generalization, and ultimately a decrease in responding over time. With the initiation of extinction, there may be a brief and dramatic increase in responding. This is described as an *extinction burst* (Wilder et al., 2006). Practitioners should be especially careful in using

extinction with severe behaviors, as the "burst" can result in even more severe aggressive or self-injurious behavior. The extinction burst may also produce response generalization. In this case, different but functionally similar responses occur when target behavior is placed on extinction (Sprague & Horner, 1994). For example, if a student uses hitting to gain attention and that response is placed on extinction, he or she may use another member of the response class (e.g., yelling) to maintain access to attention. Some behaviors can be very resistant to extinction, and the time required to achieve a decrease in the behavior can be very long if extinction is used in isolation. As such, it is critical to always combine teaching and reinforcement for the desired alternative behavior (Carr et al., 1999).

Intermittent schedules of reinforcement build strong resistance to extinction, especially with lean variable ratio (VR) and variable interval (VI) schedules. The less predictable reinforcement has been in the past, the stronger the resistance to extinction. For example, if a student raises his or her hand to gain attention but it doesn't often work, he or she may resort to using problem behaviors because they work more consistently. Problem behaviors can be hard to ignore, and that is why both prompting and teaching the replacement behavior can increase the efficiency and effectiveness of extinction.

As previously indicated, most BSPs attempt to place problem behavior on extinction and provide differential reinforcement for the desired behavior (Janney, Umbreit, Ferro, Liaupsin, & Lane, 2013). When designing support, it is necessary to define the current schedule of reinforcement for the problem behavior. It is ideal to attempt to place the problem behavior on total extinction; otherwise, you are likely to create an intermittent schedule. By teaching a replacement behavior, you establish a concurrent schedule of reinforcement, which is covered in the next section.

Complex Schedules of Reinforcement

Once a basic understanding of simple reinforcement schedules is achieved, it is critical to understand how these schedules function when arrayed simultaneously or concurrently with other schedules. We refer to these as *multiple* or *concurrent* schedules, described in Table 9.3.

Multiple Schedules When using a multiple schedule strategy, one response or behavior will involve two schedules of reinforcement, each with a specific antecedent stimulus associated with it. Typically, only one schedule operates at a time. For example, if Teacher A provides a rich schedule of praise for on-task behavior and Teacher B gives little or no attention for the same behavior, we would expect to see different rates of on-task behavior, depending on the teacher (antecedent stimulus).

Concurrent Schedules Concurrent schedules provide the best description of what is operating when we are attempting to replace one behavior (or class of behaviors) with another. Two (or more) responses must be identified (one to reduce and one to replace), along with the schedule of reinforcement that is associated with both. Both schedules will be operative at the same time, and the behavior that "competes" will show a higher rate or probability of occurrence over time (Billingsley & Neel, 1985).

Importance of Understanding Complex Schedules

Behavior support planning and implementation is nearly always a process of creating concurrent schedules of reinforcement where the schedule for one behavior competes with another (Day, Horner, & O'Neill, 1994; Sprague & Horner, 1992). We know that one behavior will compete better based on the relative efficiency of that behavior. This can be affected by the schedule of reinforcement, as shown previously. Day et al. (1994) examined the role of latency (delay)

Table 9.3.   Multiple and concurrent schedules of reinforcement

Schedule type	Example
Multiple (one behavior, two schedules)	• Samira is praised for math work 1) in small group by teacher (variable interval; VI 3), then 2) in 1:1 with tutor (variable ratio; VR 4).
Concurrent (two behaviors, two schedules)	• Betsy can get attention from the teacher by raising her hand (fixed interval; FI 5) or by making loud noises (continuous reinforcement; CRF).
	• During seat work, Dan receives attention from teacher for working (VI 15) or attention from peers for acting silly (fixed ratio; FR 1).
	• Jim gets $10 for washing his grandmother's car. Later, he gets a pat on the back for washing his mother's car.

with reinforcement and relative response effort. Thus a behavior that has a richer schedule of reinforcement, works relatively quickly, and is easier to perform will be more likely. For example, asking for help is easier than pushing papers to the floor and screaming in order to avoid a difficult task. When we provide behavior support, we also need to be sure that the behavior works well in terms of the reinforcement schedule (at least as often and as quickly as the problem behavior; Langdon, Carr, & Owen-Deschryver, 2008).

REVIEW OF CURRENT RESEARCH IN POSITIVE BEHAVIOR INTERVENTIONS AND SUPPORTS

Dunlap and his colleagues (Dunlap & Carr, 2007; O'Dell et al., 2011; Clarke & Dunlap, 2008) have provided comprehensive reviews of positive behavior interventions and supports (PBIS) for individuals with developmental disabilities (Dunlap & Carr, 2007; Clarke & Dunlap, 2008) and emotional and behavioral disabilities (Clarke, Dunlap, & Stichter, 2002), as well as comprehensive analyses of all studies published in the *Journal of Positive Behavior Interventions* (http://pbi.sagepub.com/). Their findings suggest that research has increasingly become aligned with PBIS principles in many areas, yet other areas require additional focus in the future.

O'Dell et al. (2011) used the defining features of PBS, as described by Carr and colleagues (Carr et al., 2002), for coding categories. These included nine areas that should be included in a comprehensive PBS intervention: 1) emphasis on prevention, 2) systems change and multicomponent intervention, 3) comprehensive lifestyle change and quality of life, 4) life-span perspective, 5) ecological validity, 6) stakeholder participation, 7) social validity, 8) multiple theoretical perspectives, and 9) flexibility with respect to scientific practices. In this chapter, generalization and maintenance research are reflected in the areas of multicomponent

intervention, lifestyle change and quality of life, and ecological validity. Multicomponent interventions should systematically achieve generalization and maintenance using the methods described in this chapter. Maintenance is also reflected in the area of intervention duration and follow-up (O'Dell et al., 2011). Interventions, including lifestyle and/or quality-of-life changes for participants or stakeholders, composed 52% of the studies reviewed by O'Dell and colleagues; 48% involved multicomponent strategies, and 80% emphasized ecological validity. Regarding follow-up and duration, 74% of the studies reported the duration of intervention, with the majority (77%) lasting 30 days or fewer.

Clarke and colleagues (Clarke et al., 2002) published a similar analysis of research on individuals with emotional and behavioral disabilities. Their analysis covered the years 1980–1990, providing a more dated but valuable data set. The authors coded studies based on participant demographics, settings, research designs, dependent and independent variables, intervention agents, and measures of ecological validity. The results showed similar trends across interventions with students with emotional and behavioral disabilities (EBD) and participants with developmental disabilities (DD). The majority of articles for participants with EBD employed interventions that were consequence based, followed closely by antecedent manipulations and skill development. The second and third most reported intervention types were consequence-based and antecedent interventions. Multicomponent interventions averaged approximately one-third of the articles. Measurements of generalization and maintenance were reported in less than 30% of the published studies. From these findings, there is a clear need to provide additional focus on generalization and maintenance of learned behavior, including more studies assessing the mechanisms of generalization, and a focus on collecting follow-up data, including longer intervention durations where needed.

PROGRAMMING FOR GENERALIZATION AND MAINTENANCE: HOW TO DO IT

Generalization

The beginning of this chapter outlined the "technology of generalization" as presented by Stokes and Baer (1977). While this paper was seminal and very influential, others have expanded our theoretical and practical understanding of interventions to promote generalization and maintenance. Like Stokes and Baer, Becker and colleagues (Becker, Engelmann, & Thomas, 1975; Engelmann & Carnine, 1982) agreed with the need to use multiple examples but asserted that simply teaching with more examples would not in itself reliably produce generalized responding. They indicated a need to select multiple examples that systematically sample the range of stimulus and response variation in the class of stimulus situations where responding is desired (i.e., "the instructional universe"). This approach was adapted for use with focus individuals with significant disabilities and documented as an effective strategy for teaching generalized behavior change (Horner et al., 1982, 1984); it is known as *general case programming*. The sequence of programming steps is outlined as follows, including application examples.

The application of the general case guidelines involves 1) defining the responses required for desired performance (also known as the instructional universe), 2) defining the discriminative stimuli (SD) that should control or occasion each response, 3) defining SD variations across all possible performance examples in the instructional universe, 4) defining how the response demands of each of the responses vary (e.g., response topography), 5) selecting a set of examples that sample the full range of stimulus and response variation for each SD and response required, and 6) carefully sequencing the introduction and review of those teaching examples to ensure acquisition of the generalized skill. In an early demonstration of this method, Sprague and

Horner (1984) tested the effectiveness of this strategy while teaching six young men a generalized skill (vending machine use). The instructional goal was for the learners to use any vending machine they might encounter in the community. The responses required included selecting an item, inserting the correct amount of quarters, and activating the machine. The stimuli targeted to occasion vending machine use included the price of the item, a range of items to choose from, and the type of machine (e.g., buttons, knobs, and numbers). Across a wide range of machines, the variation in stimuli (e.g., range of prices from $0.20 to $1.00) and the needed response variation (e.g., putting in different amounts of quarters based on the price and using different motor movements required to activate the machine) were specified. Finally, the examples were selected and sequenced to teach vending machine use and generalized use across a full range of possible vending machine types. Sprague and Horner (1984) demonstrated that generalized responding was only achieved with careful selection and sequencing of instructional examples, and not simply by teaching with multiple examples. The logic of general case programming and programming for maintenance will be illustrated in greater detail in the following sections, with examples from Carr et al. (1999) and Iovannone et al. (2009).

Maintenance

Strategies to achieve maintenance of behavior change include those focused on the level or strength of initial stimulus control (i.e., how well the individual can respond), the opportunity to perform the skill over time (Horner, Williams, & Knobbe, 1985), ongoing reinforcement, and the strength of competing alternative behaviors (Ferro & Dunlap, 1993; Horner et al., 1988; Kennedy, 2002). Research findings would suggest that instruction and behavior support include multiple opportunities to use the new skill over time, analyze and introduce the individual to "natural" reinforcers, make the response(s) resistant to extinction by using intermittent schedules of reinforcement, and prevent competing contingencies from overcoming the new learning. The next section will illustrate how these generalization and maintenance strategies are applied in a practical context.

APPLYING GENERALIZATION AND MAINTENANCE STRATEGIES

Example 1: In the Community

The late Edward Carr and colleagues (Carr et al., 1999) published a paper describing a practical, five-component, assessment-based (description, categorization, and hypothesis verification), hypothesis-driven strategy consisting of rapport building, functional communication training (FCT), tolerance for delay of reinforcement, choice, and embedding. This multisituational approach included a functional behavioral assessment (FBA). Their strategy also included programming for generalization, assessing and intervening in new settings, and focusing on maintaining behavior change.

In the Carr et al. (1999) study, three individuals with developmental disabilities (Val, 14 years; Gary, 17 years; and Juan, 38 years) were selected for support based on a history of severe behavior performance (and resulting exclusion from community participation) and their respective abilities for some form of communication, such as simple speech, sign language, gestures, or use of Mayer-Johnson's Picture Communication Symbols. The assessment involved three major phases, which are described next. They then implemented the five-component behavior support process.

Describe   For a 2- to 3-week period, parents, teachers, job coaches, and community residence staff all participated in functional assessment interviews (Carr et al., 1994), and direct observation sessions were scheduled based on those interviews. All results were summarized in an antecedent, behavior, and consequence (ABC) summary statement format on index cards. More than 100 cards per individual were generated.

Categorize   Once the cards were completed, the researchers began to formulate hypotheses about behavioral function for each behavior (or group of behaviors). The categories were *attention, escape, tangible,* or *other.* The social reactions to problem behavior included task removal (escape), contingent lengthy reprimands (attention), and reinstitution of television time (access to tangible/activity).

Verify   The verification phase was intended to confirm that the situations identified during description and categorization actually did evoke problem behavior. For example, the authors used the descriptive FBA data to present a similar physical context, interpersonal context, and social reaction to verify that aggressive and self-injurious behavior did indeed occur for Gary within the situation identified in the descriptive phase. On a given day, they maintained the demand situation (i.e., sandwich making) for 15 minutes, during which time data were collected. Thus one example drawn from one theme (i.e., prompted completion of an ongoing series of tasks) was used to verify information from the *describe* and *categorize* phases.

Intervention   The comprehensive multicomponent approach consisted of building rapport, providing FCT, building tolerance for reinforcement delay, providing choices, and embedding stimuli that prompt problem behavior with others that are less challenging to the individual. These approaches were applied continuously throughout the 5 years of the intervention portion of the study, as needed. Each is described briefly as follows.

Building Rapport   The purpose of this component was to increase the general level of positive interaction between the individual with disability and her or his caregivers.

Increased positivity between people is both a stated value and a functional, evidence-based strategy (Fredrickson, 2009; Shores et al., 1993) and yet often overlooked. Caregivers provided a variety of positive reinforcers to the individuals, and they took steps to support them in improving their personal hygiene and clothing to reduce the possibility of social rejection by others. The caregivers and individuals also shared activities (e.g., jogging or going out to eat).

Functional Communication Training   The purpose of the FCT component was to teach the individuals a variety of communicative responses that were functionally equivalent to their problem behaviors, making further display of such behavior unnecessary, ineffective, and inefficient (Durand, 1991; Horner & Billingsley, 1998). For example, Gary used self-injury and property destruction to escape from difficult tasks. Gary was taught to say, "I need a break," and his request was honored. This was repeated for each individual and each function that was revealed during the assessment.

Building Tolerance for Reinforcement Delay   Carr et al. (1999) noted that once the FCT procedure was successful, the individuals used the skill at a very high rate. The caregivers were concerned that too many breaks would interfere with work completion, that too much attention would compete with the teacher's ability to attend to other students in a classroom setting, or that requests for tangibles could become excessive or impossible to provide. Tolerance for delay is also related to maintenance of behavior change. In this procedure, when the individual requests a particular reinforcer, the caregiver acknowledges the request and then gives a "delay" statement, such as, "Sure, Gary, you can have a break but first you need to finish making the sandwich." This method is effective because the communication strategy is acknowledged and the individual is simply asked to delay access to the reinforcer for an increasingly longer period of time.

Using Embedding   In this procedure, stimuli that are discriminative for problem behavior (e.g., task demands) are interspersed with stimuli that are discriminative for positive behavior. This method has also been called *task interspersal* (Dunlap & Morelli-Robbins, 1990; Horner, Day, Sprague, O'Brian, & Tuesday-Heathfield, 1991) or *behavior momentum* (Mace, Mauro, Boyajian, & Eckert, 2006). For example, a series of "easy" instructions might precede the presentation of a "difficult" task. Carr et al. (1999) also demonstrated that by presenting a choice of tasks (e.g., vacuum, wash the car, or sweep the floor) and then playing some favorite music, Gary would request to have the music turned back on, and then the choice was presented again until he initiated one of the choices.

Generalization   Two strategies were employed to achieve generalization: programming generalization and conducting additional descriptive assessments and interventions in situations in which a problem behavior continued or reemerged (Horner et al., 1982). Carr et al. (1999) identified interventions that were successful in one situation and then systematically introduced these interventions into other, similar situations (Stokes & Baer, 1977). For example, when Gary learned to use, "I want a break," during sandwich making and vacuuming, his caregiver applied the teaching and prompting to other activities, such as hand washing and making the bed. The intervention team continued to conduct descriptive assessments across all valued environments and activities and adjusted their teaching and behavior support strategies to solve any remaining failures of generalized responding.

Maintenance   Consistent with the recommendation to maintain "opportunity to perform" (Horner et al., 1985), the teaching team visited important performance sites and routines about 1 day per month and also made phone contact in order to assess maintenance of behavior change and assist caregivers with problem solving.

Example 2: At School

Iovannone et al. (2009; Dunlap et al., 2010) developed and tested a five-step "prevent, teach, reinforce" (PTR) tier-3 behavior support model for use in schools. This effective model uses FBA (O'Neill et al., 1997) and FCT (Durand, 1991) to achieve acquisition, generalization, and maintenance of functionally equivalent replacement behaviors. The five-step process was facilitated by a PTR consultant and included team development, goal setting, assessment, intervention and coaching, and evaluation. The following section outlines how this process was used to support José, an elementary-age student with a disability.

In order to effectively design and deliver targeted supports to students, it is generally recognized and recommended that a school-based behavior support team be formed to complete the steps necessary for successful implementation (Crone, Hawken, & Horner, 2010). The purpose of team development (Step 1) is to evaluate the strengths and weaknesses of the behavior support team functioning, outline roles and responsibilities, and determine a consensus-making process. Team members should include people with knowledge of the student (e.g., classroom teacher, instructional assistant, and parent), someone with expertise in FBA principles (e.g., a PTR consultant or other school-based consultant), and someone with knowledge of the school context (e.g., a school administrator or designee). In case of José, his classroom teacher and father joined the PTR consultant and school administrator as members of the team.

The purpose of Step 2 (goal setting) was to identify behaviors of greatest concern to the team and possible replacement behaviors (teach). The team used an FBA to identify, prioritize, and operationally define the behaviors of concern, and those that would be targeted to replace them through direct teaching. To program for generalization of these skills, the team targeted problem behaviors for reduction and social and academic skills to teach and use across the school day. For José, the team identified a broad goal that he would communicate his wants and needs appropriately. They then identified a behavior to decrease (José will decrease screaming, hitting, and getting out of his seat) and a behavior to increase (José will ask for a break or for attention when needed).

The team also developed a teacher-friendly baseline data collection system. They used direct behavior rating (DBR; Christ, Riley-Tillman, Chafouleas, & Boice, 2010), a hybrid assessment combining features of systematic direct observations and rating scales. Problem behaviors included screaming (any loud, high-pitched noise) and hitting (any time José touches peers or adults with an open hand, fist, foot, or object while screaming or protesting). Replacement behaviors included expressing frustration appropriately using words, pictures, or signs to ask for a break or attention.

In Step 3, the FBA was continued to confirm the initial behaviors and goals in Step 1. Each team member independently answered a series of questions related to observed antecedents/triggers of problem behaviors and possible functions of the problem behaviors (including consequences typically associated with the problem behaviors). The PTR facilitator summarized the input and developed draft hypotheses about the function of José's behaviors. This process also served to identify the range of stimulus and response variation needed for teaching and generalization. For José, antecedent stimuli included nonpreferred tasks (reading, math); other students being upset or mad; the teacher attending to others; transitions from preferred to nonpreferred tasks; changes in schedule; and when he was denied and item, told no, or asked to fix something. The team selected multiple examples of each to target for selection and sequencing of teaching examples. Targeted skills included peer interaction, raising a hand to elicit attention, sharing attention, making conversation, taking turns, waiting, and asking for a break.

In Step 4, a detailed plan for teaching and reinforcing the new replacement behaviors across multiple contexts was designed. The plan also included strategies for preventing the problem behavior(s) from resulting in reinforcement. One of the strategies included giving José a "wait card" on his desk to assist him in remembering to wait his turn. Prior to group work, José was told, "Remember, when it is someone else's turn, you sit quietly and wait," while pointing to his card. If José called out, teachers would point to his card to remind him what to do and used a verbal prompt if the point prompt did not work. To promote the wait card's generalized use, the team utilized it in a wide range of situations in school. This process was repeated for all target behaviors. When the plan was complete, the PTR coach provided preimplementation training and was present on the first day of implementation to provide support in the classroom, model the procedures, and provide feedback as needed.

Finally, in Step 5, the team conducted an evaluation of the plan to see if it was working and if any modifications needed to be made. The DBRs were graphed, and decisions about the plan were based on continuous review of these data. The team discussed if the procedures should be modified or expanded and planned for generalization and maintenance. The team asked questions about José's generalized use of his new skills in different settings, with different people, and with different instructional examples. The team continued to conduct the support plan and modify components of the plan, providing maintenance as needed.

CONCLUSION

The aim of the chapter is to allow the reader to understand and use methods for promoting generalization and maintenance of skills (an APBS standard of practice). Key terms, concepts, and strategies for promoting generalization and maintenance were provided, with illustrations based on published research studies (Carr et al., 1999; Dunlap et al., 2010). A brief review of the research literature on generalization and maintenance suggests that much more research is needed in these critical areas. There is much research suggesting that these strategies *can* be effective (Clarke et al., 2002; Dunlap & Carr, 2007; Iovannone et al., 2009), yet additional research is needed regarding typical practitioners' willingness and ability to adopt and implement strategies to promote these critical outcomes (Clarke & Dunlap, 2008).

Problem behavior continues to be the primary reason children and young adults are excluded from school, home, recreation, community, and work. In their seminal article defining PBS (Carr et al., 2002), Edward G. Carr and his colleagues laid out a vision for behavior support that lays out the core values to guide what we address, how we intervene, and how we determine if we are successful. We are also called to support individuals within the context of their families and to honor the guidance and support provided *from* their families. One way to incorporate these values is to work to build and maintain valued lifestyles for the individuals we support, and generalization and maintenance of learned behavior should be at the forefront of our efforts.

REFERENCES

Baer, D.M., & Wolf, M.M. (1970). The entry into natural communities of reinforcement. In R. Ulrich, T. Stachnik, & J. Mabry (Eds.), *Control of human behavior* (Vol. 2, pp. 319–324). Glenview, IL: Scott Foresman.

Becker, W., Engelmann, S., & Thomas, D.R. (1975). *Teaching 2: Cognitive learning and instruction.* Chicago, IL: Science Research Associates.

Billingsley, F.F., & Neel, R.S. (1985). Competing behaviors and their effects on skill generalization and maintenance. *Analysis and Intervention in Developmental Disabilities, 5,* 357–372.

Carr, E.G., Dunlap, G., Horner, R.H., Koegel, R.L., Turnbull, A.P., Sailor, W., . . . Fox, L. (2002). Positive behavior support: Evolution of an applied science. *Journal of Positive Behavior Interventions, 4*(1), 4–16, 20.

Carr, E.G., Levin, L., McConnachie, G., Carlson, J.I., Kemp, D.C., & Smith, C.E. (1994). *Communication-based intervention for problem behavior: A user's guide for producing positive change.* Baltimore, MD: Paul H. Brookes Publishing Co.

Carr, E.G., Levin, L., McConnachie, G., Carlson, J.I., Kemp, D.C., Smith, C.E., & McLaughlin, D.M. (1999). Comprehensive multisituational intervention for problem behavior in the community: Long-term maintenance and social validation. *Journal of Positive Behavior Interventions, 1*(1), 5 25. doi:10.1177/109830079900100103

Charlop, M.H., & Walsh, M.E. (1986). Increasing autistic children's spontaneous verbalizations of affection: An assessment of time delay and peer modeling procedures. *Journal of Applied Behavior Analysis, 19*(3), 307–314. doi:10.1901/jaba.1986.19-307

Christ, T.J., Riley-Tillman, T.C., Chafouleas, S.M., & Boice, C.H. (2010). Generalizability and dependability of direct behavior ratings (DBR) across raters and observations. *Educational and Psychological Measurement, 70*, 825–843. doi:10.1177/0013164410366695

Clarke, S., & Dunlap, G. (2008). A descriptive analysis of intervention research published in the *Journal of Positive Behavior Interventions*: 1999 through 2005. *Journal of Positive Behavior Interventions, 10*(1), 67–71. doi:10.1177/1098300707311810

Clarke, S., Dunlap, G., & Stichter, J.P. (2002). Twenty years of intervention research in emotional and behavioral disorders: A descriptive analysis and a comparison with research in developmental disabilities. *Behavior Modification, 26*, 659–683.

Crone, D.A., Hawken, L., & Horner, R.H. (2010). *Responding to problem behavior in schools: The behavior education program* (2nd ed.). New York, NY: Guilford Press.

Crone, D.A., Horner, R.H., & Hawken, L.S. (2004). *Responding to problem behavior in schools: The behavior education program.* New York, NY: Guilford Press.

Day, H.M., Horner, R.H., & O'Neill, R.E. (1994). Multiple functions of problem behaviors: Assessment and intervention. *Journal of Applied Behavior Analysis, 27*, 279–289.

Dunlap, G., & Carr, E.G. (2007). Positive behavior support and developmental disabilities: A summary and analysis of research. In S.L. Odom, R.H. Horner, M. Snell, & J. Blacher (Eds.), *Handbook of developmental disabilities.* New York, NY: Guilford Press.

Dunlap, G., Iovannone, R., English, C., Kincaid, D., Wilson, K., Christiansen, K., & Strain, P. (2010). *Prevent-teach-reinforce: A school-based model of individualized positive behavior support.* Baltimore, MD: Paul H. Brookes Publishing Co.

Dunlap, G., & Morelli-Robbins, M. (1990). *A guide for reducing situation-specific behavior problems with task interspersal.* Tampa, FL: Florida Mental Health Institute, University of South Florida.

Durand, V.M. (1991). *Functional communication training: An intervention program for severe problem behaviors.* New York, NY: Guilford Press.

Engelmann, S., & Carnine, D. (1982). *Theory of instruction: Principles and applications.* New York, NY: Irvington Publishers.

Ferro, J., & Dunlap, G. (1993). Generalization and maintenance in behavior modification. In M. Smith (Ed.), *Behavior modification for exceptional children and*

youth (pp. 190–211). Boston, MA: Andover Medical Publishers.

Ferster, C.B., & Skinner, B.F. (1957). *Schedules of reinforcement.* New York, NY: Appleton-Century-Crofts.

Fredrickson, B. (2009). *Positivity: Top-notch research reveals the 3 to 1 ratio that will change your life.* New York, NY: Three Rivers Press.

Harvey, M.T., Lewis-Palmer, T., Horner, R.H., & Sugai, G. (2003). Trans-situational interventions: Generalization of behavior support across school and home environments. *Behavioral Disorders, 28*, 299–313.

Horner, R.H., Bellamy, T.G., & Colvin, G.T. (1984). Responding in the presence of nontrained stimuli: Implications of generalization error patterns. *Journal of The Association for Persons with Severe Handicaps, 9*(4), 287–295.

Horner, R.H., & Billingsley, F.F. (1998). The effect of competing behavior on the generalization and maintenance of adaptive behavior in applied settings. In R.H. Horner, G. Dunlap, & R.L. Koegel (Eds.), *Generalization and maintenance: Lifestyle changes in applied settings* (pp. 197–220). Baltimore, MD: Paul H. Brookes Publishing Co.

Horner, R.H., Day, M., Sprague, J.R., O'Brian, M., & Tuesday-Heathfield, L. (1991). Interspersed requests: A nonaversive procedure for reducing aggression and self-injury during instruction. *Journal of Applied Behavior Analysis, 24*(2), 256–278.

Horner, R.H., Dunlap, G., & Koegel, R.L. (Eds.). (1988). *Generalization and maintenance: Lifestyle changes in applied settings.* Baltimore, MD: Paul H. Brookes Publishing Co.

Horner, R.H., Sprague, J., & Wilcox, B. (1982). General case programming for community activities. In B. Wilcox & G.T. Bellamy (Eds.), *Design of high school programs for severely handicapped students* (pp. 61–98). Baltimore, MD: Paul H. Brookes Publishing Co.

Horner, R.H., Williams, J.A., & Knobbe, C.A. (1985). The effect of "opportunity to perform" on the maintenance of skills learned by high school students with severe handicaps. *Journal of The Association for Persons with Severe Handicaps, 10*(3), 172–175.

Iovannone, R., Greenbaum, P., Wang, W., Kincaid, D., Dunlap, G., & Strain, P. (2009). Randomized controlled trial of the Prevent-Teach-Reinforce (PTR) tertiary intervention for students with problem behaviors: Preliminary outcomes. *Journal of Emotional and Behavioral Disorders, 17*, 213–225.

Janney, D.M., Umbreit, J., Ferro, J.B., Liaupsin, C.J., & Lane, K.L. (2013). The effect of the extinction procedure in function-based intervention. *Journal of Positive Behavior Interventions, 15*(2), 113–123. doi:10.1177/1098300712441973

Kennedy, C.H. (2002). The maintenance of behavior change as an indicator of social validity. *Behavior Modification, 26*(5), 594–604. doi:10.1177/014544502236652

Kuhn, S.A.C., Lerman, D.C., Vorndran, C.M., & Addison, L. (2006). Analysis of factors that affect responding in a two-response chain in children with developmental disabilities. *Journal of Applied Behavior Analysis, 39*(3), 263–280.

Langdon, N.A., Carr, E.G., & Owen-Deschryver, J.S. (2008). Functional analysis of precursors for serious problem behavior and related intervention. *Behavior Modification, 32*(6), 804–827.

Mace, F.C., Mauro, B.C., Boyajian, A.E., & Eckert, T.L. (2006). Effects of reinforcer quality on behavioral momentum: Coordinated applied and. basic research. *Journal of Applied Behavior Analysis, 39*(4), 468–468.

Mesmer, E.M., Duhon, G.J., & Dodson, K.G. (2007). The effects of programming common stimuli for enhancing stimulus generalization of academic behavior. *Journal of Applied Behavior Analysis, 40*(3), 553–557.

O'Dell, S.M., Vilardo, B.A., Kern, L., Kokina, A., Ash, A.N., Seymour, K.J., . . . Thomas, L.B. (2011). JPBI 10 years later: Trends in research studies. *Journal of Positive Behavior Interventions, 13*(2), 78–86. doi:10.1177/1098300710385346

O'Neill, R.E., Horner, R.H., Albin, R.W., Sprague, J.R., Newton, S., & Storey, K. (1997). *Functional assessment and program development for problem behavior: A practical handbook* (2nd ed.). Pacific Grove, CA: Brookes/Cole.

Redd, W.H., & Birnbrauer, J.S. (1969). Adults as discriminative stimuli for different reinforcement contingencies with retarded children. *Journal of Experimental Child Psychology, 7*(3), 40–47.

Rincover, A., & Koegel, R.L. (1977). Classroom treatment of autistic children: II. Individualized instruction in a group. *Journal of Abnormal Child Psychology, 5*(2), 113–126. doi:10.1007/BF00913087

Rooney, E.F., Poe, E., Drescher, D., & Frantz, S.C. (1993). I can problem solve: An interpersonal cognitive problem-solving program. *Journal of School Psychology, 31*(2), 335–339. doi:10.1016/0022-4405(93)90017-D

Schuster, J.W., Gast, D.L., Wolery, M., & Guiltinan, S. (1988). The effectiveness of a constant time-delay procedure to teach chained responses to adolescents with mental retardation. *Journal of Applied Behavior Analysis, 21*(2), 169–178. doi:10.1901/jaba.1988.21-169

Shores, R.E., Jack, S.L., Gunter, P.L., Ellis, D.N., DeBriere, T.J., & Wehby, J.H. (1993). Classroom interactions of children with behavior disorders. *Journal of Emotional and Behavioral Disorders, 1,* 27–39.

Sprague, J.R., & Horner, R.H. (1984). The effects of single instance, multiple instance, and general case training on generalized vending machine use by moderately and severely handicapped students. *Journal of Applied Behavior Analysis, 17*(2), 273–278.

Sprague, J.R., & Horner, R.H. (1992). Covariation within functional response classes: Implications for treatment of severe problem behavior. *Journal of Applied Behavior Analysis, 25*(3), 735–745.

Sprague, J.R., & Horner, R.H. (1994). Covariation within functional response classes: Implications for treatment of severe problem behavior. In T. Thompson & D. Gray (Eds.), *Destructive behavior in developmental disabilities: Diagnosis and treatment* (pp. 213–242). Thousand Oaks, CA: Sage Publications.

Stokes, T.F., & Baer, D.M. (1977). An implicit technology of generalization. *Journal of Applied Behavior Analysis, 10*(22), 349–367. doi:10.1901/jaba.1977.10-349

Terrace, H.S. (1966). Stimulus control. In I.W.K. Honig (Ed.), *Operant behavior: Areas of research and application* (pp. 274–334). Englewood Cliffs, NJ: Prentice-Hall.

Wilder, D.A., Chen, L., Atwell, J., Pritchard, J., & Weinstein, P. (2006). Brief functional analysis and treatment of tantrums associated with transitions in preschool children. *Journal of Applied Behavior Analysis, 39*(1), 103–107.

Defining, Measuring, and Graphing Behavior

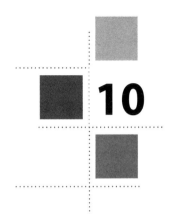

10

Matt Tincani and Elizabeth R. Lorah

In the previous chapters, you learned about a variety of proactive, individualized, positive behavior support (PBS) strategies to reduce challenging behavior and improve quality of life. Collecting data is critical in evaluating how your PBS strategies are working and, if they are not working, to change them. In this chapter, we overview strategies for defining target behaviors, developing accurate and reliable data collection systems, and converting target behavior data to graphs for visual analysis. We begin with vignettes about two focus people with challenging behavior whose teams must begin the PBS process by defining their target behaviors. We revisit these vignettes later in the chapter as the teams develop measurement and recording systems to accompany their function-based PBS interventions.

disabilities who spends his afternoons working at a nearby convenience store through a community-based vocational program. Until recently, Colin's manager considered him a model employee. He performed his job with minimal supervision, was pleasant and sociable with customers, and worked well with colleagues. Recently, Colin experienced several outbursts on the worksite that have placed his job in jeopardy. Colin's manager often asks him to stop stocking shelves to make coffee or perform other duties during busy times in the convenience store. Colin, who dislikes deviations from his routine, has refused to comply with instructions several times and on two occasions screamed at his manager and walked off the jobsite. Colin's manager informed his job coach that if Colin has any further outbursts, he will be terminated from his job.

Colin

Colin is a 17-year-old student with autism spectrum disorder (ASD) and mild intellectual

Shenile

Shenile, a fifth grader diagnosed with conduct disorder, attends a local charter school. For the past 2 years, she's spent most of her school day in a self-contained classroom for students with emotional or behavioral disorders. This year, Shenile is moving to inclusive math and reading classes. She is performing at or above grade level in all areas of reading and math; however, in the past, Shenile was frequently sent to the principal's office because of disruptive behaviors, including aggression toward teachers and students. Given her history of challenging behavior, Shenile's team wants to do everything possible to ensure she is successful in these new classroom settings.

....

WHY ARE DATA IMPORTANT?

Before we explore the process for defining, measuring, and graphing behavior, it is essential to understand the definition of *data* and why they are integral to positive behavior support (PBS). Data are "the numerical results of measuring some quantifiable aspect of behavior" (Mayer, Sulzer-Azaroff, & Wallace, 2012, p. 130). We collect data as we observe a person's behavior, record its occurrence, including characteristics of the behavior, and then convert the numerical results into a graph that we use for instructional decision making. Data provide valuable information about a person's behavior over time. This information enables us to develop and evaluate the effectiveness of interventions and modify them if necessary. Ultimately, our goal in collecting data is to increase prosocial behavior and enhance the focus person's quality of life.

In PBS, data serve three critical functions. First, as the bedrock of evidence-based practice, data allow us to make objective assessments about the focus person's progress and help us avoid subjective, "shoot from the hip" decisions that lead to poor outcomes. Programming decisions made in the absence of data are unlikely to help the individual achieve his or her behavioral goals and, even worse, can harm the individual. Data also enhance accountability of team members, as they provide a record of

the focus person's behavior and whether he or she is making adequate progress in the PBS program. Finally, at the systems level, data allow us to evaluate the success of the overall program across multiple individuals and promote positive behavior change across individuals and settings (Farkas et al., 2012). Accordingly, data-based decision making involves the following important steps: 1) defining behavior, 2) measuring behavior, and 3) graphing behavior. In the next section, we discuss procedures for the first step, defining target behavior.

DEFINING TARGET BEHAVIOR

At its most basic level, *behavior* is any activity of an individual that we can observe and record. In PBS, we are interested in operant behaviors, which are learned behaviors of the individual that are maintained by consequences that have followed them in the past (Cooper, Heron, & Heward, 2007). For example, Amy, a student with ASD who cannot speak, uses her speech-generating device because, in the past, this has been a very good way to get the teacher's attention and gain access to desired items and activities. Operant behaviors can take almost an infinite variety of forms, such as greeting a friend, writing a poem, or riding a bicycle. In addition, problem behaviors such as vocal protests, aggression, and noncompliance with teacher requests are all examples of operant behaviors, as they are learned behaviors that are maintained by the consequences that follow them. PBS interventions focus on strengthening communicative, social, academic, and other prosocial behaviors while reducing challenging behaviors that interfere with a person's quality of life and inclusion in typical environments (Carr et al., 2002).

There are three steps involved in defining target behavior: 1) identify the target behavior, 2) operationally define the target behavior, and 3) develop behavioral objectives/goals for treatment based on our operational definition.

Identify the Target Behavior

The first component in defining target behavior is to identify each behavior that will be the focus of the individual's behavior change program. In PBS, identifying target behavior is a collaborative process that involves attaining input from critical stakeholders, including staff, family members, and in some cases, the focus person, to decide which behaviors must be changed to improve the person's quality of life (Cameron, Shapiro, & Ainsleigh, 2005). Identifying target behaviors is the collective responsibility of the team, who considers factors such as 1) the unique strengths and needs of the individual; 2) which behaviors are most important to stakeholders, including teachers, parents, and the focus person; 3) which behaviors could be increased or decreased to enhance the focus person's quality of life and inclusion; and 4) which behaviors the team can reasonably expect to change given constraints of setting(s) in which the focus person behaves. The team may need to prioritize behaviors or reduce the number of behaviors selected for intervention, given practical constraints of the setting, including staffing resources (see Chapter 3).

Finally, it is critical that each behavior targeted for change be *observable* and *measurable*—that is, the behavior should be something that we can see the individual doing (e.g., writing, speaking) as opposed to covert behaviors that we cannot directly see (e.g., thinking, perceiving).

Operationally Define the Target Behavior

Once we have identified the target behavior, the next step is to operationally define the behavior. An *operational definition* describes the behavior in precise, observable, and measurable terms so that two or more people can observe the behavior and agree on its occurrence (Alberto & Troutman, 2012). The operational definition provides an unambiguous description of the behavior

so that all members of the team can readily identify the behavior's occurrence and record it. The behavior's *topography* is what it looks like in observable and measurable terms—for example, the topography of hitting a baseball includes "swinging the bat in a forward motion with enough force to make contact with the baseball while gripping the lower portion of the bat with both hands." The topography of communicating with a speech-generating device could be "selecting the appropriate symbol from an array, and touching the appropriate symbol with sufficient force to activate a voice message."

Though the process of creating an operational definition might seem straightforward, creating a good operational definition is not always easy. Consider the phrase *on-task behavior.* By itself, *on-task behavior* is not an operational definition because this behavior can include many different topographies. For instance, in a preschool classroom, on-task behavior during circle time might be sitting cross-legged with eyes on the teacher and responding verbally or nonverbally to every instruction presented by the teacher. In a high school math class, on-task behavior could be sitting at the desk, responding to each teacher question with a raised hand while refraining from noninstructional talk with peers. Therefore, it is critical that team members come to a consensus about the precise topography of the target behavior as they create an operational definition.

Develop a Behavioral Objective

Once you have identified a target behavior and created an operational definition, the final step in defining target behavior is to write a *behavioral objective.* The behavioral objective is a statement that specifies the outcome of PBS programming and clearly identifies what you expect the individual to do after successful completion of the intervention (Scott, Anderson, & Spaulding, 2008; Tincani, 2011). Behavioral objectives should include desirable skills that we want the individual to increase, in addition to challenging behaviors that we want the individual to decrease.

Behavioral objectives include four necessary and critical components. These are the learner, the conditions, the behavior, and the criteria for performance (Alberto & Troutman, 2012). The *learner* is simply the name of the person whose behavior is targeted for change. In some cases, the learner can be a group of individuals, such as a class or instructional grouping. The *conditions* specify in clear terms which stimuli will be present when the learner is expected to perform the target behavior. The conditions, or stimuli, can include the setting, such as the worksite or classroom; teacher instructions; and materials, such as worksheets, writing utensils, or technology. The *behavior* is an observable and unambiguous definition of the target behavior, as we discussed in the previous section. Finally, the *criteria* for performance clearly describe the level of proficiency for the learner to acquire the behavioral objective. For example, we could specify that we wish the learner to write answers to 90% of questions correctly; independently ask for help on four out of five opportunities; or perform an appropriate, alternative communicative response during every opportunity for 5 consecutive days.

The following examples show each of the components of behavioral objectives separately and then combined into a statement. Notice how each objective specifies the learner, the conditions in which the behavior is to be performed, an observable and measurable definition of the target behavior, and criteria for acquisition of the objective:

- *Learner:* Sofia

- *Conditions:* Presented with her speech-generating device and a preferred food or drink item in the classroom

- *Behavior:* Will touch the corresponding symbol on her speech-generating device to request the food or drink item

- *Criteria:* Independently on 8 out of 10 opportunities, for 2 consecutive days

- *Sofia's behavioral objective:* When presented with a preferred food or drink item in the classroom, Sofia will independently touch the corresponding symbol on her speech-generating device to request the food or drink item on 8 out of 10 opportunities, for 2 consecutive days.

- *Learner:* James

- *Conditions:* Given a daily written schedule of job tasks

- *Behavior:* Will point to and then complete each task on his daily schedule

- *Criteria:* Without prompting for 90% of assigned tasks for 1 week

- *James' behavioral objective*: When given a daily written schedule of job tasks, James will point to and complete each task on his daily schedule without prompting for 90% of tasks for 1 week.

- *Learner:* Jasmine

- *Conditions:* Given a written math assignment containing difficult problems

- *Behavior:* Will raise her hand to request help from the teacher with a difficult problem

- *Criteria:* Without prompting at least once per class period for 3 consecutive days

- *Jasmine's behavioral objective:* When given a written math assignment containing difficult problems, Jasmine will raise her hand to request help from the teacher with a difficult problem without prompting at least once per class period for 3 consecutive days.

Stages of Learning

When writing behavioral objectives, it is important to consider four different stages of learning and how these are relevant to each objective: acquisition, fluency, maintenance, and generalization (Woolery, Bailey, & Sugai, 1988). *Acquisition* is the initial stage of learning. At the beginning of the acquisition stage, we assume that the learner cannot perform the target behavior under any circumstances. The focus of intervention during acquisition is to teach the learner to perform the behavior accurately and without any errors. *Fluency,* the next stage, describes the extent to which the learner can perform the behavior "smoothly and without hesitation" (Mayer et al., 2012, p. 346). For example, if James is able to independently follow a written schedule but takes 15 minutes per class period to locate his schedule, find the correct page, find the task, and then begin the task, clearly his performance is not yet fluent and therefore fluency should be the focus of his behavioral objective. *Maintenance* is the degree to which the desired behavior change continues after some or all the formal intervention procedures have been withdrawn. At some point, the goal of our behavioral program is to fade away teaching procedures so the learner can perform the skill independently with natural supports. Finally, *generalization* is the extent to which the learner performs the skill under differing conditions, including various settings, materials, times of day, and people found in the natural environment. For instance, Sofia should request food and drink from not just her teachers at school but also her parents at home and during breakfast, lunch, dinner, and snack times.

Colin

Colin's teacher, job coach, and behavior analyst convene to determine a plan of action to help Colin keep his job and be successful in community employment. With assistance from the team, Colin's behavior analyst conducts a functional behavioral assessment (FBA; Chapter 14) and determines that Colin's disruptive behavior is most likely during busy times of day and when Colin is interrupted from his current work task and asked to do something different. His disruption is reinforced by escape or avoidance of the different task. After discussing potential intervention strategies with Colin and his manager, the team decides to create a job-based activity schedule for Colin. The activity schedule contains the normal sequence of tasks that Colin is expected to perform in a typical workday; busy times (i.e., breakfast and lunch) are highlighted on the schedule with the expectation that Colin may be asked to do something different

during these times. His job coach and manager will use precorrections (De Pry & Sugai, 2002) to remind Colin that he may be asked to perform different job duties during busy times. Colin will receive the reinforcer of his choice at the end of the day if he completes all required work tasks without disruption.

Shenile

Shenile's individualized education program (IEP) team convenes to develop a behavior plan to help her to be successful in math, reading, and other classes. The team reviews her records, including a previous FBA and function-based intervention plan, and determines that in the past her disruptive behavior was maintained by attention from peers and teachers and escape from work demands. Consulting with her general education teachers, they devise a plan in which each teacher will offer help and attention to Shenile once every 10 minutes during class, and she will have three opportunities per class period to take a break or request assistance if she needs help.

MEASURING AND RECORDING BEHAVIOR

As noted, data are "the numerical results of measuring some quantifiable aspect of behavior" (Mayer et al., 2012, p. 130). Data collection is critical to evaluate the focus person's success in his or her PBS program. In this section, we discuss the different dimensions of behavior that are captured with data collection systems, the types of data collection systems available, how to assess reliability of data and reduce threats to reliability, and finally, how to successfully train accurate observers.

Dimensions of Behavior

Before you select a data collection system, you must determine which dimension of behavior you wish to capture. As we evaluate our focus person's PBS program, we are interested in capturing at least one dimension of each target behavior. The seven dimensions of behavior are frequency, rate, duration, latency, topography, locus, and force.

Frequency *Frequency* is the number of behaviors performed during a specific time period. Frequency is perhaps the most straightforward dimension of behavior, as it represents a simple count of responses. For example, Colin followed his manager's instructions five times during the workday. An important assumption of frequency as a dimension of behavior is that the number of opportunities to perform the behavior are the same from session to session or from day to day. For example, frequency is the appropriate dimension of Colin's behavior to consider if the manager presents the same number of instructions during each observation period. If the manager presents a different number of instructions to Colin from session to session, then rate would be the most appropriate dimension or the behavior could be converted to a percentage of questions answered correctly.

Rate *Rate* is related to frequency in that we must count the number of behaviors during a particular time period; however, rate is the frequency of behavior divided by unit of time. In the previous example, if the workday is 6 hours and Colin complied 10 times during the workday, then his rate of complying with manager instructions was approximately 1.6 per hour (i.e., $10/6 = 1.6$). Rate is the preferred dimension of behavior when we are interested in capturing fluency of responses or whether the learner can perform the behavior quickly, accurately, and smoothly. Rate is also a useful measure when observation times vary or when the number of opportunities to perform the behavior varies from session to session and therefore frequency must be converted to rate in order to accurately reflect how often the behavior is occurring. Rate is the most relevant dimension of behavior in measuring

oral reading, as we are interested in knowing how accurately and quickly children can orally read. Specifically, a child who can orally read 120 words per minute is a more fluent reader than a child who can orally read only 50 words per minute.

Duration *Duration* describes how long the learner engages in a particular behavior or, more technically, the time period between the beginning and end of the behavior. Duration is the most critical dimension for behaviors such as tantrums or outbursts, as these responses can last for several minutes or longer and thus it is important to know how long they are happening. For example, duration would be an appropriate measure of Colin's outbursts. Frequency or rate would not be an appropriate measure, as Colin may demonstrate one outburst that lasts 10 minutes in duration. Duration would be a more appropriate measure because it provides a better quantification of the target behavior of outbursts.

Latency Like duration, *latency* is a time-based dimension of behavior. With latency, however, we consider the time period between when an instructional stimulus is presented and when the behavior begins. Latency is often the dimension of choice when there is an unacceptable lag between the instructional cue and onset of the behavior. For example, Colin may take 10 minutes to transition from one activity to the next following a cue from his manager (e.g., "Make coffee"). Shenile, who takes 10–20 seconds to respond to greetings from others, would also likely benefit from a latency measure.

Locus and Force *Locus and force,* the two remaining dimensions of behavior, are typically considered in addition to one of the dimensions described previously. Locus describes where the behavior occurs. For example, if we are interested in capturing the frequency of a Shenile's hitting, we also may want to know the location of the body where hitting typically occurs (e.g., the face, torso). Locus can also describe the location in the student's house, classroom, school, or community store where the behavior can or should occur. Force, in contrast, describes the amount of effort required to perform the behavior or the relative intensity of the behavior. For instance, the force of Colin's outburst may be a dimension of his behavior that is of interest.

Data Collection Systems

Once you have identified the dimension(s) of behavior that you wish to capture, the next step is to select a data collection system. Table 10.1, adapted from Tincani (2011), summarizes seven data collection systems, the

procedures for each system, considerations for whether the system is appropriate for a particular behavior, and examples of behaviors that could be measured with each system. The seven systems are event recording, permanent product recording, rate recording, duration recording, latency recording, interval recording (whole and partial), and momentary time sampling.

Event Recording Event recording involves recording each time the learner performs a behavior, typically using tally marks on a data collection sheet. Event recording yields a frequency of behavior per observation period (e.g., class period, school day, week). In one example, Lorimer, Simpson,

Table 10.1. Overview of data collection strategies

System	Procedure	Appropriate application	Examples
Event recording	Record each time the student performs a behavior, and count the number of behavior products.	Discrete behaviors; behaviors that leave a permanent product that can be counted	Hand raising; hitting; writing numbers
Permanent product recording	Count the permanent product left by the behavior.	Behaviors that leave a permanent product that can be counted	Math quiz; handwriting worksheet; writing numbers
Rate recording	Record each time the student performs a behavior and divide frequency of behavior by unit of time.	Behaviors for which speed and accuracy is important; observation periods that are variable in duration	Typing on a keyboard; oral reading; assembling packages
Duration recording	Record the amount of time the student engages in a behavior.	Behaviors where time is an important dimension; behaviors that have a definite beginning and end	Silently reading; playing with peers; crying
Latency recording	Record the time period between an instructional cue and when the student begins to perform a behavior.	Situations in which the student takes a long time to respond to a cue or instructions	Responding to teacher directions; leaving the building after a fire alarm; exiting the classroom after the bell
Interval recording (whole and partial interval)	Divide an observation period into equal intervals, and then record whether the behavior has occurred during each interval.	Behaviors that do not have a definite beginning or end; high-rate behaviors	Self-stimulatory behavior; on-task or off-task behavior; disruptive behavior
Momentary time sampling	Divide an observation period into equal intervals, and then record whether the behavior is occurring at the end of each interval.	Behaviors that do not have a definite beginning or end; high-rate behaviors	Self-stimulatory behavior; on-task or off-task behavior; disruptive behavior

From Tincani, M. (2011). *Preventing challenging behavior in your classroom: Positive behavior support and effective classroom management.* Waco, TX: Prufrock Press; adapted by permission.

Myles, and Ganz (2002) used event recording to evaluate if Social Stories reduced the daily frequency of interrupting vocalizations uttered by a 5-year-old boy with autism. Event recording is most appropriate for discrete behaviors—that is, behaviors that have a definite beginning and end. Hand raising, asking for a break, and hitting are examples of discrete behaviors that can be measured with event recording. Figure 10.1 shows an event recording data sheet for direction following. Notice how the data sheet includes an operational definition of the target behavior and spaces for the instructor to record the specific direction given to the student.

Permanent Product Recording Permanent product recording is a related strategy that involves counting the number of products resulting from a response. The difference between permanent product and event recording is that, with permanent product, you do not have to be present at the time the behavior occurs, as there is a product available to review and analyze at a later time. A common example of permanent product recording is when we count the number of correct written answers to math facts or count the number of written words a student spells correctly. For example, Kinney, Vedora, and Stromer (2003) evaluated the effects of computer-presented video models on the number of correctly spelled words of a first grader with ASD.

Rate Recording Rate recording is similar to event recording in that we tally the frequency of responses. However, with rate recording, we divide the frequency of responses by unit of time. For example, if Joanna types 400 words in 5 minutes, we record that her rate of typing is 80 words per minute (400 words/5 minutes = 80 words per minute). As mentioned, rate recording is appropriate when we are concerned with documenting the fluency of students' responses. Rate recording is also appropriate when capturing the frequency of responding during observational periods of differing durations.

Duration Recording Duration recording involves recording the amount of time the focus person engages in the target behavior, usually by activating a timer at the onset of the response and then stopping the timer when the response stops. Duration recording is appropriate for behaviors that have a definite beginning and ending, such as sitting at circle time, where time is a critical dimension of responding. There are two duration measures available. Total duration is the total amount of time the learner engages in a response during the observation period. It is obtained by starting and stopping the timer each time the response starts and stops and then noting the total duration of all responses at the end of the observation period. For instance, Delano and Snell (2006) evaluated the effects of Social Stories on the total duration of appropriate social engagement of children with autism with their peers. Average duration, in contrast, involves recording the total duration of responses as described but also recording the frequency of responses (as in event recording) and then dividing frequency by the total duration of responses to yield an average duration of responding. Figure 10.2 shows a duration data recording sheet. The data sheet also has spaces for the data collector to tally the number of instructor prompts (event recording; see Chapters 6 and 7).

Historically, duration recording was accomplished via paper and pencil by noting the start and stop times of behavior on a data sheet, as you see in Figure 10.2. With the advent of smartphones and tablet computers, inexpensive software is available for duration recording and other types of recording on mobile devices that most people carry. For instance, "Duration, an ABA Duration Recording App," is a low-cost application available through iTunes that allows duration recording across multiple behaviors and individuals on the Apple iPhone and iPad (Mays, 2011).

EVENT RECORDING DATA SHEET

Student name _____   Date _____

Instructor initials _____

Operational definition: *Direction following*—Responding to a teacher instruction within 5 seconds during individual or group lessons.

Record data for 10 group instructions and 10 individual instructions throughout the school day.

Instruction	During group?	Instruction	During individual?
1	Y/N	1	Y/N
2	Y/N	2	Y/N
3	Y/N	3	Y/N
4	Y/N	4	Y/N
5	Y/N	5	Y/N
6	Y/N	6	Y/N
7	Y/N	7	Y/N
8	Y/N	8	Y/N
9	Y/N	9	Y/N
10	Y/N	10	Y/N

Figure 10.1.   Event recording data sheet.

DURATION RECORDING DATA SHEET

Student name _____   Date _____

Instructor initials _____

Operational definition: *Playing with peers*—Record the name of the play activity, list the total duration that the student plays during the activity, and tally the number of prompts given for the student to play.

Activity _____	Activity _____	Activity _____
Duration _____	Duration _____	Duration _____
Prompts	Prompts	Prompts
Activity _____	Activity _____	Activity _____
Duration _____	Duration _____	Duration _____
Prompts	Prompts	Prompts

Figure 10.2.   Duration recording data sheet.

Latency Recording Latency recording, like duration recording, is a time-based measure of behavior. However, in latency recording, we note the time period between an instructional cue and when the student performs the target behavior. Latency recording is most appropriate for behaviors in which the student takes an unacceptably long time to respond to a cue or instructions. In one example, Hupp and Reitman (2000) evaluated effects of a parent-implemented training package on latency of responses to parent questions (e.g., "What was the last television show you watched?") of an 8-year-old boy with pervasive developmental disorder. Though parents provided reinforcement for eye contact only, they found that the boys' latency of responses to their questions reduced substantially below baseline levels.

Interval Recording Interval recording occurs as we divide an observation period into equal intervals and then record whether the behavior has occurred during each interval. Interval recording is most appropriate for behaviors that occur for extended period of time without a definite beginning or end and for very high-rate behaviors. For instance, it would be hard to accurately record the frequency of out-of-seat behavior for a student who gets out of his or her seat dozens of times during a 45-minute class period. Thus interval recording would be a viable alternative. Interval recording would also be appropriate for a student who engages in self-stimulatory rocking and hand waving during most of the class period, since the behavior lacks a definite beginning and end and may occur during most of the class period.

There are two variations of interval recording, *whole interval recording* and *partial interval recording*. In whole interval recording, the behavior must occur throughout the entire interval to be recorded. In partial interval recording, the behavior is recorded if it happens during any portion of the interval. In general, whole interval recording is most appropriate for prosocial behaviors that we are attempting to increase, such as on-task behaviors. Since the behavior must occur during the entire interval, whole interval recording provides us with the most conservative measure of improvement. In contrast, partial interval recording is preferred when we are measuring challenging behaviors that we wish to decrease. Because the behavior can happen during any part of the interval, partial interval recording will provide us with the most conservative measure of improvement. Figure 10.3 depicts a whole interval data recording sheet. Note that the student must engage in the behavior during the entire interval for the data collector to record it.

Although interval recording systems are very common in the PBS literature (e.g., Nuzzolo-Gomez, Leonard, Ortiz, Rivera, & Greer, 2002; Randolph, 2007) a couple of precautionary statements about these systems are worth mentioning. First, unlike event, duration, and latency recording, interval recording systems yield *discontinuous* and *indirect* measures of behavior—that is, rather than capturing all instances of each target behavior, interval recording systems yield only an approximation of each target behavior. For this reason, event, duration, and latency recording systems are preferred unless the conditions for these systems are not met. Second, interval recording tends to be more accurate when intervals are shorter (e.g., 5 second, 10 second) rather than longer (e.g., 30 second, 1 minute). Therefore, you should select the shortest interval possible when implementing interval recording systems.

Momentary Time Sampling Momentary time sampling is a variation of interval recording in which the target behavior is recorded only if the behavior is happening at the *end* of each interval. For instance, Liso (2010) used 10-second momentary time sampling to compare the effects of child-chosen and interventionist-chosen toys on engagement, nonengagement, teacher involvement,

WHOLE INTERVAL RECORDING DATA SHEET

Student name _____   Date _____

Instructor initials _____

Operational definition: *Appropriate sitting*—Student sits while participating in the current activity. Student must sit throughout the entire 30-second interval.

Activity 1			Activity 2			Activity 3		
Interval	**Yes**	**No**	**Interval**	**Yes**	**No**	**Interval**	**Yes**	**No**
1			1			1		
2			2			2		
3			3			3		
4			4			4		
5			5			5		
6			6			6		
7			7			7		
8			8			8		
9			9			9		
10			10			10		
11			11			11		
12			12			12		
13			13			13		
14			14			14		
15			15			15		
16			16			16		
17			17			17		
18			18			18		
19			19			19		
20			20			20		

Figure 10.3.   Whole interval recording data sheet.

and fussiness or crying of three preschool children with disabilities and limited mobility. Momentary time sampling is advantageous because it requires the observer to record only at the end of each interval, and thus it is easier to measure behaviors of multiple students and/or multiple behaviors. On the other hand, because target behaviors are recorded only if they are happening at the end of each interval, momentary time sampling yields the least continuous and least direct data of any of the recording systems we have discussed. Thus momentary time sampling should be avoided unless it is practical and necessary to observe multiple behaviors or multiple students simultaneously.

Observer Training and Reliability

In this section, we discuss how to train observers to collect reliable data, how to establish that your data are reliable through interobserver agreement (IOA), common threats to reliability, and how to prevent and reduce threats to reliability.

In PBS, the reliability of data collection systems is most commonly established by calculating IOA, or the extent to which two observers who collect data on the same behavior at the same time obtain the same results. IOA is typically represented numerically as a percentage of agreement. Your method of calculating percentage agreement will differ depending on the kind of data collection system you use. The following is a summary of strategies for calculating IOA for each of the data collection systems we have discussed.

Total Agreement (Event Recording)
For event recording, in which you tally each time the student performs a behavior, the method for calculating IOA is *total agreement*. To calculate total agreement, you first determine the total frequency of behavior recorded by the first observer and the total frequency of behavior recorded by the second observer. Then you divide the smaller total by the larger total and multiply by 100.

For example, if Francis records that James smiles 8 times and Lupe records that James smiles 7 times, their percentage of agreement would be calculated as follows: 7/8 × 100 = 87.5%. If James records that Lilly says hello 14 times and Mandy records that Lilly says hello 12 times, their percentage of agreement would be calculated as follows: 12/14 × 100 = 86% agreement.

Duration and Latency Agreement
Duration and latency recording are time-based measures of behavior. To calculate IOA for duration and latency recording, divide the smaller duration/latency obtained by one observer by the larger duration/latency obtained by the other observer and then multiply by 100. For instance, if Shane records that Josh sits at circle time for 9 minutes and Hannah records that Josh sits at circle time for 10 minutes, the percentage of IOA would be calculated as follows: 9/10 × 100 = 90%.

Amy records that Joey plays for 42 seconds, while Declan records that Joey plays for 38 seconds. Their percentage of agreement would be calculated as follows: 38/42 × 100 = 90.4%.

Interval-by-Interval Agreement
For partial interval recording, whole interval recording, and momentary time sampling, the simplest method for calculating IOA is *interval-by-interval agreement*. With this method, you first determine the number of intervals for which both observers agree and then the number of intervals for which both observers disagree. Finally, you divide the agreement intervals by the total number of intervals (i.e., the agreement intervals plus the disagreement intervals) and then multiply by 100.

Consider the on-task behavior data collected by Observer 1 and Observer 2 depicted in Figure 10.4. Each observer recorded the occurrence (+) or nonoccurrence (o) of the behavior during ten 30-second intervals. The observers had eight agreements and two disagreements, so we would calculate their

Observer 1: On task									
0:00–0:30	0:30–1:00	1:00–1:30	1:30–2:00	2:00–2:30	2:30–3:00	3:00–3:30	3:30–4:00	4:00–4:30	4:30–5:00
+	o	+	+	o	o	o	+	o	+
Observer 2: On task									
0:00–0:30	0:30–1:00	1:00–1:30	1:30–2:00	2:00–2:30	2:30–3:00	3:00–3:30	3:30–4:00	4:00–4:30	4:30–5:00
+	o	+	+	+	o	o	o	o	+

Figure 10.4. Sample interval recording data for on-task behavior.

percentage of agreement as follows: $8/(2 + 8)$ × 100 = 8/10 × 100 = 80%. The percentage of interval-by-interval agreement for the data depicted in Figure 10.5 would be calculated as follows: $7/(3+7)$ × 100 = 7/10 × 100 = 70% agreement.

Acceptable Levels of IOA In general, 80% or better is considered to be the minimally acceptable percentage for IOA (Cooper et al., 2007). If the IOA falls below 80%, the observers may need to be retrained by reviewing the operational definition of the target behavior(s), discussing examples and nonexamples of each behavior, and conducting additional practice sessions recording the behavior(s) (discussed in more detail later). If your IOA continues to fall below 80%, you may need to consider selecting a different recording system. For instance, if it is difficult to accurately tally the frequency of behavior with event recording, interval recording or momentary time sample recording may be viable alternatives.

When and How Much IOA Data to Collect Your IOA data should be representative of all the data you collect on each target

behavior. If you are conducting a research study, at minimum you should collect IOA data for 25%–30% of your data collection sessions. In nonresearch situations, however, it may be difficult to collect that much data for practical reasons (e.g., secondary observers are not available). Generally, you should collect IOA data at least once during each phase of evaluation (e.g., at least once during baseline, at least once during intervention). Distributing IOA data randomly across your data collection sessions will increase the likelihood that your IOA data are representative of your overall data set. Collecting IOA data may be inconvenient and a little time consuming; however, it is the best way to ensure that your data are accurate and representative of the learner's performance.

Observer training is the process of teaching data collectors to accurately and reliably record behavior. Observer training should occur before data collection begins; if we wait to conduct observer training until after data collection starts, the resulting data may be inaccurate, unreliable, and a poor representation of the focus person's behavior in the natural environment. The amount of observer training you do will vary according

Observer 1: Asking for break									
0:00–0:30	0:30–1:00	1:00–1:30	1:30–2:00	2:00–2:30	2:30–3:00	3:00–3:30	3:30–4:00	4:00–4:30	4:30–5:00
o	o	o	+	+	o	o	o	o	+
Observer 2: Asking for break									
0:00–0:30	0:30–1:00	1:00–1:30	1:30–2:00	2:00–2:30	2:30–3:00	3:00–3:30	3:30–4:00	4:00–4:30	4:30–5:00
o	o	o	+	o	+	o	o	+	+

Figure 10.5. Sample interval recording data for asking for a break.

to variables such as the experience of data collectors and their familiarity with target behaviors and/or focus people, as well as the complexity of your behavior measurement system. A well-designed data collection system with appropriately selected measures, as previously discussed, should minimize the amount of necessary training. Observer training involves the following key steps:

- Review the data collection sheet, including where to fill in necessary information such as the data collector's name or initials, the date, the student's name, and location (e.g., classroom). Do not presume that data collectors know how to complete the data sheet; explain where all information on the data sheet should go.

- Describe the operational definition(s) of each behavior. Provide several examples and nonexamples of each target behavior. Allow the data collector to ask clarifying questions about what each target behavior looks like.

- Describe the data collection strategy (e.g., event, duration, interval) and how to collect the data (e.g., "Each time the behavior occurs, make a tally mark in this space"). Provide a rationale for why data are collected with this particular strategy (e.g., "The behavior has a clear beginning and ending, so we are using event recording").

- Provide at least one opportunity for the data collectors to practice collecting data on the target behavior, either from video recordings or in vivo (i.e., as the behavior occurs in the natural setting).

- Collect IOA data with the data collector to ensure that the data are reliable.

- Review the collected data, including any IOA data, to verify reliability and accuracy. If the data are not reliable, allow clarifying questions about the data sheet, operational definitions, and data collection strategy. In many cases, you will need to "tweak" the operational definitions of behaviors to increase reliability of your system. Repeat IOA data collection as necessary.

Perhaps the most important element of observer training is establishing *reliability* of

your data collection system. A data collection system is reliable if it is "repeatable, i.e., remains standard, or consistent, regardless of who does the measuring, on what occasions" (Mayer et al., 2012, p. 108). For example, if John records that Abigail raises her hand six times during the class period and Lisa also records that Abigail raises her hand six times during the class period, we could say that John's measure is reliable because it is the same as Lisa's. Establishing that your data collection system is reliable is one way of showing that the system is *accurate*—that is, it yields a true measure of behavior as it occurs in the natural environment.

Threats to Reliability

Even a well-designed data collection system can sometimes be inaccurate. Several threats to reliability may compromise the accuracy of your data collection system. Four prominent threats to reliability are discussed in this section, followed by suggestions about how to reduce the likelihood of each threat.

Observer Drift *Observer drift* occurs when observers gradually shift the way they record behavior over time. For example, Allison's target behavior of destroying work materials is operationally defined as "forcefully tearing or crumpling worksheets or other work related materials"; however, after several weeks of data collection, staff begin to record only when Allison forcefully tears her worksheets but not when she crumples them. To prevent observer drift, you should periodically review your observation system with staff, including examples and nonexamples of target behaviors, and retrain as needed. Randomly collecting IOA data to evaluate if data collectors are continuing to agree in their observations, as previously discussed, will also counter the potential effects of observer drift.

Reactivity When an individual whose behavior is being recorded acts differently because he is being observed, this is *reactivity.* For instance, when data collectors enter the play area of the classroom, Nate is more likely to share toys with his classmates than when he is not being observed. To prevent reactivity, you should collect data as unobtrusively as possible. For example, position yourself in an area of the classroom where students are less likely to be aware of your presence. If students are unfamiliar with data collectors, it may be beneficial for them to spend time in the observation area prior to formal data collection so that students get used to the area and data collectors and are less likely to behave differently when being observed.

Complexity   The accuracy of your data collection system may be compromised because it is too complex. *Complexity* is particularly a risk if you are recording multiple behaviors or multiple students simultaneously. To reduce the likelihood of complexity as a threat to reliability, be sure to first review your data collection system with staff, including your data sheet(s), and allow them the opportunity to ask questions about the system. Moreover, you should try to simplify your system by recording the fewest number of behaviors or students possible.

Expectancy   Finally, *expectancy* is a threat to reliability when observers alter the way they record because they want a particular outcome. It is not unreasonable to expect that data collectors will record differently because they want the PBS program to work; after all, we all want our focus people to be successful and to please supervisors, parents, focus individuals, and others who may benefit the program. In fact, expectancy may cause data collectors to record differently even though they are not aware of it. To prevent expectancy as a threat to reliability, you should thoroughly review the system with observers, including examples and nonexamples of target behaviors, periodically retrain observers as needed, and randomly collect IOA data to assess if observers are continuing to reliably collect data.

GRAPHING DATA

The final step in using data to evaluate your PBS plan is to convert your raw data into graphs. *Graphs* are a visual representation of behavior across time. Visual analysis allows you to organize your data and evaluate the results of your PBS plan for individuals and groups. The primary benefit of a graphic display is that it allows you to communicate changes in behavior without the use of text (Gast, 2010). Data should be graphed and analyzed frequently. Analyzing graphic depictions of data allows you to determine what effect your PBS plan has on the behavior of an individual and/or group and make data-based decisions such as adjusting your PBS plan according to changes in the behavior. Before discussing the different methods of graphing and how to analyze a graph, you should be familiar with the components of a graph.

Figure 10.6, adapted from Tincani (2011), shows a hypothetical AB design graph (see Chapter 11) to evaluate the effects of functional communication training (FCT) and precorrections, plus a token economy system for a student's total duration of tantrums. "Baseline" depicts the duration of tantrums before intervention, while "FCT + Precorrections + Token" shows the duration of tantrums after intervention. A graph contains several components that allow us to understand how the program is working.

A.   Y-*axis:* The y-axis (also known as the ordinate) shows the behavior's level and has a descriptive label that describes the behavior and how it was measured (e.g., total duration of hitting).

B.   X-*axis:* The x-axis (also known as the abscissa) depicts the passage of time and shows the unit measurement (e.g., school days, class periods, hourly sessions).

C.   *Data points:* Data points represent the level of behavior for each observation period with lines to connect the data points.

D.   *Condition labels:* Each condition is labeled with a descriptive term so that it

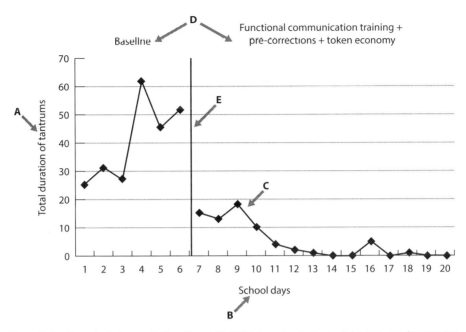

Figure 10.6. Elements of a line graph. (From Tincani, M. [2011]. *Preventing challenging behavior in your classroom: Positive behavior support and effective classroom management.* Waco, TX: Prufrock Press; adapted by permission.)

is easy to understand the comparison of baseline to the intervention.

E. *Condition change line:* A change line is drawn between the conditions (e.g., baseline and intervention) to indicate when the change of conditions occurred. The data points on either side of the condition line are not connected. Change lines allow an easy visual analysis of the success of the program.

The first step to graphing data is to determine which method of graphing will provide the most useful depiction of the data. There are two main types of graphs—line graphs and bar graphs. In PBS, we typically use line graphs to evaluate a focus individual's progress during baseline and intervention phases. (See Chapter 11 on single-case designs.) Line graphs are the best way to visually determine if a PBS plan is working and what, if any, changes are necessary to increase the likelihood that the plan will be successful, thereby allowing you to make data-based decisions. Figure 10.6 shows how a line graph can be used to depict data.

Another method of graphing data is creating a bar graph. The bar graph is a useful tool for graphing comparison data over time (Gast, 2010). For example, if you wanted to compare a student's math scores from one semester to the next, a bar graph would provide you with a meaningful way to interpret such behavior. Alternatively, if you wanted to depict duration of out-of-seat behavior before and after the implementation of your PBS plan, the bar graph could provide you with a meaningful depiction of those data, including whether the behavior had decreased from week to week or month to month. An advantage of bar graphs is that they simplify your interpretation of behavior by summarizing the learner's performance over a fixed time period. Figure 10.7 shows how a bar graph can be used to depict hypothetical data across semesters, following the introduction of a PBS plan for math. Conversely, because bar graphs represent a summary (e.g., average) of behavior during a particular time period, they do not depict the learner's performance of the behavior on a continuous basis. For example, Figure

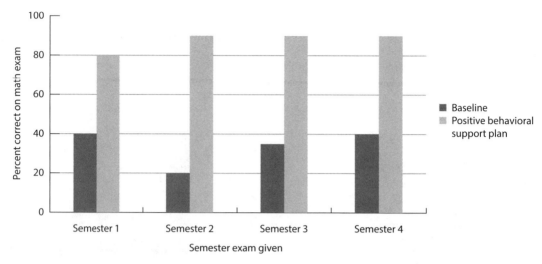

Figure 10.7. Sample bar graph.

10.7 tells us little about the learners' performance in math from day to day. For this reason, bar graphs are more appropriate for summative evaluations, such as determining how much the student has learned by the end of the semester, while line graphs are more appropriate for formative evaluation, or understanding how the learner is performing daily.

Once you have chosen the appropriate method of depicting your data, you can begin to analyze those data to determine what changes, if any, are needed to your PBS plan. When analyzing data from line graphs, it is important that you have enough data to accurately depict the learner's performance of the behavior over time. Generally, at least three separate data points are necessary (Gast, 2010). The next step is to determine the level and trend of your data. *Level* primarily refers to the amount of variability in your data. A good way to measure level is to determine what percentages of your data are falling within a specific range. Data are generally considered level if 80% of the data points are falling within a 20% range (Gast, 2010). Typically, your baseline data should be level prior to the introduction of your PBS plan so that you can predict the behavior will not improve without intervention. This is important so that it can be easily determined that

any changes in the behavior were the results of your plan and not something else that was occurring in the learner's environment.

Trend refers to the direction of your data path. There are three directions in which data may trend. These include accelerating (increasing over time), decelerating (decreasing over time), and zerocelerating (remaining level). The direction in which you want your data to trend depends on the target behavior. For example, if you were attempting to decrease aggression, as is the case with Shenile's PBS plan, decelerating would be preferred. Alternatively, if you were attempting to increase compliance, as is the case with Colin's PBS plan, accelerating data would be preferred.

Detecting level and trend within a graphic depiction of data allows you to determine the effectiveness of your PBS plan. For example, as depicted in Figure 10.6, if you were graphing the frequency of Shenile's aggression and the data depicted a zerocelerating data path (no change from baseline to the introduction of the PBS plan), a graph would provide an easy way to detect that the PBS plan is not effective and needs revision. Alternatively, as depicted in Figure 10.8, the deceleration of your data indicates that your PBS plan has been effective at decreasing the duration of tantrums, and no revisions to your PBS plan are necessary at that time.

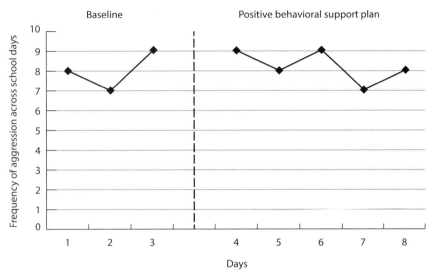

Figure 10.8.   Sample graph of zerocelerating and level data path.

CONCLUSION

Data, the numerical results of measuring behavior, are integral to the implementation and evaluation of PBS. Data-based decision making involves identifying target behaviors, operationally defining target behaviors, and writing behavioral objectives. There are several data collection systems available, depending on which dimension of behavior we wish to capture. These are event recording, permanent product recording, rate recording, duration recording, latency recording, interval recording, and momentary time sampling. Observers must be well trained to collect accurate and reliable data. The reliability of data is established through IOA. Once we have collected data, it is critical to convert data into graphs for visual analysis to evaluate how each focus person is progressing in his or her PBS program.

REFERENCES

Alberto, P., & Troutman, A. (2012). *Applied behavior analysis for teachers* (9th ed.). Upper Saddle River, NJ: Pearson.

Cameron, M.J., Shapiro, R.L., & Ainsleigh, S.A. (2005). Bicycle riding: Pedaling made possible through positive behavioral interventions. *Journal of Positive Behavior Interventions, 7,* 153–158. doi:10.1177/10983007050070030401

Carr, E.G., Dunlap, G., Horner, R.H., Koegel, R.L., Turnbull, A.P., Sailor, W., . . . & Fox, L. (2002). Positive behavior support evolution of an applied science. *Journal of Positive Behavior Interventions, 4,* 4–16.

Cooper, J.O., Heron, T.E., & Heward, W.L. (2007). *Applied behavior analysis* (2nd ed.). Columbus, OH: Prentice Hall/Merrill.

Delano, M., & Snell, M.E. (2006). The effects of social stories on the social engagement of children with autism. *Journal of Positive Behavior Interventions, 8,* 29–42. doi:10.1177/10983007060080010501

De Pry, R.L., & Sugai, G. (2002). The effect of active supervision and precorrection on minor behavioral incidents in a sixth grade general education classroom. *Journal of Behavioral Education, 11,* 255–267.

Farkas, M.S., Simonsen, B., Migdole, S., Donovan, M.E., Clemens, K., & Cicchese, V. (2012). Schoolwide positive behavior support in an alternative school setting: An evaluation of fidelity, outcomes, and social validity of Tier 1 implementation. *Journal of Emotional and Behavioral Disorders, 20,* 275–288. doi:10.1177/1063426610389615

Gast, D.L. (2010). Single subject research methodology in behavioral sciences. New York, NY: Routledge.

Hupp, S.A., & Reitman, D. (2000). Parent-assisted modification of pivotal social skills for a child diagnosed with PDD: A clinical replication. *Journal of Positive Behavior Interventions, 2,* 183–187. doi:10.1177/109830070000200308

Kinney, E.M., Vedora, J., & Stromer, R. (2003). Computer-presented video models to teach generative spelling to a child with an autism spectrum disorder. *Journal of Positive Behavior Interventions, 5,* 22–29. doi:10.1177/10983007030050010301

Liso, D.R. (2010). The effects of choice making on toy engagement in nonambulatory and partially ambulatory preschool students. *Topics in Early Childhood Special Education, 30,* 91–101.

Lorimer, P.A., Simpson, R.L., Myles, B., & Ganz, J.B. (2002). The use of Social Stories as a preventative behavioral intervention in a home setting with a child with autism. *Journal of Positive Behavior Interventions, 4,* 53–60. doi:10.1177/109830070200400109

Mayer, G.R., Sulzer-Azaroff, B., & Wallace, M. (2012). *Behavior analysis for lasting change* (2nd ed.). Cornwall-on-Hudson, NY: Sloan.

Mays, C. (2011). Duration, an ABA duration recording app. Downloaded at https://itunes.apple.com/us/app/duration-aba-duration-recording/id452984136?mt=8

Nuzzolo-Gomez, R., Leonard, M.A., Ortiz, E., Rivera, C.M., & Greer, R. (2002). Teaching children with autism to prefer books or toys over stereotypy or passivity. *Journal of Positive Behavior Interventions, 4,* 80–87. doi:10.1177/109830070200400203

Randolph, J.J. (2007). Meta-analysis of the research on response cards: Effects on test achievement, quiz achievement, participation, and off-task behavior. *Journal of Positive Behavior Interventions, 9*(2), 113–128.

Scott, T., Anderson, C., & Spaulding, S. (2008). Strategies for developing and carrying out functional assessment and behavior intervention planning. *Preventing School Failure, 52,* 39–49.

Tincani, M. (2011). *Preventing challenging behavior in your classroom: Positive behavior support and effective classroom management.* Waco, TX: Prufrock Press.

Wolery, M., Bailey, D., & Sugai, G.M. (1988). *Effective teaching: Principles and procedures of applied behavior analysis with exceptional students.* Boston, MA: Allyn and Bacon.

Single-Case Designs and Data-Based Decision Making

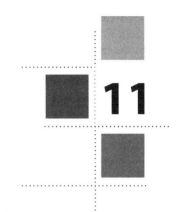

John McDonnell, Robert E. O'Neill, and Breda V. O'Keeffe

A core principle underlying positive behavior support (PBS) is that interventions must be tailored to the specific needs of the individual. This requires the practitioner to make data-based decisions on the effectiveness of an intervention in a timely manner. Achieving this goal dictates that the practitioner 1) regularly collects data on the individual's performance of the target behavior and 2) systematically analyzes a graphic display of the data to determine if the intervention is having the desired effect. The continuous analysis of the graphically displayed data allows the practitioner to judge the efficacy of the intervention and adjust it as necessary to meet the individual's needs.

Single-case designs provide the framework for systematically analyzing graphically displayed data to confirm whether a functional relationship exists between the target behavior and the intervention. A variety of single-case designs have been described

in the research literature (Cooper, Heron, & Heward, 2007; Gast & Ledford, 2009; O'Neill, McDonnell, Billingsley, & Jenson, 2011). However, we will focus on five designs that are particularly useful for PBS practitioners who are working in applied settings. These include the case study design, the multiple baseline design (MBD), the withdrawal design, the multiple treatment design (MTD), and the alternating treatment design (ATD). In addition, we will describe how to conduct the visual analysis of the data and how this information can be used to make data-based decisions.

SINGLE-CASE DESIGNS

Single-case designs can be structured to allow practitioners to answer a number of questions about an intervention: Does the intervention lead to the desired change in the target behavior? Is the intervention effective under different conditions (e.g., behaviors, settings, people)? Is Intervention X more effective than Intervention Y? As discussed throughout this chapter, the specific type of design used by the practitioner to evaluate an intervention is driven by the question or questions he or she wants to answer.

In addition, the design selected by a practitioner should enhance the ability to clearly demonstrate a functional relationship between the intervention and the target behavior. Put simply, the design should increase the practitioner's confidence that it is the intervention rather than other contextual variables changing the target behavior. For example, if a practitioner implemented a self-monitoring system to help a fifth grader increase assignment completion during independent seat work, he or she would want to select a design to show that the self-monitoring system, rather than other variables (e.g., who the student was sitting next to during the work period or the difficulty of the assignments), led to his or her improved rate of assignment completion. Clearly establishing this functional relationship allows the practitioner to draw valid and reliable conclusions about the efficacy of the intervention.

Beyond selecting an appropriate design, practitioners also need to adhere to several key principles and procedures in order to make good decisions about the effectiveness of an intervention. First, the practitioner must repeatedly gather data on the individual's performance of the target behavior over time and across all phases of an intervention. This allows for a systematic analysis of the impact of the intervention as it is changed or modified. Second, it is generally recommended that data on the target behavior be collected before and after the implementation of the intervention. The initial preintervention assessment of the individual's performance is called *baseline*. These data provide a description of the individual's performance before the implementation of the intervention. Baseline also provides a basis for predicting how the individual would have performed if the intervention had not

been implemented. The comparison of the observed changes in the behavior with the predicted level of performance helps the practitioner decide whether a functional relationship exists between the intervention and the target behavior. Data should also be collected across changes in the intervention in order to determine whether modifications or changes in an intervention have the desired effect on the target behavior.

Third, in order to clearly demonstrate that a functional relationship has been established, the practitioner must replicate the impacts of an intervention across at least three different points in time and/or across three different conditions (Horner et al., 2005). Replicating the effects of the intervention in this way affirms that the intervention is changing the target behavior. Replication also enhances the validity of the decisions that a practitioner may make about the continued use of the intervention with the individual.

Fourth, the practitioner should regularly assess the reliability of the data collection procedures used to track the target behavior. The focus here is to ensure the data collection system that is being used is accurate and reliable (see Chapter 10). Often, this is accomplished by having a second person simultaneously code the individual's performance and then comparing their codes with those taken by the practitioner (i.e., interrater reliability). The more agreement between the two sets of codes, the more confidence the practitioner can have in the accuracy of the data that he or she is collecting.

Fifth, the practitioner should also regularly assess the fidelity of implementation of the intervention. Essentially, the practitioner is trying to determine whether the intervention is being implemented the way it was designed in the intervention plan. If there is significant variation in the way the intervention is being implemented across people, settings, or time, then establishing a functional relationship between the intervention and the target behavior is difficult, if not impossible. In other words, the practitioner won't know whether it was the intervention or other factors that led to the change or lack of change in the target behavior. This kind of "procedural drift" is not uncommon in applied settings, especially when multiple people implement an intervention or when the intervention is being implemented across different contexts or settings.

Finally, the practitioner should assess the social validity of the observed changes in the target behavior. The question here is, Are these changes meaningful, and do they have a positive impact on the individual's quality of life (Carr et al., 2002)? The best way of determining this is to simply ask the individual, family, friends, peers, or other community members to confirm whether the observed change in the target behavior has had a meaningful impact on the individual and their family's daily life.

Describing the Structure of Single-Case Designs

As described in Chapter 10, there are widely accepted conventions and terminology for displaying data on a graph. Similarly, there are also established conventions and terminology for describing the structure of single-case designs. These conventions allow practitioners and researchers to communicate clearly about the design and accurately describe the intended sequence of conditions or phases of the behavior support plan.

The various phases of a design are noted through the use of capital letters (i.e., A, B, C). The capital letter A refers to the baseline condition. The first intervention applied to the target behavior is denoted with the capital letter B. Each subsequent intervention would be assigned a different capital letter (e.g., C, D, E). The letter assigned to an intervention is repeated in the series if it applied more than once to the target behavior (e.g., A-B-A-B-C-B).

This notation is used to describe the proposed phases of the intervention plan for an individual. When the plan is actually being implemented and data are being graphed for the individual, the letters are replaced with descriptive labels for each intervention included in the plan.

Case Study Design (A-B Design)

The most basic single-case design structure is a case study, or A-B design. This involves two phases—an initial baseline (A) phase and an intervention (B) phase. This is also sometimes referred to as a preexperimental design, since it does not allow practitioners to rule out various explanations for the outcomes that are obtained (O'Neill et al., 2011). For example, a supervisor in a residential home setting for adults with developmental disabilities could collect data on the frequency of aggressive behaviors exhibited by one of the home's residents. After several days of baseline data collection, the home staff could implement an intervention procedure in which the resident is taught an alternative appropriate communication skill (e.g., using sign language to indicate the need for a break from activities) and given more tangible rewards for periods of time in which he or she does not engage in aggressive acts (i.e., a differential reinforcement of other behavior, or DRO procedure). After the implementation of the intervention strategies, the staff would continue to collect data to determine if there is a decrease in the frequency of individual's aggressive behavior and an increase in the individual's break requests. After a couple of weeks of implementing the intervention, the individual's aggressive behavior substantially decreases and the appropriate communicative behavior increases.

Campbell and Skinner (2004) studied a classroom of 30 sixth graders whose teacher was concerned about the amount of time being consumed by transitions between activities (e.g., coming and going from recess and lunch). During the baseline phase, the number of seconds required for these transitions was recorded and a daily average was calculated. During the intervention phase, the research staff worked with the teacher to implement the "Timely Transitions Game"

(TTG), a procedure in which the class could qualify for rewards (e.g., popcorn party, class movie) for each transition that was accomplished in less time than a prespecified benchmark. Figure 11.1 presents the average daily time for transitions (in seconds) during the baseline and intervention phases. There was a clear and consistent reduction in the amount of transition time during the intervention (TTG) phase.

In both our hypothetical residential home example and in the Campbell and Skinner (2004) study, the data in the intervention phase were positive with regard to a desired reduction in problem behavior. However, in both cases it is not possible to confidently conclude that the decrease is due to the intervention procedures. An A-B case study design can only document change at a single point in time. Therefore, such demonstrations are vulnerable to many of the possible threats to internal validity (e.g., historical events, maturation, measurement error). In our hypothetical example, the resident in question may have experienced a change in medications or his or her work setting, which would be alternate explanations for observed changes in behavior. Similarly, in the situation described by Campbell and Skinner (2004), the school principal may have implemented some type of schoolwide behavior program that had an impact on the students' behavior without the teacher's or researchers' knowledge.

Given that such A-B comparisons are likely (and hopefully) a common evaluation approach implemented in educational and clinical settings (Hayes, Barlow, & Nelson-Gray, 1999), it is worth considering what characteristics may enhance the internal validity of such investigations and the ability to draw conclusions from them. Kazdin (1981, 1982) described a set of factors that should be considered in assessing the threats to validity of A-B or case study designs. Case study investigations that involve more objective measures (e.g., direct observation), repeated measures over time, stable data in the baseline and intervention phases, immediate and substantial effects when intervention is implemented, and demonstration of effects across multiple participants will provide more convincing evidence regarding the effects of an intervention.

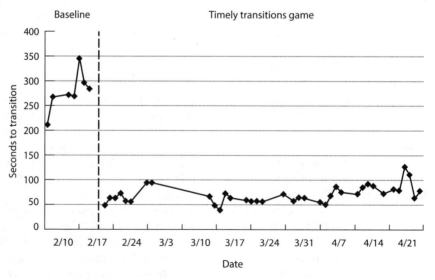

Figure 11.1. Example of a case study design (A-B). (From Campbell, S., & Skinner, C.H. [2004]. Combining explicit timing with an interdependent group contingency program to decrease transition times: An investigation of the timely transitions game. *Journal of Applied School Psychology, 20*[2], 21; reprinted by permission of the publisher [Taylor & Francis Ltd, http://www.tandf.co.uk/journals].)

A-B designs may be adequate in many applied/clinical situations. However, there may be cases where clinicians and researchers wish to eliminate alternate explanations for changes in the target behavior. The easiest way to do this is to repeatedly contrast a participant's behavior under baseline conditions (A) with their behavior during intervention (B). Withdrawal/reversal designs provide a mechanism for accomplishing this.

Withdrawal/Reversal Designs (A-B-A and A-B-A-B Designs)

In order to more clearly demonstrate the effect of an intervention, a great deal can be achieved by adding an additional baseline and potentially an additional intervention phase to a design (resulting in an A-B-A or A-B-A-B sequence). One of the critical questions with A-B-A and A-B-A-B designs is whether the behavioral performance is *reversible* or not. To assess the effects of an intervention, changes in behavioral performance must be evident each time a change is made from a baseline to an intervention condition (or vice versa). In some cases, such a change may not be very likely to occur. For example, consider a situation in which three individuals are trained to make a microwave meal. Once they learn and become fluent with the procedure, they are not likely to "forget" how to prepare such a meal; thus a return to baseline would not likely show a change in performance. An additional limitation of A-B-A-B designs is that in situations involving potentially harmful behaviors (e.g., self-injurious behavior), it may not be desirable to go back to baseline conditions that might involve higher levels of such behaviors. In particular, parents, teachers, and other caregivers may be reluctant to withdraw an intervention that is proving to be effective.

In the A-B-A-B design, the practitioner implements an additional baseline (A) and intervention conditions (B) in order to replicate the effects of the intervention on the target behavior. An example of such a design was provided by Rasmussen and O'Neill (2006). This study involved three elementary school students attending a classroom in a psychiatric day treatment setting. They engaged in verbally disruptive behavior (e.g., talking out without raising their hands), which interfered with classroom instruction. An initial functional behavior assessment (see Chapters 14–16; O'Neill et al., 1997) indicated that the students were doing this to obtain social attention, particularly from their teacher. During the initial baseline phases, data were collected on the percentage of intervals during which verbal disruptions occurred. The intervention involved *noncontingent*, or *fixed-time reinforcement* (FTR), schedules (Arnzen, Brekstad, & Holth, 2005). In such a procedure, regardless of behavior, the participant is provided with their desired reinforcement on an ongoing periodic basis, in an attempt to *preempt* the need to engage in problem behavior to obtain reinforcement. Initially, reinforcement is provided on a more frequent schedule than the participant appears to want according to his or her baseline rate of problem behavior (Rasmussen & O'Neill, 2006).

The data in Figure 11.2 represent the percentage of intervals with verbal disruptions for the three students. During the initial baseline phases, all three students were exhibiting verbal disruptions at a high rate. When FTR was provided in the form of social attention and interaction from the classroom teacher, the rate of verbal disruptions substantially decreased. The baseline and FTR phases were repeated with similar results, thus demonstrating a functional relationship between the use of the reinforcement intervention and measures of verbal disruption. In the final, or *fading*, phase, the frequency of FTR was gradually decreased (i.e., every 60–90 seconds versus every 10–20 seconds), and the low rates of behavior were maintained until the students left the day treatment program. One aspect of this study worth noting is that the three students attended the day treatment program at different times—that

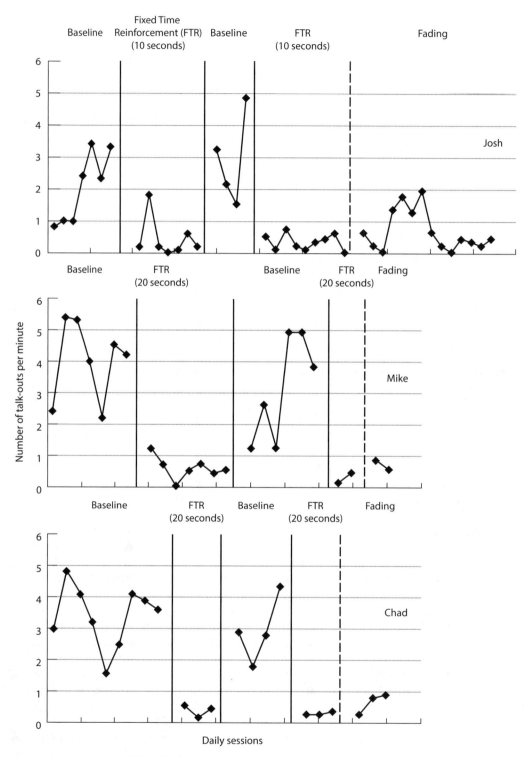

Figure 11.2. Example of a withdrawal/reversal design (A-B-A). (From Rasmussen, K., & O'Neill, R.E. [2006]. The effects of fixed-time reinforcement schedules on problem behavior of children with emotional and behavioral disorders in a day treatment classroom setting. *Journal of Applied Behavior Analysis, 39*[4], 455. Copyright 2006 by the Society of the Experimental Analysis of Behavior, Inc.)

is, their stays in the program did not overlap. This allowed the researchers to demonstrate a replication of effects not only within participants in the context of an A-B-A-B design but also across participants at different points in time (Kazdin, 1982).

Multiple Baseline Design

The MBD is a useful design to employ when support providers and researchers are 1) concerned about withdrawing interventions (e.g., due to aggressive behaviors) and 2) working with behaviors that are going to be acquired by participants and won't "reverse" when the training or intervention is withdrawn (Johnston, 2011). The basic structure of an MBD involves simultaneously collecting baseline data across a set of people, behaviors, or settings, and then sequentially introducing the intervention across those people, behaviors, or settings. That is, after collection of stable baseline data, the intervention is implemented with the first person, behavior, or setting. The remaining nonintervention baselines provide a control or comparison that behavior changes only when the intervention is implemented. Once an intervention effect is evident with the first baseline, the intervention is then sequentially implemented across the remaining longer baselines. For example, consider a situation in which a practitioner is interested in reducing self-injurious behavior (SIB) exhibited by a child diagnosed with Down syndrome in three settings. The providers have determined that the SIB is maintained by escape from non-preferred tasks/activities, and want to assess the effects of teaching alternative communicative responses (e.g., using graphic symbol cards to request a break from the task). In a typical MBD, the practitioners would first collect baseline data on communicative responses and SIB for each of the three settings. They would then train the child on the alternative response in the first setting and assess the effects on his communication and SIB. Once positive effects were observed the

intervention would then be implemented in the second setting, and then in the third setting. The intervention would continue to be implemented in the previous settings as it is introduced in each subsequent setting. Control by the intervention is demonstrated by the fact that the child's behavior changes in each setting only after the intervention is implemented.

The most common form of this design is a MBD across people. As an example, Schreibman, O'Neill, and Koegel (1983) trained siblings of children with autism to conduct training sessions to teach appropriate skills (e.g., expressive labeling of letters/numbers). They collected data on the correct performance of training procedures by the siblings and correct responses by the children with ASD. Figure 11.3 presents the data on correct performance by the children with ASD and their siblings. The solid lines represent performance by the siblings, and the dashed lines represent performance by the children with autism. The open circles with dots represent performance by the siblings in a generalization setting, and the crosses represent performance by the children with autism in a generalization setting. The siblings and children with ASD demonstrated inconsistent levels of performance during the baseline phase. As the training intervention was implemented across each of the sibling pairs, the levels of correct performance increased for both the siblings and the children with ASD.

Multiple Treatment Designs

The MTD is structured to allow practitioners to compare the effects of two or more interventions on one target behavior. The interventions are alternately applied to the target behavior over time. The effects of each intervention on the target behavior are compared across adjacent phases in the graph. The assumption underlying the MTD is that each intervention will have a consistent and differential effect on the target behavior. The most effective intervention is

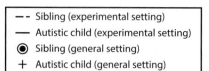

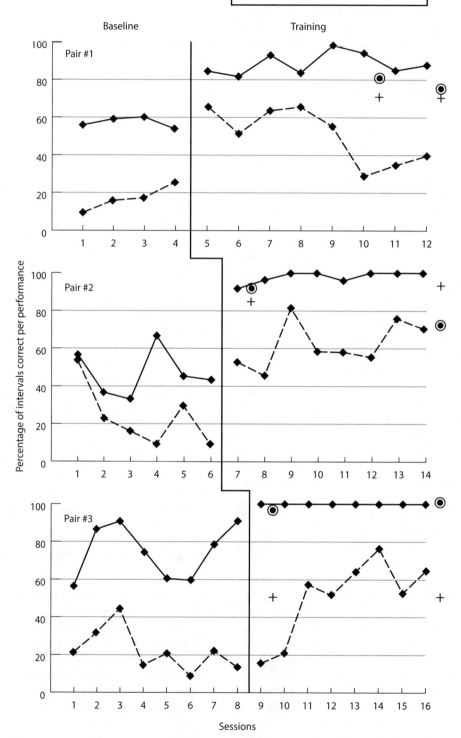

Figure 11.3. Example of a multiple baseline design (MBD). (From Schreibman, L., O'Neill, R.E., & Koegel, R.L. [1983]. Behavioral training for siblings of autistic children. *Journal of Applied Behavior Analysis, 16*[2], 135. Copyright 1983 by the Society of the Experimental Analysis of Behavior, Inc.)

the one that produces the largest sustained change in the target behavior.

There are two common structures for the MTD design. The first is the MTD without baseline: B-C-B-C-B-C. In this option, the first intervention is applied to the target behavior until the individual's performance is stable. Then the second intervention is introduced and is implemented until a consistent pattern in the individual's performance is established. For example, a practitioner might be interested in the comparing the number of social initiations by a particular student with the number of social initiations by other children during free time when support is being provided by a paraprofessional or a peer. The practitioner would begin collecting data on the number of social initiations by the student when support was provided by a paraprofessional (B). When the frequency of social initiations was stable during this condition, the practitioner would introduce the intervention in which support was provided by a peer (C). Ideally, the practitioner would reverse the interventions at least three times in order to convincingly demonstrate a differential effect between the interventions. Although reversing the interventions this many times in applied settings may not be practical, a minimum of two reversals of the interventions is required in order to demonstrate that one intervention is superior to the other in achieving the desired change in the target behavior. This is a particularly useful design when the practitioner is interested in comparing an intervention that an individual is currently receiving with a new intervention that has not been used before.

The second structure is the MTD with baseline: A-B-C-B-C-B-C. In this design, the practitioner collects baseline data on the individual's performance of the target behavior until stable performance of the target behavior is established. Following baseline, the first (B) and second (C) interventions are alternately applied to the target behavior over time. Because data can only be compared between adjacent phases in a design, the baseline (A) can only serve as a general referent about the individual's performance before the implementation of the interventions. One intervention is considered more effective than the other when there are consistent and differential effects on the target behavior across the reversals of the interventions.

While the MTD can be a powerful tool in determining the relative effectiveness of two or more interventions, the design also has several inherent weaknesses, similar to those of the A-B-A-B design. First, it is not an appropriate design when trying to compare interventions to establish the performance of nonreversible behaviors. For example, it would not be appropriate to compare interventions for teaching an individual how to button his coat, because if the first intervention led to the acquisition of the behavior, it is unlikely that the introduction of a second intervention would be necessary. A second problem with the MTD is that the alternate presentations of the interventions create the possibility of sequence and/or carry-over effects. For example, observed changes in the target behavior could be due to the fact that the interventions followed one another in a specific sequence, rather than their unique impact on the target behavior (i.e., paraprofessional support followed by peer support). So it might be difficult to determine whether it was the sequence of the interventions rather than the effectiveness of one of the interventions that produced the differential effect. In addition, observed differences in the performance of the target behavior could result from the effects of the first intervention introduced to the individual "carrying over" to the individual performance in the second intervention. The carry-over effect might lead to an overestimate of the impact of one intervention over the other.

Ingram, Lewis-Palmer, and Sugai (2005) used an MTD to compare the relative effects of behavior intervention plans based on the analysis of the function of a problem behavior and plans that were not based on the function of the problem behavior (see Figure 11.4). The

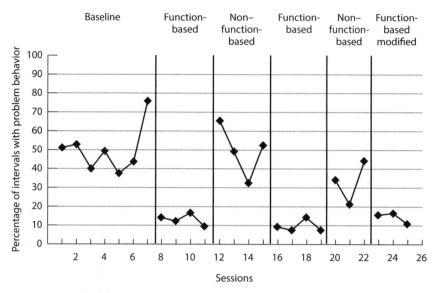

Figure 11.4.   Example of a multiple treatment design (MTD). (From Ingram, K., Lewis-Palmer, T., & Sugai, G. [2005]. Function-based intervention planning: Comparing the effectiveness of FBA function-based and non-function based intervention plans. *Journal of Positive Behavior Interventions, 7*[4], 230; reprinted by permission of SAGE Publications. Copyright 2005 by SAGE Publications.)

study was implemented with two sixth-grade boys who were enrolled in general education classes. The behaviors targeted for intervention included playing with toys, not being ready for class, and being off task. Figure 11.4 shows data for one of the students. As shown in the figure, the authors collected baseline data to establish the operational level of performance of the target behaviors. Then they alternated the presentation of the function-based and nonfunction-based behavior intervention plans over time with the student. The patterns in the data clearly show that the function-based behavior intervention plans had more effect in reducing the rates of the target behaviors than the nonfunction-based plans. A similar pattern was observed for the second student. Based on the visual analysis of these data, the authors concluded that function-based interventions were more effective for these two students.

Alternating Treatment Designs

ATDs are also structured to allow practitioners to compare the relative efficacy of

two or more interventions. Similar to the MTD, the interventions are alternated and then the practitioner examines the graphed data to determine if the interventions have differential effects. The ATD differs from the MTD in that interventions are alternated rapidly (and often randomly) within the same intervention phase. The advantage of the ATD is that it allows for immediate implementation of the interventions being examined rather than "lagging" the interventions sequentially over time.

There are two common structures for ATDs, including the traditional ATD and the adapted alternating treatment design (AATD). The ATD is organized to compare the differential effects of two or more interventions on a single target behavior. The ATD can be structured with or without a baseline phase. In the ATD without baseline, the interventions are applied alternately to the target behavior. The interventions are alternated quickly, commonly in the same session (e.g., B during the first 5 minutes of the session, C during the next 5 minutes, B during the next 5 minutes), in multiple sessions in a single day (e.g., B during the morning session and C during the afternoon session), or every other day (e.g., B on Monday, C on Tuesday, B on Wednesday).

The ATD with baseline consists of two phases—A-baseline and B-alternating treatments—in which the interventions are implemented with the target behavior in alternating fashion as described previously. This option also allows for a return to baseline (A-B-A) or for the addition of a third phase (A-B-C) in which the "best" intervention is applied to the target behavior.

The AATD allows the practitioner to compare the effects of two or more interventions on two or more separate but equivalent target behaviors. For example, the AATD would be appropriate to examine whether constant time delay or the system of least-to-most prompts is more effective in teaching an individual to read functional sight words. The practitioner would identify two sets of sight words that were considered of equal difficulty and then would use constant time delay to teach one word set and the system of least-to-most prompts to teach the second word set.

In both the ATD and the AATD, the interventions are continuously tracked across sessions and the data for each intervention are plotted in separate data paths on the graph. An intervention is considered more effective if it produces more change or more rapid change than the comparison intervention.

While the ATD and AATD offer a number of potential advantages to practitioners for comparing interventions, they also have several weaknesses that must be taken into consideration. First, similar to the MTD, these designs are also susceptible to potential sequencing and carry-over effects (i.e., least-to-most prompting following constant time delay). Second, the rapid alternation of interventions may not be compatible with the typical organization of schools or other community settings. It may not be logistically feasible or socially acceptable to alternate interventions within short periods of time. It would be problematic in the previous example if the alternation of the constant time delay and system of least-to-most conditions prevented the student from participating fully in reading lessons provided by his or her teacher. Third, in order to draw firm conclusions about whether one intervention is more effective than the other, the practitioner must control a number of procedural variables such as the amount of time that the individual is exposed to the two interventions, the individuals who are implementing the interventions, and the location and time of the interventions. If there are significant differences between the interventions, it becomes difficult to determine whether any observed differences in the effectiveness of interventions are due to the interventions themselves or other contextual variables.

A study by Park, Singer, and Gibson (2005) demonstrates the utility of a traditional ATD without baseline to compare the effectiveness of two interventions (see Figure 11.5). The researchers examined the impacts of teacher affect during instruction on "student happiness" when teaching discrete trial tasks to four elementary-age students with severe disabilities. The first intervention consisted of the teacher having a positive affect on the student during instruction (e.g., exaggerated positive tone of voice, smiling, body movements that communicated enthusiasm). The second intervention the teacher presented a neutral affect during instruction (e.g., flat voice tones, expressionless faces, body movements that communicated low enthusiasm). The students were taught to match shapes, match coins, or sign "more" to request the continuation of a preferred activity. Students were presented six instructional trials during each instructional session. The two interventions were alternated across instructional sessions. The target behavior was "student happiness" during instruction. The measure used to summarize student performance was the percentage of intervals during observations in which the students laughed and/or smiled.

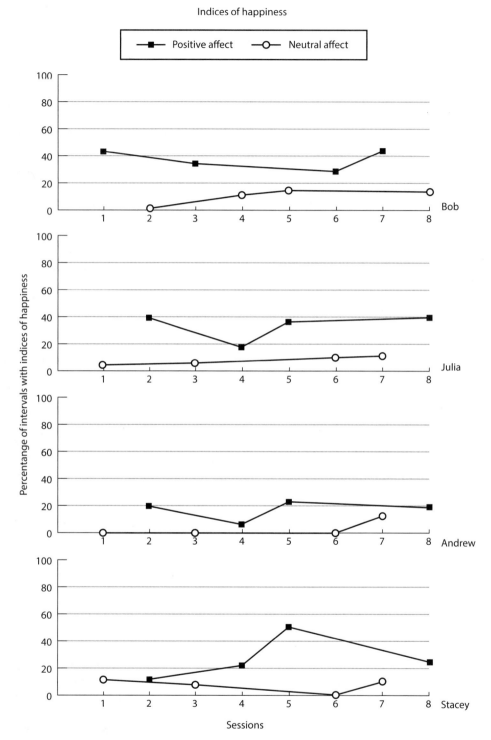

Figure 11.5. Example of an alternating treatment design without baseline. (From Park, S., Singer, G.H.S., & Gibson, M. [2005]. The functional effect of teacher positive and neutral affect on the task performance of students with significant disabilities. *Journal of Positive Behavioral Interventions, 7*[4], 242; reprinted by permission of SAGE Publications. Copyright 2005 by SAGE Publications.)

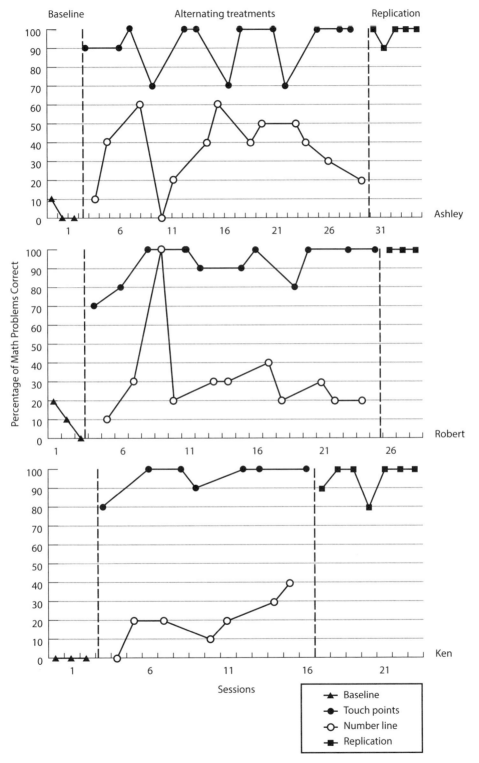

Figure 11.6. Example of an adapted alternating treatment design (AATD) with baseline. (From Fletcher, D., Boon, R.T., & Cihak, D.F. [2010]. Effects of TOUCHMATH® program compared to a number line strategy to teach addition facts to middle school students with moderate intellectual disabilities. *Education and Training in Autism and Developmental Disabilities, 45*[3], 455; reprinted by permission.)

As illustrated in Figure 11.5, Park et al. (2005) used an ATD without baseline. The researchers counterbalanced the introduction of the positive- and neutral-affect inventions across students to rule out that it was the order in which the interventions were introduced that changed the target behaviors. The patterns in the data suggest that the positive-affect intervention resulted in higher rates of student happiness during instruction than the neutral-affect intervention. The visual analysis of the data led the researchers to conclude that the teachers' positive-affect intervention was superior.

Fletcher, Boon, and Cihak (2010) used the AATD to compare the effectiveness of *TOUCHMATH* (a multisensory math program that embeds visual touch points into numerals from 1 to 9 to teach basic calculations) and the use of a number line to teach students with moderate and multiple disabilities to solve single-digit addition problems (see Figure 11.6). These two interventions were alternated across instructional sessions. The target behavior was the percentage of single-digit addition problems solved correctly during a session.

Fletcher et al. (2010) used an AATD with a replication phase. They began with an A-baseline phase to establish the operational level of students' performance before the introduction of the two interventions. Once students' baseline performance was stable, they introduced the B-alternating treatments phase, in which students used either the *TOUCHMATH* or a number line strategy during instruction to learn to add two different groups of single-addition problems. When students met a prespecified mastery criterion with one of the interventions, the researchers implemented a C-replication phase that applied the most effective treatment to both groups of single-addition problems. Based on these data, the researchers concluded that the *TOUCHMATH* strategy was the most effective approach in teaching these students single-digit additional problems and that the students were able to maintain their performance of the strategy over time.

INTERPRETING DATA FROM SINGLE-CASE DESIGNS

The graphically displayed data from single-case designs tell the story about whether the intervention(s) have been successful in producing change in the target behavior. To make this determination, the practitioner must develop skills to evaluate the characteristics of the data within and across phases of the design. This section will provide guidance for developing these skills; however, practitioners should gain experience interpreting graphically displayed data with feedback from other practitioners with expertise in interpreting data from single-case designs (Fisher, Kelley, & Lomas, 2003).

An advantage of using single-case designs is the ability to collect, graph, and interpret data in "real time"—that is, as the intervention is being conducted. Decisions about and adjustments to the intervention can be made quickly to enhance the efficiency of behavior change for target individuals. Data should be monitored closely during each phase in order to make any needed changes as soon as possible. Although statistical methods exist for interpreting data in single-case designs, visual analysis is recommended before the application of supplemental statistical methods (Horner, Swaminathan, Sugai, & Smolkowski, 2012; Kratochwill et al., 2010). This section will focus on procedures for the visual analysis of single-case data. With the exception of an A-B design, the goal of visual analysis is to determine if a functional relationship exists between the application of the intervention(s) and change(s) in the individual's behavior. Interpreting the data entails first analyzing the data patterns within each phase and then comparing data patterns across phases and sometimes analyzing data patterns across cases (e.g., in a MBD). Specific differences in the data patterns that correspond with the introduction or withdrawal of an intervention may suggest a functional relationship between the intervention and the behavior change.

Visual Analysis of Data within Phases

The purpose of visually analyzing data *within* each phase is to understand the data pattern in order to predict future responding. First, the practitioner should summarize the data pattern within each phase along the following dimensions: 1) number of data points, 2) level, 3) trend, and 4) variability. This summary will allow the practitioner to predict future responding. This prediction will then be compared with actual responding in the following phase. For example, Figure 11.7 shows a baseline phase with 10 data points, a low level, no trend, and relatively low variability. This pattern is used to predict a similar pattern in the following phase, assuming no changes were made (see the open circle, dashed-line data path in the "intervention" phase for Graphs A–D).

Number of Data Points Needed No commonly accepted standard exists for the number of data points that should be collected in each phase. A general rule of thumb is that the practitioner should try to conduct at least three to five measures of the target behavior during each phase (Horner et al., 2005; Kratochwill et al., 2010). However, factors such as the stability of the data, the number of times that the effects of an intervention have been replicated, or the potential harm that a behavior may cause to the individual or others may argue for collecting fewer measures of the target behavior. The practitioner should gather a sufficient number of data points within a phase to establish stability in the individual's performance, while maintaining the individual's and others' safety.

Level The data "level" can be thought of as the average (e.g., mean or median) performance of an individual across data points within a phase. The mean or median level of performance is usually summarized as well

as the range of the data points. For example, in Figure 11.7, the mean value of the baseline data points in each graph is 26.6 and the median is 27, suggesting a relatively low level of responding. As the mean or median level of performance increases on the scale on the vertical axis, the level of performance is "higher." When the mean or median level of performance decreases on the scale, the level of performance is "lower." The data level should be considered in relationship to the variability of the data around the mean or median level and trend (slope) of the data points. In Figure 11.7, the range of the baseline data points is 15 and the trend is flat. When the data points within a phase vary substantially around the mean or median or trend is present, the interpretability of the data level is more limited.

Trend The trend is the direction and slope of the data path within the phase. Trend is characterized by the direction (positive or negative), magnitude of the slope, and variability around the trend line (Cooper et al., 2007). In Figure 11.7, the baseline of each graph shows no trend, and the actual responding in intervention (solid circles and line) in Graphs B and D show positive trend. The desired direction of the trend will be based on the intended outcome of the intervention. In teaching new behavior, we would generally expect the trend to go up across time. In reducing problem behavior, we would expect the trend to go down across time. The slope of the trend also indicates the power of an intervention. A steeper slope suggests that the intervention is more effective than a gradual slope. Within an intervention phase, a neutral slope or a slope that goes in the opposite direction of what is predicted may suggest that the intervention is not effective. The level of the data needs to be interpreted together with the direction and magnitude of the slope of the data path.

Variability Variability occurs in the data path when repeated measures of the target behavior result in substantially different

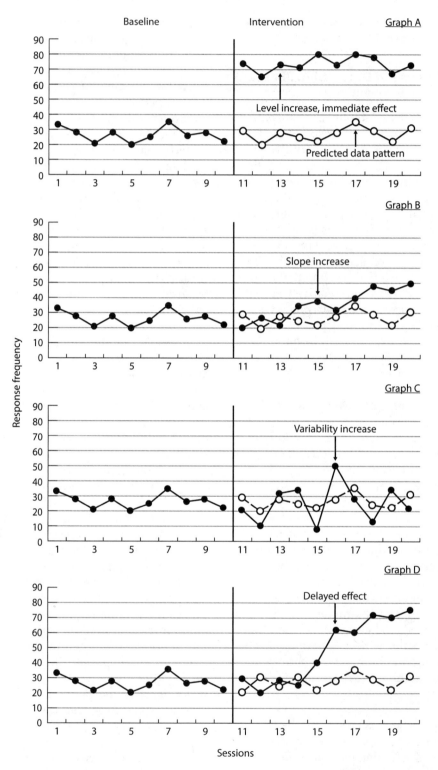

Figure 11.7. Hypothetical data patterns comparing predicted data pattern (open circles, dashed line) with intervention data pattern (solid circles and line). Graph A shows an immediate level change with no overlapping data points. Graph B shows a gradual slope change. Graph C shows a change in variability. Graph D shows a delayed effect.

values (i.e., a large range around the mean level or slope). Low variability within a phase makes the prediction of the data path much easier. For example, Figure 11.7 shows relatively low variability in the baseline phases of each graph, which is projected into each intervention phase (open circles, dashed line). When the data are "jumping around" within a phase, additional factors may be influencing the individual's performance. Graph C in Figure 11.7 shows high variability in the actual response to intervention (solid circles and line). Prediction about the direction of the data path is made more difficult with higher variability.

Once the level, trend, and variability of the data within each phase are analyzed, the next step is to compare these data patterns across phases of the design within the context of the intervention goals and type of design.

Visual Analysis of Data Across Phases

The analysis of data paths *across* phases allows practitioners to answer the primary questions of whether a functional relationship has been established and the overall efficacy of the intervention. The first guideline for carrying out visual analysis across phases is that only adjacent phases can be compared. For example, in a MTD that includes the phases A-B-C, the A phase can only be compared with the B phase and the B phase can be compared with the C phase, but the C phase may not be compared with the A phase. The features of level, trend, variability, overlap, and immediacy of effects are compared across adjacent phases (Horner et al., 2005; Kratochwill et al., 2010).

Level In comparing data paths across phases, the change in the *level* from the end of the data path in one phase should be compared with the beginning of the data path in an adjacent subsequent phase. For example, Graph A in Figure 11.7 shows a substantial level change in the actual responding during intervention (solid circles and line), with

no changes in trend or variability. A substantial change in level provides evidence of the effectiveness of the intervention. The greater the change in level, the more powerful the intervention is in changing the target behavior. Smaller changes suggest the intervention is less powerful.

Trend Another factor that must be examined in comparing adjacent phases is the direction and slope of the trend. In practice, level and trend must be considered together in order to make a reasoned judgment about whether a functional relationship has been established between the intervention and changes in the target behavior. Data paths in adjacent phases that have visible changes in level and/or slope in the desired direction suggest that the intervention is effective. For example, Graph B in Figure 11.7 shows a gradual increase in the slope of the actual responding during intervention (solid circles and line). This change in slope also results in a slight level change during intervention. Greater changes in these characteristics suggest more powerful intervention effects. Data paths in adjacent phases that have little change in level, have the same general direction, and have similar slopes suggest that the intervention has little impact on the target behavior.

Overlap The practitioner should be concerned with the number of data points in adjacent phases that fall within the same range. The number of data points in adjacent phases has been used as an indicator of a functional relationship as well as a characteristic of the strength of the intervention (e.g., effect size). When there are no or very few overlapping data points across phases (see actual responding in intervention on Graph A, Figure 11.7), this suggests that the intervention is more effective than when there are a large number of data points falling in the same range (see predicted data pattern in intervention on Graph A, Figure 11.7). Numerous strategies have been recommended in the literature for quantitatively evaluating this characteristic, such as percentage of nonoverlapping data points (PND; Parker, Hagan-Burke, & Vannest, 2007; Scruggs & Mastropieri, 2001; White, 1987), percentage of data exceeding the mean (PEM; Ma, 2006), percentage of all nonoverlapping data (PAND; Parker et al., 2007), and improvement rate difference (IRD; Parker & Hagan-Burke, 2007). However, there is no universally accepted way to quantitatively summarize the overlap of data in adjacent phases. Methods of quantitatively summarizing overlap have limitations to interpretability, particularly in the presence of trend or outlying data points (Wolery, Busick, Reichow, & Barton, 2010).

Latency   The immediacy of the onset (latency) of a change in level and trend between phases is evaluated in visual analysis (Horner et al., 2005; Kazdin, 2011). When an immediate change in level and/or trend occurs, the practitioner can be more confident that the intervention was responsible for the change in the target behavior (e.g., actual responding in intervention in Graph A, Figure 11.7, which shows an immediate level change). Longer latency in observed effects between phases decreases the practitioner's confidence that a functional relationship exists between the intervention and the target behavior (e.g., actual responding in intervention in Graph D, Figure 11.7, which shows a delayed effect).

Simultaneous Review of the Characteristics

In determining whether a functional relationship has been established between the target behavior and the intervention, the practitioner must consider all the characteristics simultaneously. The within-phase analysis allows the practitioner to predict what would occur if there were no changes in the intervention conditions (Horner et al., 2012). This prediction must be compared with the actual trend, level, and variability in the adjacent phase. It is the difference or lack of difference

between what would be predicted and what actually occurred that allows practitioners to draw conclusions about the effectiveness of the intervention (Horner et al., 2005; 2012; Kratochwill et al., 2010).

Replication of Effects

Experimental effects between phases must be documented for more than just an A-B phase comparison. For each experimental design (e.g., withdrawal design, MBD, ATD), replication of the effects should be demonstrated for a minimum of three phase comparisons at three different points in time (Horner et al., 2005; 2012). For a withdrawal design or MTD, at least four phases would need to be included, and effects would need to be found in the first A-B comparison, the B-A comparison, and the second A-B comparison. For example, Ingram et al. (2005) compared function-based and nonfunction-based interventions in a MTD. Replication of effects in level, trend, and variability were clearly demonstrated for the phase comparisons between the two types of interventions at three points in time (see Figure 11.4). For an MBD, at least three participants or conditions need to be included, with the introduction of the intervention staggered over time. Effects need to be seen for each A-B comparison and *not* in the other legs at the time of the change in one leg (Horner et al., 2012). For example, when Schreibman et al. (1983) introduced training to the first pair of siblings, the target behavior increased for both children, whereas the target behavior across the other two sibling pairs did not increase substantially (see Figure 11.3). For an ATD, separation in the data paths suggests a functional relationship between the treatment and change in the client behavior (Kennedy, 2005). Fletcher et al. (2010) showed clearly that students correctly completed a higher percentage of single-addition math problems when taught using *TOUCH-MATH* than when taught using a number line (see Figure 11.6).

CONCLUSION

PBS is focused on improving the quality of life of individuals with problem behavior. In order to do that, practitioners must efficiently assess whether the interventions they include in behavior support plans are effective. Single-case designs, along with systematic visual analysis of graphed data, provide the structure and procedures necessary for practitioners to do the following:

- Make valid and reliable decisions about the effectiveness and efficiency of an intervention.

- Provide the information necessary to guide continuous program improvement in meeting the individual's goals.

- Communicate effectively with the individual, their family, friends, community members, and other professionals about the individual's program needs and the best strategies for meeting them.

Finally, the field of PBS involves a strong commitment to the use of evidence-based practices. While an understanding of single-case designs and visual analysis of graphed data are critical to meeting the needs of the individuals we serve, it also can assist practitioners in evaluating the potential effectiveness and utility of new interventions presented in the research literature. The guidelines and recommendations presented in this chapter provide an initial foundation for practitioners to become critical consumers of the research literature.

REFERENCES

Arnzen, E., Brekstad, A., & Holth, P. (Eds.). (2005). Special issue on noncontingent reinforcement. *European Journal of Behavior Analysis, 6*(1), 1–8.

Campbell, S., & Skinner, C.H. (2004). Combining explicit timing with an interdependent group contingency program to decrease transition times: An investigation of the Timely Transitions Game. *Journal of Applied School Psychology, 20,* 11–27.

Carr. E.G., Dunlap, G., Horner, R.H., Turnbull, A.P., Sailor, W., Anderson, J.L., . . . Fox, L. (2002). Positive behavioral support: Evolution of an applied science. *Journal of Positive Behavior Intervention, 4,* 4–16.

Cooper, J.O., Heron, T.E., & Heward, W.L. (2007). *Applied behavior analysis* (2nd ed.). Upper Saddle River, NJ. Pearson.

Fisher, W.W., Kelley, M.E., & Lomas, J.E. (2003). Visual aids and structured criteria for improving visual inspection and interpretation of single-case designs. *Journal of Applied Behavior Analysis, 36*(3), 387–406.

Fletcher, D., Boon, R.T., & Cihak, D.F. (2010). Effects of *TOUCHMATH* program compared to a number line strategy to teach addition facts to middle school students with moderate intellectual disabilities. *Education and Training in Autism and Developmental Disabilities, 45,* 449–458.

Gast, D.L., & Ledford, J. (2009). *Single subject research methodology in behavioral sciences.* New York, NY: Routledge.

Hayes, S.C., Barlow, D.H., & Nelson-Gray, R.O. (1999). *The scientist practitioner: Research and accountability in the age of managed care* (2nd ed.). Boston, MA: Allyn and Bacon.

Horner, R.H., Carr, E.G., Halle, J., McGee, G., Odom, S.L., & Wolery, M. (2005). The use of single-subject research to identify evidence-based practice in special education. *Exceptional Children, 71,* 165–179.

Horner, R.H., Swaminathan, H., Sugai, G., & Smolkowski, K. (2012). Considerations for the systematic analysis and use of single-case research. *Education and Treatment of Children, 35*(2), 269–290.

Ingram, K., Lewis-Palmer, T., & Sugai, G. (2005). Function-based intervention planning: Comparing the effectiveness of FBA function-based and non-function based intervention plans. *Journal of Positive Behavior Intervention, 7,* 224–236.

Johnston, S. (2011). Multiple baseline designs. In R.E. O'Neill, J. McDonnell, F.F. Billingsley, & W.R. Jenson (Eds.), *Single case research designs in educational and community settings.* Upper Saddle River, NJ: Pearson.

Kazdin, A.E. (1981). Drawing valid inferences from case studies. *Journal of Consulting and Clinical Psychology, 49,* 183–192.

Kazdin, A.E. (1982). *Single-case research designs: Methods for clinical and applied settings.* New York, NY: Oxford University Press.

Kazdin, A.E. (2011). *Single-case research designs: Methods for clinical and applied settings* (2nd ed.). New York, NY: Oxford University Press.

Kennedy, C.H. (2005). *Single-case designs for educational research.* Upper Saddle River, NJ: Pearson.

Kratochwill, T.R., Hitchcock, J., Horner, R.H., Levin, J.R., Odom, S.L., Rindskopf, D.M., & Shadish, W.R. (2010). *Single-case designs technical documentation.* Retrieved from http://ies.ed.gov/ncee/wwc/pdf/wwc_scd.pdf

Ma, H.H. (2006). An alternative method for quantitative synthesis of single-subject researches: Percentage of data points exceeding the median. *Behavior Modification, 30*(5), 598–617. doi:10.1177/0145445504272974

O'Neill, R.E., Horner, R.H., Albin, R.W., Sprague, J.R., Storey, K., & Newton, J.S. (1997). *Functional assessment and program development for problem behavior: A practical handbook* (2nd ed.). Belmont, CA: Wadsworth.

O'Neill, R.E., McDonnell, J., Billingsley, F.F., & Jenson, W.R. (2011). *Single case research designs in educational and community settings*. Upper Saddle River, NJ: Pearson.

Park, S., Singer, G.H.S., & Gibson, M. (2005). The functional effect of teacher positive and neutral affect on the task performance of students with significant disabilities. *Journal of Positive Behavioral Interventions, 7*, 237–246.

Parker, R.I., & Hagan-Burke, S. (2007). Median-based overlap analysis for single case data: A second study. *Behavior Modification, 31*(6), 919–936. doi:10.1177/0145445507303452

Parker, R.I., Hagan-Burke, S., & Vannest, K. (2007). Percent of all non-overlapping data (PAND): An alternative to PND. *Journal of Special Education, 40*, 194–204.

Rasmussen, K., & O'Neill, R.E. (2006). The effects of fixed-time reinforcement schedules on problem behavior of children with emotional and behavioral disorders in a day treatment classroom setting. *Journal of Applied Behavior Analysis, 39*, 453–457.

Schreibman, L., O'Neill, R.E., & Koegel, R.L. (1983). Behavioral training for siblings of autistic children. *Journal of Applied Behavior Analysis, 16*, 129–138.

Scruggs, T.E., & Mastropieri, M.A. (2001). How to summarize single-participant research: Issues and applications. *Behavior Modification, 22*, 221–242.

White, O.R. (1987). Some comments concerning "The quantitative synthesis of single-subject research." *Remedial and Special Education, 8*, 34–39.

Wolery, M., Busick, M., Reichow, B., & Barton, E.E. (2010). Comparison of overlap methods for quantitatively synthesizing single-subject data. *Journal of Special Education, 44*(1), 18–28.

Systematic Instruction

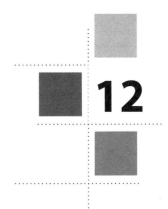

Angel Lee, Leah Wood, and Diane M. Browder

One of the most important forms of positive behavior support (PBS) is instruction of new skills for navigating current and future environments. Students with challenging behavior sometimes develop socially inappropriate behaviors or develop an overreliance on others because they have a lack of skills to cope with their contexts. Applied behavior analysis offers a wide range of strategies for shaping new skills. This chapter focuses on the systematic prompting and feedback strategies that have been used with students with challenging behavior so they can acquire a wide range of skills. These strategies are referred to as *systematic instruction*.

Systematic instruction is used to help the student learn a specific observable, measurable behavior or set of behaviors. The target behavior may be a discrete response (e.g., communicating "need a break," selecting the correct definition of a science term, reading a word) or a chain of responses (e.g., putting on a coat, crossing the street, solving a math problem, identifying the elements of a story). Each of these target responses has some naturally occurring discriminative stimulus (*SD*). For example, the printed phrase *b-u-s s-t-o-p* sets the occasion to read (or locate) *bus stop*. When the naturally occurring *SD* does not set the occasion for the target response, the instructor pairs it with a stimulus that does (the prompt). For example, if the student can imitate a model, the teacher might point at and model while reading *bus stop*. When the student reads *bus stop*, the instructor provides reinforcement (e.g., "Terrific—that is 'bus stop'!"). The instructor might also add some further instruction with this feedback (e.g., "This is where the bus picks you up."). The word is presented for multiple opportunities for the learner to respond (trials), which may occur together (massed) or across time (distributed). To transfer stimulus control from this prompt to the naturally occurring stimulus *SD*, the instructor uses some method of prompt fading. This chapter will describe several of these prompt fading methods. When the target response is chained, this prompting is applied to each response in the chain until the learner completes the entire chain (e.g., completes the steps to solve a math problem or use a vending machine). The teacher may reinforce every response in the chain, especially early in learning, or some number of responses within the chain of responding, or wait to reinforce at the end of the chain of responding. (See Chapter 8 for more on reinforcement.)

For decades, systematic instruction has been used successfully to teach daily living skills (Cuvo, Jacobi, & Sipko, 1981; Sarber & Cuvo, 1983; Mechling, 2004), leisure skills (Collins, Hall, & Branson, 1997; Tawney & Gast, 1984), and vocational skills (Browder & Minarovic, 2000). Systematic instruction has been applied to academic skills such as counting (Xin & Holmdal, 2003), recognizing sight words (Shelton, Gast, Wolery, & Winterling, 1991), solving linear equations (Jimenez, Browder, & Courtade, 2008), and comprehension of shared stories (Browder, Lee, & Mims, 2011). In fact, systematic instruction has been identified as an evidence-based practice for reading (Browder, Wakeman, Spooner, Ahlgrim-Delzell, & Algozzine, 2006), mathematics (Browder, Spooner, Ahlgrim-Delzell, Harris, & Wakeman, 2008), and science (Spooner, Knight, Browder, Jimenez, & DiBiase, 2011). An evidence-based practice is one for which there is a sufficient body of research of acceptable quality. Because systematic instruction is an evidence-based strategy, it is likely to increase student learning when applied with fidelity.

PLANNING SYSTEMATIC INSTRUCTION

To use systematic instruction, it is important to make decisions about what and how to teach prior to beginning intervention. It is difficult to be "systematic" if there is no specific target for what the student will learn or a consistent plan for prompting and feedback. Without a plan, instructors may

find themselves inadvertently promoting prompt dependency or confusing students with prompts that change across trials. Three areas to plan include 1) the target behavior, 2) prompting and feedback, and 3) generalization and maintenance. Figure 12.1 provides an example of a guide for planning systematic instruction.

Target Behavior, Objective, and Context

To begin planning, the instructor identifies a specific target behavior. Then a complete behavioral objective is written that includes the conditions, behavior, and criterion for mastery.

Burt

Consider how an objective might be written for a 12-year-old student named Burt. He has moderate intellectual disability and attention-deficit/hyperactivity disorder (ADHD). The condition the teacher selects is for Burt to learn to identify story elements using stories of high interest to Burt (sports) that he chooses daily. Because Burt tends to engage in attention-seeking behavior during independent reading times in his language arts class, this peer instruction will give him attention focused on learning a skill important to his overall academic engagement. The plan shown in Figure 12.1 focuses on a set of discrete responses that Burt makes after hearing his chosen story read aloud by a peer. The peer helps Burt use a computer tablet (e.g., iPad) set up with response boards with one page per story element and four response options per page. The peer asks Burt to identify a story element (e.g., "Who is the main character?"). Burt selects the correct response by tapping the tablet. Figure 12.2 provides an example of a simple data collection sheet that may be used by the peer or a member of the teaching team.

· ·

If the lesson illustrated in Figure 12.1 proves to be too difficult for Burt, the objective might be just for him to identify the main character (a single discrete response). Then the instructor might give him five *massed* trials to tap the character's name. Once Burt

Learner's name	Burt Capello
Target behavior: (discrete responses, chain of responses)	Identify elements of a story (use high interest sports stories that Burt selects). Burt taps to select the answers from responses shown on a computer tablet. These are discrete responses.
Objective: (condition, behavior, criterion)	After selecting a sports story and hearing it read aloud by peer or technology, Burt will identify the key story elements for 2/2 days.
Context for instruction: (small group or 1:1; settings)	Burt works on this with a peer during his language arts class independent reading time.
Presentation of trials: (massed, distributed, embedded)	These responses are embedded into independent reading time; only do for one story (all responses one time)
Method or prompting/ fading: (time delay, simultaneous prompting, least intrusive prompting, most-to-least intrusive prompting, stimulus fading, stimulus shaping)	Constant time delay
Specific prompt(s) to be used:	Model tap of correct answer
Schedule to fade prompts:	Zero delay for first two days; then 4-second delay
Reinforcement if correct:	Praise each response Burt gets correct with prompting during zero delay; then praise corrects without prompting during 4-second delay
Error correction:	Say, "No, this one" and show correct. Have Burt correctly tap the answer.
Plans for generalization:	Have the language arts teacher ask Burt for a story element he has mastered during whole-class instruction on a passage the class reads aloud. Also, have Burt apply this skill to other content (e.g., short stories, science, social studies).

Figure 12.1. Guide for planning systematic instruction.

masters identifying the main character, he might focus on a second story element (e.g., setting). While these comprehension responses are discrete, other behaviors targeted for Burt might be *chained* responses. For example, to type out his name, Burt would produce a series of responses (*B-u-r-t*). Sometimes learning trials are *distributed* across the day in naturally occurring routines. If Burt were learning to use a daily schedule, the instructor might deliver one instructional trial just prior to each transition to the next class or activity, so Burt could read the schedule one step at a time.

Sam

Sam is an 8-year-old student who sometimes engages in aggression to escape undesired tasks.

As shown in Figure 12.3, Sam is learning to locate materials with his name. This would also likely be taught using trials distributed across the day. Although Sam could be asked to locate his name with massed trials, this could set the occasion for him to seek escape. Instead, using distributed trials reduces the demand on Sam and gives him a reason for acquiring this new skill (e.g., find the box of supplies with his name on it).

One of the exciting developments in research is that systematic instruction trials can be *embedded* in general education lessons (McDonnell, Johnson, & McQuivey, 2008). While Burt's plan includes embedding his peer-tutored sessions into an independent reading time, it would also be possible for the language arts teacher to embed some additional trials during the whole-class

Task: Identify the elements of a nonfiction (e.g., sports) story
Scoring: + independent, M correct after model prompt, – error

Steps					
5. Identify the outcome	M				
4. Identify the event	M				
3. Identify the main character	+				
2. Identify the setting	M				
1. Identify the topic	+				
Percent correct	40%				
Dates	11/4	11/5	11/6	11/7	11/8

Figure 12.2.   Example of data collection for systematic instruction.

lesson (e.g., by asking Burt to identify the main character).

Prompting and Feedback

In order to promote the efficient acquisition of skills, instructional procedures used in systematic instruction promote errorless learning. *Errorless learning* is designed to increase the opportunity for a student to learn a skill making few to no incorrect responses (Mueller, Palkovic, & Maynard, 2007). By making fewer errors, the student may acquire the new skill more quickly. The purpose of prompting is to help students make correct responses without error. In

Constant time delay	
Objective: When given materials identified with names (e.g., shelves, folders, bins), Sam will find his name for ¾ trials across 2 days.	
Initial trial(s)	
Secure attention	"Listen, Sam."
Task direction	"Find your name."
Delay	0 seconds
Controlling prompt	Teacher immediately touches "Sam."
Delivery of consequences	Correct response: "Great job finding your name, Sam!" Incorrect/no response: "This is 'Sam.'" (Physically guide student to find "Sam.")
Subsequent trials	
Secure attention	"Listen, Sam."
Task direction	"Find your name."
Delay	4 seconds
Controlling prompt	Teacher touches "Sam" following delay.
Delivery of consequences	Correct response with or without prompt: "Great job finding your name, Sam!" Incorrect/no response: "This is 'Sam.'" (Physically guide student to touch "Sam.")

Figure 12.3.   Example of constant time delay.

contrast, the end goal of instruction is that the student will be able to make the response *independently* (without any prompting). As described earlier, prompt fading strategies are used to transfer *stimulus control* from the prompt to the target *SD*. There are two primary prompting strategies—response prompting and stimulus prompting. Response prompts are provided by the instructor *during* instruction to show, tell, or guide the student to make the correct response. Stimulus prompts are developed *before* instruction by modifying the materials to show the student how to respond.

Sam

For example, in teaching Sam to find his name, the teacher could gesture toward the correct response (e.g., point to his supplies box) and then let him find it (response prompt). Alternately, the teacher might color code his name in blue (response prompt).

....

Frequently used response prompts include gestures, verbal directions, models, and physical guidance. There are several prompting systems instructors may use to introduce and fade these prompts. In *time delay*, the instructor typically selects one prompt (e.g., model). The instructor promotes errorless learning by immediately providing the student with the model together with the *SD* (zero-second delay); the student's correct response is then reinforced.

Burt

On the first day Burt's peer tutor provides instruction on the story elements, he shows Burt the correct answer while asking the question. For example, while pointing to an image of a basketball, the peer asks, "What is the topic of this story?" This prompt is then faded with the insertion of small amounts of time between the SD and the prompt. Burt's peer now asks the question "What is the topic of the story?" and waits 4 seconds for Burt to anticipate the correct

response before pointing to the correct answer. If Burt makes an error, the peer will go back to the zero-delay model.

....

In *constant time delay*, a fixed amount of time (e.g., 4 seconds) is given between the presentation of the *SD* and the prompt. In *progressive time delay*, the time given between *SD* and prompt is gradually increased (e.g., 2 seconds, 4 seconds, 6 seconds). Figure 12.3 shows a sample script of constant time delay instruction. An alternative is to use *simultaneous prompting*, in which the instructor always delivers the controlling prompt immediately after the stimulus at zero delay. To determine if learning has occurred, the instructor conducts a probe session where data are recorded and no prompting is provided. If the data show that learning has occurred, then the instructor discontinues the prompt.

Another prompt fading option is *least intrusive prompts* (i.e., a least to most prompt system or a system of least prompts). In this strategy, the instructor chooses multiple prompts (around three) and arranges them in order of intrusiveness. For example, the instructor may first tell the student what to do (verbal prompt), then demonstrate the response to the student (model prompt), and then physically guide responding (physical prompt). During instruction, after the *SD* is provided, the student is given an opportunity to respond independently. If the student does not respond within a predetermined wait time (e.g., 3–5 seconds), the first-level prompt is delivered (e.g., verbal) and the instructor waits for the student to respond. If no response occurs within the predetermined wait time, then the next-level prompt is delivered (e.g., model) and the instructor again waits for a response. This continues until the student responds or the most intrusive level of prompt is delivered (e.g., full physical). If the student begins to make an error, the instructor moves to the next level of prompting (e.g., full physical). Least intrusive prompting is considered to be self-fading because less assistance is provided as the student begins to respond correctly. Figure 12.4 provides a script for least intrusive prompting.

It is important that the prompts chosen help to develop stimulus control in the most efficient manner possible. When choosing the number of prompt levels and the types of prompts, consideration must be given to the characteristics of the student (Neitzel & Wolery, 2009). For example, when planning instruction, Burt's teacher knows that he does not like a lot of physical contact. She also knows that Burt has a short attention span and that he may not engage in lengthy instruction. When planning the number of levels and types of prompt that would be most effective for Burt, she may choose a prompt hierarchy that includes verbal prompts and then visual prompts. Sam, on the other hand, may require more physical assistance and will benefit from a prompting hierarchy that includes physical guidance. A prompt hierarchy for Sam may begin with visual prompts, then a model prompt, then a partial physical prompt, and finally, a full physical prompt. As is generally the case in teaching, continuous evaluation of teaching

strategies is necessary. In Sam's case, his tendency for escape behavior may make the number of prompts impractical. If escape behaviors begin to occur, his teacher may have to adjust the number of prompts.

Most-to-least prompts (i.e., system of most prompts or the most intrusive prompts system) is the opposite of the system of least prompts in that the instructor chooses a hierarchy of prompting that moves from the most support necessary for a correct response to the least. Most-to-least prompts works well when teaching a skill where the student will benefit from physical guidance when the skill is introduced or when safety is a concern. For example, Batu, Ergenekon, Erbas, and Aknomoglu (2004) used most-to-least prompts to teach individuals with disabilities pedestrian skills related to crossing the street. Instruction began with full physical prompting together with verbal instruction for six sessions, then shifted to partial physical prompting for six sessions, and then, finally, shifted to verbal prompts only. Unlike least intrusive prompts, most-to-least prompting is not self-fading, so the instructor must decide how many sessions to assign each level of prompting. For example,

Least intrusive prompting			
Objective: When given price (e.g., $4.56), Burt will count next dollar amount (e.g., $5.00) for 8/10 prices for 2 consecutive days.			
Teacher direction: "Count the dollars for this price." (Wait for independent response.)			
Student response	Correct: Independent (no prompt needed)	No response or begins in error	Correct after prompt
Teacher feedback (1)	"Terrific! You counted four and one more—five dollars."	*Verbal prompt:* "Count out four dollars and one more."	"Good. That's four and one more. Five dollars."
Student response		No response or begins in error	Correct after prompt
Teacher feedback (2)		*Model prompt:* "Count out four dollars and one more. Like this . . ." (models counting).	"Yes. That's four and one more. Five dollars."
Student response		No response or begins in error	Correct after prompt
Teacher feedback (3)		*Physical prompt:* "Count out four dollars and one more. Let me help you do it . . ." (guide to count).	"Okay. We counted out four and one more. Five dollars."

Figure 12.4.   Example of least intrusive prompting.

after 2 days of physical guidance when the student performs the response correctly, the teacher fades to a model; after 2 more days, if the student responds correctly with the model, the teacher fades to verbal direction only and then eventually uses no prompts.

Graduated guidance is a response-prompting system that provides degrees of physical assistance and is useful when teaching motor skills. Graduated guidance has been used successfully to teach functional skills such as self-feeding (Denny et al., 2000) and requesting assistance (Dotto-Fojut, Reeve, Townsend, & Progar, 2011). As demonstrated by Dotto-Fojut, Reeve, Townsend, and Progar (2011), graduated guidance can also be used in a least-intrusive format in which the instructor shadows the student and adds more assistance on a moment-to-moment basis as needed for any part of the response (e.g., approaching the instructor to make a request). In this study, an instructor shadowed the participant's movements closely and gradually increased the distance of her hands from the participant. Another way to use this strategy is for the instructor to provide the maximum amount of physical

assistance (e.g., hand-over-hand or full physical assistance) needed for the student to perform the skill and then gradually fade the physical assistance until the instructor is simply shadowing the learner. For example, when teaching self-feeding skills, Denny et al. (2000) used a hand-over-hand prompt, followed by a hand-to-elbow prompt, a shadow prompt, and finally no prompt. Movement to the next prompt is determined by the learner demonstrating some ability to perform the response with less guidance. Reinforcement should be provided any time the learner appears to be increasing their independence.

Sometimes the instructor can modify the materials to include the prompting and then use stimulus fading or shaping to fade this assistance. *Stimulus shaping* involves using an easy-to-hard discrimination. First, the target stimulus is paired with highly divergent distracters. For example, the choice "Pam" in Figure 12.5 is paired with symbols that are not words. Over instructional trials, the distracters become more similar to the target stimulus (see Figure 12.5). Another example involves teaching the student to answer comprehension questions. In early instruction,

Level 1		
***	Pam	***
Pam	***	***
***	***	Pam
Level 2		
Pam	K	A
B	Pam	X
S	N	Pam
Level 3		
Hut	Sit	Pam
Ask	Pam	Get
Bob	Dog	Pam
Level 4		
Pam	Sue	Am
Put	Pam	Mam
Cam	Pat	Pam

Figure 12.5. Example of stimulus shaping.

the distracters might be clearly implausible. For example, after asking, "Who was the main character?," the picture options might be a picture of the boy Clarence (correct), a stapler, a shoe, and a garden. Only one of these answers "who." Over time, the distracters may be other names that do not appear in the story and eventually other names that do appear in the story.

Stimulus fading involves adding features (e.g., color, size, shape, position) to the materials to make the correct answer more salient. The salience is then faded over teaching trials. An example is shown in Figure 12.6 for the science term *volcano,* in which a small volcano picture is used to highlight the initial *v* and then faded, making it dimmer. Stimulus fading has disadvantages. The materials can be time consuming to create and the student may inadvertently focus on the wrong component of the stimulus.

Sam

To teach Sam to identify his name, the teacher began by color coding it in blue. As Sam became successful in finding his name throughout the day, his teacher made the blue darker until it eventually was black like the other names. Sam did well until his name was no longer blue. Then he seemed to lose the skill. The teacher changed her strategy by enlarging the *S* in his name so he would focus on this relevant feature. Over time, she faded the size of the *S* until it was the same as the other letters. This worked for Sam, but if it had not, she was ready to try some response prompting by gesturing to the correct name and fading this with time delay.

....

No matter which prompting and fading strategy is selected, it needs to be paired with

a reinforcement of the target response. A consequence only serves as reinforcement if it increases the likelihood that the response will occur in the presence of the *SD*. Praise is an important form of reinforcement to use during systematic instruction but should be worded so that it is motivational for that student. The words used for praise can be varied (e.g., *super, terrific, good, awesome, wow*) and, if needed, paired with a motivational social exchange (e.g., high five, brief dance, clapping). Sometimes tangible reinforcers are needed during instruction, such as tokens that are exchanged later for a leisure activity or snack. As described in Chapter 8, reinforcement may need to be continuous in the acquisition phase of learning (e.g., praise every correct response) and then faded over time (e.g., only praise unprompted responses; then only praise intermittently). Another form of feedback sometimes used in systematic instruction is error correction. If using a system with another level of prompt (e.g., least intrusive prompting), the best correction may simply be to give the next prompt. In time delay when only one prompt is used, the instructor may need to give feedback that the response is incorrect ("No") and state the correct response ("This word is *women*"). Because time delay should be near errorless, errors may mean the prompt is being faded too quickly. Reintroducing zero-delay trials may be warranted. If errors occur after the prompt, the prompt may be ineffective (e.g., the student cannot imitate a model) and another prompt may need to be used (e.g., physical guidance). An error after a prompt may indicate that the student is being reinforced by error correction (e.g., "no" is acting as a reinforcer). If the student is reinforced by error correction, it may be

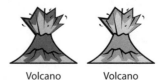

Volcano   Volcano   Volcano

Figure 12.6.   Example of stimulus fading.

better to ignore errors and give the next trial with an opportunity for reinforcement for a correct response.

Generalization and Maintenance

Response maintenance is the student's ability to perform the target behavior over time, after instruction has ceased. A key aspect of a learner's ability to maintain a learned skill is the opportunity to use that skill often. For example, Sam will likely continue to have opportunities to find materials with his name daily. In contrast, Andrea (in Figure 12.5) may need to be given opportunities to use her "next dollar" purchasing skill. Generalization is the student's ability to perform the skill under a variety of conditions (e.g., different people, materials, and settings). Burt can also learn to generalize his identification of story elements if given opportunities to use this skill with different instructors (e.g., peers, special education teacher, language arts teacher) and content (e.g., language arts; leisure interests like sports, science, and social studies). It also is important to train across multiple exemplars (Dotto-Fojut, Reeve, Townsend, & Fogar, 2011; Reeve, Reeve, Townsend, & Poulson, 2007). As a third grader who is attending general education math class, Sam is learning measurement skills. During instruction, it is important that Sam gets the opportunity to practice with a range of tools and objects to be measured. Consider the following example of Rasheeka.

Rasheeka

Rasheeka is in the tenth grade, and her school-based job is to put away school supplies in the teacher's workroom when new orders arrive. Rasheeka has autism spectrum disorder (ASD) and typically benefits from picture symbol supports when learning new vocabulary words. Her special education teacher, Ms. Copeland, realizes Rasheeka needs generalization training to learn the different types of supplies that must be sorted and put away. Initially, Ms. Copeland labeled each

area of the workroom with one picture symbol to represent each type of material (e.g., pens, pencils, paper). She quickly noticed that Rasheeka was only able to sort the materials that closely resembled the pictures she had selected for the picture symbol vocabulary cards. To encourage generalization of each material, Ms. Copeland used constant time delay to teach multiple examples of the same material. First, Ms. Copeland surveyed the types of material that were typical in the workroom. She took pictures of the various types of each item (e.g., printer paper, colored paper, notebook paper, poster board). She labeled each photograph with the same category label (e.g., paper). After developing a set of different examples of materials for each of her six target words, Ms. Copeland collated the sets to create six piles of vocabulary words, each containing one of each target word. In the zero-delay round, Ms. Copeland arranged the six cards on a table in front of Rasheeka. She presented the corresponding picture symbol currently used in the workroom and asked, "Show me ____," while immediately pointing to the target word on the table. After each request, she shuffled the order of the cards on the table. This process continued for all six words. When Rasheeka responded with 100% accuracy for two instructional sessions, Ms. Copeland incorporated a 3-second delay between the directional prompt (i.e., showing and saying the picture symbol card) and the *SD* (i.e., pointing to the corresponding picture of the item on the table). Rasheeka quickly learned to identify the different types of materials in the workroom, increasing her accuracy putting them away.

APPLYING PRINCIPALS OF POSITIVE BEHAVIOR SUPPORT DURING SYSTEMATIC INSTRUCTION

Systematic instruction can help students learn alternatives to problem behavior. As Sam learns to find his own belongings using his name, he may be less likely to grab others' materials. By learning to engage with a sports story with a peer, Burt is less likely to yell and throw materials to gain attention during independent reading time. In addition, as Burt learns that counting out money produces the opportunity to buy a desired item, he may be less likely to avoid math instruction. Systematic instruction can also be enhanced by applying some specific PBS strategies like self-determined learning, inclusive instruction, enhanced educational opportunities, and building communicative competence.

Self-Directed Learning

While there are numerous ways for students to take more of the lead in the learning experience (e.g., by making choices, setting goals, self-monitoring performance), self-instruction is especially applicable when planning systematic instruction. Agran, King-Sears, Wehmeyer, and Copeland (2003) have described the research on several models of self-instruction. One of these models is the self-determined learning model of instruction (SDLMI; Wehmeyer, Palmer, Agran, Mithaug, & Martin, 2000). In this model, teachers guide and instruct students to 1) identify the problem ("I need help to add these numbers"), 2) state a solution ("I can get a calculator"), 3) apply and evaluate the action ("I got the answer"), and 4) self-reinforce ("Way to go!"). Teachers prompt students to answer a series of problem-solving questions in order to develop goals and plans for achievement. As students increase their ability to self-regulate and self-direct their own learning, students also gain self-determination (Wehmeyer et al., 2012). Another form of self-instruction is to use some type of pictures or written instructions to perform a sequence of steps. For example, a student might use step-by-step pictures to get the materials needed to make popcorn or some other snack. Students have used technology such as video self-modeling for this self-instruction (e.g., Graetz, Mastropieri, & Scruggs, 2006). In either of these strategies, systematic prompting and feedback are used to teach the student the responses for solving a problem or following an instruction booklet. For example, least intrusive prompting might be used to teach the student to turn to each page of the instruction booklet and begin the action shown.

Burt

Burt is learning to follow picture instructions to use the computer. The teacher took screenshots of each step to find a web page he needs to access for science. The teacher then highlighted what to click on that screen to get to the next step. He self-instructs by performing each step shown on the screenshot. To teach Burt the steps, the teacher used least intrusive prompting. The teacher selected three prompts to deliver in order of least to most intrusion: 1) verbally stating the step, 2) verbally stating the step and pointing to the equipment or area on the screen needed to complete the step, and 3) verbally stating the step and modeling for Burt how to complete the step. After showing Burt each new screenshot (the SD for performing each step), the teacher waits 4 seconds before delivering the first prompt. The teacher delivers each additional prompt after additional 4-second delays as needed until Burt performs the target step.

....

Embedding self-advocacy instruction into systematic instruction can also promote self-determination and positive classroom behaviors. Self-advocacy can be as simple as providing a student with a "help" picture symbol or word in print. The teacher can instruct the student to touch the "help" card as needed throughout a lesson. Initial "help" instruction might consist of explaining things: "Sometimes I need help. When I need help, I ask someone else. If you need help, you can ask me. If you don't know the answer, touch this card to ask for help. Watch me." The instructor then models touching the card and says, "Your turn." The student then practices asking for help. The "help" symbol is then made available during ongoing instruction with reminders for the student to use it when unable to do a task or get an answer. Students also can be involved in setting goals and tracking their progress. For instance, during a social studies lesson on Native Americans, the student might set a goal for how many new vocabulary words to learn (e.g., *mesas, kiva, buffalo*). The students can self-monitor their own progress by marking a chart with a check mark, stamp, or sticker.

Sam

Sam is learning to make sets of objects using a graphic organizer to solve single-digit math equations. Sam's teacher provides a self-monitoring graph to support Sam's self-determination. The teacher models how to use a stamp to mark a square on a simple graph each time Sam correctly solves a math problem. In each lesson, Sam has five opportunities to solve addition problems, and 1 week's worth of sessions is represented on the graph. Sam records the number of math problems he completes by stamping one box on the graph. At the end of each lesson, Sam's teacher asks, "Sam, how many math problems did you solve today?" After giving Sam a 5-second wait time to respond, the teacher provides a model prompt of counting and stating the number of stamps: "Great job! You solved ___ problems today, Sam!"

....

Inclusive Contexts

Because systematic instruction has been highly effective for students with challenging behavior, it is important to realize that these strategies can be used to teach academic content in general education classes (Hudson, Browder, & Wood, 2013). Teachers, paraprofessionals, or peers can embed systematic instruction in inclusive contexts to teach a variety of academic skills. In research, constant time delay has been used to teach students vocabulary definitions across content areas (Collins, Evans, Creech-Galloway, Karl, & Miller, 2007; Jameson, McDonnell, Polychronis, & Riesen, 2008). Peers might also use systematic instruction to help the student keep track of key information in the general education lesson. For example, in a study by Jimenez, Browder, Spooner, and DiBiase (2012), peers helped students keep track of science content by using a *KWHL* graphic organizer, similar to the teacher's model. KWHL stands for what we *k*now (K), what we *w*ant to know (W), *h*ow to find out

(H), and what we *learned* (L). Systematic instruction can also be used to help students comprehend passages of text. In a study by Hudson, Browder, and Jimenez (forthcoming), students learned to answer comprehension questions about science and social studies with peers who read the passage aloud and then used a system of least intrusive prompting to help students answer the questions. These prompts included rereads of selectively smaller passages of text until the student located the answer.

Full Educational Opportunity

Systematic instruction can also be used to promote full educational opportunities like the opportunity to learn the academic content typical of the student's age and grade level. Rather than having a student who is in a middle school algebra class (i.e., age-appropriate class) working on early elementary math concepts (e.g., counting), these skills can often be embedded in adaptations of the grade-level content. For example, Jimenez, Browder, and Courtade (2008) used time delay and task-analytic instruction to teach algebraic equations to high school students with moderate developmental disabilities. Using a number chart (for numbers 1–9), a template for creating an algebraic equation ($\_\_\_ + x = \_\_\_$), colored place markers, and manipulatives, the special education teacher modeled concrete examples of solving linear equations and used constant time delay with systematic fading of praise to teach the steps of a task analysis. Real-world applications were infused in the lessons; students were solving equations in order to determine the number of materials required to complete a particular job task (e.g., number of paper clips needed). Students may also be able to engage with grade-level textbooks and novels, if the material is summarized and presented in read-aloud opportunities. For example, the peers in Hudson et al. (forthcoming) read short summaries of the science text aloud. The lesson planned for Burt (see Figure 12.1) could be expanded to

Table 12.1.   Error correction options

When an error occurs after instruction . . .	Examples
Ignore the error, do not provide reinforcement; repeat the trial at the same prompt level.	*Use a system of least prompts to teach comprehension:* The teacher asks the student to select the correct response to a literal recall question from an array of three responses. The student intentionally selects an incorrect response to get a reaction. The teacher ignores the error, does not provide any feedback (e.g., "No, you know that's not the answer"), and repeats the question.
Deliver the controlling prompt.	*Use time delay to preteach science vocabulary words:* During a delay round, the teacher shows the student four words and asks, "Which word is 'conduction'?" If the student makes an error, the teacher tells/shows the student the correct word and says, "This word is 'conduction.' Show me 'conduction.'"
Deliver the next, more intrusive prompt.	*Use a system of least prompts to teach a student to measure using a ruler:* The teacher says, "Use the ruler to measure one side of a box." The student places the ruler in the middle of the box, thus making an error. The response to the error would be to move to the next predetermined level of prompt (e.g., "Remember to line ruler up with the edge of the box.").
Insert a new level of prompt or add additional information.	*Use time delay to teach consonant-vowel-consonant (CVC) words:* During the delay round, the teacher shows the student one word at a time and asks the student to read each word. The first word is "sat." The student makes an error and says "bat." Instead of providing the controlling prompt (e.g., "This word is sat"), the teacher provides additional information by adding, "Look at the first sound /s/. This letter makes an /sss/ sound."

address additional language arts standards as he moves to higher grades. For example, a similar format might be used to teach the author's point of view, tone, and purpose.

Burt

Consider Burt's experiences in a sixth-grade language arts class. Burt is able to identify and produce all phonemes, and he is beginning to decode consonant-vowel-consonant (CVC) words independently. He enjoys reading and listening to stories about sports, particularly basketball. Burt's decoding skills are easier for him than comprehension. When asked to do comprehension work, he often becomes frustrated and says, "No." During these times, Burt will frequently leave his seat and wander around the room. This is especially distracting in his sixth-grade language arts class. His special education teacher, Ms. Fulmer, decides to use a form of the SDLMI to help Burt comprehend texts he reads or hears in his class. Burt chooses texts about animals to learn this process. First, Ms. Fulmer guides Burt to solve a series of problems across the three phases of the model: What is my problem? What is the solution? How did it work? She writes these questions on a problem-solving guide and

uses a model prompt with constant time delay to teach Burt to read each question. She then teaches him to answer each question. To answer the question "What is my problem?" Burt completes the sentence "I can't___." To generate a solution, Burt fills in "I need___." And to self-evaluate, Burt chooses "Now I can!" or "I still can't___." For the answers, Ms. Fulmer gives Burt a response board with some vocabulary for some potential problems (*can't read it, can't answer it, can't find it*) and some potential solutions (*I need a summary, I need a reader, I need to read again,* or *Show me how*). She waits for Burt to fill in the problem without help. If Burt does, she praises him. If not, she uses a verbal prompt: "Find the problem on your response board." (See Table 12.1 for examples of other error correction options.) If Burt does, she praises him. If not, she provides a model: "Find the problem. This one says, 'can't read it'; now you point to this one." Burt never needs more than a model prompt, so physical guidance is not used. This prompting system is then repeated for the solution. Once Burt communicates what he needs, the teacher provides it. After the lesson, Burt self-evaluates if the solution worked. The teacher then has Burt generalize his problem solving with a peer partner and a paraprofessional. He also begins to use his system with all his language-arts work. After Burt develops his strategies, he self-monitors his progress using a small self-monitoring chart he keeps in his desk.

·····································

Communication Competence

Systematic instruction can be especially effective to teach students communication objectives. For example, the instructor might use a model with time delay to show the student how to use a picture to make a request. Then the student might learn to indicate a choice from several pictures to make this request. One critical need is for students to have a response mode to communicate what they know during instruction. This type of communication differs from making a request or indicating a choice because there is one correct answer.

Browder et al. (2011) taught students who used either eye gaze, object selection, or touching a symbol to demonstrate comprehension during a read aloud. A model prompt was provided as needed during instruction. The model prompt for the student who used eye gaze was to tap the correct answer. For a student who was blind and using objects to respond, the model prompt was to place the student's hand on the correct object and then put it back in a neutral position so the student had the opportunity to find the object. Prompting can also be used to teach students to use a picture response board or other assistive technology. Some communication devices only require a discrete response (e.g., point to picture). Others require a response chain (e.g., scan to find topic, find subtopic, locate answer, press button). Either a system of least intrusive prompting or graduated guidance might be used to teach the student to make these responses. Johnston, Davenport, Kanarowski, Rhodehouse, and McDonnell (2009) taught letter-sound correspondence and CVC combinations to students who use augmentative and alternative communication (AAC). Constant time delay was used to teach students to identify letter sounds

and spell CVC words on an array with eight response options of lowercase letters (*a, m, t, s, i, f, d, r*). Students received instruction during literacy centers, and correct responses were reinforced with participation in engaging activities. For example, contingent on independent correct or correct prompted responses, students threw beanbags into a trashcan decorated to resemble a monster.

Students will often use some combination of communication options. Consider the following example of Rasheeka.

Rasheeka

Although Rasheeka can verbalize about 20 words, which helps her ask for basic needs and engage with peers in simple conversations, her skills are not adequate for the demands of her high school classes, more age-appropriate conversations, and future job expectations. Rasheeka is learning to use a computer tablet (e.g., iPad) that has a software program that provides a framework for arrays of vocabulary (e.g., GoTalk NOW; Attainment Company Inc., 2012). She has pages in her tablet developed by her special education teacher for each of her high school classes that contain vocabulary related to the big ideas of her current units (e.g., chemical reactions). She has some entertaining pages that her peers help her create related to current trends (e.g., singers, school events). She also has some pages she uses to deal with challenging situations that she faces at school and may face in the future on the job (e.g., requesting assistance to complete a task, inquiring about the location of materials, asking for directions to be repeated). Figure 12.7 gives an example of the symbols on one of Rasheeka's pages.

·····································

CONCLUSION

Systematic instruction is an evidence-based practice that can be used to promote skills acquisition for students with moderate and challenging behavior. In systematic instruction, the target behavior is operationally defined and may involve either discrete or chained responses. Then a method

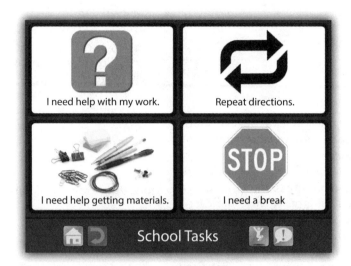

Figure 12.7. Example of Rasheeka's communication pages. (Image created using GoTalk NOW app; adapted by permission of Attainment Company, Inc. www.attainment company.com/gotalk-now)

of systematic prompting and feedback is planned. Systematic instruction can be an important component of any PBS plan. By learning adaptive skills, students do not need to rely as much on challenging behaviors to meet their needs and preferences. The principles of PBS can be promoted further when used in inclusive educational contexts that promote the full educational opportunities of the general curriculum, when students are involved in their own instruction, and when systematic instruction is applied to promote communicative competence.

REFERENCES

Agran, M., King-Sears, M.E., Wehmeyer, M.L., & Copeland, S.R. (2003). *Teachers' guide to inclusive practices: Student-directed learning.* Baltimore, MD: Paul H. Brookes Publishing Co.

Attainment Company, Inc. (2012). *Go Talk NOW* (computer application). Verona, WI.

Batu, S., Ergenekon, Y., Erbas, D., & Aknomoglu, N. (2004). Teaching pedestrian skills to individuals with developmental disabilities. *Journal of Behavioral Education, 13*(3), 147–164.

Browder, D.M., Lee, A., & Mims, P.J. (2011). Using shared stories and individual response modes to promote comprehension and engagement in literacy for students with multiple, severe disabilities. *Education and Training in Autism and Developmental Disabilities, 46,* 339–351.

Browder, D.M., & Minavoric, T.J. (2000). Utilizing sight words in self-instruction training for employees with moderate mental retardation in competitive jobs. *Education and Training in Mental Retardation and Developmental Disabilities, 35,* 78–89.

Browder, D.M., Spooner, F., Ahlgrim-Delzell, L., Harris, A.A., & Wakeman, S. (2008). A meta-analysis on teaching mathematics to students with significant cognitive disabilities. *Exceptional Children, 74,* 407–432.

Browder, D.M., Wakeman, S.Y., Spooner, F., Ahlgrim-Delzell, L., & Algozzine, B. (2006). Research on reading instruction for individuals with significant cognitive disabilities. *Exceptional Children, 72,* 392–408.

Collins, B.C., Evans, A., Creech-Galloway, C., Karl, J., & Miller, A. (2007). Comparison of the acquisition and maintenance of teaching functional and core content sight words in special and general education settings. *Focus on Autism and Other Developmental Disabilities, 22,* 220–233.

Collins, B.C., Hall, M., & Branson, T.A. (1997). Teaching leisure skills to adolescents with moderate disabilities. *Exceptional Children, 63,* 499–512.

Cuvo, A.J., Jacobi, L., & Sipko, R. (1981). Teaching laundry skills to mentally retarded students. *Education and Training of the Mentally Retarded, 16,* 54–64.

Denny, M., Marchand-Martella, N., Martella, R.C., Reilly, J.R., Reilly, J.F., & Cleanthous, C.C. (2000). Using parent delivered graduated guidance to teach functional living skills to a child with Cri du Chat syndrome. *Education and Treatment of Children, 23,* 441–454.

Dotto-Fojut, K.M., Reeve, K.F., Townsend, D.B., & Progar, P.R. (2011). Teaching adolescents with autism to describe a problem and request assistance during simulated vocational tasks. *Research in Autism Spectrum Disorders, 5,* 826–833.

Graetz, J.E., Mastropieri, M.A., & Scruggs, T.E. (2006). Show time: Using video self-monitoring to decrease inappropriate behavior. *TEACHING Exceptional Children, 38,* 43–48.

Hudson, M.E., Browder, D.M., & Jimenez, B. (forthcoming). Effects of a peer-delivered system of least prompts with adapted text read-alouds on listening comprehension for students with moderate intellectual disability. *Education and Training in Autism and Developmental Disabilities.*

Hudson, M.E., Browder, D.M., & Wood, L. (2013). Review of experimental research on academic learning by students with moderate and severe intellectual disability in general education. *Research and Practice for Persons with Severe Disabilities, 38,* 17–29.

Jameson, J.M., McDonnell, J., Polychronis, S., & Riesen, T. (2008). Embedded, constant time delay instruction by peers without disabilities in general education classrooms. *Intellectual and Developmental Disabilities, 46,* 346–363.

Jimenez, B.A., Browder, D.M., & Courtade, G.R. (2008). Teaching algebraic equation to high school students with moderate developmental disabilities. *Education and Training in Developmental Disabilities, 43,* 266–274.

Jimenez, B.A., Browder, D.M., Spooner, F., & DiBiase, W. (2012). Inclusive inquiry science using peer-mediated embedded instruction for students with a moderate intellectual disability. *Exceptional Children, 78,* 301–317.

Johnston, S., Davenport, L., Kanarowski, B., Rhodehouse, S., & McDonnell, A. (2009). Teaching sound-letter correspondence and consonant-vowel-consonant combinations to young children who use augmentative and alternative communication. *Augmentative and Alternative Communication, 25,* 123–135.

McDonnell, J., Johnson, J.W., & McQuivey, C. (2008). *Embedded instruction for students with developmental disabilities in general education classrooms.* Arlington, VA: Council for Exceptional Children.

Mechling, L.C. (2004). Effects of multimedia, computer-based instruction on grocery shopping fluency. *Journal of Special Education Technology, 19,* 23–34.

Mueller, M.M., Palkovic, C.M., & Maynard, C.S. (2007). Errorless learning: Review and practical application for teaching children with pervasive developmental disabilities. *Psychology in the Schools, 44,* 691–700.

Neitzel, J., & Wolery, M. (2009). *Steps for implementation: Least-to-most prompts.* Chapel Hill, NC: National Professional Development Center on Autism Spectrum Disorders, Frank Porter Graham Child Development Institute, The University of North Carolina.

Reeve, S.A., Reeve, K.F., Townsend, D.B., & Poulson, C.L. (2007). Establishing a generalized repertoire of helping behavior in children with autism. *Journal of Applied Behavior Analysis, 40,* 123–136.

Sarber, R.E., & Cuvo, A.J. (1983). Teaching nutritional meal planning to developmentally disabled clients. *Behavior Modifications, 7,* 503–530.

Shelton, B.S., Gast, D.L., Wolery, M., & Winterling, V. (1991). The role of small group instruction in facilitating observational and incidental learning. *Language, Speech, and Hearing Services in Schools, 22,* 123–133.

Spooner, F., Knight, V., Browder, D., Jimenez, B., & DiBiase, W. (2011). Evaluating evidence-based practice in teaching science content to students with severe developmental disabilities. *Research and Practice for Persons with Severe Disabilities, 36,* 62–75.

Tawney, J.W., & Gast, D.L. (1984). *Single subject research in special education.* Columbus, OH: Merrill.

Wehmeyer, M.L., Palmer, S.B., Agran, M., Mithaug, D.E., & Martin, J.E. (2000). Promoting causal agency: The self-determined learning model of instruction. *Exceptional Children, 66,* 439–453.

Wehmeyer, M.L., Shogren, K.A., Palmer, S.B., Williams-Diehm, K.L., Little, T.D., & Boulton, A. (2012). The impact of self-determined learning model of instruction on student self determination. *Exceptional Children, 78,* 135–153.

Xin, J.E., & Holmdal, P. (2003). Snacks and skills: Teaching children functional counting skills. *TEACHING Exceptional Children, 35*(5), 46–51.

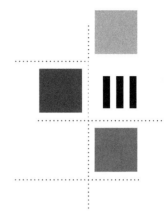

Comprehensive Function-Based and Person-Centered Assessments

 STANDARDS ADDRESSED IN THIS SECTION

I. B. Positive behavior support (PBS) practitioners adhere to the following basic assumptions about behavior:

   1. Challenging behavior serves a function.
   2. Positive strategies are effective in addressing the most challenging behavior.
   3. When positive behavior intervention strategies fail, additional functional assessment strategies are required to develop more effective PBS strategies.
   4. Features of the environmental context affect behavior.
   5. Reduction of challenging behavior is an important—but not the sole—outcome of successful intervention; effective PBS results in improvements in quality of life, acquisition of valued skills, and access to valued activities.

I. E. Practitioners of PBS understand the following legal and regulatory requirements related to assessment and intervention regarding challenging behavior and behavior change strategies:

   1. Requirements of IDEA with respect to PBS
   2. The purpose of human rights and other oversight committees regarding behavior change
   3. Works within state/school/agency regulations and requirements

(continued)

V. A. Practitioners understand the importance of multielement assessments, including the following:
1. Person-centered planning
2. Quality of life
3. Environmental/ecology
4. Setting events
5. Antecedents and consequences
6. Social skills/communication/social networks
7. Curricular/instructional needs (e.g., learning style)
8. Health/biophysical

V. B. Comprehensive assessments result in information about the focus individual in at least the following areas:
1. Lifestyle
2. Preferences and interests
3. Communication/social abilities and needs
4. Ecology
5. Health and safety
6. Problem routines
7. Variables promoting and reinforcing challenging behavior, including the following:
   a. Preferences/reinforcers
   b. Antecedents
   c. Setting events
   d. Potential replacement behavior
8. Function(s) of behavior
9. Potential replacement behaviors

V. C. Practitioners who apply PBS conduct person-centered assessments that provide a picture of the life of the individual, including the following:
1. Indicators of quality of life comparable to same-age individuals without disabilities (e.g., self-determination, inclusion, friends, fun, variety, access to belongings)
2. The strengths and gifts of the individual
3. The variety and roles of people with whom they interact (e.g., family, friends, neighbors, support providers) and the nature, frequency, and duration of such interactions
4. The environments and activities in which they spend time, including the level of acceptance and meaningful participation; problematic and successful routines; preferred settings/activities; the rate of reinforcement and/or corrective feedback; and the age appropriateness of settings, activities, and materials
5. The level of independence and support needs of the individual including workplace, curricular and instructional modifications, augmentative communication and other assistive technology supports, and assistance with personal management and hygiene
6. The health and medical/biophysical needs of the individual
7. The dreams and goals of the individual and his or her circle of support
8. The barriers to achieving the dreams and goals
9. The influence of this information on challenging behavior

V. D. PBS practitioners conduct functional behavior assessments that result in the following:
1. Operationally defined challenging behavior
2. The context in which challenging behavior occurs most often

3. Identification of setting events that promote the potential for challenging behavior
4. Identification of antecedents that set the occasion for challenging behavior
5. Identification of consequences maintaining challenging behavior
6. A thorough description of the antecedent behavior consequence relationship
7. An interpretation of the function(s) of behavior
8. Identification of potential replacement behavior

V. E. PBS practitioners conduct the following indirect and direct assessment strategies:
1. Indirect assessments: file reviews, structured interviews (e.g., person-centered planning), checklists, and rating scales (e.g., MAS)
2. Direct assessments: scatterplots, anecdotal recording, ABC data, and time/activity analyses
3. Summarize data in graphic and narrative formats

V. F. PBS practitioners work collaboratively with the team to develop hypotheses that are supported by assessment data:
1. All assessment information is synthesized and analyzed to determine the possible influence of the following on the occurrence or nonoccurrence of challenging behavior:
    a. Setting events (or establishing operations)
    b. Antecedents/triggers
    c. Consequences for both desired and challenging behaviors
    d. Ecological variables
    e. Lifestyle issues
    f. Medical/biophysical problems
2. Hypotheses statements are developed that address the following:
    a. Setting events
    b. Antecedents
    c. Consequences for both desired and challenging behaviors
    d. Function(s) challenging behavior serves for the individual

V. G. PBS practitioners utilize functional analysis of behavior as necessary on the basis of an understanding of the following:
1. The differences between functional assessment and functional analysis
2. The advantages and disadvantages of functional analysis
3. support (PBS) planning and implementation

Section III includes four chapters that examine person-centered and function-based assessments. The authors build on content presented in previous sections and the extensive literature that supports these approaches and their use as part of comprehensive positive behavior support (PBS) planning and implementation. The reader will learn about a wide variety of approaches to the assessment of challenging behavior, but a common thread across all four chapters is on methods for collaboratively understanding the purpose of the behavior and providing evidenced-based strategies that ultimately increase the quality of life for the person of concern. Each of the chapters in this section provides case examples that help illustrate major points.

Chapter 13, "Integrating and Building on Best Practices in Person-Centered Planning, Wraparound, and Positive Behavior Support to Enhance Quality of Life," describes how person-centered planning and wraparound services are provided within the context of PBS. The authors illustrate the integration of these strategies by sharing a model called Life Outcomes Through Integrated Systems (LOTIS) that embeds this discussion within a three-tiered model of PBS. Chapter 14, "Conducting Functional Behavioral Assessments," provides a historical and research basis for understanding functional behavioral assessment and includes numerous examples of its application in applied settings. In addition, the authors review a variety of indirect and direct observation methods for collecting functional assessment data. Chapter 15, "Using Functional Behavioral Assessment Data," extends the discussion started in Chapter 14 by focusing on strategies for summarizing functional assessment data; focusing on strategies for examining data, including data that are unclear or inconsistent; and outlining a process for the development of hypothesis statements that support intervention planning and implementation. Finally, Chapter 16, "Conducting Functional Analyses of Behavior," provides a concise history of the use of functional analysis and then describes a wide variety of innovative applications of this approach in both home and school settings.

Randall L. De Pry

Integrating and Building on Best Practices in Person-Centered Planning, Wraparound, and Positive Behavior Support to Enhance Quality of Life

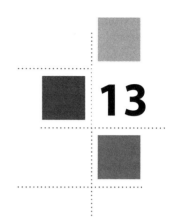

13

Rachel Freeman, Matt Enyart, Kelcey Schmitz,
Pat Kimbrough, Kris Matthews, and Lori Newcomer

Person-centered planning (PCP) refers to a set of assessment and action-planning processes that are used to improve the quality of life (QOL) of children and adults with disabilities across home, work, and community settings (Claes, Van Hove, Vandevelde, Fan Loon, & Schalock, 2010). PCP is a collaborative, strengths-based process that results in the identification of goals for establishing positive relationships, building community participation, and facilitating self-determination of individuals with a variety of abilities. The purpose of PCP is to assist individuals in designing their current preferred lifestyles, creating a vision for a meaningful future, and making a positive social contribution to society.

Wraparound planning, another person- and family-centered strategy, was developed in the 1980s during the same time period as PCP. This approach was first designed to provide person-centered and family-centered planning for children and youth with emotional and behavioral disorders (Stroul & Friedman, 1986). Wraparound planning is a process that builds on an individual's and family's strengths and establishes a set of natural and community supports and services for a child or young adult in order to improve his or her life outcomes (Winters & Metz, 2009). The wraparound process was developed as a response to expert-driven, deficit-based models that placed children in categorical services irrespective of the unique needs of each individual child. Wraparound planning has been implemented collaboratively within the context of schoolwide positive behavior intervention and support (SWPBIS) efforts across the United States (Eber, Hyde, & Suter, 2011).

Positive behavior support (PBS) is an applied science that shares the historical time line and evolution of both PCP and wraparound planning. The term *PBS* refers to a set of strategies that are used to assist individuals across the life span in increasing their self-determination and QOL while eliminating or decreasing the occurrence of problem behaviors and the future likelihood of those behaviors (Carr, 2007). Essential features of PBS include evidence-based practices that incorporate the principles of behavior, biomedical and physiological interventions, and value-based practices that fit the needs of the individual and his or her team and the tenets of systems-change implementation (Carr et al., 2002). A goal of PBS is to encourage social and communication-based solutions and redesign environmental settings that are associated with problem behavior.

The purpose of this chapter is to describe how both PCP and wraparound assessment strategies are used within the context of PBS. In the last section of the chapter, we propose a model teams can use to integrate the assessment and measurement of QOL outcomes using PCP, wraparound, and PBS. Although the Association for Positive Behavior Support (APBS) has embedded PCP within their PBS individual standards of practice, both PCP and wraparound are also considered strategies that are independent of PBS with a rich publication history (Holburn & Vietze, 2002). Therefore, an introduction to PCP and wraparound planning is shared in this chapter before discussing how all three of these strategies may be integrated when supporting individuals with challenging behavior.

PERSON-CENTERED PLANNING

PCP creates a foundation from which an individual, with assistance from his or her team, gradually builds a satisfying and meaningful life. Feedback from individuals and the people who are important in their lives guides the PCP process. The PCP planning team makes a commitment to meet collaboratively with an individual as he or she begins to take a leading role in making decisions about his or her current and future lifestyle preferences. A facilitator works with the individual and family to prepare for the meeting and provides guidance during each step of PCP. PCP is a meeting process that occurs over an extended period of time, starting with an individual and his or her team establishing an initial vision or dream for the future (Holburn, Gordon, & Vietze, 2007).

Traditional planning methods have often focused on placing individuals into already existing services and supports. In PCP, there is an emphasis on first assessing what is needed and then creating tailored services and supports that will meet the individual's needs. The team identifies a person's vision for the future and then brainstorms ways in which to achieve that vision. Over time, PCP is modified and updated as an individual has new life experiences. New PCP team members may be added while others are no longer needed. These changes are based on an individual's stage of life, developmental growth, new routines and settings experienced, and new dreams and preferred lifestyles that are identified.

TYPES OF PERSON-CENTERED PLANNING STRATEGIES

There are many forms of PCP available, each one containing helpful tools and strategies. Common forms of PCP include the McGill Action Planning System (MAPS; Vandercook, York, & Forest, 1989), essential lifestyle planning (Smull & Burke Harrison, 1992), and the PICTURE method (Holburn et al., 2007). Although there are some differences across these PCP models, most strategies include common characteristics and outcomes that are expected no matter what particular organizational approach is used. Table 13.1 contains a list of these common value-based statements and assumptions that are evident in effective person-centered and wraparound planning processes. Clearly stated values documented during meetings helps create a unified vision and assists the team in maintaining a focus on important outcomes.

Visual graphics convey information about a person via pictures or images in PCP meetings. This assists the team in articulating an emerging vision without the use of complex verbal interactions. Although the types

Table 13.1.   Value-based characteristics of person-centered planning

Essential characteristics of person-centered and wraparound planning

1. Individuals and family members are encouraged to direct meetings and select team members.
2. Meeting length, location, and processes are tailored to the preferences of the individual and family.
3. Assessment and goal development focus on strengths and team-based problem solving.
4. The team identifies natural supports, rather than overrelying on existing services.
5. Interventions focus on community-based services that help individuals make valuable contributions to society.
6. Choice making and the expression of self-determination are embedded in meetings.
7. Goals include creating a positive future as well as a preferred lifestyle.
8. Interagency collaboration is valued, with attention to service coordination.
9. Services are provided to the individual and family in an unconditional manner.
10. Developing and maintaining significant relationships with others are important parts of life.

Sources: Eber and Nelson (1997); Kincaid and Fox (2002).

of PCP strategies differ, the main outcomes expected of PCP processes are similar (Kincaid & Fox, 2002). These outcomes include 1) increasing the person's participation in the community, 2) identifying new and enhancing existing meaningful relationships, 3) expanding the opportunity for an individual to express and make choices, 4) creating a dignified life based on mutual respect, and 5) developing team skills and areas of expertise in order to improve QOL (Kincaid, 1996). Figure 13.1 shows an example of a document used to gather information during a PCP meeting.

One of the first steps involved in the PCP process is to schedule a meeting individually with the focus person. The length and format of PCP meetings are adjusted to meet the needs of each individual. Facilitators may adjust the ways in which they guide a team through the PCP process based on the unique characteristics of each person. The length of time allocated for meetings, the types of collaborative activities used, and the ways in which individuals participate in the process are modified to meet the needs of each person. An individual's age, interests, team members, and other unique characteristics guide the PCP development.

For example, Clark and Hart (2009) describe how the PCP process was modified to meet the needs of young adults with emotional and behavioral disorders. Some youth are not interested in participating in meetings with older adults asking them a lot of personal questions. To address this problem, Clark and Hart describe the importance of first establishing an unconditional positive relationship between a young person and one adult mentor called a *transition facilitator*. The transition facilitator is a young adult who works on a one-to-one basis with the youth to gather details related to PCP. Together, the transition facilitator and the young person present the young person's PCP assessment and ideas for implementation to family members, service providers, educators, and other team members in a series of smaller meetings.

It is important to consider the types of PCP meeting environments and interaction processes that will increase the level of comfort and enjoyment for both the individual and his or her team. The length of the meetings; locations; themes addressed; and the inclusion of food and drinks, music, and other individualized touches can set the stage for success.

Because of the individualized nature of PCP and the subjective characteristics of the process, there has been a great deal of debate about the role of evaluation and measurement of PCP goals (Bambara, Lohrmann, & Brown, 2002). The subjective nature of what constitutes an "ideal" QOL makes evaluation a challenging task. Some professionals question the contribution that

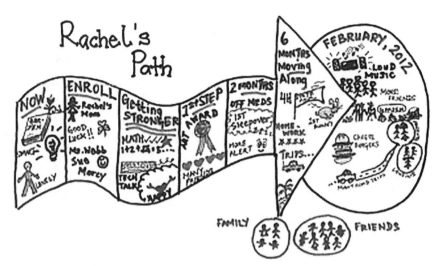

Figure 13.1. Visual example of a person-centered plan (PCP). (From Moore, M., Freeman, R., Kimbrough, P., Tieghi, M., Rosdahl, D., Smith, C., . . . & Zarcone, J. [2007]. *Person-centered and wraparound planning, version 5.0* [Online]. Lawrence: University of Kansas Center on Developmental Disabilities; reprinted by permission.)

measurement systems make in PCP since there is a strong emphasis on the subjective experience throughout the planning process (O'Brien, 2002). Other professionals in the field do advocate for the use of evidence-based evaluation methods in both QOL and PCP (Holburn et al., 2007). These strategies help provide a way to evaluate how effective the planning processes are in making significant changes in an individual's life. However, a review of PCP studies conducted by Claes and her colleagues (2010) reported only moderate evidence for the efficacy of PCP. Further research and evaluation related to QOL and PCP are needed in order to demonstrate the effectiveness of this type of planning process.

Quality of Life and Person-Centered Planning

Most people in today's society are familiar with the basic definition of the phrase *quality of life* (Schalock & Verdugo, 2002). Since the earliest times in history, human beings have searched for happiness, a sense of well-being, and the "good things" in life (Evans, 1994). QOL refers to the extent to which a person is achieving self-selected major life goals in home, school, work, and community settings. Other features of QOL include the degree to

which a person achieves ideal health and wellness and optimal life experiences. Although there are many different definitions of QOL, the literature suggests that QOL is the same for individuals with and without disabilities (Lyons, 2010). Leading QOL experts believe that the way in which QOL is conceptualized, assessed, and measured is universal and should be applied to the general population (Schalock, 1996; Turnbull & Brunk, 1990).

Researchers studying QOL break down the concept into domains (Schalock, Brown, et al., 2002). Although the names given to these different domains vary, there is a great deal of similarity across the different terms that are used. The eight QOL domains described in Table 13.2 are used for identifying multiple measures that will comprehensively evaluate QOL. Wraparound planning uses the same concept of domains in a slightly different manner. The next section describes wraparound and the domains used in the implementation process.

WRAPAROUND PLANNING

Parents of children and adults with mental health needs and challenging behavior are often expected to communicate with

Table 13.2.   Quality-of-life (QOL) domains and associated indicators

Domain	Common QOL indicator
Emotional well-being	Enjoyment of life Self-concept Stress levels
Interpersonal relations	Quality/number of interactions with others Quality/number of relationships with others Informal and formal supports for relationships
Material well-being	Financial status Type and preference for employment Quality of housing
Personal development	Educational opportunities Personal competence at home/school/work/community Performance in important activities
Physical well-being	Health status Activities to encourage exercise, stimulation, and relaxation Leisure activities: quality and number
Self-determination	Autonomy: Extent to which person has control over important life experiences Opportunities for decision making every day Goals and personal values acknowledged, followed, and respected by others
Social inclusion	Community integration and participation Community roles that bring respect and social equity Social supports necessary for community involvement
Rights	Extent to which person experiences fair and equitable treatment in the home and community Extent to which legal supports are available

Sources: Schalock and Verdugo (2002).

numerous service systems, including juvenile justice, children and family services, special education, mental health, and developmental disabilities. When these services are not coordinated, parents must make their way through additional meetings, duplicative paperwork, and multiple plans of support written about and for their children. Families have historically faced these types of fragmented and disconnected services (Knitzer, 1982). Systems-of-care meetings and wraparound planning were created in response to these challenges to assist families who were advocating for their children (Winters & Metz, 2009).

The complex task of service coordination across human and education agencies can be achieved via systems-level meetings, referred to as systems-of-care (SOC) meetings, implemented at local, regional, and/or state levels (Kutash, Duchnowski, & Lynn, 2006). These SOC meetings include team members representing administrators, state professionals,

agency directors, commissioners, as well as the individual (e.g., family, advocates). In fact, in many states, SOC and wraparound planning are now viewed as essential processes for the effective delivery of services to children with emotional and behavioral challenges across child welfare, mental health, education, special education, and juvenile justice settings (Clark & Clark, 1996).

Table 13.1 summarizes the most common values and characteristics that are reported in the wraparound and PCP literature. To implement wraparound effectively, teams must address a wide range of natural and formal supports involving different practitioners, teams, organizations, and systems (Bruns, Sather, Pullman, & Stambaugh, 2011). During the wraparound process, the team assesses a child's social strengths and the family's needs across a variety of life domains (see Table 13.3). The common life domains assist teams during the assessment process by prompting

Table 13.3.   Wraparound planning domains

- Family support (information about strengths and needs)

- Legal (the extent to which anyone in the family is involved in judicial proceedings and/or custody-related actions)

- Health/medical (the person's health status and medications, their family's health and wellness needs, and extent to which access to medical assistance is available)

- Safety (the degree to which individual family members are not in danger)

- Behavioral needs (the quality and frequency of positive social behaviors used in families)

- Educational/vocational (family access to education and jobs, transition to work supports)

- Social/recreational (access to positive social groups, meaningful family interactions)

- Emotional (ability to express feelings among family members, experience of emotional well-being, access to counseling/psychological support)

- Cultural (cultural knowledge of family and larger community)

- Spiritual (ability to access and experience spiritual leadership, mentorship, and growth)

- Substance abuse (the extent to which chemical substances are used within the family unit)

Source: Vandenberg and Grealish (1996).

discussion about supports and services across home, recreation, education, and/or work settings and financial, emotional, cultural, physical, and spiritual well-being. Whereas in traditional planning, children are placed in already existing services and systems, wraparound planning provides teams with an opportunity to think differently about the supports that meet the child's and family's needs (Eber, Nelson, & Miles, 1997). The goal of wraparound is to assist the individual in living an independent, fulfilling, law-abiding, and constructive life in the community using formal and informal supports.

Systems of care and wraparound facilitators recommend that definitions of the wraparound process be reported in a manner that allows an individual and his or her team to evaluate the fidelity of implementation (Walker & Petr, 2011). *Fidelity of implementation* refers to the evaluation of whether key features of an intervention are actually implemented in the manner intended. Measurement tools are available for guiding team problem solving and evaluating wraparound fidelity (Bruns, Suter, & Leverentz-Brady, 2008).

The evaluation of wraparound planning as an evidence-based practice is still in a relatively early stage. In fact, researchers have reported challenges in documenting wraparound outcomes that are similar to those

expressed by their PCP colleagues. While there is research reporting the efficacy of wraparound (Suter & Bruns, 2009), more studies are needed to establish wraparound planning as an evidence-based practice (Bruns et al., 2010). In the next section of the chapter, the integration of wraparound and PCP are described within the context of PBS.

INTEGRATING PERSON-CENTERED PLANNING, WRAPAROUND, AND POSITIVE BEHAVIOR SUPPORT PLANNING

PCP and wraparound models have unique strengths and tend to use slightly different strategies to empower individuals and their families. Since each child or adult is unique, we believe that there are times when a combination of PCP and wraparound strategies can be useful. For instance, a child with emotional and behavioral disorders may be part of a family in which English is a second language for some family members. The visual strategies and tools used in PCP (see Figure 13.1 for an example) can provide a way for the team to avoid language barriers by communicating via visual pictures and drawings instead of relying only on the use of the English language or on the use of translators during assessment and action planning.

PCP or wraparound is often integrated with PBS in situations where an individual is in need of intensive supports due to problem behaviors that are severe or chronic in nature (Kincaid & Fox, 2002). There are a number of benefits associated with integrating PCP and wraparound into PBS. The implementation of person-centered strategies helps the team emphasize the focus person's and the family's strengths throughout each meeting. Implementing PCP or wraparound before more intensive behavior support planning helps ensure the team is focusing on improving an individual's QOL throughout the PBS process. A facilitator can use the information from person-centered or wraparound planning to unify a team that has become distracted or off task by reviewing the positive outcomes that everyone agreed on during person-centered or wraparound planning.

Individuals who benefit from PBS often engage in problem behaviors that serve a communicative need or function. When person-centered approaches are implemented, problem behaviors may decrease naturally because an individual's needs are being met via QOL goals (Smull, 2002), making a PBS plan unnecessary. One of the great benefits of starting PBS with a person-centered approach is that a great deal of information about the environmental events preceding problem behaviors and the consequences maintaining problem behavior can be gathered (Moore et al., 2007). This information is documented in an FBA (see Chapters 14 and 15; O'Neill et al., 1997).

Bambara and Knoster (2009) describe two types of FBA information that are gathered: 1) broader contextual information about an individual's preferences, social and communication-based strengths, health, history, and goals and overall aspects of his or her QOL; and 2) specific details used to pinpoint the variables that occasion and maintain problem behavior. Person-centered or wraparound planning provides a systematic way in which teams can gather the larger contextual details while simultaneously contributing to the information regarding specific details related to problem behavior. We believe that integrating the best elements of PCP, wraparound, and PBS provides teams with the ability to tailor the assessment and planning processes for the unique needs of each individual and his or her team in a more synergistic manner.

The timing and order in which PCP, wraparound, and PBS is implemented varies across facilitators, providing training and technical assistance tailored to the needs of each person receiving support. For instance, some people describe PBS as a process that is used as part of the person-centered or wraparound-planning process. Once the person-centered or wraparound plan begins, the team chooses to focus on behavior as one of the life domains that need to be addressed. In this case, PBS begins after PCP or wraparound has already begun. On the other hand, Bambara and Knoster (2009) describe PCP as something that is included within the PBS process as "another avenue for gathering broad information about a student" (p. 33). PBS is identified first as a need, and person-centered strategies are then included in the planning process.

The differences in timing can be influenced directly by the needs of an individual and his or her family. For instance, a child or adult may already have a person-centered or wraparound plan in place when life circumstances lead to the occurrence of problem behavior. If an individual is experiencing challenges within his or her life that have resulted in the occurrence of problem behavior, we recommend that, when possible, PCP or wraparound occurs prior to the PBS plan.

PERSON-CENTERED ASSESSMENT AND INFORMATION GATHERING

The assessment and information gathering that occurs within PCP and wraparound can be improved when facilitators consider in advance: 1) the types of preparation and information that is needed prior to the first meeting, 2) details related to an individual's unique personal and cultural characteristics,

3) information about the focus person's QOL strengths and needs, and 4) the family context as well as the larger environmental and social contexts in the person's life.

Person-Centered Meeting Preparation

Early preparation by the individual facilitating the person-centered meetings can increase the effectiveness of the PCP or wraparound plan. In fact, the success of the facilitation process relies in large part on early preparation. Team meetings are more likely to be tense when problem behaviors are occurring in one or more settings. Emotional responses such as frustration, anger, and anxiety can impede progress when the facilitator is attempting to help the team focus on positive strengths. Separate meetings composed of the facilitator and individual participants before the PCP or wraparound process allows everyone to express his or her concerns or anxiety about certain topics. This, in turn, provides the facilitator with information that can be used for problem solving and early training opportunities that can be explored before or at the first meeting.

The most effective facilitators come to meetings prepared to share engaging stories that help individuals and their teams personally identify with key person-centered values and concepts (see Table 13.1). It can be challenging to assist team members in identifying meaningful and unified goals in situations where one or more team members may disagree. The cultural norms for individual team members may vary, and these cultural variations may result in differences of opinion about how to proceed with problem solving (Carr, 2007). Diffusing tension, encouraging people to "think outside of the box," and assisting individuals to creatively explore ideas while they suspend personal beliefs or judgments are a few examples of skills that an effective facilitator cultivates over time. The following story provides an example of one facilitator's assessment strategies that were implemented before the first

meeting and how the facilitator used the information to explore the underlying meanings related to the child's dream.

Andrew

Andrew, a young man with an intellectual and developmental disability living in the community, was about to experience his first integrated wraparound and PCP meeting. Andrew was beginning the planning process as a first step in PBS. Since Andrew moved to his new job, his problem behaviors had increased. At home, Andrew refused to get out of bed in the morning. He was in danger of losing his job because he was late to work almost every day. Andrew was responding to requests at work by mumbling how stupid work was while turning away from the person making the request. The team began the planning process by learning more about Andrew across each of the wraparound life domains.

Andrew's facilitator, Jackie, had spoken to Andrew and other team members before the first integrated PCP and wraparound meeting. In those preparatory meetings, Jackie learned that Andrew hated his current job and had already told a number of people that his real dream is to become an astronaut. Andrew's work coach and his mother are concerned about reinforcing this dream. They are worried about the possibility that Andrew will end up disappointed. Andrew's teacher and mother believe it is unlikely that Andrew will become an astronaut since he uses a wheelchair due to paralysis in his legs. Jackie came prepared for Andrew's meeting with a number of stories about other individuals who shared their dreams. She first explained how dreams that initially appear unattainable can be broken down into the key features or elements that are desirable to the focus person. Jackie asked Andrew a number of questions about his dream in order to explore what that dream meant to him: What do you like the most about being an astronaut? What do you think it would be like to be an astronaut? Andrew responded by saying that, to him, being an astronaut represents freedom and the excitement of the unknown. Andrew indicated that he loves airplanes and the idea of flying. However, he isn't necessarily interested in learning to fly a plane. Andrew wants to visit places that are really different from his home. By focusing on the meaning of the dream, the team was able to design a long-term plan addressing the core features of what being an astronaut represented to Andrew. Andrew and his team used the information to design an implementation plan that included looking for new jobs that would incorporate the key features that Andrew described. The team began investigating jobs that involved travel, tourism, and working at a nearby airport.

....

Assessing the Individual

The goal of assessment is to collect details about the focus person's social and communication strengths, history, experiences, living conditions, physical health, important routines, opportunities for self-determination, and future life aspirations. A person's strengths are emphasized while his or her special needs are considered from a positive point of view. Assessment at the individual level helps identify strategies for encouraging empowerment, providing more opportunities for choice and self-determination, expanding relationships, and designing informal and formal supports that meet the needs of the focus person and the family. Once individualized information is gathered, the next step is to assess how this information is related to the person's and family's QOL.

Understanding Quality of Life

To fully understand and ultimately measure each QOL domain, *indicator measures* are needed. Indicators in each of the eight domains described in Table 13.2 allow teams to address specific evaluation measures that operationally define QOL. The operationally defined QOL domains provide the foundation for a personalized measurement of an individual's QOL (Schalock, 2010). Schalock and Verdugo (2002) reviewed more than 20,900 published articles in order to identify the most commonly used indicators for each of the eight domains. Table 13.2 summarizes common QOL indicators.

Most researchers encourage those interested in QOL assessment to measure domains using multiple methods that include both qualitative and quantitative forms of data (Lyons, 2010). Interviews with the focus person, direct observation of social behaviors and communication, Likert-type rating scales that assess constructs such as well-being and empowerment, and team satisfaction surveys are all examples of measures that are used to evaluate QOL. There are hundreds of QOL evaluation instruments available (Schalock & Verdugo, 2002). Some tools assess an individual and/or team member's perceptions of well-being and satisfaction, while other assessments are tailored to address a particular QOL domain (Cummins, Lau, Davey, & McGillivray, 2010).

When individuals with more severe disabilities cannot communicate their opinions directly using interview or survey methods, it may be necessary for other people to share their observations of a focus person's QOL as a "proxy measure." Schalock and his colleagues (2007) recommend that in situations where a person cannot participate directly in the QOL assessment, two individuals are asked to respond on that person's behalf *as if they were the person.* The idea is to help the individuals participating in the assessment to think about the question not from their own viewpoints but through the eyes of the person they are representing. Including multiple viewpoints helps to increase the likelihood that an individual's QOL is assessed in a more accurate manner. The average of these two responses is used for the final summary score. Direct observation measures of individual behavior, simplification of the instructions and response formats, and using self-advocates trained to be surveyors are also ways in which we can evaluate QOL (Bonham et al., 2004).

THE ROLE OF CONTEXT: ASSESSMENT OF ORGANIZATIONAL AND SOCIAL SYSTEMS IN PERSON-CENTERED PLANNING AND WRAPAROUND

Although QOL assessment is applied at the individual level, to fully understand an individual's experience, one must gather information about what Bronfenbrenner (1986) called the *microsystem* (the immediate family, home, and workplace), the *mesosystem* (the neighborhood, organization, and greater community), and *macrosystem* (the overall cultural, sociopolitical, and economic context). This assessment is considered essential since a systems assessment of home, school, and community settings provides information that can be used to prevent or reduce the frequency of an individual's problem behavior (Freeman et al., 2002).

Bronfenbrenner (1986) described the family systems approach as a way in which to view dynamic family interactions. When an individual within a family is engaging in problem behaviors, knowing more about these dynamic interaction patterns can result in interventions for increasing or decreasing the likelihood that these problem behaviors will continue. Family members form a set of available systems and subsystems for serving the needs of each person. As the most proximal system for an individual, each family has interdependencies, special routines, and cultural patterns. This information is used to ensure that the interventions selected are a "good fit" for the individuals implementing the PBS plan.

Families are "nested" in their larger community subsystems. A number of varying smaller subsystems are "nested" within an entire community. Formal community subsystems include educational services, early childhood organizations, and governmental services. Informal community subsystems may include religious organizations, extended family units, neighbors, and recreational groups (Freeman et al., 2009). The information gathered about community systems assists teams in designing natural supports for individuals within home, school, work, and community settings. PCP or wraparound goals are set to allow an individual to make a meaningful contribution to his or her community.

Assessing the Microsystem

Assessing the microsystem includes interviews with the family to learn more about their strengths, needs, and unique cultural characteristics. A survey given to family members to evaluate overall family QOL is a helpful way to conduct an environmental assessment, especially prior to PBS planning (Smith-Bird & Turnbull, 2005). At school, reviewing a child's individualized education program (IEP) during the person-centered meeting assists team members in learning more about educational activities that could be generalized and practiced both at home and in the community.

Assessing the Mesosystem

Assessing the mesosystem level involves gathering information about the neighborhood in which an individual lives, the services available within the community, and the opportunities to participate in communal activities. Community mapping activities (Freeman, Hearst, & Anderson, 2008) can help team members assess the formal services that are available, the informal ways in which individuals in the community come together, and opportunities for spiritual connections and camaraderie. These details can be extremely helpful when the team is ready to start building natural supports around an individual person and address important goals implemented in the community. Interventions to increase community involvement and assist the individual in contributing to society in a meaningful way can only occur when an individual and his or her team knows the neighborhood and larger social network.

Assessing the Macrosystem

Teams facilitating PCP or wraparound need to assess state- and national-level resources and policies. At times, these national or statewide services are implemented in isolation with partner agencies that are unaware of resources that are available for individuals and their families. In some states, training opportunities or additional resources offered by one agency are not known by individuals from other agencies. Teams actively assessing the macrosystem level may discover resources that will assist an individual or his or her family.

Many states are now implementing three-tiered PBS models (Barrett, Bradshaw, & Lewis-Palmer, 2008; Muscott, Mann, Gately, Bell, & Muscott, 2004) that are based on a public health prevention model for disease control (Gordon, 1983). Three-tiered PBS strategies are currently implemented in schools, alternative settings for children and youth in early childhood, and juvenile justice settings, as well as in organizational settings that support adults with disabilities. Although there are variations in the application of this prevention model based on the unique person and systems variables that are present in each type of organization, most PBS efforts include the following: Tier 1 or universal interventions for teaching important social skills and behavioral expectations to all children or adults within a system, reinforcing individuals for appropriate behaviors, and increasing consistent responses to minor problem behaviors by individuals within the system; Tier 2, including both targeted and group interventions that are used to increase the intensity of social-skills teaching and reinforcement for individuals at risk for engaging in more serious problem behavior who do not respond to universal interventions; and Tier 3, or intensive, individualized systems and planning for individuals who engage in chronic or severe problem behavior that puts them at risk for exclusion from their home or community (Walker et al., 1996).

Many trainers encourage the use of PCP or wraparound planning, especially at the third, most intensive and individualized level of the PBS process (Freeman et al., 2006). Three-tiered implementation efforts within a given region should be investigated

as part of the broader contextual assessment during the PCP or wraparound and PBS plan for individuals who engage in problem behavior. The stage of implementation these organizations have reached provides information about how much training will be needed to support an individual's team effectively. Information about the level of implementation within a setting is used by the facilitator as part of a contextual fit assessment regarding the values, skills, and resources of team members. The next section of this chapter describes a tool and process that teams can use to assess family, school, work, and community systems and how an individual's QOL is addressed across these settings.

PROBLEM SOLVING USING PERSON-CENTERED PLANNING, WRAPAROUND, AND POSITIVE BEHAVIOR SUPPORT

Life Outcomes Through Integrated Systems

The life outcomes through integrated systems (LOTIS) wheel is a tool teams can use to integrate PCP or wraparound with PBS for a child or adult. The purpose of this informal assessment tool is to prompt the individual and his or her team during the planning process to engage in discussion related to 1) QOL outcomes across each domain, 2) the degree to which organizations supporting an individual are implementing three-tiered PBS, 3) interagency service coordination and collaboration related to an individual's plan, and 4) environmental settings important to the person and his or her family. The LOTIS wheel is an interactive tool that is constructed in a manner that allows for dynamic assessment and problem solving. The individual for whom person-centered and PBS approaches are being assessed can be seen in the middle of Figure 13.2, with an arrow pointing from the person toward the outside of the wheel. In Figure 13.2, when the circle is turned, the arrow points to *school/work, home,* or *community* settings. The outer circle moves as well, with the arrow in Figure 13.2 pointing to each of the QOL domains in turn. In Figure 13.2, the arrow is pointing from the person to the environmental setting *school/work* and the QOL domain of *personal development (PD)*. The next step is to move the LOTIS wheel in a clockwise fashion so that a new domain is introduced, in this case *social inclusion (SI)*, while the arrow still points to *school/work*. Once all domains are discussed in the *school/work* setting, the arrow is moved clockwise to the *home* setting, and the domains are moved again accordingly. Teams use the LOTIS wheel to prompt discussions related to QOL domains across each setting in an individual's life.

The extent to which systems-change efforts are implemented in schools, family support organizations and family environments, or in the community are addressed within the LOTIS model using colors associated with a tiered prevention process. The

red, yellow, and green areas within each setting in Figure 13.2 are meant to prompt a discussion by the individual and his or her team about the types of tiered prevention-based strategies that are implemented in each of the areas of an individual's life. Organizations implementing a three-tiered prevention model often use colors to represent the different tiers (e.g., green is associated with primary prevention, yellow with secondary prevention, and red with tertiary prevention). It is important for a team to know whether an organization supporting an individual is only just beginning to implement three-tiered PBS strategies. Many of the staff members may not be aware of the key features of PCP, wraparound, or PBS for individual students when organizations are new to PBS. During the early implementation stages, more training will be needed for the staff members within an organization, in order to support the interventions implemented within an individual PBS plan.

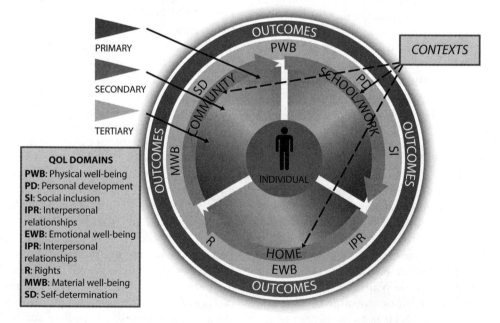

Figure 13.2.   Life outcomes through integrated systems (LOTIS) wheel. (From Enyart, M., & Freeman, R. [2011]. *Life outcomes through integrated systems [LOTIS©] WHEEL CONCEPTUAL FRAMEWORK.* Lawrence: University of Kansas Center on Developmental Disabilities; reprinted by permission. Copyright 2011 by the University of Kansas.)

For example, if a child in special education is participating in a PCP and PBS plan at a school implementing SWPBIS, it is important for the child and his or her team to discuss the schoolwide social expectations for all students and how the child's problem behavior is related to the school's expectations. The assessment includes the extent to which the child is participating in the social-skills instruction that occurs as part of primary prevention for all students. Teams should assess whether the child is receiving opportunities to practice the social expectations along with his or her peers and whether any additional instruction is needed. This additional training and support for the student while learning the school's expectations can be included in the child's IEP. Clear guidelines for implementing instruction within the IEP will help provide the structure needed to support both the child as well as his or her teachers. Writing social-skill goals linked to primary prevention also provides the SWPBIS team with another source of data for decision making and evaluation.

Teams implementing primary and secondary prevention often begin teaching school staff members how to facilitate simple FBA procedures. Each PBS plan implemented within a school provides an opportunity for expanding the experience and knowledge of PBS across more school personnel. If a child beginning the PBS process attends a school that is implementing all three prevention tiers, the school may have a larger number of staff who are familiar with PCP, wraparound, and PBS. In this scenario, school team members may volunteer to lead training and technical assistance efforts for key interventions within a student's PBS plan.

The LOTIS wheel stimulates discussion related to the broader assessment of an individual's life. The purpose of the LOTIS is to begin gathering lifestyle information that can be included in a person-centered or wraparound plan or as part of FBA. At the planning stage, the LOTIS may be used to evaluate the status of the planning processes with respect to the QOL domains.

We recommend that the team identify the most important QOL domains that need immediate attention using the LOTIS wheel to discuss each area of an individual's life. QOL assessment and evaluation measures should then be used to address these domains via indicators and outcomes to assess the success of each goal. A time line for addressing other QOL domains not yet measured can be recorded in the meeting minutes with the date of the follow-up meeting (e.g., within 6 months, 1 year) to review the remaining domains. Short- and long-term action plans for measuring all QOL domains will ensure that an individual's QOL is comprehensively evaluated.

As an individual grows older and develops more sophisticated social and communication skills, the importance of any one QOL domain may shift. Teams can use the LOTIS wheel to prompt a review of QOL domains and make corresponding adjustments to formal and informal support systems.

John

John was a 14-year-old boy in special education who engaged in inappropriate interactions with others and off-task behavior while in his classes. Anita, the school psychologist, met with John and his mother to gather information, create a list of who to invite to the first meeting, and better understand John's dreams for the future. John and Anita then had lunch together at school the next day to talk about the first meeting. Anita asked John where he wanted his meeting to occur, and they discussed how to ensure the meeting was fun and exciting. John chose the computer lab at school as the meeting location. With assistance from his art teacher, John made brightly colored postcard invitations with images of computers, and he distributed these invitations to his team. Anita met with John's English and math teachers and the school librarian, one of John's favorite people at school, who also assisted in the computer lab. Pam, the school counselor, met with two of John's peers.

Anita learned that John's mother was single and that John spent a great deal of time with his

Uncle George. George worked in the technology field and was instrumental in introducing John to computers. Uncle George offered to work with John to create a PowerPoint presentation for the meeting that highlighted John's preferences. Working with Uncle George on the presentation provided John with an opportunity to talk about his dreams with someone else before the first meeting.

On the day of the event, John and George operated the projector to display the presentation and record major messages. Anita used another computer to write down goals and actions. The team started the meeting by discussing John's strengths and needs using the wraparound life domains in Table 13.3. During the next part of the meeting, John chose *school* as the first setting and *personal development (PD)* using the LOTIS wheel (see Figure 13.2). The team reviewed the wraparound strengths and needs that had been documented earlier in the meeting and identified goals related to PD. Anita documented John's goal to explore the possibility of a career in software programming. Actions included visiting George's business and investigating whether any odd jobs might be available as a way to learn more about the organization. The math teacher shared how her class was related to John's future job interests and highlighted particular learning objectives that could be applied directly to software programming. The team moved on to each QOL domain on the LOTIS wheel as it applied to John's education before going to the next setting.

In addition to being the school counselor, Pam was also the SWPBIS coach. She shared information about SWPBIS efforts occurring at the school and described how the schoolwide social expectations were being taught to all students in the school. The team discovered that John did not have a chance to practice the expectations with his general education peers because he was attending a special education class when the instruction was presented to the students across the school. This led to a discussion about how to ensure all students have the same experiences learning the school's expectations. Pam volunteered to bring this issue to the SWPBIS team. When John moved the LOTIS wheel to the *home* setting, Pam shared how the same social expectations at school could be used within family settings and the community. John's mother and uncle suggested to John that, as a family, they work on social expectations at home. Pam offered to assist the family with this process.

Later, during a discussion about safety, John's mother expressed concern that John was unsupervised after school because she couldn't leave work until early in the evening. The team discussed the different after-school activities that were available throughout the week. John's friend mentioned some free computer classes at the public library and said that his parents were taking him to the library after school twice a week. Anita recorded in the meeting minutes that John's mother would check to see if her son could accompany his friend to the library. Since a number of students were signed up for the public library class, Pam offered to contact the library and discuss how the computer class might incorporate the school's expectations. George offered to pick John up after school 2 other days during the week. This left only 1 day during the week that John was unsupervised. The team wrote down that everyone would continue to look for possible supervised activities for that particular day.

Universal Interventions and Person-Centered and Individualized Planning Systems

Schools and other organizations supporting individuals with disabilities are now expected to provide services that expand personal outcomes (Schalock & Verdugo, 2012). The focus on creating effective person-centered environments for individuals with disabilities has led to an expansion of the use of strategies such as PCP and wraparound planning. These planning processes are no longer considered strategies at the fringes of service systems; they have become important, often publicly funded, processes (Smull & Lakin, 2002).

PCP in particular is a process that has been of benefit to a wide range of individuals—not just people who engage in problem behaviors. For adults with disabilities living in residential and community settings, person-centered strategies can help ensure that everyone has a chance to experience making meaningful choices, living independently, and contributing to society in ways that build respect within the community. Since the implementation of person-centered strategies may reduce the need for more intensive interventions (e.g., PBS plans), we recommend that PCP be considered as a way to support individuals with disabilities across schools and other organizations implementing PBS.

Unfortunately, in many cases, only one educator or service provider attends a person's PCP meeting on behalf of a school or organization. Therefore, only one person within a system may be aware of the goals and activities within a person's plan. If the staff member attending the PCP is not involved in his or her schoolwide or organization-wide team problem solving, the possibility for integrating universal PCP goals into a plan may be lost. Strategies for encouraging integrated planning across support systems for an individual with a disability require communication and service coordination.

Earlier we described how a team might integrate social expectations for all students within a school into a child's IEP. Children with disabilities often need additional opportunities to learn and practice new skills. The IEP provides a way in which primary prevention can be integrated into supports for children receiving special education services. The LOTIS wheel is a tool that can be used to address these communication issues by creating a structure for discussing broader microsystem-, mesosystem-, and macrosystem-level issues and by systematically addressing both QOL and environmental assessment within an interdisciplinary and interagency team context.

Ongoing Assessment and Problem Solving

Fidelity-of-implementation strategies allow professionals to document the important features of PCP, wraparound, and/or PBS interventions and evaluate the extent to which full implementation is occurring (Fixsen, Naoom, Blasé, Friedman, & Wallace, 2005). Fidelity of implementation for

each type of planning process (e.g., PCP, wraparound, PBS, or an integrated combination of these planning strategies) should be directly connected to the APBS standards of practice. QOL is a global construct that is influenced by a great many variables within an individual's life. Some QOL measures may be directly related to the person-centered process, while others may be linked to a student's IEP or PBS plan.

PBS plans contain both direct and indirect QOL measures, since interventions often involve 1) direct observation of social and communication behaviors, 2) documentation of physical health and wellness variables, and 3) environmental interventions related to decision making, self-determination, predictability, or other important QOL issues. The goal of the team is to make sure that the QOL domain indicators are discussed and relevant evaluation measures are established across the settings in an individual's life.

CONCLUSION

Education and human service professionals are constantly faced with the challenge of providing intensive and long-term person-centered supports with limited time and resources. As a result, the pressure to coordinate services across different educational and organizational settings while conducting in-depth QOL assessment can be challenging. New tools and strategies are needed that will allow team members to "work smarter, not harder" by integrating QOL assessment, action planning, and outcome measures across PCP, wraparound strategies, and PBS plan evaluation. State and regional systems that foster a common language across agencies may be able to provide more effective service coordination for children and adults with disabilities (Smull & Lakin, 2002). Data, systems, and practices are needed to encourage interagency dialogue; communication strategies that are braided across PCP, wraparound, and PBS; as well as other evidence-based interventions. Combining the strengths of each implementation effort will result in more effective services for individuals with and without disabilities.

REFERENCES

Bambara, L., Lohrmann, S., & Brown, F. (Eds.). (2002). *Research and Practice for Persons with Severe Disabilities, 27*(4), 250–275.

Bambara, L.M., & Knoster, T.P. (2009). *Designing positive behavior support plans* (2nd ed.). Washington, DC: American Association on Intellectual and Developmental Disabilities.

Barrett, S., Bradshaw, C.P., & Lewis-Palmer, T. (2008). Maryland statewide PBIS initiative: Systems, evaluation, and next steps. *Journal of Positive Behavior Interventions, 10*(2), 105–114.

Bonham, G.S., Basehart, S., Schalock, R.L., Marchand, C.B., Kirchner, N., & Rumenap, J.M. (2004). Consumer-based quality of life assessment: The Maryland Ask Me! Project. *Mental Retardation, 42*, 338–355.

Bronfenbrenner, U. (1986). Ecology of the family as a context for human development: Research perspectives. *Developmental Psychology, 22*, 723–742.

Bruns, E.J., Sather, A., Pullmann, M.D., & Stambaugh, L.F. (2011). National trends in implementing wraparound: Results from the state wraparound survey. *Journal of Child and Family Studies, 20*, 726–735. doi:10.1007s10826-011-9535-3

Bruns, E.J., Suter, J.C., & Leverentz-Brady, K.M. (2008). Is it wraparound yet? Setting quality standards for implementation of the wraparound process. *Journal of Behavioral Health Services & Research, 35*, 240–252.

Bruns, E.J., Walker, J.S., Zabel, M., Matarese, M., Estep, K., Harburger, D., . . . Pires, S.A. (2010). Intervening in the lives of youth with complex behavioral health challenges and their families: The role of the wraparound process. *American Journal of Community Psychology, 46*(3), 314–331.

Carr, E.G. (2007). The expanding vision of positive behavior support: Research perspectives on happiness, helpfulness, hopefulness. *Journal of Positive Behavior Interventions, 9*, 3–14.

Carr, E.G., Dunlap, G., Horner, R.H., Koegel, R.L., Turnbull, A., . . . Fox, L. (2002). Positive behavior support: Evolution of an applied science. *Journal of Positive Behavior Interventions, 4*(1), 4–16.

Claes, C., Van Hove, G., Vandevelde, S., Fan Loon, J., & Schalock, R.L. (2010). Person-centered: Analysis of research and effectiveness. *Intellectual and Developmental Disabilities, 48*(6), 432–453.

Clark, H.B., & Clark, R.T. (1996). Research on the wraparound process and individualized services for children with multi-system needs. *Journal of Child and Family Studies, 5*, 1–6.

Clark, H.B., & Hart, K. (2009). Navigating the obstacle course: An evidence-supported community transition system. In H.B. "Rusty" Clark & D.K. Unruh (Eds.), *Transition of youth and young adults with emotional or behavioral difficulties: An evidence-supported*

handbook (pp. 47–113). Baltimore, MD: Paul H. Brookes Publishing Co.

Cummins, R.A., Lau, A.L.D., Davey, G., & McGillivray, J. (2010). Measuring subjective well-being: The personal wellbeing index—intellectual disability. In R. Kober (Ed.), *Enhancing the quality of life of people with intellectual disabilities* (pp. 33–60). New York, NY: Springer.

Eber, L., Hyde, K., & Suter, J.C. (2011). Integrating wraparound into a schoolwide system of positive behavior supports. *Journal of Child and Family Studies, 20*, 782–790.

Eber, L., & Nelson, C.M. (1997). Integrating services for students with emotional and behavioral needs through school-based wraparound planning. *American Journal of Orthopsychiatry, 67*(3), 385–395.

Eber, L., Nelson, C.M., & Miles, P. (1997). School-based wraparound for students with emotional and behavioral challenges. *Exceptional Children, 63*, 539–555.

Evans, D.R. (1994). Enhancing quality of life in the population at large. *Social Indicators Research, 33*, 47–88.

Fixsen, D.L., Naoom, S.F., Blasé, K.A., Friedman, R.M., & Wallace, F. (2005). *Implementation research: A synthesis of the literature.* Tampa, FL: University of South Florida.

Freeman, R.L., Baker, D., Horner, R.H., Smith, C., Britten, J., & McCart, A. (2002). Using functional assessment and systems-level assessment to build effective behavioral support plans. In R.H. Hanson, N. Wieisler, & K.C. Lakin (Eds.), *Crisis: Prevention and response in the community* (pp. 199–224). Washington, DC: American Association on Mental Retardation.

Freeman, R., Eber, L., Anderson, C., Irvin, L., Bounds, M., Dunlap, G., & Horner, R.H. (2006). Building inclusive school cultures using school-wide PBS: Designing effective individual support systems for students with significant disabilities. *Research and Practice for Persons with Severe Disabilities, 31*(1), 4–17.

Freeman, R., Hearst, A., & Anderson, S. (2008). *Community self-assessment and action planning tool.* Lawrence, KS: University of Kansas.

Freeman, R., Perrin, N., Irvin, L., Vincent, C., Newcomer, L., Moore, M., . . . Farr Bond, K. (2009). *Positive behavior support across the lifespan: Expanding the concept of statewide planning for large-scale organizational cultural change* (PBS-Kansas Monograph No. 1). Lawrence, KS: University of Kansas, Schiefelbusch Institute for Lifespan Studies.

Gordon, R.S. (1983). An operational classification of disease prevention. *Public Health Reports, 98*, 107–109.

Holburn, S., Gordon, A., & Vietze, P.M. (2007). *Person-centered planning made easy: The PICTURE method.* Baltimore, MD: Paul H. Brookes Publishing Co.

Holburn, S., & Vietze, P.M. (Eds.). (2002). *Person-centered planning: Research, practice, and future directions.* Baltimore, MD: Paul H. Brookes Publishing Co.

Kincaid, D. (1996). Person-centered planning. In L.K. Koegel, R.L. Koegel, & G. Dunlap (Eds.), *Positive behavioral support: Including people with difficult behavior in the community* (pp. 439–465). Baltimore, MD: Paul H. Brookes Publishing Co.

Kincaid, D., & Fox, L. (2002). Person-centered planning and positive behavior support. In S. Holburn, & P.M. Vietze (Eds.), *Person-centered planning: Research, practice, and future directions* (pp. 29–49). Baltimore, MD: Paul H. Brookes Publishing Co.

Knitzer, J. (1982). *Unclaimed children: The failure of public responsibility to children and adolescents in need of mental health services.* Washington, DC: The Children's Defense Fund.

Kutash, K., Duchnowski, A., & Lynn, N. (2006). *School-based mental health: An empirical guide for decision-makers.* Tampa, FL: University of South Florida, The Louis de la Parte Florida Mental Health Institute, Department of Child & Family Studies, Research and Training Center for Children's Mental Health.

Lyons, G. (2010). Enhancing the quality of life of people with intellectual disabilities: From theory to practice. In R. Kober (Ed.), *Social indicators research series* (Vol. 41). New York, NY: Springer.

Moore, M., Freeman, R., Kimbrough, P., Tieghi, M., Rosdahl, D., Smith, C., . . . Zarcone, J. (2007). *Person-centered and wraparound planning* (v. 5.0). Lawrence, KS: University of Kansas Center on Developmental Disabilities. Retrieved from http://www.kipbs.org/

Muscott, H.S., Mann, T.B., Gately, S., Bell, K.E., & Muscott, A.J. (2004). Positive behavioral interventions and supports in New Hampshire: Preliminary results of a statewide system for implementing schoolwide discipline practices. *Education and Treatment of Children, 27,* 453–475.

O'Brien, J. (2002). The ethics of person-centered planning. In S. Holburn & P.M. Vietze (Eds.), *Person-centered planning: Research, practice, and future directions* (pp. 399–414). Baltimore, MD: Paul H. Brookes Publishing Co.

O'Neill, R.E., Horner, R.H., Albin, R.W., Sprague, J.R., Storey, K., & Newton, J.S. (1997). *Functional assessment and program development for problem behavior: A practical handbook* (2nd ed.). Pacific Grove, CA: Brooks.

Schalock, R.L. (1996). Reconsidering the conceptualization and measurement of quality of life. In Schalock (Ed.), *Quality of life:. Vol. 1. Conceptualization and measurement* (pp. 123–139). Washington, DC: American Association on Mental Retardation.

Schalock, R.L. (2010). The measurement and use of quality of life-related personal outcomes. In R. Kober (Ed.), *Enhancing the quality of life of people with intellectual disabilities* (pp. 3–16). New York, NY: Springer.

Schalock, R.L., Brown, I., Brown, I., Cummins, R.A., Felce, D., Matikka, L., . . . Parmenter, T. (2002). Conceptualization, measurement, and application of quality of life for persons with intellectual disabilities: Results of an international panel of experts. *Mental Retardation, 40*(6), 457–470.

Schalock, R.L., Gardner, J.F., & Bradley, V.J. (2007). *Quality of life for people with intellectual and other developmental disabilities: Applications across individuals, organizations, communities, and systems.* Washington

DC: American Association on Intellectual and Developmental Disabilities.

Schalock, R., & Verdugo, M.A. (2002). *Handbook on quality of life for human service practitioners.* Washington, DC: American Association on Mental Retardation.

Schalock, R., & Verdugo, M.A. (2012). *A leadership guide for today's disabilities organizations: Overcoming challenges and making them happen.* Baltimore, MD: Paul H. Brookes Publishing Co.

Smith-Bird, E., & Turnbull, A.P. (2005). Linking positive behavior support to family quality of life outcomes. *Journal of Positive Behavior Interventions, 7,* 174–180.

Smull, M., & Burke Harrison, S. (1992). *Supporting people with severe reputations in the community.* Alexandria, VA: National Association of State Mental Retardation Program Directors.

Smull, M., & Lakin, K.C. (2002). Public policy and person-centered planning. In S. Holburn & P.M. Vietze (Eds.), *Person-centered planning: Research, practice, and future directions* (pp. 379–397). Baltimore, MD: Paul H. Brookes Publishing Co.

Smull, M.W. (2002). Responding to behavioral crises by supporting people in the lives that they want. In R.H. Hanson, N.A. Wiesler, & K.C. Lakin (Eds.), *Crisis: Prevention and response in the community* (pp. 225–241). Washington DC: American Association on Mental Retardation.

Stroul, B., & Friedman, R.M. (1986). *A system of care for children and youth with severe emotional disturbances* (Rev. ed.). Washington, DC: Georgetown University, Child Development Center.

Suter, J.C., & Bruns, E.J. (2009). Effectiveness of the wraparound process for children with emotional and behavioral disorders: A meta-analysis. *Clinical Child and Family Psychology Review, 12,* 336–351. doi:10.1007/s10567-009-0059-y

Turnbull, H.R., & Brunk, G. (1990). Quality of life and public policy. In R.I. Schalock (Ed.), *Quality of life: Application to persons with disabilities.* Washington, DC: American Association on Mental Retardation.

Vandenberg, J.E., & Grealish, E.M. (1996). Individualized services and supports through the wraparound process. *Journal of Child and Family Studies, 5*(1), 7–21.

Vandercook, T., York, J., & Forest, M. (1989). The McGill Action Planning System (MAPS): A strategy for building the vision. *Journal of The Association for Persons with Severe Handicaps, 14,* 205–214.

Walker, H.M., Horner, R.H., Sugai, G., Bullis, M., Sprague, J., . . . Kaufmann, M. (1996). Integrated approaches to preventing antisocial behavior patterns among school-age children and youth. *Journal of Emotional and Behavioral Disorders, 4,* 193–256.

Walker, U.M., & Petr, C.G. (2011). Best practices in wraparound: A multidimensional view of the evidence. *Social Work, 56*(1), 73–80.

Winters, N.C., & Metz, W.P. (2009). The wraparound approach in systems of care. *Psychiatric Clinics of North America, 32,* 135–151. doi:10.1016/j.psc.2008.11.007

Conducting Functional Behavioral Assessments

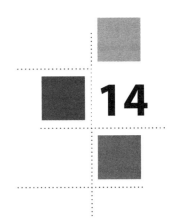

14

Robert E. O'Neill, Leanne S. Hawken, and Kaitlin Bundock

Conducting functional behavioral assessments (FBAs) in situations involving challenging behavior has become an expected professional standard (Sailor, Dunlap, Sugai, & Horner, 2009). This chapter provides the reader with a basic background in this area and describes some of the methods for conducting such assessments and their use in planning intervention and support strategies. First, however, we will consider some examples of situations involving challenging behavior.

Natalia

Ms. Sandoval prides herself on her excellent behavior management skills in her mathematics classes. Natalia is a 12-year-old student in one of her sixth-grade classes who is classified to receive special education services under the disability category of emotional disturbance (ED). Natalia is functioning academically at a third-grade level in both reading and mathematics. She is able to follow the majority of behavior expectations in a classroom and usually interacts well

with peers by engaging in conversations, working cooperatively, and complimenting other students, although she does not have any close friends. Natalia interacts respectfully with adults most of the time, as evidenced by her following directions, raising her hand to provide comments during class, and using language such as "excuse me," "please," and "thank you." However, when adults attempt to redirect Natalia when she is off task or not completing her work, Natalia often refuses to follow their directions, says verbal insults, and swears.

Natalia is able to express her feelings and emotions but usually has to be coaxed to discuss personal things, such as her feelings toward her academic strengths and weaknesses, family life, and social experiences at school with peers. She is able to follow verbal directions given by her teacher approximately 80% of the time, when restated in simple terms and with the addition of prompts. Natalia can perform three-step functional tasks with minimal prompting but struggles with multistep tasks involving four or more steps.

Natalia has been engaging in chronic misbehavior in class, such as leaving class without permission for up to 15–20 minutes, refusing to begin quizzes or exams, and arguing and swearing. Ms.

Sandoval usually responds by sending Natalia to the office. Natalia refuses to make up the quizzes and tests she misses and is failing the class as a result. Ms. Sandoval has requested assistance in addressing Natalia's behavior.

....

Trevor

Abigail works at a residential group home for adults with developmental delays. Included in her responsibilities is supervision of the residents at their worksites during 3-hour shifts twice a week. Abigail supervises three residents, Trevor, Cassie, and Michael, while they landscape different residential and commercial areas. Abigail enjoys her job most of the time but has been unsure about how to handle Trevor's intermittent but dangerous behavior of throwing objects at the worksites. Trevor is a 30-year-old adult male who is identified as having a severe intellectual disability. Trevor is usually well behaved, as long as he is given a variety of activities and a lot of choices.

Trevor is able to express his immediate physical wants, needs, and feelings using short phrases and sentences. He is able to follow short verbal directions and can follow multistep verbal directions with prompts and redirects. Trevor uses a picture communication board to support his communication ability. Trevor is able to complete multistep tasks at work that he is familiar with and for which he has pictorial reminders. At his worksite, Trevor is responsible for picking up trash and leaves off lawns. Trevor typically requires prompts to facilitate his work completion.

Abigail has requested assistance in approaching Trevor's behavior of throwing objects such as leaves, gloves, rakes, and other work items. Trevor throws objects a few times per week, typically when he is working by himself and not with a supervisor. Abigail has tried reprimanding Trevor as well as ignoring his throwing behavior. Trevor's behavior of throwing things at work has increased in response to Abigail's attempts to make him stop.

....

THE HISTORICAL CONTEXT OF FUNCTIONAL BEHAVIORAL ASSESSMENT

In many respects, the emphasis on and adoption of FBA strategies comes from the early roots of the field of applied behavior analysis. Initial examples of the implementation and evaluation of behavioral strategies to manage challenging behaviors, especially with people with disabilities, began to appear in the 1960s (e.g., Lovaas, Freitag, Gold, & Kassorla, 1965; Risley, 1968; Wolf, Risley, & Mees, 1964). These early efforts typically involved a conceptualization of the contingencies maintaining the challenging behavior as a basis for developing and implementing intervention strategies. For example, a child who repeatedly engaged in tantrums might have been assumed to be doing so to gain social attention from peers or adults. These conceptualizations were sometimes based on data and sometimes on more anecdotal observations. This so-called functional perspective was considered by some to be receiving less attention by the field in the late 1970s and early 1980s (e.g., Pierce & Epling, 1980). However, in 1977, Ted Carr published an influential paper in which he presented some theories about possible social and other functions of self-injurious behavior (Carr, 1977). This conceptual framework set the stage for the influential work of Brian Iwata and his colleagues (Iwata, et al., 1982/1994). In this initial seminal article (and in many since), they described a methodology for conducting rigorous experimental analyses of challenging behavior. Such analyses provided guidance for identifying and implementing relevant intervention strategies.

Since then, there has been a virtual explosion of research and procedural books and manuals providing guidance on conducting FBAs (e.g., Dunlap & Kincaid, 2001). (Note that we consider *FBA* an umbrella term for many different types of assessment strategies. *Functional analysis* refers to specific procedures in which environmental and contingency manipulations are conducted to empirically determine their influence on a person's behavior, as described in Chapter 16.) As mentioned previously, conducting FBAs has become integral to a variety of educational and human service fields. Language referring specifically to FBAs was included in the 2004 reauthorization of the Individuals with Disabilities Education Act (IDEA; PL 108-446). Standards requiring the competent use of a range of FBA procedures have been put forth by a variety of professional organizations, including the Council for Exceptional Children (CEC), Association for Positive Behavior Support (APBS), and the Behavior Analyst Certification Board (BACB).

Research Bases for Functional Behavioral Assessment

Since the early 1980s, a large number of research publications have documented the reliability and treatment validity of a broad range of FBA procedures and tools. (See Hanley, Iwata, & McCord [2003] and Matson [2012] for examples of periodic reviews of this voluminous research.) Some issues that have remained relatively constant topics of research include 1) the reliability and validity of indirect and direct FBA measures (e.g., interviews, rating scales, antecedent-behavior-consequence [ABC] observations), 2) the most efficient and effective combinations of procedures that produce desired outcomes, and 3) the implementation of experimental functional analysis procedures in more applied settings (e.g., classrooms). These issues are addressed in the sections that follow with regard to particular procedures.

EXPECTED OUTCOMES OF FUNCTIONAL BEHAVIORAL ASSESSMENT

The basic goal of an FBA process is to identify 1) the full range of behaviors that are of concern for an individual and how those behaviors may co-occur or be related as response classes or escalating sequences, 2) the broader setting events and more immediate antecedents that appear to increase the likelihood of their occurrence, 3) the consequences that appear to maintain the behavior(s) (i.e., their functions), and 4) hypotheses that pull all this information together into succinct statements that can be used as a basis for developing behavior

support plans (BSPs; O'Neill et al., 1997). An example of such a summary statement (hypothesis) would be, "When Maria hasn't had much sleep and is asked to do difficult academic tasks, she will curse, destroy materials, and attempt to hit the instructor in order to avoid those task demands." Such statements/hypotheses include information about setting events (lack of sleep), immediate antecedents (difficult task demands), challenging behaviors (curse, destroy, aggression), and maintaining reinforcers (avoidance of task demands/negative reinforcement).

Some Additional Critical Issues with Regard to Functional Behavioral Assessment

One major issue with regard to FBA is that practitioners need to be prepared to *think functionally* on an ongoing basis and be able to consider the necessary assessment procedures appropriate for a particular situation. When considering a challenging behavior situation, a teacher, consultant, or other practitioner who is familiar with that situation should be able to 1) generate a summary statement, such as the previous statement regarding Maria, off "the top of his or her head" (the very brief approach) and 2) employ a variety of functional assessment and analysis procedures during a more extended period to clearly identify the factors operating in a challenging behavior situation, which may take several days or multiple weeks (Borgmeier & Horner, 2006).

Another critical issue that practitioners must keep in mind is that FBA is a potentially ongoing and repetitive process (O'Neill et al., 1997). Just like any individual, children and adults with lengthy and complex histories of challenging behavior often may display changing patterns and functions of behavior over time. Therefore the FBA process may need to be periodically revisited to make sure that the analysis/understanding of situations is up-to-date and accurate, especially if the challenging behavior appears to be increasing or getting worse.

FUNCTIONAL BEHAVIOR ASSESSMENT METHODS

There are a variety of methods for gathering FBA data, and the extent to which teachers or care providers implement one, two, or a combination of the methods typically depends on the severity of the challenging behavior as well as the training/expertise of the person conducting the FBA. These different FBA methods are typically classified as 1) indirect methods (e.g., interviews, questionnaires), 2) systematic direct observations, and 3) experimental functional analysis.

Indirect Methods

Indirect methods are procedures that allow practitioners to gather function-based information from teachers, caregivers, and others without necessarily directly observing the individual in a given setting. Indirect methods are often used as a starting point for developing hypotheses about challenging behavior (O'Neill et al., 1997). While gathering information via indirect methods, it is important to work with the teachers, parents, and/or staff who are most familiar with the individual and can comment on when and where problem behavior is occurring.

Functional Behavioral Assessment Interviews FBA interviews are a widely used method (Herzinger & Campbell, 2007). Either alone or in conjunction with other FBA methods (e.g., direct observation, experimental functional analysis), the outcomes of FBA interviews should include 1) an operational definition of the challenging behaviors; 2) identification of setting events, antecedents, and consequence events, as well as problematic routines throughout the day; and 3) hypotheses about why the challenging behaviors are occurring. A variety of different FBA interviews has been published, and several of these are described in the sections that follow.

Functional Assessment Checklist for Teachers and Staff Functional Assessment Checklist for Teachers and Staff FACTS

(March et al., 2000) is a semistructured interview that was developed to help identify problematic routines throughout a day. (See Figures 14.1 and 14.2 for examples of completed FACTS forms for the case studies described at the beginning of the chapter.)

Setting events (if known), antecedents, behaviors, and consequences are identified during the interview process, which aids in the development of a behavior intervention plan or can be used as a part of a more comprehensive FBA process. FACTS is composed of two sections, Part A and Part B. Part A involves gathering background information on the individual, identification of problem behavior as well as a list of the daily activities/routines that either increase or decrease the likelihood of problem behavior. Part B involves gathering specific information about antecedents and consequences, and the final section involves developing a summary statement (hypothesis) as to why the problem behavior is occurring. A behavior specialist or coach interviews teachers or caregivers who interact frequently with the individual; this interview typically takes between 10 and 15 minutes.

Functional Assessment Interview The FAI form (O'Neill et al., 1997) is a more in-depth interview form than the FACTS and typically takes 45 to 90 minutes to complete. For efficiency's sake, it is recommended that the interview be completed with two or more people who know and interact regularly with the individual. The FAI 1) describes the challenging behaviors, 2) identifies setting events and antecedents that predict the challenging behaviors, 3) identifies the potential function(s) of the behaviors, and 4) lists a summary statement that includes the setting events, antecedents, behaviors, and consequences of the challenging behaviors. The summary statements are used in the process of developing a BSP.

Additional Interview Forms There are many other types of interview forms that can be used, including a brief FBA (Crone

Efficient functional behavioral assessment: The Functional Assessment Checklist for Teachers and Staff: Part A

Step 1:

Student/grade: _Natalia/Grade 6_   Date: _3/12/12_

Interviewer: _Curtis Henderson_   Responder(s): _Ms. Sandoval_

Step 2:

Student profile: Please identify at least three strengths or contributions the student brings to school:

Natalia is usually a pleasant student who is a very talented artist. Natalia's peers often admire her drawings.

Natalia's strong graphic and visual skills allow her to make sense of more abstract concepts

Step 3:

Problem behaviors: Identify problem behaviors

____Tardy	____Fight/physical aggression	____Disruptive	____Theft
____Unresponsive	_X_ Inappropriate language	_X_ Insubordination	____Vandalism
_X_Withdrawn	____Verbal harassment	_X_ Work not done	_X_ Other
____Verbally inappropriate	____Self-injury		

Describe problem behavior: Natalia leaves the classroom without permission for 15-25 minute periods when instructed to take assessments. When she returns, Natalia refuses to complete the assessments, argues with the teacher, and uses a lot of swear words.

Step 4:

Identifying routines: Where, when, and with whom problem behaviors are most likely.

Schedule (times)	Activity	Likelihood of problem behavior		Specific behavior
		Low	High	
11:00	Mathematics assessments	1 2 3	4 5 6	Leaves w/out permission
11:25	Mathematics assessments	1 2 3	4 5 6	Refuses to do work
11 30	Redirect to math assessments	1 2 3	4 5 6	Argues with teacher
11:35	Redirect to math assessments	1 2 3	4 5 6	Swears
11:35	Referred to office	1 2 3	4 5 6	Leaves the room

Step 5

List the routines in order of priority for behavior support: Select routines with ratings of 5 or 6. Only combine routines when there is significant (a) similarity of activities (conditions) and (b) similarity of problem behavior(s). Complete the FACTS-Part B for each of the prioritized routine(s) identified.

	Routines/activities/context	Problem behavior(s)
Routine # 1	Mathematics assessment	Leaves room, work refusal
Routine# 2		
Routine # 3		

Efficient functional behavioral assessment: The Functional Assessment Checklist for Teachers and Staff: Part B

Step 6: Routine/activities/context: Which routine (only one) from the FACTS-Part A is assessed?

Routine/activity/context	Problem behavior(s)
Mathematics assessments	Leaves room, work refusal, outbursts

Figure 14.1.   Information from the Functional Assessment Checklist for Staff and Teachers (FACTS) for Natalia. (*Source:* March et al., 2000.)

(continued)

Figure 14.1. *(continued)*

Step 7: Provide more detail about the problem behavior(s):

What does the problem behavior(s) look like? Natalia leaves the room without permission whenever there is a mathematics assessment. When she returns and is redirected to complete her work, she refuses to do so, argues with the teacher, and uses a lot of swear words directed at the assessments and the teacher.

How often does the problem behavior(s) occur? Every time a mathematics assessment is given, which is usually once every two weeks.

How long does the problem behavior(s) last when it does occur? Approximately 35 minutes. After that amount of time, Natalia is usually sent to the office.

What is the intensity/level of danger of the problem behavior(s)? Natalia's behavior is not dangerous to peers or adults, but it is incredibly distracting. The intensity of Natalia's work refusal, arguing, and swearing is severe compared with Natalia's typical behavior. The arguments and swearing usually involve Natalia yelling, waving arms, and stomping feet.

Antecedents: Triggers and setting events

What are the events that predict when the problem behavior(s) will occur? (Predictors).

Identify the trigger generally

1. In this routine, what happens most often just before problem behavior? <u>Natalia and the rest of her classmates are told to complete a mathematics assessment.</u>
2. If you put this trigger in place 10 times, how often would it result in problem behavior? <u>10 times</u>
3. Does problem behavior ever happen when (opposite of trigger or trigger absent)? <u>No</u>

Triggers		
_X_ Tasks	____ Unstructured time	_X_ Reprimands
____ Structured/nonacademic activities	____ Transitions	____ Isolated, no one around

Identify specific features of the trigger:

If task (e.g., group work, independent work, small-group instruction, lecture)	Describe the task in detail (e.g., duration, ease of task for student). What features of it likely are aversive to the student and why is this hypothesized?	Mathematics assessments usually involve 15-50 problems that are based on the material learned in class. The student is expected to sit quietly and complete the assessment individually. The assessments typically involve more difficult problems than those provided in class or for homework. It is hypothesized that the individual work expectation, in addition to the more difficult math problems, may be aversive to Natalia because she tends to work with a peer during class, has low confidence in her mathematical ability, and has expressed hating tests.
If unstructured time . . .	Describe the setting, activities, and who is around.	
If reprimanded . . .	Describe who delivers the reprimand, what is said, and what the purpose of the correction is.	
If structures, nonacademic activities . . .	Describe the context, who is around, what activities are going on, and what behaviors are expected.	
If transitions . . .	Describe the activity that is being terminated and the one that is being transitioned to. Identify whether any of the activities are highly preferred or nonpreferred and which are structured versus nonstructured.	
If isolated . . .	Where did the behavior occur? What features of the environment might be relevant.	

Step 9: Are setting events relevant?

1. Is there something that, when present makes it more likely that the trigger identified above sets off the behavior? _No_

2. If yes, is this event present sometimes and absent others? Does the behavior occur only when the event is present? _____

Setting events

____Correction/failure in previous class	____Peer conflict	____Change in routine
____Conflict at home	____Correction from adult earlier in day	
____ Homework/assignment not completed	____Hunger	____Lack of sleep
____ Medication (missed or taken)		

Step 10: Consequences

What consequences appear most likely to maintain the problem behavior(s)?

Identify the consequence generally

In the routine identified, when the trigger occurs and problem behavior happens, what occurs next?

1. What do you do? What do other students do? What activities happen or stop happening? I (the teacher) scold Natalia for leaving the room without permission, and tell her that she has to complete the assessment before she can leave for the day. The other students sit quietly and watch. Natalia starts arguing with me, swearing, and stomping her feet. Sometimes the students stare. I send her to the office so she will stop distracting the students who are trying to focus on their assessments.

2. Narrow it down: Take each consequence identified above:

a. Would the behavior still happen if that consequence couldn't occur (e.g., if peer attention, no other students were around? If your attention, would the behavior still occur if you were not around? If escape, would the behavior still occur if the task was easier?) I think it is likely that if the assessment was easier, Natalia might not leave the room without permission. I think that if I did not scold her, and let her not complete the assessment, she would not argue, swear, or stomp her feet.

b. Of the last 10 times you saw the behavior, how often did this consequence occur? The consequence occurred 9 times out of 10.

Things that are obtained	Things avoided or escaped from
____Adult attention; other: _____	_X_ Hard tasks; other: _____
____Peer attention	_X_ Reprimands
____Activity	____ Peer negatives
____Money/things	____ Physical effort
	____ Adult attention

Identify specific features of the consequence

| If adult or peer attention is obtained or avoided. | Define who delivers attention, what they say, and how long the attention typically lasts. What does the student do following this attention? Is there a back-and-forth that occurs? Does behavioral escalation occur? | I (Ms. Sandoval) provide negative attention for approximately 10 minutes while I tell Natalia she shouldn't have left the room without permission and tell her she needs to take the assessment. Natalia engages in a back and forth with me, arguing, swearing, and stomping. Behavioral escalation occurs, as Natalia usually gets louder and uses more swear words until I finally send her to the office. |

(continued)

Figure 14.1.   (*continued*)

If an activity or request follows or is removed	Describe the specific activity including who else is present, what the activity consists of, and how long it lasts.	The activities Natalia tries to escape from are mathematics assessments. The mathematics assessments usually last about 30–40 minutes. The other students are present during this activity.
If tangible items are obtained or removed	Describe the specific item(s) obtained including who else is present and how long the student has access to the item	
If sensory stimulation possibly occurs or is removed	Describe the context, who is around, what activities are going on and what behaviors are expected.	

Summary of behavior

Identify the summary that will be used to build a plan of behavior support

Setting events	→	Trigger	→	Behavior	→	Consequence
Mathematics class	→	Mathematics assessment	→	Leaves room/outbursts	→	Avoids mathematics assessment (sent to office/not in room)

How confident are you that the Summary of behavior is accurate?

Not very confident			Very confident		
1	2	3	4	5	6

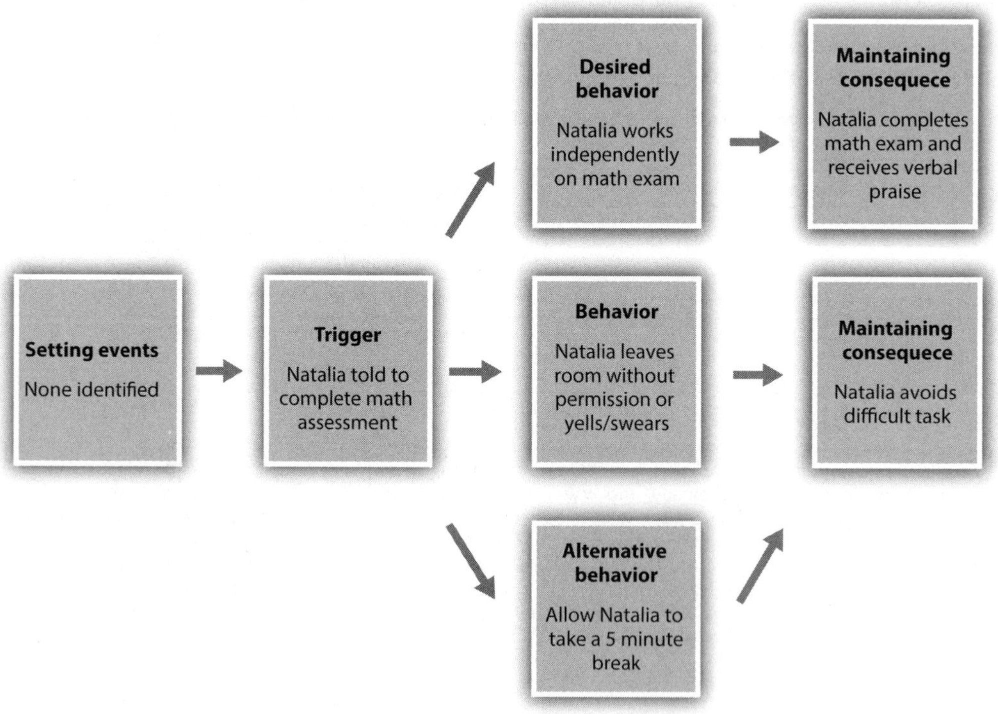

Efficient functional behavioral assessment: The Functional Assessment Checklist for Teachers and Staff: Part A

Step 1:

Student/grade: _Trevor_   Date: _10/17/12_

Interviewer: _Devin Smith_   Responder(s): _Abigail_

Step 2:

Student profile: Please identify at least three strengths or contributions the student brings to school:
Trevor is usually a very cheerful individual who often helps his peers and workers at his work site and group
home. Trevor shows a lot of compassion for animals and people.

Step 3:

Problem behaviors: Identify problem behaviors

____Tardy	____Fight/physical aggression	____ Disruptive	____Theft
____Unresponsive	____Inappropriate language	_X_ Insubordination	_X_ Vandalism
____Withdrawn	____Verbal harassment	_X_ Work not done	____Other
____Verbally inappropriate	____Self-injury		_____

Describe problem behavior: _Trevor throws objects at his work site. The objects Trevor usually throws include trash,_
leaves, gloves, and rakes.

Step 4:

Identifying routines: Where, when, and with whom problem behaviors are most likely.

Schedule (times)	Activity	Likelihood of problem behavior						Specific behavior
		Low			High			
2:00 (midway through 2 hour shift that occurs twice a week)	Raking leaves & trash while supervised by Abigail	1	2	3	4	5	6	Throws objects
		1	2	3	4	5	6	
		1	2	3	4	5	6	

Step 5

List the routines in order of priority for behavior support: Select routines with ratings of 5 or 6. Only combine routines when there is significant (a) similarity of activities (conditions) and (b) similarity of problem behavior(s). Complete the FACTS-Part B for each of the prioritized routine(s) identified.

	Routines/activities/context	Problem behavior(s)
Routine # 1	2 hour yard work shift	Throws objects
Routine# 2		
Routine # 3		

Efficient functional behavioral assessment: The Functional Assessment Checklist for Teachers and Staff: Part B

Step 6: Routine/activities/context: Which routine (only one) from the FACTS-Part A is assessed?

Routine/activity/context	Problem behavior(s)
Yard work (raking leaves and trash)	Throwing objects

Figure 14.2.   Information from the Functional Assessment Checklist for Staff and Teachers (FACTS) for Trevor. (*Source:* March et al., 2000.)

(continued)

Figure 14.2. *(continued)*

Step 7: Provide more detail about the problem behavior(s):

What does the problem behavior(s) look like? Trevor throws the objects that are near him at the work site, which include rakes, leaves, trash, gloves, and other gardening tools.

How often does the problem behavior(s) occur? Twice per week, which is every yard work shift. The previous supervisor never reported any similar behavior.

How long does the problem behavior(s) last when it does occur? For approximately 15-30 minutes

What is the intensity/level of danger of the problem behavior(s)? There is a high level of danger of the problem behaviors because gardening tools, such as rakes, are very dangerous when thrown for both Trevor and people in the surrounding area. The level of intensity is high because Trevor is throwing objects away from himself, rather than just on the ground. He does not seem to take into consideration whether he is throwing objects towards people, buildings, or other objects.

Antecedents: Triggers and setting events

What are the events that predict when the problem behavior(s) will occur? (Predictors).

Identify the trigger generally

1. In this routine, what happens most often just before problem behavior? _Abigail is helping other residents_

2. If you put this trigger in place 10 times, how often would it result in problem behavior? _9_

3. Does problem behavior ever happen when (opposite of trigger or trigger absent)? _Trevor does not throw objects when Abigail is helping him or communicating with him._

Triggers		
____ Tasks	____Unstructured time	_X_ Reprimands
_X_ Structured/nonacademic activities	____Transitions	____ Isolated, no one around

Identify specific features of the trigger:

If task (e.g., group work, independent work, small-group instruction, lecture)	Describe the task in detail (e.g., duration, ease of task for student). What features of it likely are aversive to the student and why is this hypothesized?	
If unstructured time . . .	Describe the setting, activities, and who is around.	
If reprimanded . . .	Describe who delivers the reprimand, what is said, and what the purpose of the correction is.	
If structures, nonacademic activities . . .	Describe the context, who is around, what activities are going on, and what behaviors are expected.	
If transitions . . .	Describe the activity that is being terminated and the one that is being transitioned to. Identify whether any of the activities are highly preferred or nonpreferred and which are structured versus nonstructured.	
If isolated . . .	Where did the behavior occur? What features of the environment might be relevant.	

Step 9: Are setting events relevant?

1. Is there something that, when present makes it more likely that the trigger identified above sets off the behavior? <u>No</u>

2. If yes, is this event present sometimes and absent others? Does the behavior occur only when the event is present? ____

Setting events

____ Correction/failure in previous class	____ Peer conflict	____ Change in routine
____ Conflict at home	____ Correction from adult earlier in day	
____ Homework/assignment not completed	____ Hunger	____ Lack of sleep
____ Medication (missed or taken)		

Step 10: Consequences

What consequences appear most likely to maintain the problem behavior(s)?

Identify the consequence generally

In the routine identified, when the trigger occurs and problem behavior happens, what occurs next?

1. What do you do? What do other students do? What activities happen or stop happening? I (Abigail) yell at Trevor to stop throwing things. The other residents try to get out of Trevor's way and also yell at him to stop. To make sure he doesn't start throwing things again, I work with Trevor for the rest of the shift.

2. Narrow it down: Take each consequence identified above:

a. Would the behavior still happen if that consequence couldn't occur (e.g., if peer attention, no other students were around? If your attention, would the behavior still occur if you were not around? If escape, would the behavior still occur if the task was easier?) I (Abigail) tried to ignore Trevor twice when he started throwing things, but he started throwing bigger objects and continued for 20 minutes. I yelled at him and worked with him for the rest of the shift after 20 minutes because it didn't seem like he was going to stop.

b. Of the last 10 times you saw the behavior, how often did this consequence occur? The consequence occurred 9 times out of 10.

Things that are obtained	Things avoided or escaped from
_X_ Adult attention; other: _____	____ Hard tasks; other: _____
____ Peer attention	____ Reprimands
____ Activity	____ Peer negatives
____ Money/things	____ Physical effort
	____ Adult attention

Identify specific features of the consequence

If adult or peer attention is obtained or avoided.	Define who delivers attention, what they say, and how long the attention typically lasts. What does the student do following this attention. Is there a back-and-forth that occurs? Does behavioral escalation occur?	Abigail delivers the attention by yelling at Trevor, "Stop throwing things, you are going to get hurt or hurt someone!" The yelling usually lasts 2-5 minutes. Abigail then works with Trevor for the remainder of the shift, which is approximately 1 hour. Behavioral escalation does not occur once Abigail is helping Trevor. Trevor doesn't argue with Abigail, but he does ask her to help him after she yells at him

(continued)

Figure 14.2.   *(continued)*

If an activity or request follows or is removed	Describe the specific activity including who else is present, what the activity consists of, and how long it lasts.	
If tangible items are obtained or removed	Describe the specific item(s) obtained including who else is present and how long the student has access to the item	
If sensory stimulation possibly occurs or is removed	Describe the context, who is around, what activities are going on, and what behaviors are expected.	

Summary of behavior

Identify the summary that will be used to build a plan of behavior support

| Setting events | → | Trigger | → | Behavior | → | Consequence |
| Mathematics class | → | Abigail helps other residents | → | Trevor throws object | → | Abigail yells at Trevor and then helps him (adult attention) |

How confident are you that the Summary of behavior is accurate?

Not very confident			Very confident		
1	2	3	4	5	6

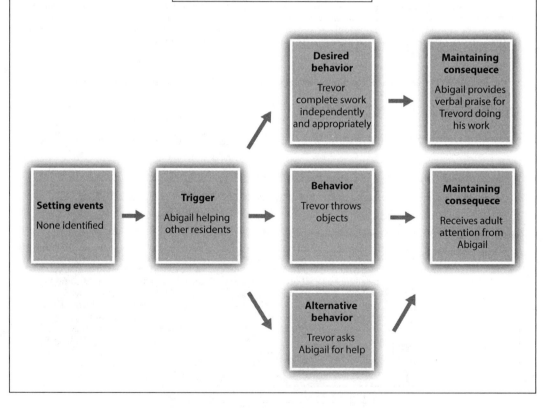

& Horner, 2003). In some circumstances, it may be appropriate to interview not only the teacher, caregiver, or parent but also the individual. Depending on the age of the individual and his or her level of skills, information about setting events that may not be observable can be obtained from the individual, including factors that may not be known to teachers and caregivers (e.g., bullying on the playground). Also, a list of potential reinforcers can be identified to aid with intervention development. Many of the FBA interview forms can be used with individual, but there are also specific forms, such as the student-directed FAI (O'Neill et al., 1997).

Questionnaires/Rating Scales Using questionnaires or rating scales is an additional, time-efficient way to help teachers/ care providers gather FBA data. These are completed by a care provider, teacher, or family member who is very familiar with the individual. He or she is typically asked to rate challenging behavior on a Likert-type scale (e.g., 0–2 or 1–5) to help determine when challenging behavior is most likely to occur. As with FBA interviews, the purpose of using rating scales is to identify antecedent and consequence events that are maintaining the challenging behavior. A few questionnaires that have been cited in the literature are the Motivation Assessment Scale (MAS; Durand & Crimmins, 1992), the functional analysis screening tool (FAST; Iwata, 1996), and the problem behavior questionnaire (PBQ; Lewis, Scott, & Sugai, 1994). Some sample items from these can be found in Table 14.1.

Motivation Assessment Scale The MAS (Durand & Crimmins, 1992) is a 16-item questionnaire that asks teachers/care providers to rate on a scale from 0 (never) to 6 (always) the extent to which challenging behavior occurs under different conditions (e.g., during instructional activities, in isolation). Once the form is completed, scores are summarized and ranked by the following four functions: 1) sensory, 2) escape, 3) attention, and 4) tangible.

Durand and Crimmins (1992) state that the tool can be used to assist in the development of interventions as well as selection of potentially effective reinforcers.

Functional Analysis Screening Tool The FAST (Iwata, 1996) is a 27-item questionnaire that asks teachers/care providers to respond using a *yes/no* format the extent to which challenging behavior occurs across different contexts or situations. Once completed, the questionnaire is summarized into the following functions: 1) social reinforcement (attention, tangible, or escape) and 2) sensory (self-stimulation or pain attenuation). Iwata (1996) recommends that several informants who frequently interact with the individual complete the FAST; then the information should be used to help guide direct observations to either confirm or disconfirm the hypotheses.

Problem Behavior Questionnaire The PBQ (Lewis, Scott, & Sugai, 1994) is a 15-item questionnaire that asks respondents to rate on a Likert-type scale from 0 (never) to 6 (always) points the extent to which challenging behavior occurs in different contexts. The PBQ also includes questions regarding possible setting events that may be influencing the occurrence of challenging behavior. Unlike the MAS and the FAST, the PBQ does not identify challenging behaviors maintained by sensory or tangible reinforcement. Rather, it identifies the following functions: escape (peer or adult) and attention (peer or adult). Lewis, Scott, and Sugai (1994) indicate that the PBQ was designed to help develop hypotheses regarding challenging behavior in general education settings (Lewis et al., 1994).

Issues and Limitations with Indirect Methods Although indirect methods are frequently used to help determine behavior function (Herzinger & Campbell, 2007), several issues and limitations should be taken into account. To begin with, all the data gathered using interviews and questionnaires are

Table 14.1.   Items from some commonly used functional behavioral assessment (FBA) questionnaires/rating scales

Name	Sample items	Response format
Motivation Assessment Scale (MAS; Durand & Crimmins, 1992)	• Would the behavior occur continuously if this person was left alone for long periods of time? • Does the behavior occur when any request is made of this person? • Does the behavior occur when you take away a favorite food, toy, or activity? • Does this person seem to do the behavior to upset or annoy you when you are trying to get him or her to do what you ask?	0 (never) to 6 (always)
Functional Analysis Screening Tool (FAST; Iwata, 1996)	• The behavior occurs frequently when the student is alone or unoccupied. • The behavior occurs when the student has not received much attention. • The behavior often occurs during training activities or when asked to complete tasks.	Yes/no
Problem Behavior Questionnaire (PBQ; Lewis et al., 1994)	• Does the challenging behavior occur and persist when you make a request to perform a task? • When the problem behavior occurs, do peers verbally respond or laugh at the student? • If the student engages in the problem behavior, do you provide one-to-one instruction to get the student back on task?	0 (never) to 6 (always)

MAS items from Durand, V.M. & Crimmins, D.B. (1992). *The Motivation Assessment Scale (MAS) administration guide.* Topeka, KS: Monaco & Associates; reprinted by permission. FAST items from Iwata, B. (1996). *Functional Analysis Screening Tool (FAST).* Gainesville: Florida Center on Self Injury, University of Florida. PBQ items from Lewis, T.J., Scott, T.M., & Sugai, G.M. (1994). The problem behavior questionnaire: A teacher-based instrument to develop functional hypotheses of problem behavior in general education classrooms. *Diagnostique, 19,* 103–115. Copyright © 1994 by SAGE Publications. Reprinted by Permission of SAGE Publications.

based on teacher/caregiver perception and thus may be subject to bias or misinterpretation. This may be particularly true if the care provider has little experience identifying environmental factors that influence and predict challenging behavior. When gathering information from multiple informants (e.g., different teachers/staff or staff and parents), there may be disagreement as to the events that are maintaining and/or triggering the challenging behavior. In these situations, direct observation is critical, as it may be difficult to discern which information is accurate for hypothesis development. Disagreement among informants may be related to the fact that, for some individuals, the same challenging behavior can serve multiple functions. For example, a student in one class may be disrupting the class by making loud noises/using obscene language to get out of a difficult math assignment, whereas in another class, he may be engaging in the challenging behavior to get access to peer attention (e.g., peers laugh/cheer him on when he engages in the behavior). On the other hand, during high-preference

activities, the individual does not engage in challenging behavior at all.

Overall, research is clear that indirect methods alone may not be as effective for identifying behavior function when compared with combining interviews and other methods (Cunningham & O'Neill, 2007). To increase the validity of functions identified using indirect methods, it's important to gather direct observation data and, if appropriate, conduct a functional analysis (Iwata, DeLeon, & Roscoe, 2013).

Direct Observation

Systematic direct observation is the process of observing an individual in his or her setting to determine the setting events (if possible), antecedents, and consequences that are maintaining challenging behavior (Bijou, Petersen, & Ault, 1968). Indirect methods such as interviews and questionnaires provide initial information to help with hypothesis development, and direct observation can be used to either confirm this hypothesis or develop alternative hypotheses for behavior functions. Subjective information about which settings or times of day result in increased challenging behavior can be obtained during the interview process. In order to establish a pattern of behavior, it has been recommended that at least 10 to 15 occurrences of the challenging behavior be observed prior to analyzing behavior function (O'Neill et al., 1997). In addition to observing settings where problem behavior occurs, it's important to observe settings/situations in which the problem behavior does not occur. This provides additional evidence regarding the triggers for the problem behavior as well as examples of routines/contexts that support appropriate behavior for the individual.

Antecedent-Behavior-Consequence Observation Form
An ABC observation form is one of the most commonly used observation tools for gathering FBA data (Bijou, Peterson, & Ault, 1968). A sample completed ABC observation form related to Natalia's case study is presented in Figure 14.3.

Observers complete the top portion related to the individual's name, who is conducting the observation, as well as the setting

in which the observation occurs. There is also a section for observation start and stop time. During the interview process, the challenging behaviors are operationally defined in observable and measurable terms. During the observation, the observer, typically using very brief statements/phrases, documents instances of the challenging behavior and provides details on what immediately occurred prior to the behavior (antecedents) and what events followed the challenging behavior (consequences). Observations should take place during the times that were identified during the FBA interview as most problematic and likely to evoke challenging behavior.

Functional Assessment Observation Form
The FAO form (O'Neill et al., 1997) is similar to the ABC form described previously but provides a more streamlined data collection system to gather ABC and event data. An example of a completed FAO form for Trevor's case study is presented in Figure 14.4.

To complete the FAO form, observers are asked to determine time periods for observation (e.g., for secondary students, time

---

Child's name: __Natalia__   Observer: __Curtis Henderson__   Date: __3/12/12__

Setting: __Mathematics class__   Observation start time: __10:50__   Observation stop time: __12:00__

Antecedent events	Behaviors	Consequent events
Ms. Sandoval hands out math assessment and tells students to work on it individually	Natalia gets out of her seat and walks out of the classroom without permission.	Ms. Sandoval monitors students taking exam. She ignores Natalia's behavior by not leaving the room to find her.
Natalia returns to the room after 25 minutes.	Natalia sits at her desk with her head down.	Ms. Sandoval tells Natalia to do work on her test.
Ms. Sandoval prompts Natalia to work on the test.	Natalia refuses to do work and argues.	Ms. Sandoval tells Natalia that she needs to work on her test or else she will be sent to the office.
Ms. Sandoval prompts Natalia to work on the test.	Natalia argues with Ms. Sandoval and swears at her, waves her arms, and stomps her feet.	Ms. Sandoval tells Natalia to go to the office.
Ms. Sandoval tells Natalia to go to the office.	Natalia leaves the room.	Natalia avoids the math assessment.

Figure 14.3. ABC data collection form example for Natalia. (*Source:* Bijou, Peterson, & Ault, 1968.)

Functional assessment observation form

Name: Trevor

Starting date: 10/15/12 Ending Date: 10/17/12

Time	Throwing objects	Off-task behavior	Work refusal	Instigating others	Demand/request (B)	Difficult task	Transitions	Interruption	Demand/request (P)	Alone (no attention)	Abigail		Attention	Desired item/activity	Self-stimulation	Demand/request (E)	Activity (yard work)	Person	Other/don't know	Verbal redirect	Adult assistance/help	Comments/observers initials
			Behaviors					Predictors							Perceived functions (Get/obtain · Escape/avoid)					Actual consequence		
1:20																						
1:30																						
1:40																						
1:50	4									4			4							4		DS
2:00	1	5			5				5	1			1 5							1 5		DS
2:10		2	6		2 6				2 6				2 6							2	6	DS
2:20	7		3		3				3	7			3 7							7	3	DS
2:30		8			8				8				8							8		DS
2:40			9		9				9				9								9	DS
2:50																						
3:00																						
Totals	3	3	3		6				6	3			9							6	3	

Events: 1 2 3 4 5 6 7 8 9 10 11 12 13 14 15 16 17 18 19 20 21 22 23 24 25 26 27 28 29 30 31 32 33 34 35 36 37 38 39 40

Dates: 10/15 10/16 10/17

Figure 14.4. Functional assessment observation form example for Trevor. (From O'Neill/Horner/Albin/Sprague/Storey/Newton. *Functional Assessment and Program Development for Problem Behavior*, 2E. © 1997 South-Western, a part of Cengage Learning, Inc. Reproduced by permission. www.cengage.com/permissions)

periods may be broken down into class periods, and for adults, the day could be broken down into hour increments). Based on the FBA interview, a list of behaviors to observe is generated and written on the form. The FAO form has a list of common predictors (e.g., antecedents) as well as perceived functions that can be used and a section for observers to write in the actual observed consequence following the challenging behavior. Additional predictors and functions can be added to the form based on information gathered from the FBA interview. The bottom section of the FAO form allows observers to track the number of events that occur during a given day, and the event number is used when completing the section on behaviors, predictors, perceived functions, and consequences. So the number 1 is used for the first observed challenging behavior, the number 2 is used for the second observed challenging behavior, and so forth. The FAO form can be used across several days or observation sessions.

Issues and Limitations with Direct Observation Direct observation provides additional FBA data that lead to hypothesis development regarding behavior function. An issue arises when the hypothesis developed using direct observation does not match the hypothesis developed via indirect methods. This may happen when a teacher or care provider is not as aware of the environmental events that are maintaining the challenging behavior. Having an outside observer document the ABC sequence of events allows for a less biased, more direct measure of why the challenging behavior occurs.

Determining when, how long, and across how many days an individual should be observed can be complex. As mentioned previously, it is recommended that data be collected on 10–15 behavior events prior to attempting to analyze behavior function (O'Neill et al., 1997). For high-frequency behaviors, this number of recommended events could be observed in 1 day or perhaps even in 1 hour (e.g., stereotypic behavior).

For low-frequency but high-intensity behaviors (e.g., extreme aggression with property destruction), the behavior may only occur 1 to 2 times a week, which makes it difficult to reach an adequate number of events. These instances may require relying on more indirect methods such as an FBA interview for hypotheses and/or perhaps a functional analysis (described in the next section), which could be conducted to elicit more instances of challenging behavior.

As with indirect methods, direct observations may reveal that behavior serves multiple functions across environments. This may lead to more effective intervention development because the settings and conditions under which the challenging behavior occur are directly observed during behavior observation. One final limitation of direct observation is that behavior function identified during this process can only be seen as hypothetical, because no experimental manipulations of environmental variables occur (as during a functional analysis).

Functional Analysis

Functional analysis involves the process of experimentally manipulating environmental variables (either antecedents or consequences) to determine the function(s) the challenging behavior serves for an individual (Iwata, Dorsey, Slifer, Bauman, & Richman, 1982/1994). There are many different variations of how to conduct a functional analysis, but the key component involves "observation of behavior under well-defined test versus control conditions" (Iwata & Dozier, 2008, p. 5). More specifically, a hypothesis is developed using indirect methods such as interviews or rating scales, and this hypothesis is tested by exposing the individual to situations that would predict challenging behavior and those that would not. For example, we may hypothesize that an individual is engaging in physical aggression (i.e., hitting, slapping, pinching, biting) to escape demands (e.g., requests to do work). A functional analysis could experimentally evaluate this hypothesis by comparing rates of aggression under demand versus a control (e.g., no demands) condition. If rates of aggression are significantly higher under the demand versus control condition, the hypothesis has been confirmed and intervention plans can be developed to address the behavior function. (For a more detailed description of functional analysis, see Chapter 16.)

Issues and Limitations with Functional Analysis There are several issues that should be considered when determining whether a functional analysis is needed or feasible. To begin with, functional analysis typically needs to be conducted or overseen by a well-trained behavior analyst or PBS practitioner; such people may not be available in all settings (Iwata & Dozier, 2008). Second, implementing a functional analysis involves attempting to evoke the challenging behavior in order to isolate relevant antecedent and consequence variables. Teachers, care providers, and/or parents may object to any methods that will increase the challenging behavior—particularly if it poses a safety hazard (e.g., self-injurious or aggressive behavior). Finally, in more naturalistic settings such as schools and communities, it may be difficult to manipulate and/or control the variables that are maintaining the challenging behavior. For example, behavior maintained by peer attention may not always be easy to manipulate in a classroom setting.

USING FUNCTIONAL BEHAVIORAL ASSESSMENT INFORMATION TO DEVELOP BEHAVIOR SUPPORT PLANS

The primary purpose of conducting an FBA is to gather information that can be used to gather effective intervention and support strategies into a BSP. A variety of strategies have been proposed for moving from an FBA to a BSP (O'Neill et al., 1997; Umbreit, Ferrero, Liaupsin, & Lane, 2007). One such approach is a *competing behavior analysis* (O'Neill et al., 1997). This approach is exemplified in the FACTS forms presented

in Figures 14.1 and 14.2, following the summary of behavior. The competing behavior analysis identifies relevant setting events, antecedents/predictors, the problem behavior(s), desired and alternative behaviors, and relevant maintaining consequences for all behaviors.

For example, in Figure 14.1, Natalia is identified as engaging in challenging behavior to avoid difficult tasks. The desired behavior would be for Natalia to complete the task and receive some appropriate consequence (e.g., social praise, activity break, tangible item). As an alternative behavior, Natalie could request a break or help with the task, therefore avoiding the aversive difficulty. The components of Natalia's BSP would include strategies to prevent the challenging behavior and make the desired and alternative behaviors more likely to occur. For example, antecedent strategies could include 1) modifying the difficulty of tasks provided, 2) giving Natalia choices about which tasks to do and when, and 3) prompting/reminding her to ask for a break or help if she feels the need. Teaching strategies could include 1) additional instruction on the difficult task and 2) instruction on when/how to request help or a break as needed. Consequence strategies could include 1) providing desired reinforcers contingent on work completion, 2) providing a break or help when requested, and 3) not allowing Natalia to escape when she engages in challenging behavior.

Figure 14.2 provides information about Trevor that indicates that he engages in challenging behavior during work activities to obtain adult attention. The desired behavior would be for him to complete the requested activities and then receive an appropriate consequence (e.g., adult attention). An alternative behavior could be for Trevor to establish proximity to his supervisor and use appropriate communication (e.g., gesture/sign, verbal utterances) to obtain attention. The components of Trevor's BSP would include strategies to prevent the challenging behavior and make the desired and alternative behaviors more likely to occur.

For example, antecedent strategies could include 1) providing Trevor with attention more frequently on a proactive basis and 2) prompting/reminding him to ask for attention/interaction if he feels the need. Teaching strategies could include instruction on when/how to request attention as needed. Consequence strategies could include 1) providing desired reinforcers contingent on work completion without challenging behavior, 2) providing attention when requested, and 3) attempting to avoid providing attention to Trevor when he engages in challenging behavior.

Additional information on developing BSPs and specific intervention strategies of the types described here can be found in several other chapters in this book (see Chapters 7, 8, 15, 21).

CONCLUSION

This chapter provides a brief summary/overview of the principles and procedures of conducting an FBA. This technology is a major component of our currently most effective and evidence-based practices for supporting people exhibiting challenging behavior. However, a number of significant and practical questions remain for ongoing research. There is still a need for additional research on the reliability, validity, and utility of indirect methods such as interviews and questionnaires/rating scales. There are ongoing efforts to adapt more rigorous functional analysis methods that are suitable in applied settings such as classrooms (e.g., Lambert, Bloom, & Irvin, 2012). As mentioned previously, there remain critical training needs so that appropriate service providers learn basic strategies of thinking functionally and have the skills to conduct more elaborate and complex assessments/analyses as required (Durand, 1990). It may be more appropriate to consider that these basic versus more advanced skills are respectively relevant for people with different levels of training and expertise (e.g., classroom teachers, school psychologists, district/state-level behavior specialists). It is clear that these issues will remain important and inspire active areas of research and application for many years to come.

REFERENCES

Bijou, S.W., Peterson, R.F., & Ault, M.H. (1968). A method to integrate descriptive and experimental studies at the level of data and empirical concepts. *Journal of Applied Behavior Analysis, 1,* 175–191.

Borgmeier, C., & Horner, R.H. (2006). An evaluation of the predictive validity of confidence ratings in identifying functional behavioral assessment hypothesis statements. *Journal of Positive Behavior Interventions, 8,* 100–105.

Carr, E.G. (1977). The motivation of self-injurious behavior: A review of some hypotheses. *Psychological Bulletin, 84,* 800–816.

Crone, D.A., & Horner, R.H. (2003). *Building positive behavior support systems in schools: Functional behavioral assessment.* New York, NY: Guilford Press.

Cunningham, E., & O'Neill, R.E. (2007). Assessing agreement among the results of functional behavioral assessment and analysis methods with students with emotional/behavior disorders (E/BD). *Behavioral Disorders, 32,* 211–221.

Dunlap, G., & Kincaid, D. (2001). The widening world of functional assessment: Comments on four manuals and beyond. *Journal of Applied Behavior Analysis, 34,* 365–377.

Durand, V.M. (1990). *Severe behavior problems: A functional communication training approach.* New York, NY: Guilford.

Durand, V.M., & Crimmins, D.B. (1992). *The Motivation Assessment Scale (MAS) administration guide.* Topeka, KS: Monaco Associates.

Hanley, G.P., Iwata, B.A., & McCord, B.E. (2003). Functional analysis of problem behavior: A review. *Journal of Applied Behavior Analysis, 36,* 147–185.

Herzinger, C.V., & Campbell, J.M. (2007). Comparing functional assessment methodologies: A quantitative synthesis. *Journal of Autism and Developmental Disorders, 37,* 1430–1445.

Individuals with Disabilities Education Improvement Act (IDEA) of 2004, PL 108-446, 20 U.S.C. §§ 1400 et seq.

Iwata, B. (1996). *Functional analysis screening tool (FAST).* Gainesville: Florida Center on Self Injury, University of Florida.

Iwata, B.A., DeLeon, I.G., & Roscoe, E.M. (2013). Reliability and validity of the functional analysis screening tool. *Journal of Applied Behavior Analysis, 46,* 271–284.

Iwata, B.A., Dorsey, M.F., Slifer, K.J., Bauman, K.E., & Richman, G.S. (1982/1994). Toward a functional analysis of self-injury. *Journal of Applied Behavior Analysis, 27,* 197–209.

Iwata, B.A., & Dozier, C. (2008). Clinical application of functional analysis methodology. *Behavior Analyst, 1,* 3–9.

Lambert, J.M., Bloom, S.E., & Irvin, J. (2012). Trial-based functional analysis and functional communication training in an early childhood setting. *Journal of Applied Behavior Analysis, 45,* 579–584.

Lewis, T.J., Scott, T.M., & Sugai, G.M. (1994). The problem behavior questionnaire: A teacher-based instrument to develop functional hypotheses of problem behavior in general education classrooms. *Diagnostique, 19*, 103–115.

Lovaas, O.I., Freitag, G., Gold, V.J., & Kassorla, I.C. (1965). Experimental studies in childhood schizophrenia: Analysis of self-destructive behavior. *Journal of Experimental Child Psychology, 2*, 7–84.

March, R., Horner, R., Lewis-Palmer, T., Brown, D., Crone, D., Todd, A., . . . Carr, E. (2000). *Functional assessment checklist for teachers and staff (FACTS)*. Eugene, OR: Educational and Community Supports.

Matson, J.L. (2012). *Functional assessment for challenging behaviors*. New York, NY: Springer.

O'Neill, R.E., Horner, R.H., Albin, R.W., Sprague, J.R., Storey, K., & Newton, J.S. (1997). *Functional assessment and program development for problem behavior:* *A practical handbook*. Pacific Grove, CA: Brooks/Cole.

Pierce, W.D., & Epling, W.F. (1980). What happened to analysis in applied behavior analysis? *Behavior Analyst, 3*, 1–9.

Risley, T.R. (1968). The effects and side effects of punishing the autistic behaviors of a deviant child. *Journal of Applied Behavior Analysis, 1*, 21–35.

Sailor, W., Dunlap, G., Sugai, G., & Horner, R.H. (Eds.). (2009). *Handbook of positive behavior support*. New York, NY: Springer.

Umbreit, J., Ferrero, J.B., Liaupsin, C., & Lane, K. (2007). *Functional behavioral assessment and function-based intervention: An effective practical approach*. Upper Saddle River, NJ: Pearson.

Wolf, M.M., Risley, T.R., & Mees, H. (1964). Application of operant conditioning procedures to the behavior problems of an autistic child. *Behavior Research and Therapy, 1*, 305–312.

Using Functional Behavioral Assessment Data

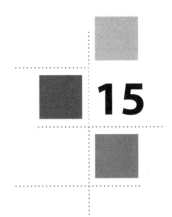

15

Lee Kern and Beth Custer

Chapter 14 describes the procedures for conducting a functional behavioral assessment (FBA). To briefly summarize the process, a comprehensive FBA relies on information collected from both indirect and direct assessments. These assessments are generally conducted across a variety of settings with multiple individuals. For instance, data may be collected across class periods, during recess or lunchtime, at a jobsite in the community, or during recreational activities. Similarly, information may be obtained from teachers, parents, job coaches, peers, friends, the individual, and others. The end purpose of the functional assessment process is to identify interventions that are linked to the data gathered and therefore have a high probability of being effective. That is, the assessment data identify antecedents or events that occur prior to problem behavior, potential replacement behaviors that an individual can use instead of problem behavior, and events that occur

after problem behavior that may be reinforcing and thereby maintaining the behavior. This information is essential for developing and implementing an effective comprehensive multicomponent behavior support plan.

Because an FBA generally yields a great deal of information, it is crucial that team members systematically organize and summarize the information in a way that will facilitate intervention development. Specifically, the data gathered can be organized and arranged in a manner that makes events associated with problem behavior evident, thereby helping to discern potentially effective interventions. This is an important step in the assessment-intervention process. However, this step is often bypassed, and teams revert to randomly selecting interventions when they are confronted with an overwhelming amount of information that they are unable to organize in a meaningful way.

In this chapter, we describe several strategies for summarizing information collected during the functional assessment process. In addition, we offer suggestions for approaching data that are inconsistent or unclear. Finally, we describe the process for developing hypothesis statements, which serve as a succinct summary of the information gathered and lead directly to intervention selection. One caveat we should note is that the process we describe is based primarily on information gathered during the functional assessment process that focuses on events immediately surrounding problem behavior. Broad information, such as lifestyle issues, preferences, and long-term goals, is critical and should be a significant part of comprehensive support planning. Although we describe specific strategies to interpret data proximal to problem behavior, we also discuss approaches for understanding the role of broad data so that lifestyle, quality of life, and long-term planning are integrated as pertinent parts of the support plan.

Before beginning, we introduce Max and Lucas, two individuals whose experiences help illustrate the process of data summarization and interpretation. Both are individuals with disabilities who exhibit significant behavior problems.

Max

Max is a fifth grader identified as having an emotional and behavioral disorder and attention-deficit/hyperactivity disorder (ADHD). He is included in the general education setting for his full school day. Max's teacher reports that he frequently disrupts the class. Specifically, he fails to complete work, wanders around the classroom, pulls books and materials from shelves and scatters them on the floor, kicks objects in the classroom, and curses. These behaviors frequently result in Max being removed from the classroom and sent to the principal's office.

Lucas

Lucas is an adult with intellectual disabilities who uses the Picture Exchange Communication System

(PECS) as his primary method of communication. He lives in an apartment with his mother and works at a restaurant where he receives support from a local agency. Each weekday morning, he is picked up by an agency staff member who takes him to the restaurant where he is employed. At the restaurant, Lucas prepares silverware by unloading clean items from the dishwasher and rolling a knife, fork, and spoon into a napkin. The support staff have indicated that there are times when Lucas "shuts down" by sitting in the corner of the dining room with his head down. During these times, he reportedly fails to engage in any form of communication (e.g., does not use or respond to PECS). The store owner is also concerned because this has resulted in a shortage of available silverware, and other restaurant employees must neglect their assigned duties to assist with preparing the silverware during these times.

EXTRACTING RELEVANT INFORMATION FROM ASSESSMENT DATA

A great deal of data and information follows individuals with disabilities throughout their school career and life in general. In addition, parents often accumulate information and reports from a variety of sources, such as pediatricians and diagnosticians. Each piece of the data may help develop an overall picture of the student in addition to long-term planning. However, not all data are relevant for developing hypotheses regarding problem behavior and constructing a related behavior support plan. For example, relying solely on the broad characteristics of a disability or reports of student performance on standardized measures of behavior are generally ineffective for developing a meaningful behavior plan (Scott, McIntyre, Liaupsin, Nelson, & Conroy, 2004; Shapiro & Kratochwill, 2000; Shriver, Anderson, & Proctor, 2001). Furthermore, behavior support team members may have significant background information after working with an individual for an extensive time period. This information, however, may be dated and not currently relevant in leading the team to accurately identify the conditions presently associated with problem behavior (Scott et al., 2004). The information collected during a functional assessment that is most important to support plan development focuses on environmental events that currently trigger or maintain problem behavior, related skills that may be capitalized on or taught to replace problem behavior, and lifestyle issues that may play a role in the occurrence of problem behavior (Association for Positive Behavior Support [APBS], 2007, V-E 1 and 2).

Because a significant amount of information is gathered during the functional assessment process from both indirect methods (e.g., parent interviews, behavior rating scales, office discipline history) and direct methods (i.e., direct observation), sorting through and extracting relevant data can be a challenge. To reduce this burden, there are three general types of information that should be considered. The first is *environmental events associated with problem behavior*. The second is *environmental events associated with desirable behavior*. The third is *quality-of-life variables* that play a broader or distal role in occurrences of problem behavior.

When examining environmental events associated with problem behavior, antecedents, consequences, and setting events to problem behavior should be identified. As described in Chapter 14, an antecedent is the event that occurs immediately before a behavior and is sometimes referred to as the *trigger*. Examples include a teacher request to begin an assignment that a student does not have the skills to complete or the request for social interaction delivered to a withdrawn or asocial individual. A *consequence* is an event or response that occurs immediately after the behavior. Data describing what happens in the environment directly following the behavior of concern often helps to identify behavioral function, or the underlying reason for the problem behavior. For example, if disruptive behavior consistently occurs during an academic subject and the classroom consequence for disruption is being sent to the office by the teacher, then the disruption might function as escape from

academic work. Behavioral functions are classified as positive reinforcement, in which the individual gains something (e.g., attention, tangible item, self-stimulation), or negative reinforcement, in which the individual avoids or escapes something (e.g., a task or person). Finally, potential setting events should be considered. Setting events are events or conditions that occur at an earlier time and indirectly influence the likelihood of problem behavior. For instance, a difficult bus ride, lack of sleep, or medication side effects can increase the likelihood of problem behavior in circumstances where it generally would not occur. Conversely, positive interactions with a teacher in the morning may reduce the likelihood of problem behaviors when this same teacher issues a request to complete schoolwork. Setting events may not always be readily apparent because they are usually difficult to directly observe and identification may rely on information from family members or others.

In addition to variables associated with problem behavior, it is important to identify variables that are associated with desired behavior. When a student engages in problem behavior, naturally much of the focus will be on the environmental variables associated with the problem. However, it is also useful to conduct observations of the individual in environments where the behavior does not occur. Detailed information about situations associated with desirable behavior can suggest interventions or environmental modifications to reduce problem behavior. For example, sometimes a particular staff member may interact with a very anxious individual in a manner that calms him or her, thereby reducing incidents of self-injury. This information may be useful for training other support staff to adopt similar styles of interaction. Likewise, a particular teacher may utilize routines or specific academic support strategies that reduce a student's problem behavior and help him or her perform well in classroom settings. These routines and strategies may be introduced in other settings where the individual is experiencing difficulty.

A final area of relevant data pertains to quality-of-life variables. It is common for practitioners to view a student's challenging behaviors as isolated incidents that need to be remedied within the immediate context. However, broad aspects of an individual's quality of life can contribute to his or her happiness, safety, and well-being and play a significant role in occurrences of problem behavior. There are several different domains of quality of life that have been proposed in the literature (Carr & Horner, 2007; Schalock et al., 2002). These differ depending on the source or type of assessment and are discussed in subsequent chapters. Among the most commonly recognized, and perhaps most important to individuals with challenging behaviors, are social inclusion, interpersonal relations, physical well-being, self-determination, and emotional well-being (Turnbull, Turnbull, Wehmeyer, & Park, 2003; Wehmeyer & Schalock, 2001).

Variables associated with quality of life can contribute to problem behavior, either directly or indirectly. For example, health problems such as infections, allergies, or other ailments may result in behavior problems, particularly if an individual has limited means of communicating that he or she is experiencing illness or pain. Also, problem behaviors often increase when an individual does not have sufficient opportunities to engage in stimulating community events. Unfortunately, as severe behavior problems increase, individuals tend to become increasingly isolated from community events—a situation that only exacerbates the likelihood of problem behavior. Data, particularly when obtained from parents, care providers, or other partners, can help identify the quality-of-life variables that may be contributing to problem behaviors so that important lifestyle events can be increased or reintroduced.

INTERPRETING DATA

In the previous section, we discussed the types of functional assessment information that contribute to support plan development. Although knowing the type of information useful for support plan development is imperative, it is important to synthesize the data in a way that will both allow for easy interpretation and facilitate the identification of linked and potentially effective interventions. In general, the best approach is to look for consistent patterns in the data. In the case of problem behavior, it is improbable that data will be crystal clear and that strategies to reduce or eliminate problems behavior will be readily evident. Problem behavior is usually shaped over long periods of time in multiple ways and may occur for a variety of reasons. Thus it is unlikely that data will perfectly align. Rather, some type of consistency or pattern emerges from the data that can be used to develop informed hypotheses or "best guesses" about the events associated with problem behavior.

To identify these consistencies or patterns, it is helpful for the support team members to summarize the data in graphs or tables (APBS, 2007, V-E 3). Such displays facilitate interpretation and comparison. Although each team member may opt to select a specific data set to analyze and summarize, it is helpful to invoke ongoing discussion to ensure there is consensus across stakeholders with respect to data interpretation.

Several types of data should be analyzed. The first is antecedent events (APBS, 2007, V-D 4). There are several key questions that should be asked when examining antecedents to problem behavior (Kern, 2005): When does the behavior occur? What activities or events occur prior to problem behavior? Which people, if any, are present when the behavior occurs? Similarly, it is important to identify times, events, and people who are associated with the absence of problem behavior. It sometimes is most helpful to begin by identifying the times of day when behavior occurs and those times when it does not occur (O'Neill et al., 1997). It may be that problem behavior occurs only during a particular time of the day (e.g., in the morning) or during a specific class (e.g., math). Problem behavior may also be absent during particular classes, at certain time periods, or with specific individuals. This information is an important first step, but is not sufficient for intervention development. For example, information that behavior problems occur during math class is a good start but does not provide information about specific variables in math class that precede problem behavior. Thus after the time of day with and without problem behaviors is determined, specific activities or events and people routinely present during those times need to be identified. For instance, specific activities during math class that result in problem behavior might be the presentation of a lengthy or difficult worksheet, teacher feedback that completed work is incorrect, or recurring teasing from a particular peer also attending the math class. This type of detailed information leads directly to antecedent interventions.

In addition to summarizing antecedents in graphic or tabular format, events that follow behavior, or consequences, should be similarly summarized (APBS, 2007, V-D 5; Kern, 2005). There are some important questions regarding consequences: Does the behavior allow the individual to escape or avoid a particular activity, event, or person? Does the behavior allow the individual to obtain a particular activity, item, or type of sensory stimulation? An analysis of the consequences that follow behavior helps generate suppositions about what maintains the behavior or the functions the behavior serves. For example, if the data show that a student is sent to the office at least half of the time following classroom disruption, the data would suggest that his or her problem behavior may be maintained by escape.

Finally, it is important to examine setting events or conditions that indirectly influence the likelihood of problem behavior increasing or decreasing, as described in Chapter 14. As with antecedents and consequences, the data should be reviewed to detect patterns. Identifying setting events,

however, is considerably more challenging because, unlike antecedents and consequences, they are generally not proximal to problem behavior and may not be directly observable. In addition, setting events may not occur regularly. For example, setting events such as negative feedback from a teacher in a previous class that is upsetting to a student, periodic lack of sleep, and various family circumstances (e.g., visits with noncustodial parent) may occur only occasionally. Therefore, it is important to rely on interviews with teachers, family, and other support staff, which may provide valuable clues about the conditions that tend to increase the likelihood of behavioral incidents (Kern, O'Neill, & Starosta, 2004).

Setting events should be considered after antecedents are examined. When the data suggest that a particular antecedent seems to be associated with problem behavior but problem behavior does not always occur when the antecedent is present, then the possibility that a setting event is influencing behavior should be considered. Direct observation data may help indicate the presence of a setting event. For example, when a student periodically comes to class angry, an employee appears tired from time to time, or a preschooler refuses to participate in morning circle on Mondays, the presence of a setting event should be explored (Horner, Vaughn, Day, & Ard, 1996).

Because data interpretation can be a challenge, it is important to reconsider team membership during this process (APBS, 2007, I-C 1). Chapter 3 discusses important considerations for building an effective team. At times, however, additional team members are needed to interpret data. Bambara, Nonnemaker, and Koger (2005) described three considerations when forming a support team. The first is to consider which individuals have the expertise necessary to make good decisions about the individual for whom the support plan is being developed. The second is to consider who will be affected by the team's decision. The third is to identify who has a vested interest in participating. Bambara et al. and others (e.g., Snell & Janney, 2005) also note that, in addition to a core team, it is often helpful to have an extended team. Extended team members include experts who are called on, as needed, to address specific issues. It is common during the data interpretation process to rely on extended team members for several reasons. First, individuals such as behavior specialists have served on teams in the past and usually have extensive experience analyzing and interpreting data. These individuals may be able to advise the team which data are important and how to graph the data for easy interpretation, saving the team a great deal of time. In addition, the data may suggest extended team members who could provide additional information critical to data interpretation. For instance, if direct observation data indicate that problem behavior occurs throughout the day at an adolescent's workplace but occurs far less frequently between 2:30 and 4:00 p.m., a coworker or employer might be able to offer additional information about activities during that time frame. Also, when setting events are suspected, extended team

members with specific expertise may be needed. For example, if lack of sleep is identified as a setting event and the team determines that a child has sleep difficulties, it may be important to include his or her pediatrician as an extended team member until the sleep problems are resolved. Similarly, if bus problems that occur periodically are identified as setting events, it may be valuable to include the bus driver or bus aide as an extended team member to determine the specific problem and assist with intervention development and implementation.

We now return to our case examples to illustrate how data collected during the functional assessment process are summarized. We begin with Max. During the functional assessment process, interviews were conducted with Max's family and teachers. In addition, direct observation data were collected across a school week. Table 15.1 shows a summary of the interview conducted with Max's mother and teacher. A few pieces of information that are noteworthy include the reported occurrence of problem behaviors during language arts, math, and independent work; Max's difficulties with math, writing,

Table 15.1.   Summary of functional behavioral assessment interviews with Max's mother and teacher

Problem behaviors

- Pulling books and materials from shelves
- Throwing items from shelf onto floor/carpet
- Kicking items on carpet
- Cursing

Important information from interviews

- Behavior is most likely to occur during language arts class and math class, when Max is expected to work independently, or when asked to clean his room in the evening.
- Max may play with his shoelaces or items near him as a signal that he is about to engage in the defined behavior.
- Teacher and parent believe function may include escape of a less preferred activity as well as gaining adult and peer attention.
- Parent believes possible setting events include parents' divorce, a recent change in medication, and seasonal allergies.
- Parent reported that Max does not participate in activities outside of the school setting, which may reduce his quality of life.
- Teacher reported that Max has academic skill impairments in writing and is a grade below his typical peers in math. Teacher and parent both reported that Max has difficulty with self-regulation, which results in impulsivity. They reported that he sometimes acts without thinking and later feels badly for what he has done. Teacher also noted that Max receives social skills instruction to improve appropriate conversations with peers.

and social skills; teacher and parent identification of escape and attention as potential behavioral functions; the presence of possible setting events; and limited outside activities that may play a role in Max's quality of life.

In addition to interviews, antecedent-behavior-consequence (ABC) data were collected. After collecting data across several days, Max's team decided first to graph incidents of problem behavior according to his daily schedule to get a big picture of times during the day that problem behavior was most and least likely to occur. Data on occurrences of problem behavior across each of Max's class periods were graphed first and are shown in Figure 15.1. This graph shows that Max is more likely to engage in problem behavior during language arts and math classes. Following this initial assessment, the team collected additional data during math and language arts for 5 school days to identify specific activities that were problematic. The data, shown in Figure 15.2, revealed that when Max is given an assignment in which he is expected to write, he is much more likely to engage in problem behavior.

After summarizing antecedents to problem behavior, consequences were then summarized and graphed in the same manner as antecedents. Figure 15.3 illustrates that the classwide consequence for the majority

of Max's problem behavior was a discipline referral, which required removing him from the class and sending him to the office. The summarized consequence data suggested that his problem behavior is maintained by escape.

Data were collected and analyzed in the same manner for Lucas. Table 15.2 shows a summary of interview information collected from his mother and job support staff. Important information that emerged from the interview is that Lucas sometimes stays up late watching movies, he sometimes fatigues easily, and problem behavior may function to communicate that he wants a break from work.

Direct observation data also were collected across 2 weeks. In light of interview information from Lucas's mother indicating that he sometimes stays up late watching movies, the team decided to monitor Lucas' sleeping patterns to see if this could be a possible setting event for the behavior, in addition to collecting ABC data. Lucas's mother checked in on him twice each night and recorded the activity taking place. The summarized raw data that were collected are reported in Table 15.3. When the team analyzed the data, they noticed that indeed there was variability in the occurrence of problem behavior across days. However, the summarized data clearly showed that that problem behavior almost always occurred when Lucas

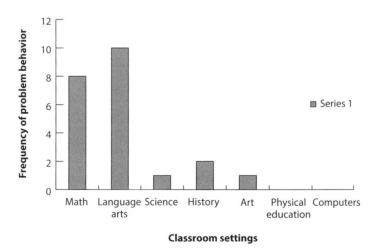

Figure 15.1. Summary of occurrences of Max's problem behavior across classes.

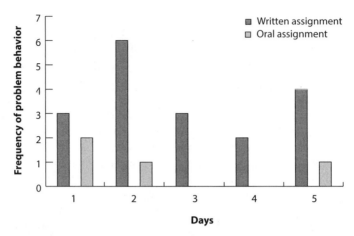

Figure 15.2. Frequency of Max's problem behavior during written and oral activities.

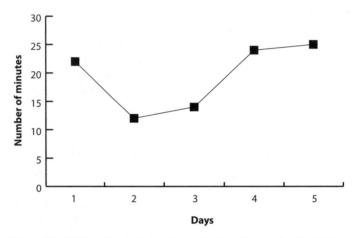

Figure 15.3. Total number of minutes Max spent in the office each day prior to intervention.

Table 15.2. Summary of functional behavioral assessment interviews with Lucas's mother and teacher

Problem behaviors

- Sitting in corner with head down
- Failing to complete job activities

Important information from interviews

- Lucas's mother reported that he likes to stay up and watch movies at night, but when he does, it is difficult to rouse him for work.
- Lucas's support staff indicated that he seems to fatigue easily and cannot persist with work tasks; however, it was noted that this does not occur every day—some days he will work for extended periods of time.
- Lucas's support staff noted that problem behavior may serve to communicate he is tired and wants a break.

Table 15.3.   Results of setting event and ABC data for Lucas

Date	Mother's report of activities the previous night		Antecedent	Behavior	Consequence
	9:00 p.m.	11:30 p.m.			
12/6	In room	Sleeping	N/A	None	N/A
12/7	In room	Watching movie	At work, no change in routine, working for 5 minutes	Turned his back to work; refused to continue	Allowed a break
12/8	Watching movie	Sleeping	N/A	None	N/A
12/9	Watching movie	Watching movie	At work, working for 20 minutes	Went to corner of restaurant and sat down	When offered the Picture Exchange Communication System (PECS) book, selected the icon for a break
12/10	Sleeping	Sleeping	N/A	None	N/A
12/13	Watching movie	Watching movie	Entered restaurant and immediately went behind door and sat down	Sat down in corner	Allowed 10-minute break and then prompted to work
			Performed task for less than 1 minute	Refused to complete job	Allowed to go home early from work
12/14	Sleeping	Sleeping	N/A	None	N/A
12/15	Sleeping	Sleeping	At home after dinner	Sat in corner and began banging on wall	Offered PECS book and selected a preferred snack
12/16	Watching movie	Watching movie	At work immediately following scheduled break	Sat in corner once at work	Prompted to continue work
			Mother called Lucas for dinner	Refused to come to dinner at home	Allowed to stay in room and dinner was brought to him in room
12/17	Watching movie	Sleeping	N/A	None	N/A

had stayed up late the previous night. Specifically, data collected over 2 weeks indicated that when Lucas was up past 11:30 p.m. watching movies, he was more likely to engage in problem behavior the following day.

DEALING WITH CONFUSING OR UNCLEAR DATA

The case examples illustrate how to summarize assessment data. Both Max and Lucas presented fairly straightforward assessment data. At times, however, data may be confusing and consistencies or patterns are not evident, even after summarizing the data in several different ways. When it is not possible to detect clear antecedents or common responses and infer behavioral function, the first question to ask is whether a sufficient amount of data has been collected. Generally, data pertaining to 15–20 occurrences of a behavior problem are ample to identify the events triggering or maintaining problem behavior. However, there is a variety of reasons that data may not be clear. One possibility is inconsistencies in an individual's life that result in variable data—that is, when an individual's schedule or activities vary from day to day or throughout the week, it is sometimes difficult to detect behavior patterns. In these cases, it may be necessary to collect additional data. For example, Seth worked at a restaurant chain located in a large city, assisting at three different restaurants. In addition, his work schedule changed daily, depending on how busy the restaurant was and its business needs. Although data were collected surrounding 15 occurrences of problem behavior, no consistent antecedents or responses could be identified. After reviewing the data, the team noticed that limited data were available across days, locations, and activities, due to the many changes in his daily and weekly schedule. Additional data were needed to get a better idea of locations, situations, and activities that were problematic.

Another circumstance where data can be difficult to interpret is when problem behaviors occur at a low frequency. Low-frequency, high-intensity behavior requires intervention, but it is usually difficult to specify consistent antecedents and consequences. A common example is a student who fights at school every few months. Gathering information on 15–20 occurrences of the behavior could take several school years, an unreasonable length of time to delay intervention. One option is to examine precursors to the problem behavior. For example, it is unlikely that a student who fights at school, albeit infrequently, has adequate social skills to negotiate difficult situations with peers. Assessment data collected on problematic peer interactions may identify precursors that lead to social difficulties, which occasionally escalate to fighting. Intervention that successfully addresses the precursor also will eliminate the more serious behavior that follows. For example, Jeanna frequently argues with peers during free time in the classroom or on the playground, which occasionally escalates to fighting. Data were collected on the precursor of arguing with

peers. The data indicated that Jeanna had difficulty with two particular peers who tended to tease her. Her fights almost always involved one of these two peers. Thus intervention focused on introducing a Tier-2 intervention within the schoolwide positive behavior support (SWPBS) system to decrease teasing and improve the social interactions of Jeanna's peers. Jeanna was also taught alternative strategies for responding when teasing occurs.

An additional strategy for interpreting low-frequency behavior is to rely on historical information. Whether at school, a worksite, or home, incidents of serious problem behavior are generally documented. This information can be reviewed to detect patterns. For example, Paulo was able to use several picture cards to communicate his daily needs. However, he periodically engaged in severe self-injury, and during those episodes, he was unresponsive to his parents' attempts to persuade him to communicate what he wanted. Paulo's parents kept detailed notes of each episode of self-injury. When his team reviewed the notes, they found that the self-injury always occurred to the cheek area of his face. When the team examined Paulo's health records, they found that he had significant oral health problems in the form of gum disease with recurring flare-ups. Because Paulo would not comply with dental cleanings, the gum disease had never been adequately treated. Paulo's team was able to find a dentist who provided mild anesthesia for dental work. Regularly scheduled cleanings addressed Paulo's dental problems and eliminated self-injury.

Behavior that is influenced by highly idiosyncratic events may also result in confusion during the assessment process. Generally, there are common events that influence problem behavior, such as the presentation of a difficult task or insufficient attention, and teams tend to look for those types of antecedents. Thus, when atypical or unusual events influence problem behavior, they may not be evident. For example, Kennedy and Itkonen (1993) conducted an FBA with Kelly, a 20-year-old student with intellectual disabilities. The assessment results indicated that multiple and severe problem behavior (e.g., falling to the ground, aggression, pulling her hair, tearing her clothing, screaming, whining) occurred following instructional demands. Intervention, consisting of eliminating nonpreferred activities and increasing reinforcement during activities that could not be eliminated, resulted in a decrease in problem behavior. However, behavior problems continued about every third or fourth school day. After several months, additional assessment data were collected and revealed that problem behavior appeared to be related to the number of stops made by her transportation vehicle on the way to school. Specifically, two routes were taken. One was a highway route with few stops, while the other was a city route with approximately 20 stops due to traffic lights and stop signs. Data indicated that the city route served as a setting event, resulting in increased problem behavior in conjunction with demands. When the city route was eliminated, problem behavior remained low each day. Given the idiosyncratic nature of this setting event, it was difficult to identify. Kelly's case illustrates the need for additional data and persistence when events associated with problem behavior are not readily identified.

Another circumstance when data may be confusing or unclear occurs when behavior is difficult to observe. Behaviors such as stealing, cutting oneself, carrying weapons, or abusing drugs generally cannot be observed. Although there is limited guidance in the literature, we believe covert problem behaviors should be addressed in the same manner as overt behaviors, identifying environmental events that appear to be associated with the problem behavior and examining lifestyle issues that could be modified to improve life quality. Similar to low-frequency behavior problems, it is important to carefully document events associated with known occurrences of the covert behavior. For example, if evidence of cutting is observed, potentially associated events or changes should be documented, such as impending exams at school, a decrease in parental supervision, or an increase in comments regarding future success and life planning. In addition, it is critical to obtain information directly from the individual in the form of self-report. Several functional assessment interviews, such as the "student-assisted functional assessment interview" and the "student-directed functional assessment interview" (Kern, Dunlap, Clarke, & Childs, 1994; O'Neill et al., 1997), can be used to obtain this critical information.

Emergent data also may be confusing when behavior serves a biological or sensory function. In this case, behavior problems are usually readily observable and a sufficient amount of data has been collected; however, no clear patterns can be discerned with respect to associated antecedent events or consequences—that is, the problem behavior appears to occur at similar frequencies, regardless of environmental events. If this pattern of data occurs, teams should consider that the behavior may not be related to the external environment. It should be noted, however, that epidemiologic studies indicate that this is unusual and that the majority of problem behavior, including severe self-injury, occurs for environmental reasons (e.g., Iwata et al., 1994). Nevertheless, at times, problem behavior is unrelated to the environment, and this may be the case more commonly in particular disability groups. For example, stereotypic behavior tends to occur more frequently among individuals with autism or severe intellectual disabilities.

In general, stimulatory or biologic hypotheses are arrived at by default; only after all potential environmental causes have been ruled out should a biologic or self-stimulatory hypothesis be considered. This is important because behavior can also occur across multiple situations and at a high rate for environmental reasons, which has implications for intervention. For example, 3-year-old Maahir's behavior was highly attention seeking, and self-injury occurred if he did not have physical contact with an adult. His high rate of self-injury across settings immediately suggested a biologic cause. However, his team fortunately collected detailed data showing the absence of self-injury when Maahir was being held. Thus a very different intervention was developed than would have been the case for biologic self-injury. His plan involved gradually and systematically fading physical contact, providing highly reinforcing activities when he had no contact, teaching him to request contact while building in a gradual delay for contact, and providing reinforcement for the absence of self-injury.

We mention one final consideration regarding self-stimulatory behavior. It is also important to note that although the purpose of self-stimulatory behavior is to provide sensory input, research shows that it occurs at a higher frequency in environments that are barren or insufficiently stimulating (Hall, Thorns, & Oliver, 2003). Consequently, self-stimulation may occur across settings but at different frequencies, making the data difficult to interpret. One important aspect of intervention involves creating environments that are interesting and stimulating.

Last, multiple problem behaviors or single problem behaviors serving multiple functions might also result in confusing or unclear data. In the case of multiple problem behaviors, each behavior should be examined individually. The data suggest two potential outcomes. One is that different types or topographies of behavior problems have different functions (e.g., Kamps, Wendland, & Culpepper, 2006). In this circumstance, supports are needed to address each function. The other possible outcome is that all topographies of behavior serve the same function. In this case, supports addressing a single function should reduce all topographies of behavior. Marie, a young child with autism, provides an example of multiple problem behaviors serving different functions. Marie engaged in both aggression and self-injury. She had very poor communication skills and was in the early phases of learning PECS. The FBA revealed that her aggression occurred primarily when she was given an instruction to complete a task that was difficult for her (e.g., pick up toys, brush her hair). Because her aggression, in the form of scratching, was severe and generally caused harm to others, her parents and preschool teacher unknowingly avoided or backed away from demands so they would not be hurt. Marie quickly learned that this type of aggression was successful at helping her avoid tasks she did not want to complete. At the same time, she incidentally found that when she banged her head, her mother ran to her to make sure she was all right. She soon learned that she was able to gain attention from others by head banging. Therefore, her support plan involved interventions to reduce both aggression that served an escape function and self-injury that served an attention function.

Elijah also engaged in multiple problem behaviors, including disruption, aggression, and tantrums. His support team believed that because of the multitude and diversity of his problem behaviors, it would be a challenge to eliminate them. The FBA data, however, revealed that they all served the same function, which was to avoid interactions with others. A look into Elijah's history revealed that he was very sick as an infant, was hospitalized for extended periods of time, and had to endure multiple and frequent invasive medical procedures. Thus he learned that the approach of others generally meant something unpleasant was impending. He had developed a repertoire of problem behaviors, one of which was almost always effective at getting an approaching person to retreat. Specifically, the topography of his problem behaviors caused others to retreat because the behaviors were either harmful or aversive. Disruption behavior, for example, consisted of throwing objects, so anyone who approached Elijah was likely to get hit with the objects. Similarly, aggression was severe and likely to cause injury. Tantrums included extremely loud screaming that was aversive to anyone nearby. As Elijah's support team summarized his FBA data, they identified the common function for behavior problems. Subsequently, they were able to develop a single intervention plan involving gradual desensitization, frequent pleasant social exchanges, and communication training, which successfully reduced all his problem behaviors.

DEVELOPING HYPOTHESIS STATEMENTS

After the functional assessment data have been interpreted and summarized, the next step is to develop a hypothesis statement (e.g., Kern, 2005). The purpose of a hypothesis statement is to provide a succinct summary of the findings from the FBA process (APBS, 2007, V-F 1). This is an important step because it links the assessment information to the support plan. In other words, it helps to ensure that the data gathered are explicitly considered and linked to intervention selection. By narrowing the events associated with problem behavior in this manner, classes of interventions can be identified that have a high likelihood of reducing problem behavior.

Hypothesis statements can be written in many different ways. The specific format is not as important as the content. A hypothesis statement should contain three pieces of information (APBS, 2007, V-F 2): First, it should describe events that occur before the problem behavior. This includes both antecedents and setting events, should they be present. Second, the hypothesis statement should describe the problem behavior of concern. In situations where there are multiple target behaviors that serve different functions, a separate hypothesis should be developed for each target behavior. Third, the hypothesis statement should state the assumed function of the problem behavior.

Generally, hypothesis statements present the antecedent, behavior, and function in sequential order. The typical format is, "When [*setting event* or *antecedent*] occurs, [*individual's name*] engages in [*problem behavior*], to [*presumed function*]." A few example hypotheses follow: When presented with a math worksheet (*antecedent*), Sara rips

her paper (*behavior*) to avoid completing the worksheet (*presumed function*). When a peer is playing with an item Jane wants (*antecedent*), she grabs it (*behavior*) to gain access to the item (*presumed function*). When Steve has not slept well and is tired (*setting event*) and the environment becomes loud and busy (*antecedent*), he screams repeatedly (*behavior*) in order to escape by having staff remove him to a quieter location (*presumed function*).

There are several guidelines for developing hypotheses that will help a team stay on track and facilitate intervention selection and support plan development (Kern & Dunlap, 1999). First, the hypothesis should specify environmental variables that can be manipulated to form an intervention. Teams sometimes draw conclusions about an individual's problem behavior because of his or her disability status or psychiatric diagnosis. For example, a team might conclude the following in a hypothesis statement: "Gia engages in self-stimulatory behavior because she has autism," or "During academic tasks, Reece exhibits off-task behavior because he has ADHD." As we noted, the purpose of an FBA is to identify environmental variables associated with problem behavior so that modifications that can be made to reduce problem behavior. Behavior characteristics associated with particular disabilities or psychiatric diagnoses do not eliminate the possibility that behavior problems occur for environmental reasons. Furthermore, environmental supports can reduce problem behaviors, even if there are biological mechanisms involved; therefore, these are not useful hypothesis statements.

A second guideline essential for hypothesis development is that the hypothesis should reflect the data collected (APBS, 2007, II-B 4 and 5). Team members have different histories with the individual exhibiting problem behavior, as well as diverse experiences and philosophies. These are immense attributes to a team; however, they sometimes interfere with a team member's ability to objectively evaluate data. For example, a child psychiatrist may strongly believe that an adolescent's depression is biological and fail to see the environmental events that trigger episodes of depression as well as settings where depressive symptoms are diminished. Regardless of a team member's presupposition about the function of behavior, the hypothesis ultimately must be consistent with the data.

The third guideline for hypothesis development is that teams should agree that a hypothesis is parsimonious and reasonable (APBS, 2007, II-B 3). If FBA data were always consistent and crystal clear, the process would be simple. However, this is rarely the case. Instead, teams almost always need to come to consensus that the hypothesis is reasonable and logical, based on the available information. If team members disagree that the hypothesis is reasonable and the most logical representation of the data, additional dialogue is needed. Generally, it is advised that teams review the data to assess whether all team members have interpreted them accurately or whether additional data are needed to clarify ambiguities. When consensus is achieved regarding the accuracy and reasonability of the hypothesis, team members can be assured they are working toward common goals.

To illustrate the procedure of developing hypotheses based on functional assessment information, we revisit our case studies for Max and Lucas. Recall that Max's assessment data indicated that his problem behaviors were associated with tasks that required writing. Thus the following hypothesis was developed: When given an assignment where Max is expected to write (*antecedent*), he throws and kicks materials and curses (*behavior*) to avoid or escape the writing task (*presumed function*).

For Lucas, the team identified a setting event that was associated with problem behavior, with the following hypothesis: When Lucas stays up past 11:30 p.m. watching movies (*setting event*) and is presented with lengthy tasks at work (*antecedent*), he sits with his head down in the corner or leaves the task (*behavior*) to escape (*presumed function*).

CONCLUSION

A thorough functional assessment often yields a great deal of information that may appear unwieldy. Therefore, an important step in the assessment and intervention development process is to systematically organize and summarize the information. Data can be summarized in graphic or tabular format. This allows the data to be easily reviewed to identify patterns associated with both challenging and appropriate behavior. There are instances, however, when data patterns are not evident. In these cases, a number of alternatives can be considered, such as reviewing historical data, examining precursors to problem behavior, and determining whether all behavioral topographies serve the same function.

After data have been summarized and interpreted, hypotheses should be developed. Hypotheses serve as a succinct summary of the assessment data and link the functional assessment to related interventions. In other words, hypotheses ensure that teams have appropriately summarized data so that events associated with behavior have been parceled out and function has been presumed. In addition, accurate hypotheses help a team readily develop a support plan. It is critical that these steps are carefully followed so that a support plan is truly linked to the functional assessment data. Support plans derived in this way are highly likely to effectively reduce problem behavior and therefore are likely to be maintained.

Finally, as we suggested, the process of conducting the functional assessment and interpreting and summarizing the data that emerge is best achieved through a team process. Data interpretation is sometimes accomplished through consensus, and respecting diverse perspectives from all key stakeholders is critical for a full understanding of the individual and the circumstances surrounding his or her problem behavior. The result will be an informed plan that is acceptable to all invested parties and offers a good contextual fit.

REFERENCES

Association for Positive Behavior Support (APBS). (2007). *Positive behavior support standards of practice: Individual level.* Retrieved from http://www.apbs.org/files/apbs_standards_of_practice_2013_format.pdf

Bambara, L.M., Nonnemaker, S., & Koger, F. (2005). Teaming. In L.M. Bambara & L. Kern (Eds.), *Individualized supports for students with problem behaviors* (pp. 71–106). New York, NY: Guilford Press.

Carr, E.G., & Horner, R.H. (2007). The expanding vision of positive behavior support research perspectives on happiness, helpfulness, hopefulness. *Journal of Positive Behavior Intervention, 9,* 3–14. doi:10.1177/1098300707009001201

Hall, S., Thorns, T., & Oliver, C. (2003). Structural and environmental characteristics of stereotyped behaviors. *American Journal on Mental Retardation, 108,* 391–402. doi:10.1352/0895-8017

Horner, R.H., Vaughn, B.J., Day, H.M., & Ard, W.R. (1996). The relationship between setting events and problem behavior: Expanding our understanding of behavioral support. In L.K. Koegel, R.L. Koegel, & G. Dunlap (Eds.), *Positive behavioral support: Including people with difficult behavior in the community* (pp. 381–402). Baltimore, MD: Paul H. Brookes Publishing Co.

Iwata, B.A., Pace, G.M., Dorsey, M.F., Zarcone, J.R., Vollmer, T.R., Smith, R.G., . . . Willis, K.D. (1994). The functions of self-injurious behavior: An experimental-epidemiological analysis. *Journal of Applied Behavior Analysis, 27,* 215–240. doi:10.1901/jaba.1994.27-215

Kamps, D., Wendland, M., & Culpepper, M. (2006, February). Active teacher participation in functional behavior assessment for students with emotional and behavioral disorders risks in general education classrooms. *Behavioral Disorders, 41,* 128–146. Retrieved from http://www.ccbd.net/behavioraldisorders/Journal/index.cfm

Kennedy, C.H., & Itkonen, T. (1993). Effects of setting events on the problem behavior of students with severe disabilities. *Journal of Applied Behavior Analysis, 26,* 321–327. doi:10.1901/jaba.1993.26-321

Kern, L. (2005). Developing hypothesis statements. In L.M. Bambara & L. Kern (Eds.), *Individualized supports for students with problem behaviors* (pp. 165–202). New York, NY: Guilford Press.

Kern, L., & Dunlap, G. (1999). Assessment-based interventions for children with emotional and behavioral

disorders. In A.C. Repp & R.H. Horner (Eds.), *Functional analysis of problem behavior: From effective assessment to effective support* (pp. 197–218). Florence, KY: Brooks/Cole.

Kern, L., Dunlap, G., Clarke, S., & Childs, K. (1994). Student-assisted functional assessment interview. *Diagnostique, 19,* 29–39.

Kern, L., O'Neill, R.E., & Starosta, K. (2004). Gathering functional assessment information. In L.M. Bambara & L. Kern (Eds.), *Individualized supports for students with problem behaviors* (pp. 129–164). New York, NY: Guilford Press.

O'Neill, R.E., Horner, R.H., Albin, R.W., Sprague, J.R., Storey, K., & Newton, J.S. (1997). Functional assessment and program development for problem behavior (2nd ed.). Pacific Grove, CA: Brooks/Cole.

Schalock, R.L., Brown, I., Brown, R., Cummins, R.A., Felce, D., Matikka, L., . . . Parmenter, T. (2002). Conceptualization, measurement, and application of quality of life for persons with intellectual disabilities: Report of an international panel of experts. *Mental Retardation, 40,* 457–470.

Scott, T., Bucalos, A., Liaupsin, C., Nelson, C., Jolivette, K., & Deshea, L. (2004, February). Using functional behavior assessment in general education settings: Making a case for effectiveness and efficiency. *Behavioral Disorders, 29,* 300–323. Retrieved from http://eric.ed.gov/?id=EJ772522

Scott, T., McIntyre, J., Liaupsin, C., Nelson, C., & Conroy, M. (2004, August). An examination of functional behavior assessment in public school settings: Collaborative teams, experts, and methodology. *Behavioral Disorders, 29,* 384–395. Retrieved from http://eric.ed.gov/?id=EJ772538

Shapiro, E., & Kratochwill, T. (2000). *Behavior assessment in schools* (2nd ed.). New York, NY: Guilford Press.

Shriver, M., Anderson, C., & Proctor, B. (2001). Evaluating the validity of functional behavior assessment. *School Psychology Review, 30*(2), 180–192.

Snell, M.E., & Janney, R. (2005). *Teachers' guides to inclusive practices: Collaborative teaming* (2nd ed.). Baltimore, MD: Paul H. Brookes Publishing Co.

Turnbull, H., Turnbull, A., Wehmeyer, M., & Park, J. (2003). A quality of life framework for special education outcomes. *Remedial and Special Education, 24,* 67–74. doi:10.1177/07419325030240020201

Wehmeyer, M., & Schalock, R. (2001). Self-determination and quality of life: Implications for special education services and supports. *Focus on Exceptional Children, 33*(8), 1–16.

Conducting Functional Analyses of Behavior

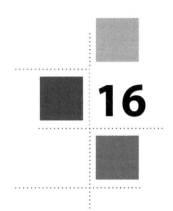

16

David P. Wacker, Wendy K. Berg, Brenda J. Bassingthwaite, Todd G. Kopelman,
Kelly M. Schieltz, Yaniz C. Padilla Dalmau, Scott D. Lindgren, and John F. Lee

In applied behavior analysis, the term *function* most often refers to the effect of behavior on the environment (Hanley, Iwata, & McCord, 2003). Thus, when describing a behavior, a behavior analyst might indicate that the behavior functions to produce consequences such as breaks from demands or access to attention or toys. In contrast to descriptions of behavior that focus on the form or topography of behavior (e.g., self-injury, aggression), a functional description provides a basis to treat the behavior using reinforcement techniques (Pelios, Morren, Tesch, & Axelrod, 1999).

Developers of positive behavior interventions and supports (PBIS) suggest this functional approach for assessing individuals who are classified at the tertiary level in their framework (Sugai et al., 2000). When behavior does not change as a result of the interventions put in place at the primary (universal) and secondary (specialized group) levels, specialized individual assessment focusing on the function of the behavior is warranted (Sugai et al., 2000). This is described as a functional behavior assessment (FBA). An FBA is a summary of the methods (e.g., interview, direct observation, and experimental analyses) used to obtain information regarding the function of a behavior (Cooper, Heron, & Heward, 2007).

Identifying the function of behavior identifies the reinforcers that most likely maintain the behavior. Thus, if behavior functions to escape demands, we might say that the behavior is reinforced by negative reinforcement in the form of escape from nonpreferred tasks (see Table 16.1).

In applied situations in which the goal is to reduce the occurrence of problem behavior, knowing the function of the behavior facilitates the development of effective reinforcement-based treatments in three ways. First, as shown in Table 16.1, identifying the function allows us to specify the reinforcers maintaining the behavior. We can develop

Table 16.1. Identified function of behavior, hypothesized reinforcement, and potential differential reinforcement procedures

Identified function	Hypothesized reinforcers	Examples of differential reinforcement procedures
Escape from demands	Negative reinforcement in the form of escaping from demands	Providing breaks contingent on requests (functional communication training; FCT) and/or task completion (differential reinforcement of alternative behavior)
Access to attention	Positive reinforcement in the form of receiving attention	Providing positive attention for specific requests and/or for playing independently for a specific period of time
Access to preferred toys/materials	Positive reinforcement in the form of receiving tangibles	Providing access to a toy (or other tangible) for an appropriate request and/or for playing with other toys (or materials) for a specified period of time

plans that provide the same reinforcer for desired behavior, such as making appropriate requests for breaks (e.g., Carr & Durand, 1985) instead of using inappropriate behaviors to get a break from completing a required task. Second, we can eliminate or reduce reinforcement following problem behavior with procedures such as noncontingent reinforcement, extinction, or punishment (e.g., Wacker, Steege, Northup, Sasso, et al., 1990). Third, we can identify the antecedent stimuli that are associated with the reinforcers maintaining problem behavior and use this information to design a treatment plan for the child. In particular, we can identify events that momentarily alter the value of a reinforcer and the occurrence of behaviors that result in the same reinforcer (*motivating operations;* Michael, 1982). For example, if we determine that a child shows problem behavior to escape schoolwork, we might alter the reinforcement for task engagement (e.g., provide high-quality attention) or the task (e.g., make it easier or more preferred) to influence the likelihood that the child will choose to complete the task rather than escape or avoid the task (Gardner, Wacker, & Boelter, 2009). Altering the reinforcers for completing a task or altering the task itself may abolish the student's motivation to escape the task and thus

reduce problem behaviors that are associated with negative reinforcement.

Being able to match treatment, especially reinforcement-based treatment, to the function of problem behavior is a major concern of behavior analysts, who emphasize the need to conduct functional analyses prior to treatment. A functional analysis should not be confused with an FBA. A functional analysis is the systematic manipulation of antecedents and consequences to test the hypothesized function through an experimental design (Cooper et al., 2007). A functional analysis may or may not be conducted as part of an FBA.

Sugai et al. (2000) suggested that a functional analysis is necessary when hypotheses are not confirmed through interviews or direct observations in the environment and when behaviors are resistant to treatment. We also support conducting a functional analysis prior to treatment when the problem behavior is severe (e.g., self-injury) and must be reduced as quickly as possible. Treatment that is implemented in a trial-and-error fashion might result in the inadvertent reinforcement of problem behavior. For example, if escape from demands is the functional reinforcer, then providing breaks (e.g., time-out) to a student who engages in problem behavior will likely reinforce or increase the future occurrence of that behavior.

In this chapter, we provide a brief historic overview of functional analysis procedures and then describe how we (as behavior analysts at the University of Iowa's Center for Disabilities and Development [CDD]) have applied functional analysis procedures to outpatient clinics, home settings, and school settings, as well as via teleconsultation. We discuss how these applications were implemented to address the needs of families and teachers in Iowa who lacked routine access to trained behavior analysts who could conduct functional analysis procedures in these settings.

OVERVIEW OF FUNCTIONAL ANALYSIS PROCEDURES

Carr (1977) provided a conceptual analysis to show how severe problem behaviors such as self-injury might function to obtain reinforcement. Carr's analysis was based on studies (e.g., Lovaas & Simmons, 1969) showing that self-injury was maintained by reinforcement. Subsequent studies (e.g., Carr, Newsom, & Binkhoff, 1980) continued to show the relation between problem behavior and reinforcement, but a systematic method for identifying the function of behavior for each individual was not available until the seminal publication by Iwata, Dorsey, Zarcone, et al. (1994).

Iwata et al. (1994) showed how different functions could be tested within a multi-element design (see Table 16.2). Test conditions for social positive reinforcement (attention), social negative reinforcement (escape from demands), and sensory reinforcement (alone time or isolation, simply indicated by the word *alone* from this point forward) were each conducted along with a control condition (free play). Conducting

Table 16.2. Example of test and control conditions in functional analysis

Condition	Purpose	Description	Conclusions
Free play	Control condition	Client is provided with non-contingent access to preferred items, activities, and attention; no demands are presented; and there are no programmed consequences for problem behavior.	If problem behavior observed, consider if free play was conducted with good integrity (e.g., Were demands presented?) or possible automatic function. If problem behavior not observed, free play serves as a control condition.
Attention	To test for social positive reinforcement	Attention is diverted from client and then is presented contingently for brief periods (e.g., 30 seconds) following problem behavior.	If problem behavior occurs at higher levels than free play, results indicate behavior is maintained by access to attention. If problem behavior not observed, behavior is not maintained by attention.
Escape	To test for social negative reinforcement	Demands are presented unless problem behavior is emitted. Problem behavior results in brief breaks (e.g., 30 seconds).	If problem behavior occurs at higher levels than free play, results indicate behavior is maintained by escape or avoidance of demands. If problem behavior is not observed, behavior is not maintained by escape or avoidance.
Alone	To test for sensory or automatic reinforcement	Client is alone or ignored and does not have access to social stimuli.	If problem behavior occurs more often in this condition than in free play, behavior may be maintained by automatic reinforcement. If problem behavior is not observed, behavior may not be maintained by automatic reinforcement.

Source: Iwata, Dorsey, Slifer, Bauman, and Richman (1982/1994).

these four conditions multiple times in a counterbalanced or random order makes it possible to identify whether problem behavior functions to obtain negative, positive, or automatic reinforcement by comparing the magnitudes and trends in behavior across sessions and conditions (Hagopian et al., 1997).

A number of early researchers using functional analysis procedures showed that treatments matched to function were often successful in reducing problem behaviors (Hanley et al., 2003; Iwata et al., 1994), and these reductions often were achieved with reinforcement-based procedures (Pelios et al., 1999). Subsequent researchers provided variations of the procedures that included analyses of antecedent variables (e.g., Carr & Durand, 1985); additional test conditions (e.g., tangible condition; Carr & Durand, 1985); brief versions of functional analyses (e.g., Northup et al., 1991); biologic variables (e.g., O'Reilly, 1995); and applications to different subgroups (e.g., typically developing children; Cooper, Wacker, Sasso, Reimers, & Donn, 1990), settings (e.g., homes; Wacker et al., 1998), and delivery systems (e.g., teleconsultation; Barretto, Wacker, Harding, Lee, & Berg, 2006). Each of these variations successfully showed that problem behaviors often produced changes in the environment that served to reinforce those behaviors. These successful applications occurred despite numerous changes in the way functional analyses were conducted (e.g., Wallace & Iwata, 1999), and they were replicated across multiple research teams working in a wide variety of settings (Neef, 1994). Hundreds of examples of functional analyses have been published (Beavers, Iwata, & Lerman, 2013), which continues to strengthen the applied merits of conducting these procedures as part of evidence-based intervention. Recent epidemiological and review articles (e.g., Beavers et al., 2013) have shown that functional analyses continue to be applied successfully across settings (e.g., public schools; Mueller, Nkosi, & Hine, 2011), subgroups (e.g., typically developing children; Gardner,

Spencer, Boelter, DuBard, & Jennett, 2012), and delivery systems (e.g., teleconsultation; Wacker et al., 2013).

CONDUCTING FUNCTIONAL ANALYSES IN OUTPATIENT CLINICS

One of the first novel applications of functional analysis was the development of brief functional analyses conducted in outpatient clinics with both children and adults with disabilities (Northup et al., 1991) and children with typical development (Cooper et al., 1990). Outpatient behavior services are typically scheduled for a one-time 90-minute to 120-minute period, which severely limits the procedures that can be conducted. Cooper et al. (1990) and Northup et al. (1991) adapted the functional analysis procedures described by Carr and Durand (1985) and Iwata et al. (1994), respectively, to assessments that could be completed within one 90-minute outpatient evaluation. The same test and control conditions used in an extended functional analysis were included, but the length of each test session was reduced to 5 minutes from 15 minutes, and each test condition was conducted only once or twice. The abbreviated procedures are referred to as *brief functional analyses*. In response to concerns regarding short session lengths and few-to-no repetitions of test conditions relative to identifying the correct function of problem behavior, Wallace and Iwata (1999) compared the results of functional analyses in which only the first 5 minutes, the first 10 minutes, and the full 15 minutes of each test session were used to identify the function of problem behavior. The results from the 10-minute sessions were identical to the results from the 15-minute sessions, and the results from the 5-minute sessions matched 93% of the analyses from the 15-minute sessions. Wallace and Iwata concluded that shorter sessions could be used to increase the efficiency of a functional analysis without reducing the accuracy of the analysis in clinical situations. Similarly, Kahng and Iwata (1999) compared results using single sessions to results of extended functional analyses and reported that the results from single session analyses corresponded with extended analyses in 66% of the cases. Derby et al. (1992) showed that the major limitation of brief functional analyses is *false negatives*—that is, problem behavior may not occur during the relevant test condition of the outpatient evaluation. When problem behavior is displayed, brief functional analyses are efficient and effective procedures for identifying reinforcers that maintain problem behavior for people with (Derby et al., 1992) and without (Gardner et al., 2012) developmental disabilities.

Outpatient Procedures and Case Example

Figure 16.1 depicts a typical sequence of activities that we follow to conduct a behavior evaluation in outpatient clinics at the CDD within a limited amount of time.

Individuals are referred to the outpatient service by their primary care physicians, parents, classroom teachers, or other support personnel. The outpatient service is staffed by a multidisciplinary team, including behavior analysts, a nurse practitioner, a social worker, and a speech and language therapist, that reviews the patient's medical records before the evaluation. Information about the specific behaviors of concern and the conditions under which the behaviors are most likely to occur is obtained from an antecedent-behavior-consequence (ABC) structured parent interview and the record review. Given the time constraints of an outpatient evaluation, this information is reviewed prior to the appointment to maximize the amount of time available for conducting the evaluation. The purpose of the ABC interview is to gather information that will lead to hypotheses about the environmental conditions under which the target behavior is likely to occur and

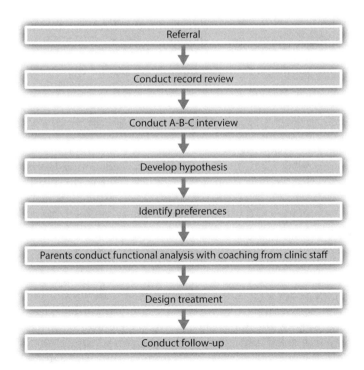

Figure 16.1. Sequence of activities conducted in outpatient clinics for severe problem behavior.

the consequences that may reinforce and therefore increase the occurrence of the target behavior. The 90-minute evaluation is devoted to testing the hypotheses and then matching the treatment to the results of the brief functional analysis (Wacker, Steege, Northup, Reimers, et al., 1990).

Each evaluation begins with a preference assessment conducted within a free-play condition (Roane, Vollmer, Ringdahl, & Marcus, 1998) to identify preferred items and at least one nonpreferred activity for the demand session. After one or two items are identified as preferred, the brief functional analysis is initiated and is usually conducted by parents with coaching provided by clinic staff. As described by Wacker, Berg, Harding, and Cooper-Brown (2004), the brief functional analysis begins with the test condition hypothesized to be correlated with problem behavior based on the ABC interview. Sessions last 5 minutes and are conducted within a multielement design. Data on the occurrence of problem behavior are recorded using a 6-second partial-interval scoring system. The 5-minute session is divided into fifty 6-second intervals. Problem behavior is recorded within the interval in which it occurs. The number of intervals scored with problem behavior is divided by the total number of intervals scored, and this number is multiplied by 100 to give us the percentage of intervals with problem behavior. The results from each session are plotted on a graph and compared with the results from the control condition and every other test condition. Test sessions that are clearly differentiated as being higher than the control condition and other test conditions are identified as the *function* for the behavior. The results of the analysis are used to select a treatment to reduce problem behavior and increase appropriate behavior.

An example of this assessment is provided in Figure 16.2. Kazi, a 20-month-old girl with developmental delay and speech delay, was referred to the outpatient service by her physician to address her self-injurious behaviors and tantrums that occurred throughout the day. Kazi showed a pattern of problem behavior that began with crying and quickly escalated to screaming and self-injury (e.g., pulling her hair and scratching herself). For the purposes of the outpatient evaluation, we used crying and screaming as the target behaviors for the functional analysis. The behaviors were part of a response chain that resulted in self-injury, and providing reinforcers contingent on these more mild forms of problem behavior averted the self-injurious behaviors. Based on information provided by Kazi's parents, we hypothesized that she engaged in problem behavior to gain or maintain parent attention. The brief functional analysis began with a play session during which Kazi received her mother's undivided attention and access to toys. As expected, no problem behavior occurred during the play condition (i.e., shown with the shaded circle on Figure 16.2). To test our hypothesis that Kazi showed problem behavior to gain adult attention, we let Kazi play with the preferred toys but had her mother turn away from her to talk with a therapist (i.e., attention condition, shown with the open squares in Figure 16.2) unless she cried or screamed. If she cried or screamed, her mother attended to her for about 20 seconds. Kazi screamed each time her mother turned away from her.

A second attention session was conducted to confirm the role of parent attention as a functional reinforcer for Kazi, and she showed similar levels of problem behavior. We returned to the control condition (i.e., play), and problem behaviors decreased as the session progressed. An escape condition was conducted next (shown with the shaded triangle in Figure 16.2). Kazi's mother directed her to complete a simple task (e.g., put a block in a tub). Each time Kazi screamed, the task was withdrawn for 20 seconds and then reintroduced. Initially, Kazi was placed on the mat next to her mother to perform the task. Kazi screamed and attempted to climb onto her mother's lap for the first few minutes of the escape session. Her behavior did

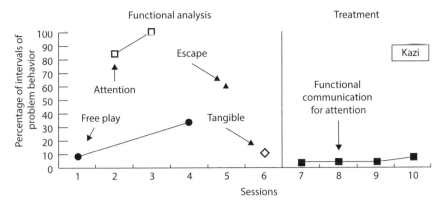

Figure 16.2. Results of brief functional analysis and treatment trials completed for Kazi during an outpatient visit, showing that behavior was maintained by attention and that functional communication training (FCT) was effective for reducing problem behavior.

not appear to be affected by the presentation or removal of the task. Kazi was allowed to sit on her mother's lap to perform the task for the final few minutes of the escape session, and she completed the remaining demands without problem behavior. Thus specific types of attention abolished her motivation to escape the task.

A tangible session was conducted last (shown with the open diamond in Figure 16.2). Kazi sat on her mother's lap and played with a preferred toy prior to the start of the session. At the start of the session, her mother set the toy on the floor and offered Kazi a less preferred toy. Kazi was cooperative with exchanging toys and showed very little problem behavior. The results of the brief functional analysis showed that the attention test condition resulted in the highest levels of problem behavior across all conditions, and we determined that Kazi showed problem behavior to gain parent attention. Problem behavior was elevated during the demand session as well, but our observations showed that problem behavior occurred when Kazi was taken off her mother's lap and her behavior did not vary with the presentation and removal of the demand.

Functional communication training (FCT) to teach Kazi a better way to gain parent attention was selected as the treatment

strategy (closed squares on Figure 16.2). The speech therapist working in the clinic showed Kazi how to use a voice output switch to ask for her mother's attention. During the first FCT session, Kazi remained on her mother's lap while the therapist prompted her to press the switch. Pressing the switch resulted in praise and a hug from her mother. Over the course of the first three FCT sessions, Kazi progressed from sitting on her mother's lap to sitting several feet away from her mother and crawling several feet to reach the switch. She consistently pressed the switch with minimal prompting and reached toward her mother after pressing the switch.

Challenges in Conducting Functional Analyses in Outpatient Settings

Conducting functional analyses in outpatient clinics can be challenging. One challenge we frequently encounter is the absence of problem behavior. Derby et al. (1992) showed that problem behavior occurred in only 63% of cases evaluated in an outpatient clinic, thus leaving 37% of cases in which problem behavior did not occur within the time-limited clinical outpatient setting. Some reasons problem behavior is not consistently observed in an outpatient setting may be that 1) the individual receives high levels of attention from caregivers en route to and during the appointment and thus the individual's motivation to engage in behavior maintained by attention is abolished; 2) the setting, people, and materials in the clinical setting are novel to the individual, which may disrupt ongoing behavior; and 3) the clinical setting does not contain one or more environmental variables that evoke or reinforce behavior (e.g., the way instructions are delivered, specific noises, access to peers). One option to address this problem is to conduct the analyses in home, school, and community settings (Durand & Carr, 1992), as discussed in the following sections.

A second challenge occurs with low-frequency behaviors. Behaviors that occur infrequently (e.g., less than once per day) are less likely to occur within the limited probes that can be conducted within a 90-minute evaluation. Behaviors that last for an extended period of time (e.g., longer than 15 minutes) are also difficult to address within an outpatient setting. The brief functional analysis requires rapid alternation between 5-minute functional analysis sessions and is best suited for behaviors with a brief onset and offset.

One alternative for evaluating the function of low-frequency or long-duration behaviors is to use a concurrent operant's assessment (COA) to identify social reinforcers for appropriate behavior. A COA uses an individual's choices from among concurrently available social reinforcers to identify the individual's relative preferences (Berg, Wacker, Harding, Ganzer, & Barretto, 2007; Harding et al., 1999), without relying on the occurrence of problem behavior. When highly preferred social reinforcers are identified, these reinforcers can be provided contingent on the occurrence of an appropriate response and withheld for problem behavior. However, this assumes that the reinforcers identified are either the same as those identified via a functional analysis or powerful enough to compete against those reinforcers. Some studies (e.g., Harding et al., 1999) have

shown that these reinforcers can compete effectively, but this is still an inference that must be made.

A COA was used for a 21-year-old man, Saunders, who was referred to an outpatient clinic following a 2-week admission to a psychiatric hospital for aggression, destruction, and vocal threats. According to group home staff, episodes of problem behavior occurred without warning and typically lasted 20 to 60 minutes. The length of individual episodes of problem behavior precluded the use of a brief functional analysis in the outpatient setting. COA sessions were presented to Saunders vocally, and he was allowed to make his selection with vocal statements. Saunders was given choices between events such as 1) working alone or hanging out with staff with preferred activities and 2) doing a work task with a staff member or doing a preferred activity alone. A clinician presented a series of four choices to Saunders and then repeated the four choices. Saunders chose the alternative that included staff attention regardless of the activity. These results showed that staff attention was very important to Saunders and could be a reinforcer for behavior. Based on these results, recommendations were made to provide positive social attention to Saunders for appropriate behavior throughout the day and to use FCT to teach him appropriate ways to request attention. Recommendations also included directions to withdraw attention to the degree possible when problem behavior occurred.

Another challenge with brief functional analyses occurs when behaviors are not maintained by social consequences. Some individuals engage in the target behavior across every assessment condition, and the behavior does not appear to be affected by the presentation or removal of social reinforcers. Other individuals may show the behavior only when they are alone or have nothing to do. The term *automatic reinforcement* (Vaughan & Michael, 1982) is used to describe the function of target behavior that is not socially mediated. The limited time available during an outpatient assessment is likely to prevent an adequate evaluation to rule out the role of social reinforcers for an individual's behavior. However, a pairwise assessment in which a free play condition is alternated with an alone condition may provide information that either supports or refutes a hypothesis of automatic reinforcement. During the alone condition, the person remains in the room alone and no consequences are provided for problem or appropriate behavior. Removing other people from the room removes discriminative stimuli associated with gaining a reaction for the behavior. Depending on the behaviors in question, leisure materials may remain in the room or be removed. If behavior continues to occur during multiple sessions of the alone condition, then the hypothesis that behavior is not socially mediated is supported. For example, a young child was referred to the outpatient service to address his behavior, which included throwing items such as toys, clothing, magazines, and anything within reach. His parents questioned if he threw items to get a reaction from them or simply because he liked to throw things. The frequency of throwing objects during a play session with parents present was compared with the frequency of throwing items when the child was alone. The child continued to throw items at similar levels across the two conditions, indicating that throwing did not serve a social function and was likely maintained by automatic reinforcement. In contrast, a young woman was referred to the outpatient service for standing next to walls and talking to herself about events that had not occurred. Care providers were concerned that the woman was delusional. The woman's comments were observed via a remote camera as she visited with her care providers to determine the frequency of concerning comments. During a subsequent session, the care providers left the woman by herself for an alone session. All comments stopped after the care providers left the room. The onset of self-talk with care providers present

and the lack of self-talk when left alone suggested that the woman's comments most likely served a social function. If behaviors occur across all the functional analysis conditions except the alone condition, then other hypotheses, such as those suggesting that the individual is not discriminating between functional analysis conditions, need to be considered and addressed.

The evolution of brief functional analyses continues to occur, in an attempt to address the many challenges of conducting these procedures. For example, several researchers (Boelter et al., 2007; Call, Wacker, Ringdahl, Cooper-Brown, & Boelter, 2004; Gardner et al., 2009) developed assessments that show the conditions under which demands lead to compliance or problem behavior. Gardner et al. (2009) conducted a brief functional analysis of problem behavior with typically developing children and showed that high-quality praise for compliance eliminated the children's motivation to escape demands.

The results of these and other studies have shown that parents can conduct functional analysis procedures with coaching provided by trained behavior analysts in clinical settings. These results suggested another application of functional analysis procedures—parents as therapists for their young children in home settings.

CONDUCTING FUNCTIONAL ANALYSES IN HOME SETTINGS

We conducted four National Institutes of Health (NIH)–funded multiyear studies (Wacker & Berg, 1992; Wacker, Berg, & Harding, 1996, 2000, 2004), from 1991 to 2010, in which parents with young children with a developmental disability (e.g., intellectual disability, autism spectrum disorders, genetic syndromes) and destructive behavior (e.g., aggression, self-injury, property destruction) conducted functional analyses in their homes (Wacker et al., 1998). The parents conducted all functional analysis procedures and received in-person coaching from a trained behavior analyst during weekly to monthly 1-hour visits (Berg et al., 2007; Derby et al., 1997; Harding, Wacker, Berg, Lee, & Dolezal, 2009; Wacker et al., 1998). The behavioral analysts were located at the CDD and the University of Iowa Children's Hospital and traveled up to 150 miles to work with the participants and their parents.

Prior to conducting the functional analyses, the behavior analysts completed indirect and descriptive assessments with the parents using procedures that were similar to those conducted in the outpatient clinics. These included a parent interview, daily behavior record, behavior rating form, and preference assessment. After completing these assessments, the behavior analysts coached the parents to implement four conditions as part of the functional analysis: free play (control), attention, escape, and tangible. A detailed description of parent coaching and functional analysis procedures can be found in Harding et al. (2009). Most conditions were repeated at least three times using 5-minute sessions that were conducted in a counterbalanced order.

Summary of Findings and Case Example

During the 19 years of these projects, parents completed a total of 95 functional analyses, and social functions for target behaviors were identified for 85% of the participants. An example of one of these functional analyses is presented in Figure 16.3. Diego was a 4-year-old boy diagnosed with a developmental delay. Diego's problem behavior consisted of self-injury (e.g., head hitting, pinching, head banging) and aggression (e.g., head butting, kicking, hitting). Diego did not engage in problem behavior during the free play or attention conditions. In comparison, Diego displayed elevated levels of problem behavior during the escape condition, suggesting that his problem behavior was maintained by escape from demands.

Findings from the in-home studies provided strong support for a model in which parents are trained to conduct functional analyses in their homes, which decreases the possibility of false negative findings (discussed previously) for brief functional analyses conducted in outpatient settings (Derby et al., 1992). For some parents, the option of conducting the evaluation at home is preferred because of the economic or practical difficulties associated with traveling to a clinical setting.

CONDUCTING FUNCTIONAL ANALYSES VIA TELEHEALTH

Despite several potential advantages, conducting functional analyses in the home presents its own set of challenges. In the studies conducted by Wacker et al. (Wacker & Berg, 1992; Wacker, Berg, & Harding, 1996, 2000, 2004), participants lived within a 150-mile radius of the project site. To serve participants who lived on the extremes of this radius, the behavior analysts spent more time traveling to and from the homes than conducting the functional analysis procedures, which increased the costs associated with the process. In many rural states such as Iowa, the number of referrals for behavior evaluations can surpass the ability of trained behavior analysts to meet the demand (Wacker et al., 2013). A model in which behavior analysts are required to travel long distances regularly to conduct functional analyses may not be sustainable because of concerns about efficiency and financial viability.

For these reasons, we began to focus on conducting functional analysis procedures through telehealth methodology. The use of telehealth to conduct functional analyses may provide benefits related to efficiency and convenience for both families and clinicians (Barretto et al., 2006). Within the field of medicine, telehealth has been used by multiple subspecialties, including psychiatry, pediatrics, cardiology, internal medicine, and obstetrics and gynecology, and

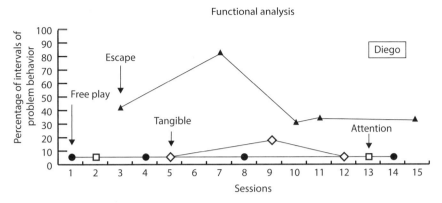

Figure 16.3. Results of functional analysis completed with Diego in his home, showing that his problem behavior was maintained by escape from nonpreferred activities.

it is also being used to deliver services in areas with limited medical resources (e.g., Holden & Dew, 2008; Singh & Das, 2010; Whitten & Buis, 2008). Telehealth has been associated with several positive outcomes, including improved access to medical care, high reported levels of patient and caregiver satisfaction, and reduced health care costs. Specific to children and adolescents, studies have indicated that telehealth can be conducted in a range of settings and is acceptable for both physicians and caregivers (Myers, Valentine, & Melzer, 2007; Nesbitt, Marcin, Dasbach, & Cole, 2005; Shore & Manson, 2005). For behavior analysts, telehealth may increase the geographical radius across which procedures such as functional analyses can be conducted and help to meet the need for services.

Previous Telehealth Studies

Barretto et al. (2006) conducted the first telehealth study in the field of applied behavior analysis. Using a fiber-optic tele-communications network, brief functional analyses were conducted with two children. During both evaluations, the behavior analysts were located at a tertiary-level hospital, and the child, care provider, and local service team were located at either a local school or a department of human services office. Through telehealth, the behavior

analysts provided ongoing consultation to the parents and local team on how to implement the functional analysis procedures. Clear social functions for the behaviors of concern were identified for both children. These results were the first to indicate that caregivers could be trained to conduct functional analysis procedures remotely through telehealth.

Machalicek et al. (2009) conducted functional analyses with two school-age children with autism using telehealth. The functional analyses were conducted in the school setting by graduate students who did not have previous experience with this procedure. The graduate students received coaching through telehealth on how to implement the functional analysis procedures from graduate students with extensive behavioral experience who were physically located in the same school building. Similar to the findings of Barretto et al. (2006), clear social functions were identified for both children. Following the telehealth functional analysis, classroom interventions were developed and implemented that led to a reduction in problem behaviors and an increase in academic engagement for both children.

Wacker and colleagues (2013) conducted functional analyses via telehealth with 20 children diagnosed with autism spectrum disorders. The functional analyses were conducted by the children's parents in regional health care clinics with remote live coaching from a behavioral consultant and on-site support from a parent assistant with no previous training in behavior analysis. The functional analysis procedures used in this study were based on those previously conducted in the home (as described by Harding et al., 2009, and as summarized in Wacker et al., 1998). Clear social functions were identified for 18 out of the 20 children. Conducting functional analyses via telehealth was found to be a more cost- and time-effective service delivery model than delivering the services in person. In addition, parents rated the acceptability of telehealth-based functional analyses as highly as when the functional analyses were conducted in home settings with coaching from therapists. This study demonstrated that parents in a clinical setting could conduct functional analyses effectively and safely without the presence of an on-site behavior analyst.

Current Telehealth Project and Case Example from 2012

Our group is currently (2011–2015) evaluating the use of telehealth in home settings to conduct functional analyses (Lindgren & Wacker, 2011). Participants in this study are young children (18 months to 6 years) with autism spectrum disorders who engage in challenging behaviors. Necessary telehealth equipment (i.e., a laptop computer, webcam, Ethernet cables) is shipped to the participant's home, and the caregivers are provided with assistance in setting up the equipment, if needed. During weekly 60-minute appointments, the caregivers receive remote coaching from behavior consultants in conducting functional analysis sessions similar to those described by Wacker et al. (2013). All functional analysis sessions are recorded, scored, and graphed. Data are also collected on variables such as the severity of the child's disruptive behavior and family factors that may influence assessment and treatment outcomes.

A case example is presented in Figure 16.4 to illustrate the results of the functional analyses conducted via telehealth in a child's home by her mother. Tera, a 6-year-old girl diagnosed with pervasive developmental disorder, engaged in aggression (e.g., hitting) and property destruction (e.g., throwing toys). The functional analysis consisted of four conditions: free play, attention, escape, and tangible. Tera did not engage in problem behavior during the free play and attention conditions. In contrast, she displayed elevated levels of problem behavior during the escape and tangible conditions, suggesting that her aggression and property destruction were maintained by access to her preferred tangible items and escape from demands.

The use of telehealth to conduct functional analyses is still in its early stages. Research conducted to date indicates that

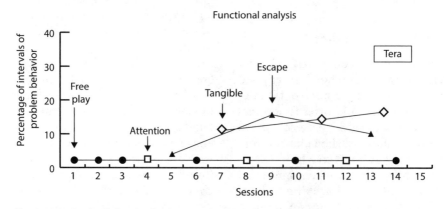

Figure 16.4. Results of a functional analysis completed with Tera via teleconsultation, showing that her problem behavior was maintained by access to tangibles and escape from demands.

parents can be coached remotely to conduct functional analyses successfully, social functions can be identified for the majority of participants, parents find the use of telehealth to be very acceptable, and telehealth is more cost effective compared with a model in which functional analyses are conducted by clinicians in the home setting. These initial findings are promising and suggest that telehealth may be a viable option for families and clinicians in the evaluation of severe problem behaviors. Behavior analysts need to ensure that they and the families possess the necessary telehealth equipment (i.e., computer, webcam, high-speed Internet) to securely and reliably conduct sessions. Even when the technology is available, it may take parents and children some time to adjust to conducting behavior sessions via telehealth. For example, in Wacker et al. (2013), additional free play sessions were conducted to allow the participants to adapt to the technology and the clinic space. Although no safety concerns have been reported in the literature, clinicians should be cautious when conducting procedures such as functional analyses remotely. Clinicians should consider the possibility that an individual will engage in behavior that places him or her or others at risk of injury and should not conduct sessions if adequate safeguards cannot be arranged. On a practical level, clinicians should consider whether parents have the support available to work with their child without distractions, such as frequent interruptions from other children.

CONDUCTING FUNCTIONAL ANALYSES IN SCHOOL SETTINGS

Another logical extension of functional analysis methods is for researchers to integrate functional analyses into school programs (Mueller et al., 2011). Schools, particularly those located in rural areas, often have very limited access to trained behavior analysts. For this reason, we have been actively involved in training school teams in Iowa to conduct functional analyses in the schools.

Mandates to conduct FBAs were one of many changes to assessment activities in educational settings that were part of the 1997 Individuals with Disabilities Education Act (IDEA; PL 105-17). Educators turned to the field of applied behavior analysis as they developed procedures to carry out these mandates and adequately address students' challenging behaviors (Barnhill, 2005). School-based FBAs are often conducted using indirect assessments (e.g., interviews, behavior-rating scales) and direct descriptive assessments (e.g., ABC observations, scatterplot analysis). In a review of 71 FBAs across the state of Wisconsin, Van Acker, Boreson, Gable, and Potterton (2005) found that 90% of the FBAs used indirect data collection methods, 49% used direct observation methods, and 15% used functional analysis methods.

Barriers to Conducting Functional Analyses in School Settings

There are several reasons more functional analyses are not conducted in school settings as part of an FBA. Following IDEA 1997 (PL 105-17), school personnel were cautioned about using functional analyses because the field of functional analysis research was perceived as narrow (Gresham, Quinn, & Restori, 1999). Cautions included the following: 1) assessments were conducted primarily in analog settings rather than natural environments; 2) assessments primarily included individuals who had severe to profound intellectual disabilities, rather than individuals who were typically developing or who had mild disabilities; and 3) the primary behavior evaluated was self-injury rather than other common behaviors (e.g., destruction, aggression, noncompliance; Gresham et al., 1999). More recent reviews of the literature (2003–2011), however, have demonstrated positive results from utilizing functional analyses in a variety of naturalistic settings; with a variety of individuals with and without developmental disabilities; and with a variety of topographies of behaviors, suggesting that cautions about a narrow evidence base for functional analysis are unwarranted. (See Hanley et al., 2003, for a general review of the literature of functional analyses; Gardner et al., 2012, for a review specific to using brief functional analysis procedures with children who are typically developing; and Mueller et al., 2011, for a summary article on conducting functional analyses in schools.)

There are numerous examples of functional analyses being conducted in school settings. Ervin et al. (2001) reviewed 100 articles published between 1980 and 1999 that described school-based functional assessment. Ninety percent of the published assessments included an experimental analysis (i.e., experimental manipulation of antecedents or consequences or both). However, Ervin et al. (2001) noted that the "experimenter" (i.e., the author) conducted the analysis in 52% of the assessments and with school personnel in 14% of the assessments. Only 21% of the school personnel implemented the procedures independently. Mueller et al. (2011) summarized 90 functional analyses that were conducted with 69 students in school settings between 2006 and 2009. In this sample, a "trained behavioral consultant" manipulated the variables in the analyses 80% of the time. Teachers, paraprofessionals, or school system behavioral specialists served as therapists 20% of the time after being trained by the consultant.

One reason that functional analyses are not conducted more often in school settings is the lack of training in functional analysis procedures by individuals who hold responsibility for conducting the FBAs (Iwata et al., 2000). Thus it should not be surprising that a 2011 survey of general education teachers' awareness of different behavior assessment and intervention procedures indicated that 56% of the teachers were not sure whether someone in their school system could conduct an FBA or develop and implement an intervention (Stormont, Reinke, & Herman, 2011).

A Training Service for School Consultants: The Challenging Behavior Service

In Iowa, professionals who provide special education support services (e.g., school psychologists, school social workers, occupational therapists) for behavior and academics are hired by nine area education agencies (AEAs). The Iowa Department of Education awarded funds to each AEA to hire two full-time employees to partake in an AEA challenging behavior team, looking to increase the number of AEA professionals trained in behavior assessment. The Iowa Department of Education also contracted with the CDD in 2009 to provide training to these challenging behavior teams. We trained these teams to conduct functional analyses so that they could consult more effectively with school teams regarding assessment and programming for students who engage in challenging behavior. Prior to this project, only three AEAs had challenging behavior teams.

We provided training to the challenging behavior teams for 4 years in skill content areas of data tools (data collection, graphing, data analysis) and behavior-assessment procedures (preference assessment, functional analyses, antecedent analyses, COA). Although didactic training through a workshop or other professional development activity and via follow-up consultation is often the method for training new methodologies to educational professionals (Crone, Hawken, & Bergstrom, 2007), this training project took a different approach. Trainees learned by observing the trainers conducting the assessments and by conducting the assessments with the trainers.

Participants (Trainees and Trainers)

Thirty trainees from eight of the nine AEAs participated in the project across 4 years. The team size of each challenging behavior team varied between 1 member and 9 members, with a median size of 3.5 members. Most trainees held master's degrees and specialist degrees (90%), were school social workers (37%) or school psychologists (37%), and had been working in their designated field for fewer than 15 years (60%). Six trainers from the CDD participated in the project across the 3 years. All trainers had extensive experience in behavior analysis through education or clinical experience, and their educational disciplines consisted of psychology, social work, and education.

Procedures During Training Sessions

From 11 to 12 training visits were scheduled for each challenging behavior team throughout an academic year. During each visit, the team was responsible for identifying one or two students with challenging behavior for whom a functional analysis procedure was appropriate. Visits occurred in a clinical setting at the CDD and in schools across Iowa.

During the training sessions, trainees were evaluated based on their levels of independence when conducting their portion of the assessment (e.g., planning the assessment, data collection, summarizing data, conducting functional analysis procedures). Task analyses were created for each skill area. Table 16.3 presents the task analysis for functional analysis. The task analysis was divided into three skill content areas: preparation for the analysis, procedures of the analysis, and decision making during the analysis. The trainees' level of independence was scored on a scale of 1 to 5:

1 = Trainer implemented or coached all procedures; trainee observed all procedures.

2 = Trainer implemented or coached procedures; trainee participated in some procedures.

3 = Trainer implemented or coached procedures; trainee implemented procedures (50/50).

4 = Trainer coached trainee in the implementation of procedures.

5 = Trainee implemented procedures independently.

The trainee needed to achieve a rating of 5 in each skill content area during two different training sessions to be considered independent. At the end of 4 years, 24 trainees (80%) became independent in all three skill content areas for conducting functional analyses.

Case Example of School-Based Functional Analysis

Henry was a 3-years-and-8-month-old boy who attended an early childhood special education program because of delays in speech and language development and cognitive development. The challenging behavior team conducted a brief functional analysis of destructive behaviors (e.g., grabbing and throwing materials) in his classroom setting with low levels of coaching from the trainers. One of the challenging behavior team members coached the teacher through the procedures in the analysis. No other children were present during the assessment. The challenging behavior team hypothesized that Henry engaged in destructive behaviors to escape instructional demands and/or gain access to preferred items. The analysis included escape and tangible conditions, and a free play condition was conducted as a control condition.

Results of Henry's brief functional analysis are displayed in Figure 16.5. Elevated levels of destructive behavior were observed during escape and tangible sessions. Results of the analysis indicated that Henry engaged in destructive behavior to both escape instructional demands and gain access to preferred tangible items. It took approximately 60 minutes to confirm the hypothesized functions of Henry's destructive behavior.

As the results in Figure 16.5 show, school staff, similar to parents, can conduct functional analyses, and those functional analyses can become part of the repertoires of school teams working with students who engage in challenging behavior. However, this is not a quick process, because the skills needed to conduct a functional analysis and to use the results to develop effective treatments are often difficult to acquire and require substantial practice.

Table 16.3.   Task analysis for brief functional analysis

Skill content area		Skill component
Preparation for the analysis		• Define problem behavior that will be reinforced. • Define communication that will be reinforced (if applicable). • Determine session length. • Determine length of reinforcement interval. • Determine order of the conditions.
Procedures for the analysis	Free play	• Identify that preferred leisure activities are available. • Ensure there is attention available to the student. • Ensure there is an absence of demands (including instruction on how to play). • Ensure there is an absence of consequences for problem behavior.
	Escape	• Identify task demands. • Provide prompts to "work" or instructions for the demand activity. • Ensure there is a consequence for target problem behaviors (removal of the demand for designated time). • Ensure there is an absence of attention and leisure items when the demand is removed. • Repeat the prompt/removal sequence.
	Attention	• Identify activities available in the room. • Provide prompt to "play." • Orient the adult away from child. • Ensure there is a consequence for target problem behaviors (attention in the form of disapproval for a designated time). • Repeat the prompt/attention sequence.
	Tangible	• Identify the preferred tangible (high-preference item). • Adult removes tangible away from child (only low-preferred items remain). • Ensure there is a consequence for target problem behaviors (adult provides tangible for designated time). • Repeat prompt/tangible sequence.
	Alone	• Ensure absence of tangible items. • Ensure absence of attention. • Ensure absence of demands. • Ensure absence of consequences for problem behaviors.
Decision making during the analysis		• Adjust session length appropriately; end session if problem behavior too severe (e.g., tissue damage). • Adjust assessment plan as appropriate; conduct free play following sessions in which a child is very upset. • Identify which condition should be tested next; provide rationale for running it next. • Identify the need for reversals in which the condition is retested. • Identify a new variable to be tested.

CONCLUSION

In this chapter, we provide multiple exemplars of how the functional analysis procedures developed by Iwata et al. (1994) can be applied to outpatient clinic, home, and school settings, as well as via teleconsultation. The overall results show that this methodology is highly adaptable and that the procedures can be implemented in a valid manner (e.g., via single-case multi-element designs) across most situations and settings. This methodology could be used as part of an individualized FBA for individuals who are categorized at the tertiary level in the PBIS framework. The future goals for behavioral analysts are to continue to apply the procedures across other situations and behaviors, continue to refine the procedures, study the conditions under which these

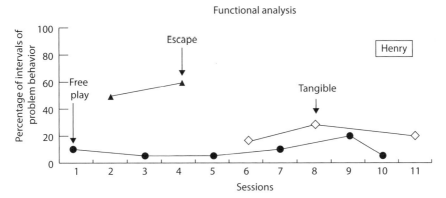

Figure 16.5. Results of a functional analysis completed with Henry in a school setting, showing that his problem behavior was maintained by escape from demands and access to tangibles.

procedures can be conducted most successfully, and study the conditions that are most likely to lead to successful interventions.

REFERENCES

Barnhill, G.P. (2005). Functional behavioral assessment in the schools. *Intervention in School and Clinic, 40*(3), 131–143. doi:10.1177/10534512050400030101

Barretto, A., Wacker, D.P., Harding, J., Lee, J., & Berg, W.K. (2006). Using telemedicine to conduct behavioral assessments. *Journal of Applied Behavior Analysis, 39*, 333–340. doi:10.1901/jaba.2006.173-04

Beavers, G.A., Iwata, B.A., & Lerman, D.C. (2013). Thirty years of research on the functional analysis of problem behavior. *Journal of Applied Behavior Analysis, 46*, 1–21. doi:10.1002/jaba.30

Berg, W.K., Wacker, D.P., Cigrand, K., Merkle, S., Wade, J., Henry, K., & Wang, Y. (2007). Comparing functional analysis and paired-choice assessment results in classroom settings. *Journal of Applied Behavior Analysis, 40*, 545–552. doi:10.1901/jaba.2006.173-04

Berg, W., Wacker, D., Harding, J., Ganzer, J., & Barretto, A. (2007). An evaluation of multiple dependent variables across distinct classes of antecedent stimuli pre and post functional communication training. *Journal of Early and Intensive Behavioral Intervention, 3*(4)–4(1), 305-333.

Boelter, E.W., Wacker, D.P., Call, N.A., Ringdahl, J.E., Kopelman, T., & Gardner, A.W. (2007). Effects of antecedent variables on disruptive behavior and accurate responding in young children in outpatient settings. *Journal of Applied Behavior Analysis, 40*, 321–326. doi:10.1901/jaba.2007.51-06

Call, N.A., Wacker, D.P., Ringdahl, J.E., Cooper-Brown, L.J., & Boelter, E.W. (2004). An assessment of antecedent events influencing noncompliance in an outpatient clinic. *Journal of Applied Behavior Analysis, 37*, 145–157. doi:10.1901/jaba.2004.37-145

Carr, E.G. (1977). The motivation of self-injurious behavior: A review of some hypotheses. *The Psychological Bulletin, 84*, 800–816. doi:10.1037/0033-2909.84.4.800

Carr, E.G., & Durand, V.M. (1985). Reducing behavior problems through functional communication training. *Journal of Applied Behavior Analysis, 18*, 111–126. doi:10.1901/jaba.1985.18-111

Carr, E.G., Newsom, C.D., & Binkhoff, J.A. (1980). Escape as a factor in the aggressive behavior of two retarded children. *Journal of Applied Behavior Analysis, 13*, 101–117. doi:10.1901/jaba.1980.13-101

Cooper, J.O., Heron, T.E., & Heward, W.L. (2007). *Applied behavior analysis* (2nd ed.). Upper Saddle River, NJ: Pearson Education.

Cooper, L.J., Wacker, D.P., Sasso, G.M., Reimers, T.M., & Donn, L.K. (1990). Using parents as therapists to evaluate appropriate behavior of their children: Application to a tertiary diagnostic clinic. *Journal of Applied Behavior Analysis, 23*, 285–296. doi:10.1901/jaba.1990.23-285

Crone, D.A., Hawken, L.S., & Bergstrom, M.K. (2007). A demonstration of training, implementing, and using functional behavioral assessment in 10 elementary and middle school settings. *Journal of Positive Behavior Interventions, 9*, 15–29. doi:10.1177/10983007070090010301

Derby, K.M., Wacker, D.P., Berg, W., DeRaad, A., Ulrich, S., Asmus, J., . . . Stoner, B. (1997). The long-term effects of functional communication training in home settings. *Journal of Applied Behavior Analysis, 30*, 507–531. doi:10.1901/jaba.1997.30-507

Derby, K.M., Wacker, D.P., Sasso, G., Steege, M., Northup, J., Cigrand, K., & Asmus, J. (1992). Brief functional assessment techniques to evaluate aberrant behavior in an outpatient setting: A summary of 79 cases. *Journal of Applied Behavior Analysis, 25*, 713–721. doi:10.1901/jaba.1992.25-713

Durand, V.M., & Carr, E.G. (1992). An analysis of maintenance following functional communication training. *Journal of Applied Behavior Analysis, 25*, 777–794. doi:10.1901/jaba.1992.25-777

Ervin, R.A., Radford, P.M., Bertsch, K., Piper, A.L., Ehrhardt, K.E., & Poling, A. (2001). A descriptive analysis and critique of the empirical literature on school-based functional assessment. *School Psychology Review, 30*, 193–210.

Gardner, A.W., Spencer, T.D., Boelter, E.W., DuBard, M., & Jennett, H.K. (2012). A systematic review of brief functional analysis methodology with typically developing children. *Education and Treatment of Children, 35*(2), 1–20. doi:10.1353/etc.2012.0014

Gardner, A.W., Wacker, D.P., & Boelter, E.W. (2009). An evaluation of the interaction between quality of attention and negative reinforcement with children who display escape-maintained problem behavior. *Journal of Applied Behavior Analysis, 42,* 343–348. doi:10.1901/jaba.2009.42-343

Gresham, F.M., Quinn, M.M., & Restori, A. (1999). Methodological issues in functional analysis: Generalizability to other disability groups. *Behavioral Disorders, 24,* 180–182.

Hagopian, L.P., Fisher, W.W., Thompson, R.H., Owen-DeSchryver, J., Iwata, B.A., & Wacker, D.P. (1997). Toward the development of structured criteria for interpretation of functional analysis data. *Journal of Applied Behavior Analysis, 30,* 313–326. doi:10.1901/jaba.1997.30-313

Hanley, G.P., Iwata, B.A., & McCord, B.E. (2003). Functional analysis of problem behavior: A review. *Journal of Applied Behavior Analysis, 36,* 147–185. doi:10.1901/jaba.2003.36-147

Harding, J.W., Wacker, D.P., Berg, W.K., Cooper, L.J., Asmus, J.A., Mlela, K., & Muller, J. (1999). An analysis of choice making in the assessment of young children with severe behavior problems. *Journal of Applied Behavior Analysis, 32,* 63–82. doi:10.1901/jaba.1999.32-63

Harding, J.W., Wacker, D.P., Berg, W.K., Lee, J.F., & Dolezal, D. (2009). Conducting functional communication training in home settings: A case study and recommendations for practitioners. *Behavior Analysis in Practice, 2*(1), 21–33.

Holden, D., & Dew, E. (2008). Telemedicine in a rural geo-psychiatric inpatient unit: Comparison of perception/satisfaction to onsite psychiatric care. *Telemedicine and e-Health, 14,* 381–384. doi:10.1089/tmj.2007.0054

Individuals with Disabilities Education Act Amendments (IDEA) of 1997, PL 105-17, 20 U.S.C. §§ 1400 et seq.

Iwata, B.A., Dorsey, M.F., Slifer, K.J., Bauman, K.E., & Richman, G.S. (1994). Toward a functional analysis of self-injury. *Journal of Applied Behavior Analysis, 27,* 197–209. doi:10.1901/jaba.1994.27-197

Iwata, B.A., Pace, G.M., Dorsey, M.F., Zarcone, J.R., Vollmer, R.T., Smith, R.G., . . . Willis, K.D. (1994). The functions of self-injurious behavior: An experimental-epidemiological analysis. *Journal of Applied Behavior Analysis, 27,* 215–240. doi:10.1901/jaba.1994.27-215

Iwata, B.A., Wallace, M.D., Kahng, S., Lindberg, J.S., Roscoe, E.M., Conners, J., . . . Worsdell, A.S. (2000). Skill acquisition in the implementation of functional analysis methodology. *Journal of Applied Behavior Analysis, 33,* 181–194. doi:10.1901/jaba.2000.33-181

Kahng, S., & Iwata, B.A. (1999). Correspondence between outcomes of brief and extended functional analyses. *Journal of Applied Behavior Analysis, 32,* 149–159. doi:10.1901/jaba.1999.32-149

Lindgren, S., & Wacker, D.P. (2011). *Behavioral treatment through in-home telehealth for young children with autism* (MCHB Autism Intervention Research Grant R40MC22644). Washington, DC: U.S. Department of Health and Human Services, Health Resources and Services Administration.

Lovaas, O.I., & Simmons, J.Q. (1969). Manipulation of self-destruction in three retarded children. *Journal of Applied Behavior Analysis, 2,* 143–157. doi:10.1901/jaba.1969.2-143

Machalicek, W., O'Reilly, M., Chan, J., Lang, R., Rispoli, M., Davis, T., . . . Didden, R. (2009). Using videoconferencing to conduct functional analysis of challenging behavior to develop classroom behavioral support plans for students with autism. *Education and Training in Developmental Disabilities, 44,* 207–217.

Michael, J. (1982). Distinguishing between discriminative and motivational functions of stimuli. *Journal of the Experimental Analysis of Behavior, 37,* 149–155. doi:10.1901/jeab.1982.37-149

Mueller, M.M., Nkosi, A., & Hine, J.F. (2011). Functional analysis in public schools: A summary of 90 functional analyses. *Journal of Applied Behavior Analysis, 44,* 807–818. doi:10.1901/jaba.2011.44-807

Myers, K.M., Valentine, J.M., & Melzer, S.M. (2007). Feasibility, acceptability, and sustainability of telepsychiatry with children and adolescents. *Psychiatric Services, 58,* 1493–1496. doi:10.1176/appi.ps.58.11.1493

Neef, N.A. (1994). Special issue on functional analysis approaches to behavioral assessment and treatment. *Journal of Applied Behavior Analysis, 27,* 196. doi:10.1901/jaba.1994.27-196

Nesbitt, T.S., Marcin, J.P., Daschbach, M.M., & Cole, S.L. (2005). Perceptions of local health care quality in 7 rural communities with telemedicine. *Journal of Rural Health, 21,* 79–85. doi:10.1111/j.1748-0361.2005.tb00066.x

Northup, J., Wacker, D., Sasso, G., Steege, M., Cigrand, K., Cook, J., & DeRaad, A. (1991). A brief functional analysis of aggressive and alternative behavior in an outclinic setting. *Journal of Applied Behavior Analysis, 24,* 509–522. doi:10.1901/jaba.1991.24-509

O'Reilly, M.F. (1995). Functional analysis and treatment of escape-maintained aggression correlated with sleep deprivation. *Journal of Applied Behavior Analysis, 28,* 225–226. doi:10.1901/jaba.1995.28-225

Pelios, L., Morren, J., Tesch, D., & Axelrod, S. (1999). The impact of functional analysis methodology on treatment choice for self-injurious and aggressive behavior. *Journal of Applied Behavior Analysis, 32,* 185–195. doi:10.1901/jaba.1999.32-185

Roane, H.S., Vollmer, T.R., Ringdahl, J.E., & Marcus, B.A. (1998). Evaluation of a brief stimulus preference assessment. *Journal of Applied Behavior Analysis, 31,* 605–620. doi:10.1901/jaba.1998.31-605

Shore, J.H., & Manson, S.M. (2005). A developmental model for rural telepsychiatry. *Psychiatric Services, 56,* 976–980. doi:10.1176/appi.ps.56.8.976

Singh, M., & Das, R. (2010). Utility of telemedicine for children in India. *Indian Journal of Pediatrics, 77,* 73–75. doi:10.1007/s12098-009-0292-x

Stormont, M., Reinke, W., & Herman, K. (2011). Teachers' knowledge of evidence-based interventions and available school resources for children with emotional and behavioral problems. *Journal of Behavioral Education, 20,* 138–147. doi:10.1007/s10864-011-9122-0

Sugai, G., Horner, R.H., Dunlap, G., Heineman, M., Lewis, T.J., Nelson, C.M., . . . Ruef, M. (2000). Applying positive behavior support and functional behavior assessment in the schools. *Journal of Positive Behavior Interventions, 2*(3), 131–143. doi:10.1177/109830070000200302.

Van Acker, R., Boreson, L., Gable, R.A., & Potterton, T. (2005). Are we on the right course? Lessons learned about current FBA/BIP practices in schools. *Journal of Behavioral Education, 14,* 35–56. doi:10.1007/s10864-005-0960-5

Vaughan, M.E., & Michael, J.L. (1982). Automatic reinforcement: An important but ignored concept. *Behaviorism, 10,* 217–227.

Wacker, D., Berg, W., Harding, J., & Cooper-Brown, L. (2004). Use of brief experimental analyses in outpatient clinic and home settings. *Journal of Behavioral Education, 13,* 213–226. doi:10.1023/B:JOBE.0000044732.42711.f5

Wacker, D., Steege, M., Northup, J., Reimers, T., Berg, W., & Sasso, G. (1990). Use of functional analysis and acceptability measures to assess and treat severe behavior problems: An outpatient clinic model. In A.C. Repp & N.N. Singh (Eds.), *Perspectives on the use of nonaversive and aversive interventions for persons with developmental disabilities* (pp. 349–359). Sycamore, IL: Sycamore.

Wacker, D.P., & Berg, W.K. (1992). *Inducing reciprocal parent/child interactions.* Washington, DC: Department of Health and Human Services, National Institute of Child Health and Human Development.

Wacker, D.P., Berg, W.K., & Harding, J.W. (1996). *Promoting stimulus generalization with young children.* Washington, DC: Department of Health and Human Services, National Institute of Child Health and Human Development.

Wacker, D.P., Berg, W.K., & Harding, J.W. (2000). *Functional communication training augmented with choices.* Washington, DC: Department of Health and Human Services, National Institute of Child Health and Human Development.

Wacker, D.P., Berg, W.K., & Harding, J.W. (2004). *Maintenance effects of functional communication training.* Washington, DC: Department of Health and Human Services, National Institute of Child Health and Human Development.

Wacker, D.P., Berg, W.K., Harding, J.W., Derby, K.M., Asmus, J.M., & Healy, A. (1998). Evaluation and long-term treatment of aberrant behavior displayed by young children with disabilities. *Journal of Developmental and Behavioral Pediatrics, 19,* 260–266. doi:10.1097/00004703-199808000-00004

Wacker, D.P., Lee, J.F., Padilla Dalmau, Y.C., Kopelman, T.G., Lindgren, S.D., Kuhle, J., . . . Waldron, D. (2013). Conducting functional analyses of problem behavior via telehealth. *Journal of Applied Behavior Analysis, 46,* 31–46. doi:10.1002/jaba.29

Wacker, D.P., Steege, M.W., Northup, J., Sasso, G., Berg, W., Reimers, T., . . . Donn, L. (1990). A component analysis of functional communication training across three topographies of severe behavior problems. *Journal of Applied Behavior Analysis, 23,* 417–429. doi:10.1901/jaba.1990.23-417

Wallace, M.D., & Iwata, B.A. (1999). Effects of session duration on functional analysis outcomes. *Journal of Applied Behavior Analysis, 32,* 175–183. doi:10.1901/jaba.1999.32-175

Whitten, P., & Buis, L. (2008). Use of telemedicine for haemodialysis: Perceptions of patients and health-care providers, and clinical effects. *Journal of Telemedicine and Telecare, 14,* 75–78. doi:10.1258/jtt.2007.070411

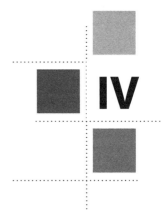

IV

Function-Driven Interventions

STANDARDS ADDRESSED IN THIS SECTION

VI. A. Positive behavior support (PBS) practitioners apply the following considerations/foundations across all elements of a PBS plan:
1. Plans are developed in collaboration with the individual and his or her team.
2. Plans are driven by the results of person-centered and functional behavioral assessments.
3. Plans facilitate the individual's preferred lifestyle.
4. Plans are designed for contextual fit, specifically in relation to (a) values and goals of the team, (b) current and desired routines within the various settings in which the individual participates, (c) skills and buy-in of those who will be implementing the plan, and (d) administrative support.

VI. B. Behavior support plans (BSPs) include interventions to improve/support quality of life in the following areas:
1. Achieving the individual's dreams
2. The individual's health and physiological needs
3. Promoting all aspects of self-determination
4. Improvement in individual's active, successful participation in inclusive school, work, home, and community settings

(continued)

5. Promotion of social interactions, relationships, and enhanced social networks
6. Increased fun and success in the individual's life
7. Improved leisure, relaxation, and recreational activities for the individual throughout the day

VI. C. PBS practitioners develop behavior support plans that include antecedent interventions to prevent the need for challenging behavior using the following strategies:
1. Alter or eliminate setting events to preclude the need for challenging behavior.
2. Modify specific antecedent triggers/circumstances based on the functional behavioral assessment (FBA).
3. Identify and address behaviors using precursors.
4. Make the individual's environment/routines predictable.
5. Build opportunities for choice/control throughout the day that are age appropriate and contextually appropriate.
6. Create clear expectations.
7. Modify curriculum/job demands so the individual can successfully complete tasks.

VI. D. PBS plans address effective instructional intervention strategies that may include the following:
1. Match instructional strategies to the individual's learning style.
2. Provide instruction in the context in which the challenging behaviors occur and in the use of alternative skills, including communication skills, social skills, self-management/monitoring skills, and other adaptive behaviors as indicated by the FBA and continued evaluation of progress data.
3. Teach replacement behavior(s) based on competing behavior analysis.
4. Select and teach replacement behaviors that can be as or more effective than the challenging behavior.
5. Utilize instructional methods of addressing a challenging behavior proactively.

VI. E. PBS practitioners employ consequence intervention strategies that consider the following:
1. Reinforcement strategies are function based and rely on naturally occurring reinforcers as much as possible.
2. Intervention strategies use the least intrusive behavior reduction strategy.
3. Emergency intervention strategies are used only where safety of the individual or others must be assured.
4. Intervention strategies consider plans for avoiding power struggles and provocation.
5. Intervention strategies consider plans for potential natural consequences. They consider when these should happen and when there should be attempts to avoid them.

VI. F. PBS practitioners develop plans for successful implementation of PBS plans that include the following:
1. Action plans for implementation of all components of the intervention
2. Strategies to address systems change need for implementation of PBS plans

VI. G. PBS practitioners evaluate plan implementation and use data to make needed modifications:
1. Implement plan and evaluate and monitor progress according to time lines.
2. Collect data identified for each component of the PBS plan.
3. Analyze data regularly to determine needed adjustments.
4. Evaluate progress on person-centered plans.
5. Modify each element of the PBS plan as indicated by evaluation data.

The five chapters in Section IV address a variety of evidence-based intervention strategies that are often components of positive behavior support (PBS) plans. The techniques covered in this section are effective when used individually. However, when used as interventions for challenging behavior, they are selected based on a functional assessment of target behavior and are often one of several components of a support plan. Examples of each intervention are provided throughout the section as is the evidence supporting the strategy. Chapter 17, "Strategies to Promote Self-Determination," describes the concept of self-determination as an individual becoming a causal factor in his or her own life. The components of self-determination, strategies for promoting/teaching these components, and the relationship to PBS are addressed. Self-management is a component of self-determination that has been found to be particularly useful and effective in dealing with challenging behavior. Chapter 18, "Strategies for Self-Management," explores the various types of self-management and their effectiveness as PBS interventions. Chapter 19, "Visual Supports as Antecedent and Teaching Interventions," presents a variety of visual supports such as picture/graphic/video schedules, story-based strategies, power cards, and contingency maps and their use as function-based components of comprehensive PBS plans.

The interrelationship between academic learning and challenging behavior is explored in Chapter 20, "Curricular Modification, Positive Behavior Support, and Change." Evidence-based instructional strategies and curricular modifications are discussed, along with suggestions for using multitiered systems of support (MTSS) that address behavior and social skills and academic learning as a framework for comprehensive education reform. Chapter 21, "Strategies for Functional Communication Training," describes the extensive evidence base for functional communication training (FCT) across populations and settings. A multistep process for FCT is provided that includes assistance with cognitive barriers to effective implementation.

As you read the chapters in this section, note that each intervention strategy and the manner of its implementation are based on a functional assessment of the target behavior of each individual. Consider whether any of these strategies would be useful for the individuals with challenging behavior with whom you interact. Reflect upon the need for individualization and the fact that although all PBS plans are multicomponent, no PBS plan would include all the strategies described in this section.

Jacki L. Anderson

Strategies to Promote Self-Determination

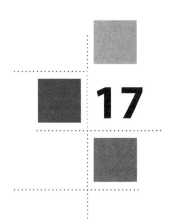

17

Michael L. Wehmeyer

Readers of this text will, no doubt, be well versed in the definition of and historical antecedents to positive behavior support (PBS). As such, it might seem redundant to revisit these issues. Yet, if one is to understand the role of self-determination in PBS, this is exactly where one must begin. Sugai and Simonsen (2012) summarized PBS as "a framework for enhancing the adoption and implementation of a continuum of evidence-based interventions to achieve academically and behaviorally important outcomes for all students" (p. 1). Sugai and Simonsen rebutted the misconception that PBS is an intervention or a practice in and of itself, pointing out that it is, instead, a "*framework* or *approach* that provides the means of selecting, organizing and implementing . . . evidence-based practices" (p. 4).

Toward what end is this framework or approach implemented? Carr and colleagues (1999) pointed out that PBS shifted the focus of behavior interventions from, primarily, reducing and controlling problem behavior to, first, enhancing quality of life and, second, reducing problem behavior. To achieve this, Carr et al. (1999) noted, PBS focuses on modifying deficient contexts to make problem behavior inefficient or irrelevant.

This important shift in focus places PBS in the broader context of paradigmatic changes in how disability is understood (Wehmeyer, 2014). Briefly, these changes have been precipitated by the abandonment of historic conceptualizations of disability as an interiorized state of pathology—essentially as a problem within the person—and by the worldwide adoption of models that view disability as a function of the fit between personal capacity and the demands of the context. Such models, most frequently referred to as *person-environment fit models,* emphasize that disability exists in the context of typical human functioning. Since disability resides only in the gap between personal capacity and the demands of the environment or context, rather than residing as a problem within the person, efforts to close the gap by enhancing personal capacity or modifying the environment or context can, if not only technically, eliminate disability and make it irrelevant (Wehmeyer et al., 2008).

Conceptualizing PBS as an approach to apply evidence-based practices to *remediate deficient contexts,* thus making problem behavior irrelevant, is in line with practices emerging from these person–environment fit models of disability. One of the implications of such practices (i.e., practices emerging from new ways of understanding disability) is that we move from creating programs based on disability types or labels to the provision of supports that enable each individual to participate in the full array of life activities. Supports are "resources and strategies that aim to promote the development, education, interests, and personal well-being of a person and that enhance individual functioning" (Luckasson et al., 2002, p. 151). Quite simply, *supports* refers to anything that enhances human functioning in the context of typical settings and activities (Thompson et al., 2009). Schalock et al. (2010) notes:

> Supports can be technologies, such as a personal digital assistant (PDA) that shows the steps to follow in completing a job task or an augmentative communication device that enhances a person's communication skills through icon input and voice output. Supports can be people, such as a bus driver who prompts a person when it is time to get off at a certain stop or a paid job coach who works one-on-one with a person in a community job. Supports can be referenced to the person or the environment. (p. 111)

In fact, the term *supports* is best defined as anything that can reduce the gap between personal capacity and successful functioning in typical environments and contexts. Receiving funds from a state developmental disability (DD) system is a form of support but so is using a smartphone to shop independently or getting assistance from

a coworker to complete a portion of a task or job. Education that enhances personal capacity is a form of support, whether that education is "specially designed instruction" (e.g., special education services), or not. In addition, relevant to this chapter, an important source of supports is the individual himself or herself. The more that professionals can do to enable people with disabilities to become self-determined, the more likely it is that the person will require less external support.

In essence, then, the "continuum of evidence-based interventions to achieve academically and behaviorally important outcomes for all students" (Sugai et al., 2000)—the adoption and implementation of which Sugai and Simonsen (2012) proposed as providing the framework for defining PBS—must include interventions to promote self-determination. Before examining efforts to promote self-determination within a PBS frame, it is worth briefly discussing what is meant by the term *self-determination* and examining the literature pertaining to the impact of promoting self-determination on outcomes important to adolescents and young adults with disabilities.

WHAT IS SELF-DETERMINATION?

There have been several theoretical models of self-determination developed from research in special education over the past 2 decades. All share common elements, though they vary as a function of how the construct is understood or framed. For purposes of this chapter, the functional theory of self-determination (Wehmeyer, Kelchner, & Richards, 1996) will be used to understand and define *self-determination.* Within this *functional model*—so called because actions are viewed as self-determined based on the function they serve for the individual—self-determination is seen as a dispositional characteristic (enduring tendencies used to characterize and describe differences among people). Self-determined behavior refers to "volitional actions that enable one to act as the primary causal agent in one's life and to maintain or improve one's quality of life" (Wehmeyer, 2005, p. 117). *Causal agency* implies that it is the person who makes or causes things to happen in his or her life—that he or she acts with the intention to accomplish a specific end or create change. Self-determined actions are identified by four essential characteristics: 1) the person acts autonomously, 2) the behavior is self-regulated, 3) the person initiates and responds to the event(s) in a psychologically empowered manner, and 4) the person acts in a self-realizing manner. People become self-determined through the acquisition and practice of component elements of self-determined behavior (discussed in detail subsequently). The functional model sees self-determination as an integral part of the process of individuation and adolescent development. This model has been empirically validated (Shogren et al., 2008; Wehmeyer et al., 1996) and operationalized by the development of an assessment linked to the theory (Wehmeyer, 1996). It has served as the foundation for intervention development, particularly with regard to the development of the self-determined learning model of instruction (discussed subsequently; Wehmeyer, Palmer, Agran, Mithaug, & Martin, 2000), and has provided an impetus for a variety of research activities (Wehmeyer, Abery, Mithaug, & Stancliffe, 2003; Wehmeyer, Agran, Hughes, Martin, Mithaug, & Palmer, 2007).

As noted, other theoretical models of self-determination have been forwarded, including an ecological model of self-determination (Stancliffe, Abery, & Smith, 2000) that defines *self-determination* as "a complex process, the ultimate goal of which is to achieve the level of personal control over one's life that an individual desires within those areas the individual perceives as important" (Abery & Stancliffe, 1996, p. 27); a model that proposes self-determination as a form of self-regulation (Mithaug, 1998); and a five-step model proposed by Field and colleagues (Field &

Hoffman, 2001; Field & Hoffman, 2005), in which self-determination is either promoted or discouraged by factors within the individual's control (e.g., values, knowledge, skills) and variables that are environmental in nature (e.g., opportunities for decision making, attitudes of others). For more information on these and other models, see Wehmeyer et al. (2003).

WHY IS PROMOTING SELF-DETERMINATION IMPORTANT?

Promoting self-determination has become an important component of recommended practice in special education for a number of reasons, but most relevantly because of the positive impact of enhanced self-determination on student academic, behavioral, and functional outcomes and quality of life. With regard to the former (positive impact of enhanced self-determination on outcomes), a number of studies established a relationship between self-determination status at the time of graduation from high school and more positive employment, independent living, and community inclusion–related outcomes (Powers et al., 1998; Wehmeyer & Palmer, 2003; Wehmeyer & Schwartz, 1997). These studies methodologically provided evidence that self-determination status predicted or was related to more positive outcomes. Wehmeyer and colleagues (Shogren, Wehmeyer, Palmer, Rifenbark, & Little, forthcoming; Wehmeyer, Palmer, Shogren, Williams-Diehm, & Soukup, 2013) conducted a randomized-trial, control-group study of the effect of interventions to promote self-determination on the self-determination of high school students receiving special education services under the categorical areas of intellectual disability and learning disabilities. Students in the treatment group ($n = 235$) received instruction using a variety of instructional methods to promote self-determination and student involvement in educational planning meetings over 3 years, while students in the control group ($n = 132$) received no such intervention. The self-determination of each student was measured using two instruments, the Arc's self-determination scale (Wehmeyer & Kelchner, 1995) and the American Institute for Research (AIR) self-determination scale (Wolman, Campeau, Dubois, Mithaug, & Stolarski, 1994), across three measurement intervals (at baseline, after 2 years of intervention, and after 3 years of intervention). Using latent growth curve analysis, Wehmeyer and colleagues found that students with intellectual disabilities who participated in interventions to promote self-determination over a 3-year period showed significantly more positive patterns of growth in their overall or global self-determination, as reflected by the scores on both measures, than students not exposed to interventions to promote self-determination.

Subsequently, in a follow-up study of the treatment- and control-group students from Wehmeyer et al. (2013), Shogren, Wehmeyer, Palmer, and Little (2012) investigated adult outcomes 1 and 2 years after leaving school. The study measured employment, community access, financial independence, independent living, and life satisfaction outcomes, utilizing a questionnaire from previous research. Results indicated that self-determination status at the end of high school predicted significantly more positive employment, career goal, and community access outcomes. Students who were self-determined were significantly higher in these areas. These two studies provided causal evidence that promoting self-determination results enhanced self-determination and that enhanced self-determination results in more positive adult outcomes, including employment and community inclusion.

With regard, then, to including interventions to promote self-determination among those interventions that frame PBS, it is important to allow students to gain greater self-determination and related skills so they can achieve more positive outcomes. Studies of individual interventions expands the evidence for the impact of promoting

self-determination to include benefits to school-related outcomes, such as academic and functional goal achievement, and access to the general education curriculum (Powers et al., 2012; Shogren, Palmer, Wehmeyer, Williams-Diehm, & Little, 2012; Wehmeyer et al., 2011, 2012).

But what about promoting self-determination makes it particularly important to include within PBS? First, promoting self-determination involves teaching skills that will be equally important for addressing problem behaviors, such as problem solving, decision making, or goal setting. Second, there is evidence that decision making, which is a component element of self-determination, is, itself, a potentially effective intervention to reduce problem behavior. Shogren, Faggella-Luby, Bae, and Wehmeyer (2004) performed a meta-analysis of 13 single-subject design studies examining the efficacy of the use of decision making as an intervention to reduce problem behavior. Overall, providing decision-making opportunities resulted in clinically significant reductions of problem behavior.

Third, as the Association for Positive Behavior Support (APBS) standards of practice (2007) emphasize, a primary focus of behavior interventions in PBS is to enhance quality of life. A number of studies have established a strong relationship between enhanced self-determination and increased quality of life (Lachapelle et al., 2005; Nota, Ferrari, Soresi, & Wehmeyer, 2007; Schalock et al., 2005; Wehmeyer & Schwartz, 1998). Fourth, the APBS standards of practice (2007) articulate other standards that clearly show the importance of efforts to promote self-determination within PBS. For example, one of the principle assumptions about PBS is that problem behavior serves a function for the person. In many cases, that function is communicative, and if one considers what a person is communicating by engaging in problem behavior, the answer is that in many, if not most, cases what is being communicated is a personal preference or a desire for greater autonomy or personal control. In many ways, people who are engaging in problem behavior are trying to exert control over their lives in some way. They are acting as causal agents in their lives—that is, they are trying to make something happen in their lives. What they need to learn, of course, are more appropriate or effective ways to communicate personal preferences and gain greater control over their lives. Next, the APBS standards require that practitioners actively engage and involve the person in the planning process, as discussed subsequently. In addition, the APBS standards for the use of antecedent manipulations to influence behavior include efforts to promote opportunities for choice and control.

In summary, one could argue that efforts to promote self-determination are at the heart of PBS, philosophically and practically. If problem behavior is communicative, reflecting issues pertaining to personal self-determination, then PBS is fundamentally about enabling people to become more self-determined; learn ways to more effectively communicate personal preferences; and learn to act on those preferences by setting goals, solving problems, making decisions, and advocating for oneself.

PROMOTING SELF-DETERMINATION WITHIN A POSITIVE BEHAVIOR SUPPORT FRAMEWORK

This section discusses research-based interventions that can be infused into PBS practices.

Person-Centered Planning and Assessment

The APBS standards of practice require that practitioners ensure "person-centered decision making" in the development of PBS supports and conduct "Person Centered Assessments that provide a picture of the life of the individual" (2007, p. 7). Person-centered planning (PCP) processes share common beliefs and attempt to put those shared beliefs into a planning framework. Schwartz, Jacobson, and Holburn (2000)

used a consensus process to define *person-centeredness*. This effort provides a useful picture of the values underlying PCP. Specifically, Schwartz and colleagues identified eight "hallmarks" of a PCP process (2000, p. 238):

1. The person's activities, services, and supports are based on his or her dreams, interests, preferences, strengths, and capacities.

2. The person and people important to him or her are included in lifestyle planning and have the opportunity to exercise control and make informed decisions.

3. The person has meaningful choices, with decisions based on his or her experiences.

4. The person uses, when possible, natural and community supports.

5. Activities, supports, and services foster skills to achieve personal relationships, community inclusion, dignity, and respect.

6. The person's opportunities and experiences are maximized, and flexibility is enhanced within existing regulatory and funding constraints.

7. Planning is collaborative, recurring, and involves an ongoing commitment to the person.

8. The person is satisfied with his or her relationships, home, and daily routine.

These hallmarks of PCP make it clear that to meet the standards articulated by APBS, practitioners will have to implement planning processes that not only invite the student to participate but engage the student to the maximum extent possible. One of the areas of focus in efforts to promote self-determination has been the development of strategies to promote student involvement in the educational planning process. Test and colleagues (2004) conducted an extensive review of the literature pertaining to student involvement and determined that students across disability categories can be successfully involved in educational planning and that a number of programs are effective in increasing student involvement. Martin, Marshall, and Sale (2004) conducted a 3-year study of middle, junior, and senior high school individualized education program (IEP) meetings and found that the presence of students at IEP meetings had considerable benefits, including increasing parental involvement and improving the probability that a student's strengths, needs, and interests would be discussed.

At least two programs to promote student involvement in educational planning and decision making can be considered evidence-based practices. Martin et al. (2006) conducted a randomized-trial, control-group study of the self-directed IEP (SDIEP; Martin, Marshall, Maxson, & Jerman, 1997). The SDIEP lessons enable students to learn the leadership skills necessary to run their IEP meeting. These lessons teach students 11 steps for leading their own meeting, from stating the purpose of the meeting and introducing participants, to reviewing past goals and performance, to identifying the support they need to be successful, and of course, identifying goals for the coming year. Martin and colleagues found that students in a treatment group—students with learning disabilities, emotional and behavioral disorders, and intellectual disabilities—who were taught the SDIEP lessons attended more IEP meetings; increased their active participation in the meetings; showed more leadership behaviors in the meetings; expressed their interests, skills, and support needs across educational domains; and remembered their IEP goals after the meeting at greater rates than students in the control group, who received no such instruction.

Second, Wehmeyer, Palmer, Lee, Williams-Diehm, and Shogren (2011) conducted a randomized-trial, placebo control group design study of the effects of the "Whose future is it anyway?" (WFA) process on self-determination and transition knowledge and skills. The WFA process (Wehmeyer et al., 2004), available online

at no cost (http://www.ou.edu/content/education/centers-and-partnerships/zarrow/trasition-education-materials/whos-future-is-it-anyway.html), consists of 36 sessions enabling students to self-direct instruction related to 1) self- and disability awareness; 2) making decisions about transition-related outcomes; 3) identifying and securing community resources to support transition services; 4) writing and evaluating transition goals and objectives; 5) communicating effectively in small groups; and 6) developing skills to become an effective team member, leader, or self-advocate. The materials are student directed in that they are written for students as end users. The level of support needed by students to complete activities varies greatly. Some students with difficulty reading or writing need one-to-one support to progress through the materials; others can complete the process independently. The materials make every effort to ensure that students retain control while at the same time receiving the support they need.

Results from Wehmeyer et al. (2011) indicate that instruction using the WFA process resulted in significant, positive effects on self-determination, compared with a control group, and those students who received instruction gained transition knowledge and skills. Palmer and colleagues (2012) conducted a randomized-trial, control-group study of the effect of the beyond high school (BHS) model, designed to actively engage students with intellectual and developmental disabilities in planning and goal setting in post–high school settings. The BHS model incorporates multiple stages, beginning with student involvement in a self-regulated planning process using the WFA process. Palmer et al. (2012) determined that students in the treatment group had greater gains in self-determination than their peers in the control group.

These two processes provide models for efforts to actively involve students in supports planning. In both, the content of the goal being discussed is flexible; students using either model have been supported to set not only academic or transition-related goals but also behavioral goals. Further, this chapter emphasizes these student-directed planning models rather than PCP models typically implemented in adult support services, such as essential lifestyle planning, the McGill Action Planning System (MAPS), Planning Alternative Tomorrows with Hope (PATH), or circles of support models. (See Holburn & Vietze, 2002, and Chapters 4 and 13 for a comprehensive treatment of these and other models.) This is because student-directed planning is linked to requirements in the Individuals with Disabilities Education Improvement Act (IDEA; PL 108-446) of 2004 for transition planning and, thus, may be more prevalent in schools. (Although, certainly, many school districts implement modified versions of PCP processes like essential lifestyle planning or MAPS.) In addition, the impact of these student-directed planning models on self-determination has been directly tested. In fact, Cross, Cooke, Wood, and Test (1999) compared the effects of the MAPS process and the SDIEP process on the self-determination of adolescents with disabilities. Both processes resulted in enhanced self-determination, but the SDIEP process had larger effects.

The particular PCP process implemented is not that important; it is more important that the process adheres to the hallmarks identified by Schwartz and colleagues (2000; previously listed). If PBS practitioners are attending to those issues, using either traditional PCP models or student-directed planning models such as WFA or SDIEP, they will be better able to meet the standards established by APBS.

Of course, assessment is an important part of planning. Readers of this volume are likely well versed in functional behavioral assessment (FBA), but such efforts should include assessing student instructional and support needs in the area of self-determination. This involves a combination of standardized and informal procedures incorporating input from multiple sources, including the student, his or her family, professionals, and others. Informal procedures will be similar to those described by Clark (1996) with regard to transition assessment. Clark identified informal assessments from which transition-related decisions can be made as those that include the following elements: 1) situational or observational learning styles assessments; 2) curriculum-based assessment; 3) observational reports from teachers, employers, and family members; 4) situational assessments in home, community, and work settings; 5) environmental assessments; 6) personal-future planning activities; 7) structured interviews with students; 8) structured interviews with parents, guardians, advocates, or peers; 9) adaptive, behavioral, or functional skill inventories; 10) social histories; 11) employability, independent living, and personal-social skills rating scales; and 12) technology or vocational education skills assessments.

In addition to these informal assessment processes, there are two widely used standardized, norm-referenced measures of self-determination, Arc's self-determination scale (Wehmeyer & Kelchner, 1995) and the AIR self-determination scale (Wolman et al., 1994), mentioned previously in the context of research documenting the impact of interventions. Both, however, were designed for use in the context of individual student planning and can provide information on areas of instructional need in self-determination. (Both are available online, free of charge, at http://www.ou.edu/content/ education/centers-and-partnerships/zarrow/ self-determination-assessment-tools/.)

Returning to the issue of FBA, Wehmeyer, Baker, Blumberg, and Harrison (2004) conducted a pilot study of a student self-report version of a widely used FBA tool. Wehmeyer and colleagues created a self-report version of the functional assessment interview (Horner & Carr, 1997), allowing students to self-report on issues pertaining to setting events, antecedents, problem behavior itself, and consequences. This pilot study determined that students were able to contribute meaningful and otherwise unidentified information to the FBA process. This would seem to be an important area for future exploration.

Self-Determination in the Context of Schoolwide Multitiered Systems of Supports

Once a plan is created that actively involves the student, and instructional needs pertaining to self-determination are assessed and identified, the focus turns to incorporating efforts to promote self-determination in each of the three tiers associated with the multitiered systems of supports. Tier-1 supports, also called primary prevention interventions, involve applying assessment and planning information to identify schoolwide expectations and design lesson plans that teach those expectations to all students. Tier-2 and Tier-3 supports, also called secondary and tertiary prevention supports, involve increasingly personalized interventions for students who need such supports. Tier-2 supports involve targeted interventions in areas such as social skills instruction, academic instruction, or higher-level prompting strategies. Tier-3 supports are the most intensive and involve the development of behavior support plans, wraparound services, and other more intensive supports.

Interventions to promote self-determination should be components of all three tiers but particularly Tier-2 and Tier-3 interventions. One presumption of effective instructional experiences for all students based on another multitiered model, response to intervention (RTI), is that all students receive instruction using high-quality strategies and interventions to promote self-determination would be among those implemented schoolwide for all students (Tier 1). With PBS, the presumption is that all students are receiving instruction that supports the development of self-determination and related skills; some students will need more

individualized and intensive instruction to enhance self-determination—hence the emphasis on Tiers 2 and 3.

In adhering to the notion that PBS involves the implementation of evidence-based practices, this chapter focuses on a small number of interventions that have evidence of sufficient level. It should be noted that there are a wider array of potential interventions and strategies that might be implemented, which, to this point, lack sufficient efficacy data to be called evidence based. Further, one class of interventions that results in enhanced self-determination involves the implementation of self-management strategies (see Chapter 18). As there is a separate chapter on those in this volume, they will not be discussed here.

Promoting Component Elements of Self-Determined Behavior In the functional model of self-determination, Wehmeyer and colleagues (1996) identified a set of component elements of self-determined behavior, including self-advocacy, goal setting and attainment, self-awareness, problem-solving skills, and decision-making skills. Instruction in these component elements or modifications to the environment or context to support these skills, perceptions, and beliefs have been shown to promote self-determination. Evidence for the effect of instruction in these component elements come not from randomized-trial, control-group studies of a particular intervention, but from meta-analyses of multiple studies of the impact of such instruction. Algozzine, Browder, Karvonen, Test, and Wood (2001) conducted group- and single-subject design meta-analyses of studies in which individuals with disabilities received some intervention to promote component elements of self-determined behavior—specifically, decision-making skills, goal-setting and attainment skills, self-advocacy knowledge or skills, problem-solving skills, and self-awareness skills. The median effect size across 100 group intervention comparisons was 1.38, interpreted as a moderate effect.

For the single-subject design studies, the median percentage of nonoverlapping data (PND) was 95%, with seven interventions with a PND of 100%. This is interpreted as a strong effect. Subsequently, Cobb, Lehmann, Newman-Gonchar, and Alwell (2009) conducted a narrative metasynthesis—a narrative synthesis of multiple meta-analytic studies—covering seven existing meta-analyses examining self-determination and concluded that there is sufficient evidence to support interventions to teach or promote problem-solving, decision-making, goal setting and attainment, and self-advocacy skills as effective practices to promote self-determination.

Alex

To illustrate the application of interventions to promote component elements of self-determined behavior in a school-based PBS context, consider Alex, a third grader with autism. Alex is working on grade-level classwork with some modifications to his work schedule to accommodate for his tendency to act impulsively. He is able to communicate with peers, though he tends to focus on details that are sometimes off topic, which seems to contribute to his distractibility. Alex's elementary school has adopted three schoolwide expectations for *all* students as part of its Tier-1 activities: Be respectful, be responsible, and be safe. Alex had no difficulty learning the expectations, but during the IEP meeting to discuss Alex's involvement in the classroom, his mother and his teacher both indicated that Alex sometimes puts himself in a position of risk, safetywise. He would frequently run toward the school bus, without consideration of oncoming traffic, and was prone to use playground equipment inappropriately. Both his mother and his teacher felt that Alex knew how to be safe but sometimes just made poor decisions about how to act. Alex's teacher talked with him about acting in ways that kept him safe, and through their discussions, Alex agreed that at times he might put himself at risk. To address these issues instructionally, Alex was involved with several other students in small-group activities to teach some basic problem-solving skills. Problem-solving instruction focused on teaching students, first, to identify when there is a problem—in this case, when a situation might pose some risk. Students were then taught how to explicate the problem—that is, to explore the problem situation in more detail to identify possible solutions to the problem (e.g., what ways of approaching the situation might reduce the risk). Finally, students chose one solution. Alex's teacher worked individually with each student to practice the problem-solving strategy in each of the higher-risk settings around the school. Eventually, Alex learned to apply his problem-solving skills when boarding the bus (stop at the curb, look both ways, proceed across the crosswalk to the bus if safe) and when on the playground (when playing on familiar or new equipment, learn how it is supposed to be used and what ways would be inappropriate). These Tier-2 interventions better enabled Alex to follow the school's expectations.

....

Self-Determined Learning Model of Instruction A specific instructional strategy with evidence of a causal impact on self-determination and other positive outcomes is the self-determined learning model of instruction (SDLMI; Wehmeyer et al., 2000). The SDLMI is based on the component elements of self-determined behavior (e.g., problem solving, goal setting, self-regulation) and research on student-directed learning. The SDLMI is a model of teaching designed to enable teachers to encourage students to set and attain goals in multiple content areas, from academic to functional to behavioral. Implementing the SDLMI consists of a three-phase instructional process: Set a goal (Phase 1), take action (Phase 2), and adjust the goal or plan (Phase 3). Each instructional phase presents a problem to be solved by the student. The student solves this problem by posing and answering a series of four questions per phase. Teachers support students to learn these questions, modify them to make them their own, and apply them to self-selected goals. Each question is linked to a set of teacher objectives and a list of educational supports that teachers can use to enable students to self-direct learning. In each instructional phase, the student is the primary causal agent for choices, decisions, and actions, even when actions are teacher directed (Wehmeyer et al., 2003).

More than a dozen quasi-experimental or single-subject design studies have shown the potential efficacy of the SDLMI to promote self-determination and goal attainment (Wehmeyer et al., 2003). Two studies establish it as an evidence-based practice. Wehmeyer et al. (2012) conducted a switching replication, randomized-trial, control-group study on the impact of intervention with the SDLMI on student self-determination. Data on self-determination using multiple measures was collected with 312 high school students with cognitive disabilities in both a control and a treatment group. Wehmeyer and colleagues examined the relationship between the SDLMI and self-determination using structural equation modeling. After determining strong measurement invariance for each latent construct, these researchers found significant differences in latent means across measurement occasions and differential effects attributable to the SDLMI. This was true across disability categories, though there was variance across disability populations. In other words, instruction using the SDLMI resulted in enhanced self-determination. Next, Shogren et al. (2012) reported findings from a cluster or group randomized-trial, control-group study examining the impact of the SDLMI on student academic and transition goal attainment and access to the general education curriculum for students with intellectual disability and learning disabilities. Students in the treatment group had significantly higher levels of goal attainment and access to the general education curriculum than their peers in the control group.

Nathan

Nathan is an eighth grader who receives special education services under the categorical areas of intellectual disability and other health impairment. Nathan has difficulty focusing his attention during his general education classroom, and his behavior outbursts have too frequently resulted in him having to leave the classroom. During the FBA, the school psychologist working with Nathan's teachers and parents noticed that there were a number of triggers to Nathan's outbursts, and that, as a setting event, he was most likely to have a behavior outburst if he had been late for class. Despite frequent discussions with Nathan about the importance of getting to class on time, Nathan often became distracted when making the transition from one class to another and, as a consequence, was late. Nathan's teacher felt that it was important that Nathan become more actively involved in addressing his lateness, so she and Nathan sat down to work through the SDLMI to set a goal related to Nathan's tardiness. Since it was, simply, the frequency of tardy arrivals that was the problem, Nathan decided, with support from his special education teacher, to set a goal to reduce his tardy behavior to no more than twice per month. He learned from his teacher's records that he had been tardy, on average, three times per week across all classes up to that point. Once Nathan set his goal, his teacher then worked with him to answer the questions in the second phase of the SDLMI and create an action plan. The action plan developed involved Nathan checking his watch immediately after he left any class to determine how much time he had to get to the next class and then creating a self-monitoring program to record when he arrived in class on time or was tardy. After 2 months of implementing his action plan, Nathan worked through the third phase of the SDLMI to self-evaluate his progress toward his goal. He determined that, in the past month, he had been tardy only three times. He knew he had not reached his goal yet but felt that if he kept to his current action plan, he would do so. His teachers noticed a concomitant drop in behavior outbursts associated with his increased on-time behavior. Nathan's experience is an example of how the SDLMI might be incorporated as a component of a comprehensive PBS plan and intervention.

....

TAKE CHARGE for the Future A second intervention model with causal evidence of its impact is TAKE CHARGE for the Future (Powers et al., 1996; Powers et al., 2001). TAKE CHARGE is a student-directed, collaborative model to promote student involvement in educational and transition planning. This intervention model uses four primary components or strategies to promote development of self-determination: 1) skill facilitation, 2) mentoring, 3) peer support, and 4) parent support. For example, TAKE CHARGE introduces youth to three major skills areas needed to take charge in one's life: 1) achievement skills, 2) partnership skills, and 3) coping skills. Youth involved in the TAKE CHARGE process are matched with successful adults of the same gender who experience similar challenges, share common interests, and are involved in peer-support activities (Powers, Turner, Westwood, Loesch, Brown, & Rowland, 1998). Parent support is provided via information and technical assistance and written materials.

Powers et al. (2001) conducted a control-group study and found that the TAKE CHARGE materials had a positive impact on student involvement in planning. Powers et al. (2012) conducted a longitudinal, randomized-trial study of the effect of the TAKE CHARGE model on self-determination and transition-related outcomes for youth in foster care receiving special education services. Assessment at baseline, postintervention, and a 1-year follow-up indicated moderate to large effects at postintervention and the 1-year follow-up for self-determination, quality of life, and utilization of community transition services. Youth in the intervention group also completed high school, were employed, and carried out independent living activities at higher rates than their peers in the control group (Powers et al., 2012, p. 2179).

Michelle

Michelle is a high school junior who receives special education services under the category of emotional and behavioral disorders. Michelle has a difficult time in school and at home, has frequent combative run-ins with her parents, and has been in and out of the juvenile justice system in her town. Michelle is a bright young woman and knows cognitively that she is heading down the

wrong path, but she is unable to control her emotions when she interacts with adults—particularly adults in authority positions. When her teacher suggests that Michelle participate in a very intensive intervention, TAKE CHARGE for the Future, she reluctantly agrees. First, Michelle learns about self-determination and about more effective ways to solve problems and make decisions. Michelle felt she knew how to solve a problem, but when she really thought about it, she realized she didn't approach potentially combative situations in a problem-solving manner. She learned, through instruction, how to think through responses that would not escalate a situation into a conflict. She liked the idea of setting her own goals for her future, and when she learned those skills through her TAKE CHARGE activities, she felt she was in charge and was willing to accept help from her teacher and other adults. Her parents utilized the parent materials to learn ways to support Michelle to engage in problem-solving activities in her daily life. Finally, as part of the TAKE CHARGE process, Michelle was paired with a mentor, a young woman named Fiona who had gone through similar difficulties in high school but had turned her life around and was working as a research scientist at a local biology company. Michelle was interested in biology and had always done well in science, so Fiona's shared experiences and her current success were of intense interest to Michelle.

Michelle continued in the TAKE CHARGE intervention through her junior and senior years in high school. Her emotional outbursts didn't disappear immediately, but by the end of her senior year, Michelle felt she could control those emotions to achieve goals that mattered to her, including her goal to go to the local community college to take courses in science and raise her grade point average so that she might be admitted to a local 4-year college.

··

CONCLUSION

The main point of this chapter is, simply, that among the most important research-based practices that should be implemented as part of PBS are interventions to promote student involvement and self-determination. In many ways, the primary intent of PBS is to do just that—to promote and enhance self-determination and thus enable students to achieve more positive outcomes in school and adulthood, increasing their quality of life.

REFERENCES

Abery, B.H., & Stancliffe, R.J. (1996). The ecology of self-determination. In D.J. Sands & M.L. Wehmeyer (Eds.), *Self-determination across the life span: Independence and choice for people with disabilities* (pp. 111–145). Baltimore, MD: Paul H. Brookes Publishing Co.

Algozzine, B., Browder, D., Karvonen, M., Test. D.W., & Wood, W.M. (2001). Effects of interventions to promote self-determination for individuals with disabilities. *Review of Educational Research, 71,* 219–277.

Association for Positive Behavior Support (APBS). (2007). *Positive behavior support standards of practice: Individual level.* Retrieved from http://www.apbs.org/files/apbs_standards_of_practice_2013_format.pdf

Carr, E.G., Horner, R.H., Turnbull, A.P., Marquis, J.G., McLaughlin, D.M., McAtee, M.L., . . . Doolabh, A. (1999). *Positive behavior support for people with developmental disabilities: A research synthesis.* Washington, DC: American Association on Mental Retardation.

Clark, G.M. (1996). Transition planning assessment for secondary-level students with learning disabilities. In J.R. Patton & G. Blalock (Eds.), *Transition and students with learning disabilities: Facilitating the movement from school to adult life* (pp. 131–156). Austin, TX: PRO-ED.

Cobb, B., Lehmann, J., Newman-Gonchar, R., & Alwell, M. (2009). Self-determination for students with disabilities: A narrative metasynthesis. *Career Development for Exceptional Individuals, 32*(2), 108–114.

Cross, T., Cooke, N.L., Wood, W.M., & Test, D.W. (1999). Comparison of the effects of MAPS and ChoiceMaker on students' self-determination skills. *Education and Training in Mental Retardation and Developmental Disabilities, 34,* 499–510.

Field, S., & Hoffman, A. (2001). *Teaching with integrity, reflection, and self-determination.* Detroit, MI: Wayne State University.

Field, S., & Hoffman, A. (2005). *Steps to self-determination* (2nd ed.). Austin, TX: PRO-ED.

Holburn, S., & Vietze, P. (2002). *Person-centered planning: Research, practice, and future directions.* Baltimore, MD: Paul H. Brookes Publishing Co.

Horner, R.H., & Carr, E.G. (1997). Behavioral support for students with severe disabilities: Functional assessment and comprehensive intervention. *Journal of Special Education, 31,* 84–104.

Individuals with Disabilities Education Improvement Act (IDEA) of 2004, PL 108-446, 20 U.S.C. §§ 1400 et seq.

Lachapelle, Y., Wehmeyer, M.L., Haelewyck, M.C., Courbois, Y., Keith, K.D., Schalock, R., . . . Walsh, P.N. (2005). The relationship between quality of life and self-determination: An international study. *Journal of Intellectual Disability Research, 49,* 740–744.

Luckasson, R., Borthwick-Duffy, S., Buntinx, W.H.E., Coulter, D.L., Craig, E.M., Reeve, A., . . . Tasse, M.J. (2002). *Mental retardation: Definition, classification, and systems of supports* (10th ed.). Washington, DC: American Association on Mental Retardation.

Martin, J.E., Marshall, L.H., Maxson, L.M., & Jerman, P.L. (1997). *The self-directed IEP.* Longmont, CO: Sopris West.

Martin, J.E., Marshall, L.H., & Sale, P. (2004). A 3-year study of middle, junior high, and high school IEP meetings. *Exceptional Children, 70,* 285–297.

Martin, J.E., Van Dycke, J.L., Christensen, W.R., Greene, B.A., Gardner, J.E., & Lovett, D.L. (2006). Increasing student participation in IEP meetings: Establishing the self-directed IEP as an evidenced-based practice. *Exceptional Children, 72*(3), 299–316.

Mithaug, D. (1998). Your right, my obligation? *Journal of the Association for Persons with Severe Disabilities, 23,* 41–43.

Nota, L., Ferrari, L., Soresi, S., & Wehmeyer, M.L. (2007). Self-determination, social abilities, and the quality of life of people with intellectual disabilities. *Journal of Intellectual Disability Research, 51,* 850–865.

Palmer, S.B., Wehmeyer, M.L., Shogren, K., Williams-Diehm, K., & Soukup, J. (2012). An evaluation of the *Beyond High School* model on the self-determination of students with intellectual disability. *Career Development for Exceptional Individuals, 35*(2), 76–84.

Powers, L.E., Geenen, S., Powers, J., Pommier-Satya, S., Turner, A., Dalton, L., . . . Swand, P. (2012). My life: Effects of a longitudinal, randomized study of self-determination enhancement on the transition outcomes of youth in foster care and special education. *Children and Youth Services Review, 34,* 2179–2187.

Powers, L.E., Sowers, J., Turner, A., Nesbitt, M., Knowles, E., & Ellison, R. (1996). TAKE CHARGE! A model for promoting self-determination among adolescents with challenges. In L.E. Powers, G.H.S. Singer, & J. Sowers (Eds.), *On the road to autonomy: Promoting self-competence in children and youth with disabilities* (pp. 291–332). Baltimore, MD: Paul H. Brookes Publishing Co.

Powers, L.E., Turner, A., Matuszewski, J., Wilson, R., & Phillips, A. (2001). TAKE CHARGE for the future: A controlled field-test of a model to promote student involvement in transition planning. *Career Development for Exceptional Individuals, 24,* 89–103.

Powers, L.E., Turner, A., Westwood, D., Loesch, C., Brown, A., & Rowland, C. (1998). TAKE CHARGE for the future: A student-directed approach to transition planning. In M.L. Wehmeyer & D.J. Sands (Eds.), *Making it happen: Student involvement in education planning, decision making and instruction* (pp. 187–210). Baltimore, MD: Paul H. Brookes Publishing Co.

Schalock, R., Borthwick-Duffy, S., Bradley, V.J., Buntinx, W.H.E., Coulter, D.L., Craig, E.M., . . . Yeager, M.H. (2010). *Intellectual disability: Definition, classification, and systems of supports* (11th ed.). Washington, DC: American Association on Intellectual and Developmental Disabilities.

Schalock, R., Verdugo, M., Jenaro, C., Wang, M., Wehmeyer, M., Xu, J., . . . Lachapelle, Y. (2005). Cross-cultural study of core quality of life indicators. *American Journal on Mental Retardation, 110,* 298–311.

Schwartz, A.A., Jacobson, J.W., & Holburn, S. (2000). Defining person-centeredness: Results of two consensus methods. *Education and Training in Mental Retardation and Developmental Disabilities, 35,* 235–258.

Shogren, K., Faggella-Luby, M., Bae, S.J., & Wehmeyer, M.L. (2004). The effect of choice-making as an intervention for problem behavior: A meta-analysis. *Journal of Positive Behavior Interventions, 6,* 228–237.

Shogren, K., Palmer, S., Wehmeyer, M.L., Williams-Diehm, K., & Little, T. (2012). Effect of intervention with the *Self-Determined Learning Model of Instruction* on access and goal attainment. *Remedial and Special Education, 33*(5), 320–330.

Shogren, K.A., Wehmeyer, M.L., Palmer, S.B., Rifenbark, G., & Little, T. (forthcoming). Relationships between self-determination and postschool outcomes for youth with disabilities. *Journal of Special Education.*

Shogren, K.A., Wehmeyer, M.L., Palmer, S.B., Soukup, J.H., Little, T., Garner, N., & Lawrence, M. (2008). Understanding the construct of self-determination: Examining the relationship between the Arc's Self-Determination Scale and the American Institute for Research Self-Determination Scale. *Assessment for Effective Instruction, 33,* 94–107.

Stancliffe, R.J., Abery, B.H., & Smith, J. (2000). Personal control and the ecology of community living settings: Beyond living-unit size and type. *American Journal on Mental Retardation, 105,* 431–454.

Sugai, G., & Simonsen, B. (2012). Positive behavioral interventions and supports: History, defining features, and misconceptions. Storrs, CT: University of Connecticut, Center for Positive Behavioral Interventions and Supports. Retrieved from http://www.pbis.org/common/pbisresources/publications/PBIS_revisited_June19r_2012.pdf

Test, D.W., Mason, C., Hughes, C., Konrad, M., Neale, M., & Wood, W. (2004). Student involvement in individualized education program meetings. *Exceptional Children, 70,* 391–412.

Thompson, J.R., Buntinx, W., Schalock, R.L., Shogren, K.A., Snell, M.E., Wehmeyer, M.L., . . . Yeager, M.H. (2009). Conceptualizing supports and the support needs of people with intellectual disability. *Intellectual and Developmental Disabilities, 47,* 235–146.

Wehmeyer, M.L. (2014). Disability in the 21st century: Seeking a future of equity and full participation. In M. Agran, F. Brown, C. Hughes, C. Quirk, & D.L. Ryndak (Eds.), *Equity and full participation for individuals with severe disabilities: A vision for the future* (pp. 3–23). Baltimore, MD: Paul H. Brookes Publishing Co.

Wehmeyer, M.L. (1996). A self-report measure of self-determination for adolescents with cognitive disabilities. *Education and Training in Mental Retardation and Developmental Disabilities, 31,* 282–293.

Wehmeyer, M.L. (2005). Self-determination and individuals with severe disabilities: Reexamining meanings and misinterpretations. *Research and Practice in Severe Disabilities, 30,* 113–120.

Wehmeyer, M.L., Abery, B., Mithaug, D.E., & Stancliffe, R.J. (2003). *Theory in self-determination: Foundations for educational practice.* Springfield, IL: Charles C. Thomas.

Wehmeyer, M.L., Agran, M., Hughes, C., Martin, J., Mithaug, D.E., & Palmer, S. (2007). *Promoting self-determination in students with intellectual and developmental disabilities.* New York, NY: Guilford Press.

Wehmeyer, M.L., Baker, D., Blumberg, R., & Harrison, R. (2004). Self-determination and student involvement in functional assessment: Innovative practices. *Journal of Positive Behavior Interventions, 6,* 29–35.

Wehmeyer, M.L., Buntinx, W.E., Lachapelle, Y., Luckasson, R., Schalock, R., Verdugo-Alonzo, M., . . . Yeager, M. (2008). The intellectual disability construct and its relationship to human functioning. *Intellectual and Developmental Disabilities, 46*(4), 311–318.

Wehmeyer, M.L., & Kelchner, K. (1995). *The Arc's Self-Determination Scale.* Arlington, TX: The Arc National Headquarters.

Wehmeyer, M.L., Kelchner, K., & Richards, S. (1996). Essential characteristics of self-determined behavior of individuals with mental retardation. *American Journal on Mental Retardation, 100,* 632–642.

Wehmeyer, M., Lawrence, M., Kelchner, K., Palmer, S., Garner, N., & Soukup, J. (2004). *Whose future is it anyway? A student-directed transition planning process* (2nd ed.). Lawrence, KS: Beach Center on Disability.

Wehmeyer, M.L., Palmer, S., Agran, M., Mithaug, D., & Martin, J. (2000). Promoting causal agency: The self-determined learning model of instruction. *Exceptional Children, 66,* 439–453.

Wehmeyer, M.L., Palmer, S., Shogren, K., Williams-Diehm, K., & Soukup, J. (2013). Establishing a causal relationship between interventions to promote self-determination and enhanced student self-determination. *Journal of Special Education, 46*(4), 195–210.

Wehmeyer, M.L., & Palmer, S.B. (2003). Adult outcomes for students with cognitive disabilities three-years after high school: The impact of self-determination. *Education and Training in Developmental Disabilities, 38,* 131–144.

Wehmeyer, M.L., Palmer, S.B., Lee, Y., Williams-Diehm, K., & Shogren, K.A. (2011). A randomized-trial evaluation of the effect of *Whose future is it anyway?* on self-determination. *Career Development for Exceptional Individuals, 34*(1), 45–56.

Wehmeyer, M.L., & Schwartz, M. (1997). Self-determination and positive adult outcomes: A follow-up study of youth with mental retardation or learning disabilities. *Exceptional Children, 63,* 245–255.

Wehmeyer, M.L., & Schwartz, M. (1998). The relationship between self-determination, quality of life, and life satisfaction for adults with mental retardation. *Education and Training in Mental Retardation and Developmental Disabilities, 33,* 3–12.

Wehmeyer, M.L., Shogren, K., Palmer, S., Williams-Diehm, K., Little, T., & Boulton, A. (2012). The impact of the *Self-determined learning model of instruction* on student self-determination. *Exceptional Children, 78*(2), 135–153.

Wolman, J., Campeau, P., Dubois, P., Mithaug, D., & Stolarski, V. (1994). *AIR Self-Determination Scale and user guide.* Palo Alto, CA: American Institute for Research.

Strategies for Self-Management

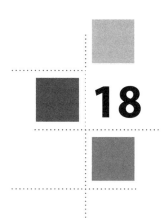

Martin Agran

As discussed by Michael Wehmeyer in Chapter 17, one area that has received much national attention in the last decade is *self-determination*. The behaviors associated with self-determination (i.e., making choices, taking risks, having control over actions to achieve desired outcomes, and assuming responsibility for personal actions) are highly valued in our society. Active student involvement in educational planning and decision making and the regulation of one's own learning are positively associated with improved learning outcomes (Agran, King-Sears, Wehmeyer, & Copeland, 2003). Although self-determination has been well researched in school, community living, and work contexts (Wehmeyer et al., 2007), its relationship to and presence in positive behavior support (PBS) plans has received limited attention, particularly for students with intellectual and developmental disabilities.

Self-management strategies, subsumed under self-determination, represent strategies students can use to modify and regulate their own behavior (Wehmeyer et al., 2007). They allow students to problem-solve; retrieve, process, and synthesize information; and manage their own behavior. As noted throughout this text, problem behaviors can be triggered by one or more antecedent events (e.g., being given a difficult task) and maintained by reinforcing consequences (e.g., getting teacher attention when acting inappropriately). Self-management instruction informs students about ways in which they can manipulate antecedents and consequences themselves and, in doing so, become less dependent on others, as well as have a direct and personal investment in their own development and learning. In this respect, the responsibility for implementing (and managing) behavior change becomes that of the student and not another individual (e.g., teacher, aide) who is referred to as an external change agent. This chapter examines various strategies that have allowed students to self-manage their own behavior change and, as a result, behave appropriately. Recommendations for promoting student self-management and self-regulation are presented.

LACK OF CONTROL
AND PROBLEM BEHAVIOR

Although theories to explain challenging behaviors are plentiful (Sigafoos, Arthur, & O'Reilly, 2003), it is widely acknowledged that problem behaviors occur when individuals do not have alternative (and socially acceptable) ways in their behavioral repertoires to express their needs and achieve desired outcomes or when their environments do not provide opportunities for them to engage in more acceptable social or communicative responses. As Bambara and Kern (2005) noted, problem behavior suggests that there is something "wrong" in the environment—that is, there is a mismatch between an individual's needs, wishes, or preferences and the conditions or characteristics of that environment. As a consequence, individuals feel that they have little or no opportunity to make choices that will allow them to achieve desired ends (Mithaug, 2005). Limited opportunities to make choices and have control over their environments can serve as either the consequence or the cause of challenging behavior (Sigafoos et al., 2003; Wehmeyer, Baker, Blumberg, & Harrison, 2004).

Clark, Olympia, Jenson, Heatherfield, and Jenson (2004) indicated that lack of control and failure to self-regulate is associated with an increased risk for mental health problems and psychiatric disorders. Psychological health can be greatly enhanced by providing more opportunities for personal control and choice. Deci and Ryan (2002) suggested that three basic psychological needs are *competence* (feeling effective in one's ongoing interactions with one's environment), *relatedness* (feeling connected to others), and *autonomy* (perceived origin or source of one's own behavior). Failure to realize one or

more of these dimensions may compromise one's well-being and ability to regulate his or her behavior. When individuals are denied opportunities to feel autonomous, they may perceive themselves as incompetent (Skinner & Edge, 2002; Skinner, Zimmer-Gembeck, & Connell, 1998), which in turn may cause them to behave hostilely, feel coerced, and experience chaos (Deci & Ryan, 1985). This may lead to anger and aggression (Skinner & Edge, 2002) or oppositional behavior (e.g., defiance, explosion; Kochanska, 1997). In contrast, individuals who have a sense of autonomy are able to access their goals and preferences and personal resources—in short, self-manage their actions and ensuing outcomes (desired behaviors).

POSITIVE BEHAVIOR
SUPPORT AND SELF-MANAGEMENT

Traditionally, a student's role in behavior management has been passive and involved responding to the cues and consequences delivered by the teacher—that is, the teacher (or team) determines how to modify the student's "problem" behavior and under what conditions, as well as the consequence-management system used. This approach has been challenged by a number of researchers who suggested that such a teacher-directed approach promotes dependency, minimizes motivation, and restricts student engagement and ownership (Mithaug, Mithaug, Agran, Martin, & Wehmeyer, 2003; Wehmeyer et al., 2007; Zirpoli, 2012). To enhance learning and skill development, it is critical that we maximize the involvement of students with disabilities in self-directed decision making and actions that have a direct impact on their learning—that is, enable students to become more self-determined and more self-regulated (Agran et al., 2003; Wehmeyer, Agran, & Hughes, 2000). This involves teaching students to use learning strategies that allow them to modify and regulate their own behavior—specifically, self-management strategies (Agran, 1997).

Scheuermann and Hall (2012) indicated that the goal of PBS is to move students from external behavior supports to self-managed supports. In a definitive article on PBS, Carr et al. (2002) indicated that it is critical that consumers have an active role in modifying their challenging behavior. By employing self-management strategies, individuals will be empowered and in turn realize they are the primary causal agents in their own lives. To promote this realization, Carr et al. recommended the use of self-management strategies. As Carr et al. noted, these strategies are integral to the values that drive PBS. An essential goal of PBS is to redesign environments to minimize external influences and shift responsibility to the individual. Self-management strategies involve teaching students to modify and regulate their own behavior (Agran, 1997). Of equal importance is the ensuing and concurrent change in the individual's environment, since he or she is manipulating (or controlling) many of the cues and consequences present in that environment—that is, the individual is delivering cues and consequences to himself or herself. This will produce a potentially more responsive environment in which salient, self-directed cues and positive consequences are available and predictable.

Problem or challenging behaviors represent a means by which individuals try to gain control, albeit in an unacceptable manner (Bambara & Kern, 2005). Individuals either lack the skills to achieve desired outcomes or are in environments that fail to provide opportunities for self-expression or control (Brown, Gothelf, Guess, & Lehr, 1998). As noted by Dunlap, Harrower, and Fox (2005), a primary goal of PBS is to teach the individual an alternative (and more socially acceptable) way to act on the environment and, in effect, create more opportunities for choice and exerting control. Self-management can serve as a potentially effective way to facilitate the acquisition of these alternative behaviors—that is, assist students in acquiring and maintaining prosocial skills (Smith & Sugai, 2000). In particular, Halle, Bambara, and Reichle

(2005) recommended that self-management skills can be of value when individuals are in particularly difficult or stressful situations. In such situations, students can use these strategies to help them cope with stressors. For example, a student may experience great stress when he or she is left out of a group activity. In the past, this student may have resorted to disruptive behavior to express his or her dissatisfaction and gain access to the activity. A self-management strategy such as self-instruction in which a student verbally cues (directs) himself or herself to behave in an acceptable way (e.g., "I will ask if I can join in") can provide the student with a means of recognizing problematic situations and developing an immediate action to resolve the problem.

SELF-MANAGEMENT STRATEGIES

Self-determination is a complex construct involving the interplay of several components. As indicated by Wehmeyer et al. (2007), most of these components involve self-management strategies that focus on specific behaviors or actions in which people exert increased control over their behaviors and in the contexts in which they are displayed (Agran & Wehmeyer, 2006; Bambara & Kern, 2005). The development and acquisition of these strategies is lifelong and begins when children are very young (e.g., expressing preferences). A variety of strategies have been used to teach students with disabilities how to manage and regulate their own behavior. Among the most commonly used strategies are choice-making, self-monitoring, self-evaluation, self-reinforcement, self-recruited reinforcement (or support), self-instruction, or a combination of two or more of these behavior interventions. Students' execution of these strategies will not automatically produce model behaviors or eliminate problem behaviors, since other factors such as reinforcement histories and environmental demands may maintain the responses. Nevertheless, as part of a multicomponent PBS plan, these strategies may provide students with a means to monitor and regulate their own behavior and achieve self-selected outcomes. Examples of the applications of these strategies in PBS plans are described in the following sections.

Choice Making

Choice making is the self-management strategy that has been most frequently reported (Wood, Fowler, Uphold, & Test, 2005) and one that has been used with some frequency in PBS plans. Indeed, it is widely acknowledged that providing students with choice-making opportunities may lessen, if not eliminate, their display of problem behavior. By serving as a positive antecedent condition, it sets the context for a successful and nonaversive behavior intervention (Carter, 2001). Promoting choice making has become an important focus of disability services and supports and is regarded as a basic component in service delivery (Wehmeyer, 2001); it serves as the foundational credo for many educational and human services (Bambara, 2004). By allowing individuals with intellectual disabilities to express their preferences, make choices based on those preferences, and act on those choices, students are provided opportunities to self-regulate and assume greater control over their behavior than allowed by externally manipulated behavior interventions. All too frequently, students with disabilities are provided little opportunity to make choices and decisions based on their preferences (Romaniuk & Miltenberger, 2001; Stancliffe & Abery, 1997; Stancliffe & Wehmeyer, 1995; Wehmeyer & Metzler, 1995). Further, many students with disabilities may not know how to express preferences or make choices. This often results in their display of problem behavior. An individual's quality of life and perception that he or she does have control over his or her life (and behavior) are integrally related to the frequency in which opportunities to make choices are provided and the degree to which these choices are supported. Effective

support plans aim to reduce the occurrence of problem behaviors by enhancing students' self-management—in this case, providing increased opportunities for choice making (Carr et al., 2002; Dunlap et al., 2005).

Romaniuk and Miltenberger (2001) reviewed the literature on the relationship of assigning tasks and providing opportunities for choice making on levels of problem behavior for individuals with developmental disabilities. They reported that incorporating preference and choice into behavioral interventions reduced problem behavior. To explain this reduction, Romaniuk and Miltenberger suggested that incorporating preferences and choices into support plans lessens the aversiveness of "other"-determined activities and, as a result, increases motivation and engagement. Also, by providing more opportunities for choice, individuals can perceive that they indeed have more control over their situations, which may result in a reduced level of problem behavior. With this increased sense of control, problem behaviors are rendered "irrelevant, inefficient, and ineffective" (Carr et al., 2002, p. 5)—a primary goal of PBS.

To assess the effects of choice making as a behavior intervention, Shogren, Faggella-Luby, Bae, and Wehmeyer (2004) reviewed 13 studies involving 30 participants. Specifically, the extent to which participants were provided opportunities to either choose task order or select an activity among several was examined. The study provided preliminary support on the benefits of providing choice-making opportunities. Choice-making interventions resulted in reductions in the frequency of problem behavior 65% of the time, and 42% of the data points stayed at zero once that level was achieved. Interestingly, although the number of participants who displayed aggressive behavior was restricted (with a number of participants excluded from the analysis because their target behaviors had not been described sufficiently in the studies reviewed), Shogren et al. reported a greater reduction in aggressive than nonaggressive behaviors as a result of the choice interventions, but an explanation of this effect was not provided. Further, interventions involving choice making were more effective in reducing problem behavior when introduced at an early age.

Cole and Levinson (2002) investigated the relationship between increased choice-making opportunities in daily instructional routines and the frequency of challenging behavior (e.g., aggression, noncompliance) of two boys with severe developmental and behavioral disabilities. The study compared the effects of a *choice* instruction condition, in which students were asked a question for each step of the task analysis, to a *no-choice* condition, in which no choices were provided and the students were given directive prompts for each step of the task. An A-B-A-B experimental design was used. The results suggested dramatic differences between the two instructional conditions. There was a marked decrease in challenging behavior from the baseline level during the first and second choice conditions and a return to a high level of challenging behavior during the second no-choice condition. As Cole and Levinson noted, simply asking choice questions resulted in a reduction of serious challenging behavior. Rather than making a single choice involving the selection of a task or reinforcer, as many choice-making studies have done, in this study, participants had multiple opportunities to make choices. This enabled students to have a more active role in their learning experiences and positive classroom participation.

Similar to the experimental design used by Cole and Levinson (2002), Carter (2001), employing an A-B-A-B design, compared the level of challenging behavior (i.e., disruptive behaviors) during choice and no-choice conditions for three children with autism and severe language delays. The disruptive behaviors included noncompliance, screaming, and tantrums. In addition, Carter examined the effect of choice making on language development (i.e., production of grammatical morphemes) and play-initiation actions. In the choice condition, the children were provided opportunities to choose toys and games they preferred and that toy or game became the naturalistic context for language intervention; in the no-choice condition, these selections were made by the interventionist. The results indicated that levels of disruptive behavior were highest during the no-choice condition, with subsequent reductions in the choice condition. Similar findings were reported for initiating play. Regarding language development, the generalization of grammatical morphemes was only facilitated when the choice condition had been provided. Carter indicated that, as suggested by Dunlap et al. (1994) and Sigafoos (1998), choice may have intrinsically reinforcing properties, as it permits greater access to a preferred object or activity and allows the child to have an active role in their own development.

Last, Kern, Mantegna, Vorndran, Bailin, and Hilt (2001) examined the differential effects on the frequency of problem behavior and level of engagement when students either were directed by their teacher to complete a task or self-selected a task. Problem behavior was lower and engagement was higher for student-selected tasks.

In summary, as Salmento and Bambara (2000) noted, the absence of choice making renders individuals powerless to control critical aspects of their lives and may lead to challenging behavior. Choice making by itself and/or in combination with other self-management strategies has been positively associated with effective PBS.

Self-Monitoring

It is widely accepted that learning to monitor one's behavior is the key or prerequisite to self-regulation (Kanfer, 1970). Students who have learned to monitor their own behavior are in a better position to identify a discrepancy between an existing performance level and a future desired level. Self-monitoring involves a student's observation of his or her own behavior and recording whether the targeted behavior has occurred. The strategy requires that a student understand how to 1) successfully discriminate whether the desired or goal behavior was or was not performed and 2) accurately record the occurrence on a monitoring card or recording device. Figure 18.1 is an example of a self-monitoring form.

Self-monitoring produces behavior change because it may serve as a discriminative stimulus to the student and, thus, cue the desired response. Utilized as a self-managed behavioral change strategy, it involves transferring data collection responsibility from the teacher (external change agent) to the student—a critical step in ensuring student ownership of problem behavior and replacing problem behaviors with more acceptable behaviors. Self-monitoring allows the student to recognize that the specific target behavior has occurred and reminds the student of present and future contingencies that exist in the environment (i.e., "If I perform this response, this will happen"). The target behavior is more likely to occur when this information is available to the student. As Mithaug (1993) suggested, the more often the student has the opportunity to monitor his or her behavior, the more competent he or she will be and the more likely he or she will appreciate the value and utility of self-monitoring.

Smith and Sugai (2000) taught a 13-year-old male student with a history of behavior problems (e.g., defiance, physical aggression) to monitor four behaviors: completing work, obtaining teacher attention, reacting to peers, and asking and responding to questions. Accessing attention was identified as the reason for displaying these problem behaviors. The student was taught to record how and if he had performed the targeted behavior. For example, the student was asked to respond to written prompts: "Did I keep my cool?" or "Did I wait and raise my hand for teacher attention?" The results indicated that self-monitoring increased the student's on-task behavior (work completion) and decreased several of the problem behaviors.

Barry and Messer (2003) studied the impact of a self-management program on five sixth-grade boys diagnosed with attention-deficit/hyperactivity disorder (ADHD) in addition to a variety of problem behaviors (e.g., disruptive behaviors, disruptive noises). The students were taught to respond to a series of questions about their behavior (e.g., "Was I in my seat?"; "Did I play or fight with my classmates?"). After responding to these questions, the students then placed a sticker on a data-collection sheet. Periodic checks were made by the teacher to ensure accuracy. An A-B-A-B-A-B design was used to compare the differential effects of the students' use and disuse of the self-monitoring procedure. The results clearly showed that

---

Self-monitoring form

Name ____John_____ Date _10/1_____

Daily goal: "I was in my seat _8_ out of 10 intervals."

1	2	3	4	5	6	7	8	9	10
+	–	+	+	+	+	–	+	+	+

Mark a "+" if you were in your seat at the end of each interval.

Mark a "–" if you were not in your seat at the end of each interval.

How many intervals was I in my seat? _8 intervals_

Did I reach my goal today?

_X_ Yes ____ No

Figure 18.1.   Example of a self-monitoring form.

self-monitoring consistently helped increase academic performance and lower disruptive behaviors. Barry and Messer noted that the intervention took a relatively short time to teach (20 minutes) and fit well into the general education class's routines.

Rock (2005) examined the effects of a strategic self-monitoring intervention on a variety of academic and problem behaviors for seven elementary-level students. The students had varying types of disabilities (e.g., autism, ADHD, learning disability) and problem behaviors (e.g., physical aggression, disruptive noise, disengagement). The self-monitoring intervention used was referred to as ACT-REACT (Rock, 2005). The strategy involved teaching the students to set goals for themselves (e.g., the number of checks they wanted to receive for work completion), monitoring their on-task behavior for a designated period of time, engaging in self-instruction or self-talk in which they would verbally prompt their behavior (e.g., "I need to have my materials ready"), and last, evaluating their overall performance relative to the goals they had previously set. An A-B-A-B design was used, in which the intervention was withdrawn in the A conditions. The results revealed that there was a consistent increase in academic engagement and a consistent decrease in problem behaviors when the students self-monitored. Rock suggested that the overall gains may have been achieved due in part to providing students with the opportunity to monitor several behaviors concurrently—that is, monitoring several behaviors may produce greater effects than monitoring a single behavior. An additional benefit was that the strategy was effective across disabilities and only slight variations had to be made.

Anderson, Fisher, Marchant, Young, and Smith (2006) described a self-monitoring procedure used in a school implementing the three-tier PBS model. Specifically, the effects of the strategy on two fourth-grade students who engaged in emotional and verbal outbursts were examined. The students were taught to respond to a *cool card* that provided prompts for managing anger: "Take a deep breath," "Count backward from 10," and "Think of something relaxing." Following this, the students were instructed to record their performance on a self-management form, which asked them to record any acts of anger in a designated time period. The effects were immediate and, except for a few outlier data points, the students maintained a 100% record (no angry outbursts) for the duration of the study. Anderson and colleagues suggested that self-monitoring serves as an important component of effective PBS.

Several studies have examined the effects of a self-monitoring program that also included a self-reinforcement component. For example, Lee, Poston, and Poston (2007) examined the effects of a self-management program involving self-monitoring and self-reinforcement on a variety of problem behaviors displayed by a student with autism. The intervention was delivered in the student's home setting. Among the problem behaviors displayed by the student were making growling sounds, not completing a nighttime routine, yelling, and putting hands over ears. The student was taught to self-monitor his performance of four target behaviors. Performance of the target behaviors gave him access to a self-selected reinforcer. The results revealed that the self-management program increased the independent performance of his nighttime routine and decreased the frequency of inappropriate behavior.

Self-Recruited Reinforcement

If newly acquired or developing behaviors are not reinforced sufficiently, they may no longer be emitted. Teacher attention or praise provides a strong means of gaining social approval, which serves as a powerful reinforcer (Alber & Heward, 2000). Because general education settings may be busy environments full of competing stimuli, a resulting problem may be either that students are not being reinforced or that such reinforcement is delayed or inconsistently delivered. As Alber and Heward (2000) noted, all too often teachers attend to disruptive students rather than students who are working quietly and productively. This of course compromises the value and quality of reinforcement in that environment. How then can a teacher be assured that students in the classroom, especially those in need of frequent and immediate reinforcement, can obtain such reinforcement?

A particularly useful approach in general education settings is to teach students to self-recruit support—that is, the student is taught to recruit praise or attention from a teacher. For example, after responding to a number of reading comprehension questions on a worksheet, the student will prompt the teacher to respond to and praise the completed assignment. Craft, Alber, and Heward (1998) taught four elementary students with intellectual disabilities to show their work to their teacher a specified number of times each session. The students were taught to walk to the teacher's desk or raise their hands, wait until the teacher recognized them, and ask the teacher about their work (e.g., "How am I doing?"; "Did I do a good job?"). Improvements in performance were reported for all participants.

For students who find teacher praise reinforcing, self-recruited reinforcement provides a win-win situation in which the student receives reinforcement for successful classroom performance, with such delivery due to the student's self-initiation and "control" of the environment. Rather than continue to depend on others (external change agents), self-recruited reinforcement provides an opportunity for students to express the support they need. An obvious advantage of this is that it provides the student with a strategy that can be used across different classrooms and learning experiences.

Combined
Self-Management Interventions

Several researchers have examined the effects of combined self-management applications, which are composed of two or more self-management strategies. For example, Koegel, Harrower, and Koegel (1999) investigated the effects of a combined self-reinforcement and self-evaluation intervention on the problem behavior of two young children. Two kindergarten-age children with severe cognitive and language disabilities participated. Problem behaviors included yelling, running around the classroom, singing loudly and out of context (for the first child), and wandering and daydreaming (for the second child). The children were taught to place a mark after each interval in which they engaged in appropriate classroom behavior (schoolwork). The children were given a wristwatch with a chronograph function that signaled when the interval ended; a support person increased the length of the intervals over time (from 5 minutes to 20 minutes). Each tally mark could be traded for a reinforcer (selected by the child). The children's self-recordings were compared with those of a support person. Prompts to self-manage were gradually faded during the course of the investigation. The results showed that appropriate classroom behavior increased for both children. Decreases in disruptive behavior were also reported. Koegel et al. noted that the self-management strategy did not make any extra demands on the general education classroom teachers, and they recommended further applications of it.

Ninness et al. (1995) employed a self-management training program to modify the aggressive behavior of four adolescent students in a junior high school. The participating students were four males identified as having serious emotional disturbances. The aggressive behavior they displayed involved striking, kicking, hitting, and shoving other students, among other behaviors. These behaviors were either self-initiated or displayed when the students were provoked by others. An A-B-A-B research design was utilized. The self-management intervention involved the following steps. First, the students were asked to assess their own behavior, specifically their prosocial (i.e., appropriate social behavior) behavior and their performance of an aggression-replacement behavior. A 4-point Likert-type scale was used in which 1 indicates "poor" and 4 indicates "excellent." The students graded and recorded their self-assessments and received bonus points if their scores were within 1 point of the teacher's assessment. Next, the students were taught a number of aggression control techniques, including the verbalization of self-instructions (i.e., self-directed verbal prompts) to guide their behavior (e.g., "I'm not going to let this person bother me"). Following the dictates of the experimental design, the intervention was alternately delivered and withdrawn. The results indicated that there were immediate and dramatic decreases in aggressive behavior when the students were instructed to use the self-management program, with a return to high levels of aggression when the training was withdrawn in the two baseline conditions. Ninness et al. recommended that self-management strategies can be of great value in aggression control packages and in situations where the students are not supervised. Also, they noted that self-management interventions—in particular, self-instruction—may be effective because they prompt students to perform more socially acceptable behavior to deal with emotional expression. In addition, they suggest that self-management interventions are most effective when a number of strategies are taught.

In summary, the available research on self-management suggests that it can potentially serve as an effective behavioral change strategy. Several benefits of self-management are apparent. First, self-management strategies remind the student of the consequences of his or her responding. Second, they are relatively easy to teach and do not appear to take any more time than any other behavior intervention. Third, these strategies may have a multifunctional capacity. For example, the primary function of self-monitoring is for the student to record the frequency of occurrence of a target behavior. However, this strategy may serve a self-evaluative (e.g., "Did

the desired behavior as defined occur?") and/or a self-reinforcing function. Fourth, it has been suggested that by transferring responsibility from the teacher to the student, much of the teacher's time will free up, as he or she does not have to be as vigilant in monitoring the student's behavior (Meadan & Mason, 2007). Self-management provides students with opportunities to, in essence, provide their own positive support—specifically, cue desired behavior, determine and deliver consequences to themselves, evaluate their performance, and if appropriate, recruit their own praise and attention from a teacher.

PERSON-LED BEHAVIOR SUPPORT PLANS

The interventions described previously provide participants with methods they can use to manipulate their environments (Wehmeyer et al., 2004). These strategies have been shown to be effective, but as noted by Wehmeyer et al., they reveal that although the participant may have a critical role in modifying his or her behavior, other aspects of what we presume to be a self-regulation are made by others—specifically, identifying the nature of and function of the problem behavior (i.e., functional assessment). Wehmeyer et al. suggest that although it is recommended that students have an integral role in the development of the functional assessment (Martin, Marshall, & De Pry, 2002; O'Neill et al., 1997), this is not always the case. Efforts must be made to ensure that students have an active role in developing the functional assessment. Such involvement allows students to engage in problem solving. Problem solving involves teaching students strategies to identify problems and determine feasible solutions to these problems (Agran & Wehmeyer, 1999). When faced with problems, many students respond impulsively, do not weigh the consequences of their actions, or take no action at all. They are easily victimized by circumstances and feel helpless in identifying a workable way to resolve their difficulty, as discussed in the

Ninness et al. (1995) study. Involving students in developing the functional assessment provides them with potential insights about why they behave as they do.

Wehmeyer et al. (2004) invited 10 students with a variety of disabilities and challenging behaviors to be interviewed for a functional behavioral assessment. The functional assessment employed was the functional assessment interview developed by O'Neill et al. (1997). The students were asked to provide input about potential setting events, antecedents, problem behaviors, and consequences. The students' responses were compared with those of school staff. The results revealed a relatively high level of agreement in identifying problem behaviors and the consequences that occurred after these behaviors were performed. Also, there was general agreement in identifying antecedent events, although there was lower agreement for setting events. Wehmeyer et al. suggest that it is critical that we involve students in all aspects of support plans and that functional assessment activities indeed be self-guided.

With a similar research goal, Ruef and Turnbull (2002) asked nine participants with intellectual disabilities or autism to share their perspectives about issues relating to their problem behaviors. Although the information they provided was not directly used in functional assessments—focus groups were conducted—the value of engaging individuals in problem-solving activities relating to their challenging behaviors was investigated. The participants had received varying degrees of support services to address a number of serious problem behaviors (i.e., self-injury, physical aggressiveness, and property destruction). In the focus groups, the participants were asked to describe their problem behaviors, how they dealt with them, what upset them most, and how they have learned to deal with their behavior, among others. A number of the participants indicated that they value being self-aware and appreciate being able to define desired outcomes and make choices. Also, the participants emphasized the importance of having control over the quality of their lives. Indeed, they suggested that problem behaviors were due to exclusion, lack of personal choice, and restricted lifestyles—outcomes very much aligned with self-determination outcomes (see Chapter 17).

INDIVIDUAL APPLICATIONS OF SELF-MANAGEMENT STRATEGIES

The following are two case studies describing the application of self-management strategies with students with serious emotional disabilities.

Casey

Casey was a fifth grader in a neighborhood elementary school. He received adult support throughout the school day. Based on the disability categories used in his school district, Casey was labeled as having an emotional disability. Casey displayed an array of aggressive behaviors, including lunging at teachers; slugging with closed fists; spitting, biting, and pushing other students; overturning tables; and destroying school materials. A functional assessment of his problem behavior suggested that he behaved this way to avoid doing nonpreferred tasks, in response to corrective feedback, and/or when he has a negative peer interaction, which results in him showing aggression toward teachers. He was not prescribed psychotropic medications.

A self-management intervention was recommended based on a failure of externally delivered consequence interventions used previously (e.g., extended time-outs, suspension). The self-management intervention included two strategies. First, Casey was involved in goal setting, in which he would indicate the "allowable" number of behavioral episodes he could have in a day. From an average of 25 events a day, decreases in frequency in units of 10 were sought. Second, every half hour, Casey was asked to evaluate his behavioral performance. At first, an electronic data collection was used by the teacher, which displayed graphs for Casey to see. Over time, Casey was taught to self-monitor. Among the questions he was to ask himself were, "How safe were you?"; "Did you avoid any conflicts?"; and "How respectful were your words?" These two strategies were taught following a sequence developed by Agran et al. (2003). First, the benefits of using the strategy were discussed. Next, the strategy was demonstrated by the teacher. Then Casey was provided guided practice in role-play situations, and feedback was delivered as needed. Following this, independent practice opportunities were presented within authentic situations and then reinforced for mastery.

Over time, consistent and positive changes were observed. The first change was the use of respectful words, followed by a decrease in higher-level aggressive behavior (e.g., punching, spitting, biting) and lower-level aggressive behaviors (e.g., destruction of school property). Casey still had episodes of problem behavior, but their severity and frequency decreased, with longer periods of stable and safe behaviors.

Jay

Jay was a seventh-grade junior high school student labeled as having multiple disabilities (e.g., intellectual disability, emotional disability). He received full adult support throughout the day. (Note his parents requested that he not be left unsupervised because they fear he may attack a classmate, but this has not happened to date.) He displayed a variety of verbally aggressive behaviors—specifically, arguing, swearing, and raising his voice. In addition, he broke his glasses purposefully several times, liked to hide under furniture, and pushed over room partitions. Although he has not been physically aggressive to staff, he has threatened to do so and has in fact attacked his mother. A functional assessment suggested that he behaved this way to avoid tasks and achieve some level of power and control. Jay was an adopted child and had strained relationships with his siblings, who were older than he was.

To allow Jay to have some control, he was taught to self-monitor his behavior. Specifically, he was taught to monitor after designated time periods when he had his hands in lap, uttered respectful words, kept his glasses on his face or handed them to an adult for safe keeping, and had an appropriate voice level. The training sequence involved the following steps. First, the benefits of performing the desired behaviors were discussed, followed by examples and

nonexamples of them. Following, the self-monitoring procedure was modeled by the teacher. Next, guided practice and feedback were provided in role play and then authentic situations. Last, after approximately 8 months, Jay was able to accurately monitor his behavior 75% of the time. Improvements across all target behaviors were reported, although the avoidance behaviors continued during stressful or demanding situations. However, the verbally aggressive behavior was reduced dramatically, and there were no further incidents with his mother.

FUTURE RESEARCH

As noted by Crimmins and Farrell (2006), self-management can serve as invaluable student-centered intervention to teach adaptive alternatives to problem behavior. Although its value has been well supported in the PBS literature, the extent to which self-management strategies are used in practice is limited. Wehmeyer et al. (2000) indicated that a foremost reason teachers do not teach self-management strategies is that they are aware of the construct of self-management but are not cognizant of the various instructional strategies subsumed within that term, which strategy provides the best "fit" for different problem behaviors, and methods to use to systematically and efficiently teach these strategies. Increased efforts to inform professionals—and of course parents and students—about self-management must be conducted.

Also, although the value of self-management is well demonstrated in the research literature, the extent to which it is used in schoolwide and individual PBS systems remains unknown. Educators and practitioners may be reluctant to give students with behavior challenges more "control," thinking that this will only exacerbate the situation. Further, they may believe that shifting responsibility to the student will only compromise the rigor of their behavior plans. Research on the extent to which teachers provide systematic instruction to their students on how to use self-management and self-regulatory strategies suggest that many students—particularly those with cognitive disabilities—receive little or no self-management instruction (Agran, Snow, & Swaner, 1999; Wehmeyer, Agran, & Hughes, 2000). Research is needed on both the extent to which self-management is a component in PBS and practices used to promote its inclusion in plans.

Last, it is generally acknowledged that the greater the involvement of a student in a self-directed behavior change process, the greater the student's sense of ownership. The extent to which the student is involved in each of the steps of developing a support plan—from providing critical input for the functional assessment to evaluating if he or she is behaving appropriately—will have a direct and positive impact on desired behavior change. In this respect, efforts must be made to fully involve the student in the process, providing support as needed. Self-management strategies are selected based on a student's preference and instructional needs. An additional consideration is that combined self-management interventions, as demonstrated in several of the studies described in this paper, appear to have greater efficacy. PBS planning committees (teams) need to examine ways in which students can have extended roles in their behavior change.

CONCLUSION

Individuals who engage in problem behaviors do so to achieve some control over their lives and circumstances. It is well acknowledged that we cannot just eliminate the problem but must teach individuals alternative ways to act in their environments and achieve desired outcomes (Bambara & Kern, 2005; Dunlap et al., 2005). Self-management serves as a potentially alternative (and effective) way to achieve this control. It can provide the student with an acceptable means to manipulate an environment that was otherwise restrictive and unresponsive.

REFERENCES

Agran, M. (Ed.). (1997). *Student-directed learning: Teaching self-determination skills.* Pacific Grove, CA: Brooks/Cole.

Agran, M., King-Sears, M.E., Wehmeyer, M.L., & Copeland, S.R. (2003). *Student-directed learning.* Baltimore, MD: Paul H. Brookes Publishing Co.

Agran, M., Snow, K., & Swaner, J. (1999). Self-determination: Benefits, challenges, characteristics. *Education and Training in Mental Retardation and Developmental Disabilities, 34,* 293–301.

Agran, M., & Wehmeyer, M. (1999). *Teaching problem solving to students with mental retardation.* Washington, DC: American Association on Mental Retardation.

Agran, M., & Wehmeyer, M. (2006). Child self-regulation. In M. Hersen (Ed.), *Clinical handbook of behavioral assessment* (pp. 181–199). San Diego, CA: Elsevier Scientific.

Alber, S.R., & Heward, W.L. (2000). Teaching students to recruit positive attention: A review and recommendations. *Journal of Behavioral Education, 10,* 177–204.

Anderson, D.H., Fisher, A., Marchant, M., Young, K.R., & Smith, J.A. (2006). The cool card intervention: A positive support strategy for managing anger. *Beyond Behavior, 16,* 3–13.

Bambara, L.M. (2004). Fostering choice-making skills: We've come a long way but still have a long way to go. *Research and Practice for Persons with Severe Disabilities, 29,* 169–171.

Bambara, L.M., & Kern, L. (2005). *Individual supports for students with problem behaviors.* New York, NY: Guilford Press.

Barry, L.M., & Messer, J.J. (2003). A practical application of self-management for students diagnosed with attention deficit/hyperactivity disorder. *Journal of Positive Behavior Interventions, 5,* 238–248.

Brown, F., Gothelf, R., Guess, D., & Lehr, H. (1998). Self-determination for individuals with the most severe disabilities: Moving beyond chimera. *Journal of The Association for Persons with Severe Handicaps, 23,* 17–26.

Carr, E.G., Dunlap, G., Horner, R.H., Koegel, R.L., Turnbull, A., Sailor, W., . . . Fox, L. (2002). Positive behavior support: Evolution of an applied science. *Journal of Positive Behavior Interventions, 4,* 4–16, 20.

Carter, C.M. (2001). Using choice with game play to increase language skills and interactive behaviors in children with autism. *Journal of Positive Behavior Interventions, 3,* 131–151.

Clark, E., Olympia, D.E., Jensen, J., Heatherfield, L.T., & Jenson, W.R. (2004). Striving for autonomy in a contingency-governed world: Another challenge for individuals with developmental disabilities. *Psychology in the Schools, 41,* 143–153.

Cole, C.L., & Levinson, T.R. (2002). Effects of within-activity choices on the challenging behavior of children with severe developmental disabilities. *Journal of Positive Behavior Interventions, 4,* 29–38.

Craft, M.A., Alber, S.R., & Heward, W.I. (1998). Teaching elementary students with developmental disabilities to recruit teacher attention in a general education classroom: Effects on teacher praise and academic productivity. *Journal of Applied Behavior Analysis, 31,* 399–415.

Crimmins, D.B., & Farrell, A.F. (2006). Individualized behavioral supports at 15 years: It's still lonely at the top. *Research and Practice in Severe Disabilities, 31,* 31–45.

Deci, E.L., & Ryan, R.M. (1985). *Intrinsic motivation and self-determination in human behavior.* New York, NY: Plenum.

Deci, E.L., & Ryan, R.M. (2002). *Handbook of self-determination research.* Rochester, NY: University of Rochester Press.

Dunlap, G., Harrower, J., & Fox, L. (2005). Understanding the environmental determinants of problem behaviors. In L. Bambara & L. Kern (Eds.), *Individualized supports for students with problem behaviors* (pp. 25–46). New York, NY: Guilford Press.

Halle, J., Bambara, L., & Reichle, J. (2005). Teaching alternative skills. In L. Bambara & L. Kern (Eds.), *Individualized supports for students with problem behaviors: Designing positive behavioral support plans.* New York, NY: Guilford Press.

Kanfer, F.H. (1970). Self-regulation: Research, issues, and speculations. In C. Neuringer & L. Michael (Eds.), *Behavior modification in clinical psychology* (pp. 178–220). New York, NY: Appleton-Century-Crofts.

Kern, L., Mantegna, M.E., Vorndran, C.M., Bailin, D., & Hilt, A. (2001). Choice of task sequence to reduce problem behaviors. *Journal of Positive Behavior Interventions, 3,* 3–10.

Kochanska, G. (1997). Mutually responsive orientation between mothers and their young children: Implications for early socialization. *Child Development, 68,* 94–112.

Koegel, L.K., Harrower, J.K., & Koegel, R.L. (1999). Support for children with developmental disabilities. *Journal of Positive Behavior Interventions, 1,* 26–34.

Lee, S., Poston, D., & Poston, A. (2007). Lessons learned through implementing a positive behavior support intervention at home: A case study of self-management with a student with autism and his mother. *Education and Training in Developmental Disabilities, 42,* 418–427.

Martin, J.E., Marshall, L.H., & De Pry, R.L. (2002). Participatory decision-making: Innovative practices that increase student self-determination. In R.W. Flexer, T.J. Simmons, P. Luft, & R. Baer (Eds.), *Transition planning for secondary students with disabilities* (3rd ed., pp. 340–366). Columbus, OH: Merrill.

Meadan, H., & Mason, L.H. (2007). Reading instruction for a student with emotional disturbance: Facilitating understanding of expository text. *Beyond Behavior, 16,* 18–26.

Mithaug, D.E. (1993). *Self-regulation theory: How optimal adjustment maximizes gain.* Westport, CT: Praeger.

Mithaug, D.E. (2005). On persistent pursuits of self-interest. *Research and Practice for Persons with Severe Disabilities, 30,* 163–167.

Mithaug, D.E., Mithaug, D.K., Agran, M., Martin, J.E., & Wehmeyer, M.L. (2003). Understanding the engagement problem. In D.E. Mithaug, D.K. Mithaug, M. Agran, J.E. Martin, & M.L. Wehmeyer

(Eds.), *Self-determined learning theory: Construction, verification, and evaluation* (pp. 3–18). Mahwah, NJ: Lawrence Erlbaum Associates.

Ninness, H.A., Ellis, J., Miller, W.B., Baker, D., & Rutherford, R. (1995). The effect of a self-management training package on the transfer of aggression control procedures in the absence of supervision. *Behavior Modification, 19,* 464–490.

O'Neill, R., Horner, R., Albin, R., Sprague, J., Storey, K., & Newton, J. (1997). *Functional assessment and program development for problem behavior: A practical handbook.* Pacific Grove, CA: Brooks/Cole.

Rock, M.L. (2005). Use of strategic self-monitoring to enhance academic engagement, productivity, and accuracy of students with and without exceptionalities. *Journal of Positive Interventions, 7,* 3–17.

Romaniuk, C., & Miltenberger, R.G. (2001). The influence of preference and choice of activity on problem behavior. *Journal of Positive Behavior Interventions, 3,* 152–159.

Ruef, M.B., & Turnbull, A.P. (2002). The perspectives of individuals with cognitive disabilities and/or autism on their lives and their problem behavior. *Research and Practice for Persons with Severe Disabilities, 27,* 125–140.

Salmento, M., & Bambara, L.M. (2000). Teaching staff members to provide choice opportunities for adults with multiple disabilities. *Journal of Positive Behavior Interventions, 2,* 12–21.

Scheuermann, B.K., & Hall, J.A. (2012). *Positive behavioral support for the classroom.* Upper Saddle River, NJ: Pearson.

Shogren, K., Faggella-Luby, M., Bae, S.J., & Wehmeyer, M. (2004). The effect of choice making as an intervention for problem behavior: A meta-analysis. *Journal of Positive Behavior Interventions, 6,* 228–237.

Sigafoos, J. (1998). Assessing conditional use of graphic mode requesting in a young boy with autism. *Journal of Developmental and Physical Disabilities, 10,* 133–151.

Sigafoos, J., Arthur, M., O'Reilly, M. (2003). *Challenging behavior and developmental disability.* Philadelphia, PA: Whurr.

Skinner, E.A., & Edge, K. (2002). Self-determination, coping, and development. In E.L. Deci & R.M. Ryan (Eds.), *Self-determination theory: Extensions and applications* (pp. 297–337). Rochester, NY: University of Rochester Press.

Skinner, E.A., Zimmer-Gembeck, M.J., & Connell, J.P. (1998). Individual differences and the development of perceived control. *Monographs of the Society for Research in Child Development, 63*(2/3), series 254.

Smith, B.W., & Sugai, G. (2000). A self-management functional assessment-based behavior support plan for a middle school student with EBD. *Journal of Positive Behavior Interventions, 2,* 208–217.

Stancliffe, R.J., & Abery, B.H. (1997). Longitudinal study of institutionalization and the exercise of choice. *Mental Retardation, 35,* 159–169.

Stancliffe, R., & Wehmeyer, M.L. (1995). Variability in the availability of choice to adults with mental retardation. *Journal of Vocational Rehabilitation, 5,* 319–328.

Wehmeyer, M.L. (2001). Self-determination and mental retardation. *International Review of Research in Mental Retardation, 24,* 1–48.

Wehmeyer,M.L.,Agran,M.,&Hughes,C.(2000).A national survey of teachers' promotion of self-determination and student-directed learning. *Journal of Special Education, 34*, 58–68. doi:10.1177/00224669003400201

Wehmeyer, M.L., Agran, M., Hughes, C., Martin, J.E., Mithaug, D.E., & Palmer, S.B. (2007). *Promoting self-determination in students with developmental disabilities.* New York, NY: Guilford Press.

Wehmeyer, M.L., Baker, D.J., Blumberg, R., & Harrison, R. (2004). Self-determination and student involvement in functional assessment: Innovative packages. *Journal of Positive Behavior Interventions, 6*, 29–35.

Wehmeyer, M.L., & Metzler, C.A. (1995). How self-determined are people with mental retardation? The national consumer survey. *Mental Retardation, 33*, 111–119.

Wood, W.M., Fowler, C.H., Uphold, N.M., & Test, D.W. (2005). A review of self-determination interventions with individuals with severe disabilities. *Research and Practice for Persons with Severe Disabilities, 30*, 121–146.

Zirpoli, T.J. (2012). *Behavior management positive applications for teachers.* Upper Saddle River, NJ: Pearson.

Visual Supports as Antecedent and Teaching Interventions

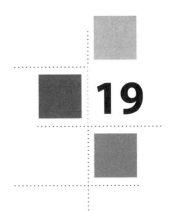

19

Pat Mirenda and Brenda Fossett

V isual supports employ real objects or graphic media, such as photographs, line drawings, or other symbols, in order to enhance comprehension and/or support the acquisition of new skills. In positive behavior support (PBS), visual supports are commonly used in the context of antecedent and instructional interventions. When used as antecedents, visual supports are designed to prevent problem behavior by enhancing the predictability of upcoming events and/or supporting an individual's ability to understand social situations and the expectations therein. When used instructionally, visual supports can be combined with various teaching techniques to support independent performance and/or teach new behaviors that are functionally equivalent to existing problem behaviors. Visual supports are related to several Association for Positive Behavior Support (APBS; 2007) standards of practice guidelines, including the use of antecedent

manipulations (standards III-B and IV-C) and the use of effective instructional intervention strategies (standard IV-D).

Most of the literature on the use of visual supports has involved individuals— primarily children—with autism spectrum disorder (ASD). This is not to say that interventions that utilize visual supports are only appropriate for individuals with ASD; for example, in a comprehensive review of story-based intervention studies, Reynhout and Carter (2011) found that approximately 30% of participants had other diagnoses. Disability labels aside, visual supports appear to be effective for several reasons. Many individuals who engage in problem behavior seem to prefer environments and activities that afford them the ability to predict future events accurately (Flannery & O'Neill, 1995). Because family, school, and community life is often impossible to arrange consistently from day to day, visual supports can be used to help these individuals to better understand

and predict their everchanging routines and schedules. In addition, visual supports utilize the relatively strong visuospatial processing abilities of some individuals—especially those with ASD—in order to compensate for auditory processing deficits that can result in language comprehension difficulties (Mitchell & Ropar, 2004; Roth, Muchnik, Shabtai, Hildesheimer, & Henkin, 2011; Siegal & Blades, 2003). Regardless of the mechanism(s) involved, visual supports appear to alleviate at least some of the confusion, anxiety, and frustration that many individuals experience when they encounter unexpected changes or events. Visual supports may also facilitate a person's understanding of social situations and cause-and-effect relationships and can assist with the acquisition of new skills and alternative replacement behaviors by depicting them in a concrete, visual form. The end result is often a reduction in problem behaviors that are used to escape from confusing and/or novel situations.

ANTECEDENT SUPPORTS: VISUAL ACTIVITY SCHEDULES

As noted previously, visual supports can be used as both antecedent and teaching interventions within comprehensive PBS plans. The most common type of visual support is the visual activity schedule (VAS), which can be used to address specific setting events and/or antecedents that are identified during a functional behavioral assessment (FBA). A VAS can be designed to depict either between-activity or within-activity events. Video-based activity schedules may be also be used in addition or as an adjunct to static VASs.

Between-Activity Visual Activity Schedules

Between-activity VASs (sometimes referred to as schedule systems; Mesibov, Browder, & Kirkland, 2002) depict a sequence of activities that occur within a specified period of time (typically, over several hours within a day). They employ object or picture symbols and/or written words that are presented in sequential order to inform the user about transitions *between* upcoming activities or events. A between-activity VAS is usually intended to enhance predictability and thus reduce problem behavior associated with changes or transitions from one activity to the next.

Jake

Jake was a 5-year-old boy who perceived only light and dark and was diagnosed with a bilateral profound sensorineural hearing loss. He was enrolled in kindergarten in his neighborhood school and engaged in severe tantrums (e.g., screaming, biting staff, and falling to the floor) whenever staff attempted to direct him from one activity to the next. Jake's FBA indicated that his tantrums enabled him to escape transitions to new tasks and maintain access to a current activity. Because of his visual impairment, Jake was unable to perceive photographs or other graphic symbols; thus his education team developed a set of tangible symbols (Rowland & Schweigert, 2000) that depicted the activities that occurred at school. Each activity was represented by an object that bore a tactile similarity to an item used in the activity. For example, recess was represented by a small piece of chain that felt similar to the chain that suspended Jake's favorite playground swing. A plastic scoop was used to represent the sandbox, as Jake used the scoop to play in the sand. A touch-and-feel book was used to represent circle time, as Jake used similar books during this time of the day. The symbols were placed in individual boxes, and the boxes were sequenced on a shelf to depict the order of activities (see Figure 19.1).

When Jake arrived at school, his support worker (a trained deafblind intervener) supported him to feel each of the symbols in their boxes, while pairing each symbol with a tactile sign. This allowed Jake to have a sense of what activities would occur during the day. Then before the first activity, the intervener provided physical guidance to help Jake remove and feel the first symbol and bring it with him to the activity. When the activity was completed, she guided Jake back to his schedule, assisted him to place the symbol in a large bin (the "finished" box), and guided him to pick up and feel the symbol for the next activity. This process was repeated for each transition across the school

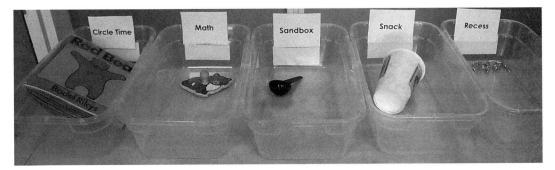

Figure 19.1.   Jake's between-activity schedule system with tangible symbols representing kindergarten activities: circle time, math, sandbox, snack, and going on the swing during recess. (Photograph courtesy of Brenda Fossett.)

day. Initially, Jake engaged in some tantrum behavior when directed toward the schedule system, but his intervener persisted in directing him to the next activity. Over several weeks, Jake's tantrums during transitions reduced in number and severity. In addition, staff noted that, upon picking up a symbol, Jake began to pull his intervener in the direction of the related activity. Over the next few months, Jake learned the associations between 25 tangible symbols and activities, and his tantrum behavior was significantly reduced.

Within-Activity Visual Activity Schedules

The second type of VAS uses pictures or symbols to represent a sequence of steps *within* an activity or task. The goal of a within-activity VAS is to increase an individual's ability to perform a single activity without assistance by depicting a series of discrete steps or skills that are required, in sequential order, resembling a task analysis of the activity. Typically, an individual is taught to refer to the within-activity schedule after completing each step in the sequence and to use the pictures as reminders of the steps that follow.

Alisa

Alisa was a young woman with a significant intellectual disability who lived in a supported home with two other women with similar disabilities.

Alisa was unable to speak but used line-drawing symbols to communicate her wants and needs. During the morning routine—especially during bath time—Alisa engaged in a number of problem behaviors, including screaming, stomping her feet, hitting support staff or the wall, and biting her hand. An FBA indicated that Alisa's problem behaviors were maintained by escape from bathing-related demands. When her support worker asked her to wash a specific body part, she engaged in problem behavior, and her worker's usual response was to provide assistance with washing, even though the motor skills required for the task were within Alisa's repertoire. This pattern, which had persisted for several years, prevented Alisa from achieving independence in a routine that, for most adults, is conducted in private.

A within-activity schedule was developed to support Alisa to understand and learn the steps for bathing. Alisa was involved in setting up the schedule each morning; this involved providing her with choices regarding the type of tool (e.g., a preferred washcloth or a body scrubber) she would use to wash each body part and the type of bubble bath she wanted to put in the tub. The schedule also depicted the order in which each body part would be washed; Alisa placed symbols representing herself or her support worker next to each pictured body part to indicate who would be responsible for washing. Initially, she was permitted to place a support worker symbol next to all except the "private" body parts, which were paired with her symbol. Over time, the number of support worker symbols that were available for the schedule were decreased gradually, to encourage Alisa to wash more parts of her body. Figure 19.2 depicts Alisa's within-activity VAS.

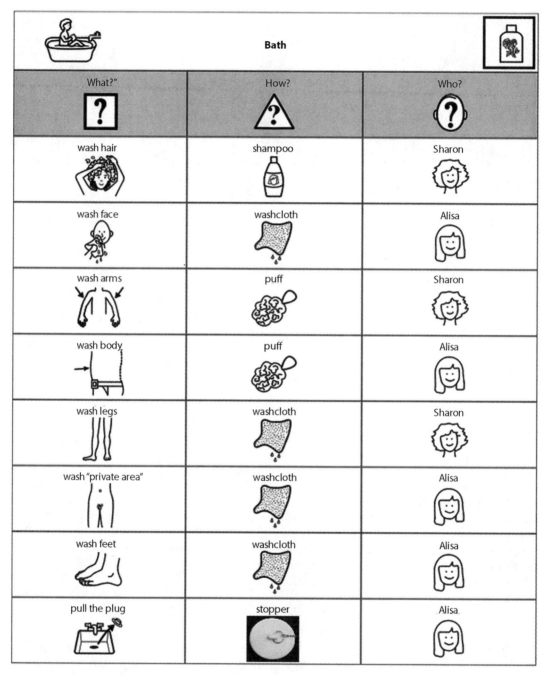

Figure 19.2. Alisa's within-activity bathing schedule, with symbols representing steps of the task, her choice of related materials, and who was responsible for each step (Alisa or her support worker, Sharon). (The Picture Communication Symbols ©1981–2010 by Mayer-Johnson LLC. All Rights Reserved Worldwide. Used with permission. Boardmaker™ is a trademark of Mayer-Johnson LLC.)

Over a 3-month period, all but three support worker symbols were faded, as Alisa gradually assumed increasing responsibility for bathing herself. Praise and access to favorite bath items continued to be used to reinforce self-bathing, and staff reported that Alisa's problem behaviors decreased in both frequency and intensity. While she continued to engage occasional problem behaviors (i.e., 1–2 times per week), they were less severe in nature and staff were able to persist with the routine. Four months after the intervention was initiated, Alisa was washing her entire body independently with no problem behavior and was requesting that staff wait outside the bathroom.

....

It is important to note that, in most cases, VASs are implemented in the context of multielement interventions that include various instructional strategies aimed at teaching the target individual to follow and use the VAS independently. Such strategies may include prompting and fading procedures (e.g., graduated guidance, least-to-most prompting, time delay) to teach the behaviors depicted in the VAS, reinforcement contingencies for following the VAS, and/or escape extinction for noncompliance (Lequia, Machalicek, & Rispoli, 2012; Waters, Lerman, & Hovanetz, 2009). For example, in Jake's example described previously, his intervener gave Jake a high-five and blew gently on his hair (a preferred activity) if he changed activities without engaging in problem behavior (i.e., differential reinforcement of other behavior, DRO). However, if Jake began to tantrum after retrieving the symbol for the next activity, the intervener gently escorted him to the activity area and helped him to begin the associated task. Although the use of instructional procedures may not be emphasized in some published descriptions of VAS interventions, they are usually required, at least in the initial stage of implementation. Once the routine associated with a VAS has been taught, the VAS then functions as an antecedent prompt to inform and/or remind the individual of upcoming events or steps in a task, much like a conventional day planner or written recipe. For example, Jake's intervener was able to fade her prompts and no longer needed to use escape extinction after 7 days, and she gradually faded the reinforcement procedures as well over a 4-week period. However, Jake continued to rely on his VAS in order to make smooth transitions at school for the remainder of the school year.

Video Activity Schedules

In the past few years, researchers have incorporated prerecorded prompts into the design of within-activity schedules to teach functional living skills such as use of an ATM (Cihak, Alberto, Taber-Doughty, & Gama, 2006) and independent cooking skills (Mechling, Gast, & Seid, 2009; Mechling & Gustafson, 2008). In these studies, participants typically watched taped task sequences on a portable DVD player (Mechling & Gustafson, 2008) or personal data assistant (Mechling et al., 2009) and were able to stop the recording after each step of a task in order to complete it. In addition, a few studies have used taped scenes in between-activity schedules to decrease tantrums and other disruptive transition behaviors (e.g., Cihak, 2011; Schreibman, Whalen, & Stahmer, 2000). For example, Schreibman et al. (2000) taped upcoming events or activities (e.g., transitions from home to the community or from the toy department of a store to the checkout counter) in which three preschool-age children with ASD typically exhibited problem behaviors such as tantrums. During intervention, the children viewed the videos prior to the target events to help them predict the transitions, much as they might view a traditional VAS with the steps of a problem routine depicted pictorially. For all three children in the study, results showed a gradual reduction or elimination of the disruptive behaviors, with generalization to novel settings and routines. Similarly, Cihak (2011) compared the use of a pictorial VAS and a video activity schedule to treat problem transitions in three older children with ASD and found positive outcomes for both types of schedules. While additional research in this area is needed, it appears that activity schedules that take advantage of modern digital technologies also hold promise as visual supports.

Research Evidence

Several reviews have examined the effectiveness of between- and within-activity VASs. Banda and Grimmett (2008) conducted a narrative review of 13 VAS studies that were published between 1993 and 2004, six of which targeted problem behaviors such as tantrums, kicking, screaming, aggression, and off-task behavior in children with ASD, ages 3–14. The results found VASs to be effective, generalizable, and socially valid for use with this population. Two subsequent systematic reviews (Lequia et al., 2012; National Autism Center, 2009) included VAS studies published up to 2007 and 2010, respectively, and employed stringent methods for evaluating the quality of the research studies. Both reviews found results that were similar to Banda and Grimmett (2008); in fact, the National Autism Center identified VAS as one of only 11 "established" behavioral/educational treatments that support self-regulation in individuals with ASD. Finally, a narrative review by Koyama and Wang (2011) examined the use of VASs across studies that were published up to 2009 and included individuals with intellectual disabilities in general (ages 3–57), not just ASD. Of the 23 studies that were included, 8 targeted decreases in disruptive or self-injurious behavior and 15 targeted increases in on-task behavior. As was the case in the other reviews, results indicated VASs to be effective for promoting the self-management skills associated with problem behavior reduction for a broad range of individuals with intellectual disabilities.

TEACHING INTERVENTIONS

Visual supports can also be combined with appropriate instructional techniques to teach new, replacement behaviors that are functionally equivalent to specific problem behaviors. The most commonly used visual supports of this type include story-based interventions, the power card strategy, and contingency maps.

Story-Based Interventions

We use the phrase *story-based intervention* in this chapter to refer to stories that are written to describe socially appropriate behaviors and the situations in which they are expected to occur. These include but are not limited to the Social Story, a tool developed by Gray (2000) for the purpose of explaining socially challenging situations. A Social Story is written according to a specific format and is often used to explain upcoming events so that misinterpretations, confusion, and unpredictability do not result in problem behavior. Several studies (e.g., Reynhout & Carter, 2006, 2009, 2011) have suggested that a majority of the story-based interventions implemented in both research and practice, including those employed in many published reports, do not adhere to Gray's recommendations for Social Story construction and implementation, which have evolved considerably over the years (Gray, 2010). Thus we have elected to use the generic term *story-based intervention* rather than Social Story when discussing the research in this section.

Story-based interventions can be designed and implemented for a wide range of purposes, such as teaching specific social skills for interaction, play, or communication and teaching self-care skills (Test, Richter, Knight, & Spooner, 2011). However, the most common purpose, explicitly identified in approximately 50%–60% of story-based research studies to date, is to teach socially appropriate behaviors as functional alternatives for problem behaviors (Kokina & Kern, 2010; Reynhout & Carter, 2011). Typically, the problem behaviors addressed in story-based interventions are mild (i.e., "tolerable") or disruptive but not dangerous. Although the story itself is meant to be the key feature of story-based interventions, most also include visual supports such as pictures, symbols, or other graphic images that are designed to complement the story and facilitate learners' comprehension and retention of the information provided (Kokina & Kern, 2010; Reynhout & Carter, 2009, 2011).

Gregg

A story-based intervention that utilized visual supports was reported by Lorimer, Simpson, Myles, and Ganz (2002). The study involved Gregg, a 5-year-old boy with ASD who participated in an early childhood special education classroom and also received speech, occupational, and behavior therapies at home several times weekly. Gregg engaged in frequent tantrums (i.e., screaming, hitting, kicking, and throwing objects) at home, which appeared to be maintained by both attention and tangible reinforcement. He also engaged in a number of "pretantrum" or precursor behaviors, including ineffective and inappropriate verbalizations when he was asked to wait or when two adults were talking to one another (e.g., Gregg would repeatedly yell, "Stop talking!"; "Listen to me!"; or "You are too loud!"). Based on the results of an FBA, the authors developed two stories that were designed to teach Gregg to wait and to raise his hand or say "Excuse me" to gain the attention of an adult. Gregg's stories also contained several suggestions for activities he could do if he had to wait, including watching a video, listening to an audio book, looking at a book, or playing a game. Because Gregg was a prereader, line drawings were paired with the written text; Figure 19.3 depicts one of Gregg's stories and the associated visual supports.

An A-B-A-B design was used to evaluate the impact of the intervention. During intervention, the stories were read to Greg prior to each of his home-based therapy sessions and at least once daily on weekends. If he engaged in pretantrum behaviors (e.g., interrupting two adults when they were talking), he was asked to review his stories to determine the correct behavior. Immediately following implementation of the story-based intervention, Gregg's pretantrum verbalizations decreased dramatically, and his tantrums were reduced to near-zero levels. This effect was

repeated after the second baseline condition, and the authors concluded that the intervention was effective in reducing both pretantrum and tantrum behavior.

A number of narrative research reviews were published between 2004 and 2006 and identified concerns with the methodological quality of much of the early story-based intervention research, as well as a need for examination of variables that moderate intervention effectiveness (Ali & Frederickson, 2006; Nichols, Hupp, Jewell, & Ziegler, 2006; Reynhout & Carter, 2006; Rust & Smith, 2006; Sansosti, Powell-Smith, & Kincaid, 2004). However, the National Autism Center (2009) identified story-based interventions as one of 11 "established" evidence-based practices for individuals with ASD.

Since the National Autism Center report was published, several meta-analyses have sought to further quantify the state of the research evidence (Kokina & Kern, 2010; Reynhout & Carter, 2011; Test et al., 2011); all three of these included published research (up to 2007–2009) and the first two also included dissertations. The unanimous conclusions of these reviews can be summarized by an excerpt from Reynhout and Carter (2011), who noted that, although story-based interventions "may be attractive to practitioners because they are easy to implement and require very limited resources. . . . [They] appear to have only a small clinical effect on behavior and practitioners should factor this consideration into decisions about appropriate intervention" (p. 897). While Reynhout and Carter applied this conclusion to story-based interventions in general, Kokina and Kern (2010) found that stories that incorporated visual supports were more effective than those that did not. Based on their review, these authors also suggested that higher effectiveness may be associated with factors such as 1) using target children as their own intervention agents; 2) reading or reviewing the story immediately prior

Page 1 Adults like to talk.	**Page 2** Sometimes they talk to each other.	**Page 3** Sometimes they talk to my brother.	**Page 4** Sometimes they talk on the phone.
Page 5 Sometimes they talk to me.	**Page 6** When adults are talking to someone else I can probably	**Page 7** watch a video, listen to a book on tape	**Page 8** look at a book, or play a quiet game
Page 9 When I want to talk, I will wait my turn.	**Page 10** If they do not see me, I can raise my hand or quietly say, "Excuse me, please."	**Page 11** Then, they will listen to me. I don't have to yell or hit.	**Page 12** I will remember to wait my turn by thinking about my ant book. The ants go marching one by one. People talk one by one.

Page 13

I like when my wait is over and it is my turn . I like when people listen.

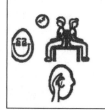

Figure 19.3. Gregg's "Talking with Adults" story. (From Lorimer, P.A., Simpson, R.L., Myles, B.S., & Ganz, J.B. [2002]. The use of social stories as a preventative behavioral intervention in a home setting with a child with autism. *Journal of Positive Behavior Interventions, 4*[1], 53–60; reprinted by permission of SAGE Publications. Copyright 2002 by SAGE Publications.)

to the target situation; 3) using stories that describe simple, singular behaviors rather than complex chains of behavior; 4) using FBA to inform the content of the intervention; and 5) using comprehension checks to determine learners' understanding of the story. Kokina and Kern's recommendations notwithstanding, practitioners who elect to employ story-based interventions should do so with caution, given the mixed reviews of research evidence related to their effectiveness. As is the case for other types of visual supports, these interventions should not be used as either the sole or even the primary element in a comprehensive behavior support plan; in fact, story-based interventions are almost always combined with additional strategies such as VASs as well as modeling, prompting, and reinforcement of appropriate behavior (Reynhout & Carter, 2009, 2011).

Power Cards

Like story-based interventions, the power card strategy (Gagnon, 2001) is used to teach functional alternatives to problem behaviors; however, this strategy is unique in that it incorporates visual supports to "connect an appropriate behavior or social skill to an individual's special interest" (Keeling, Myles, Gagnon, & Simpson, 2003, p. 104). The power card strategy utilizes a personalized script that describes 1) the target individual's hero or special interest model (e.g., Superman, dinosaurs) with relevant pictures or other graphics; 2) the problem behavior or situation of concern; 3) the hero/model attempting a solution to the problem behavior or situation using a 3- to 5-step strategy that results in a successful outcome; and 4) a recommendation that the individual try to use the same strategy that was used successfully by the hero/model (Gagnon, 2001). The script is accompanied by a separate power card, which contains a picture of the hero/model and a brief summary of the strategy described in the script. Typically, the power card script is reviewed with (i.e., read to or read by) the target individual prior to the challenging event for which it was designed, and the power card itself is made available during the event as a visual reminder of the desired strategies.

Evan

Figure 19.4 provides an example of the script and power card that was developed for Evan, an adolescent with Asperger syndrome who often engaged in problem behavior (e.g., yelling, kicking, swearing) if he was losing a game or competition (e.g., in gym class). In fact, Evan was barred from participating in his local soccer team because of frequent outbursts and "poor sportsmanship." Through his school counselor, Evan was provided with anger-management instruction that focused on teaching appropriate "sportsmanship" behaviors and self-monitoring; however, although Evan was able to describe and demonstrate the desired behaviors when asked to do so, he failed to exhibit these behaviors when they were required in real-life situations. The counselor decided to incorporate Evan's intense interest in television game shows into a power card strategy. Together, they created a script that featured game show illustrations and described how game show contestants might react appropriately to disappointing or challenging events. They also made two small power cards that summarized the strategies, along with pictures representing television game shows; Evan carried one card in his wallet and kept the second card in his gym shorts.

Every morning at school, Evan and his counselor spent a few minutes reviewing the script together, and Evan agreed to review the power card prior to each gym class as well. Within a few days, his gym teacher reported that he noticed that Evan was standing off to the side and taking a few deep breaths to calm himself when his score or that of his team was lower than that of the opposing team. He even observed Evan congratulating members of the winning team on a few occasions. The teacher acknowledged Evan's efforts at self-control by quietly praising him when he noticed these new behaviors. Over the next 2 weeks, Evan engaged in problem behavior in gym class on only one occasion, compared with almost daily occurrences before the power card strategy was introduced. One month later, the soccer coach who had refused to allow him on

People love to play game shows. Many people go to Hollywood and line up for hours to play game shows. Game shows usually have on big winner. The rest of the players lose. When people win on game shows, they may cheer, they say "alright!" or "way to go!" The people who lose on game shows usually look disappointed, but they congratulate the winner. They may say things like "good game" or "congratulations." Sometimes they will stand quietly and take a deep breath. There are a few things I can remember when I play games:

1. Games should be fun and exciting for all players.
2. If I win a game, I can cheer or say "alright!" or "way to go!"
3. If I lose a game, I can congratulate the other player. I can stand quietly and take a deep breath.

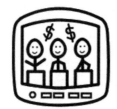

1. Games should be fun and exciting for all players.
2. If I win a game, I can cheer or say "alright!" or "way to go!"
3. If I lose a game, I can congratulate the other player. I can stand quietly and take a deep breath.

Figure 19.4. Evan's game show script and associated power card. (The Picture Communication Symbols ©1981–2010 by Mayer-Johnson LLC. All Rights Reserved Worldwide. Used with permission. Boardmaker™ is a trademark of Mayer-Johnson LLC.)

the team agreed to give him another try, and Evan successfully played on the team for the rest of the school year with only a few minor outbursts. He continued to refer to his power card before (and sometimes during) each game and even asked for new cards with images of additional game show logos on them.

. . . .

Only three published studies to date have examined the effectiveness of the power card strategy across five young children (ages 5–10) with ASD. Some of the heroes/models on which the scripts and power cards were based included the Powerpuff Girls (Keeling et al., 2003); Lightning McQueen, a character from the Disney movie *Cars* (Spencer, Simpson, Day, & Buster, 2008); and a train conductor for a boy whose special interest was trains (Campbell &

Tincani, 2011). The methodological quality of the studies varied considerably, and two of the three studies included components in addition to the basic power card strategy (e.g., a self-monitoring "score card" in Keeling et al., 2003). Nonetheless, all three studies documented a reduction in target problem behaviors and/or an increase in alternative replacement behaviors after the intervention was implemented. In one study (Campbell & Tincani, 2011), these improvements were documented for up to 8 weeks later. Although these results are promising, additional research is required to identify how to select special interests that will be most useful, which individuals are most likely to benefit from this strategy (considering its effectiveness with older individuals or with individuals not on the autism spectrum), and how it can be combined effectively with other instructional and/or visual supports.

Contingency Map

The aim of a contingency map (also referred to as a consequence map; Tobin & Simpson, 2012) is to make the contingencies that govern both problem and appropriate (i.e., alternative) behaviors transparent to the learner (Brown, 2004; Brown & Mirenda, 2006). As such, contingency maps represent the following components and the relationships between them: 1) the common antecedent that precedes both the problem and the alternative behavior, 2) depictions of both the problem and alternative behaviors, 3) the functional reinforcer that will be available contingent on alternative behavior(s), and 4) the consequence that will be available contingent on problem behavior(s).

James

Brown (2004) first described a clinical example of the use of a contingency map with James, a child with ASD who attended a regular classroom in his small suburban school. Although James's verbal skills were beginning to emerge, his primary mode of communication was through gestures and problem behaviors such as tantrums (i.e., screaming, crying, hitting, and running away). His tantrum behavior was most problematic at school and often resulted in James being removed from class and placed on a time-out chair for a short period of time. An FBA indicated that James's tantrums were maintained by escape from specific types of noises, including crying children, sirens, bells, and loud motorcycles. Based on this assessment, James's support team decided to teach him to cover his ears with his hands and ask to leave the environment by pointing to the closest door when he was confronted with a noise he found aversive. They implemented a functional communication training (FCT) intervention in order to accomplish this, using the conventional procedures described in Chapter 21. Unfortunately, though the support plan appeared to be technically sound and FCT was implemented with fidelity by James's team, meaningful change did not occur and James continued

to engage in tantrums whenever he encountered an unexpected loud noise.

Because many members of James's team believed him to be a strong visual learner, a decision was made to depict the contingencies of his support plan using a contingency map, as depicted in Figure 19.5.

Each morning at school, James's educational assistant used the pictures on the contingency map to explain to him that if he heard a loud noise, he should put his hands over his ears and ask to leave by pointing to the door. She explained that if he asked to leave, he would be allowed to move to a quiet place. Using the contingency map, she also pointed out that if James encountered a loud noise and had a tantrum, he would no longer be removed to get away from the noise. She presented the contingency map to James throughout the day before every major transition (e.g., classroom to playground and vice versa), with the same explanation. Simultaneously, the school team continued to implement the FCT intervention that had been unsuccessful previously. Within a few days, James's problem behavior was reduced to near-zero levels, and he began to place his hands over his ears and gesture to leave a noisy room or area without prompting. It appeared that the contingency map helped James learn the new behavior–environment contingency and understand the advantage of engaging in the alternative behaviors of covering his ears and pointing.

⋯⋯⋯⋯⋯⋯⋯⋯⋯⋯⋯⋯⋯⋯

The effectiveness of contingency maps was examined in two published accounts to date. In a case-study report, Tobin and Simpson (2012) described the use of contingency maps with Axel, a 6-year-old boy with emotional disturbance, attention-deficit/hyperactivity disorder (ADHD), and oppositional defiant disorder. His problem behaviors included screaming, throwing materials, and removing his clothes when he was asked to work on nonpreferred tasks and activities that he perceived to be difficult. Results suggested that problem behavior—in particular, disrobing—was reduced by about half when the contingency maps were in place. In an experimental examination that used a multiple baseline design,

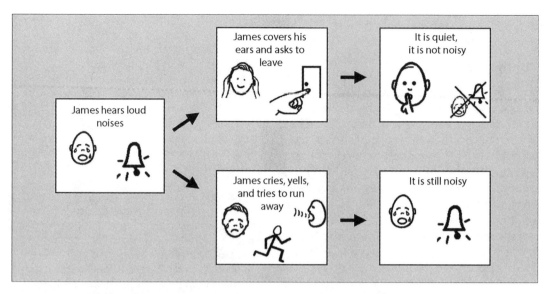

Figure 19.5.   Contingency map used to explain the contingencies for alternative behaviors (covering ears and pointing to the door) and problem behaviors (crying, yelling, running away). (From Brown, K.E. [2004]. *Effectiveness of functional equivalence training plus contingency mapping with a child with autism* [Unpublished master's thesis]. University of British Columbia, Vancouver, British Columbia, Canada; adapted by permission of Kenneth Brown. The Picture Communication Symbols ©1981–2010 by Mayer-Johnson LLC. All Rights Reserved Worldwide. Used with permission. Boardmaker™ is a trademark of Mayer-Johnson LLC.)

Brown and Mirenda (2006) compared the effectiveness of verbal explanations alone and combined with contingency maps with Kirk, a 13-year-old boy with ASD and extreme prompt dependency at school. In the study, he was first provided with only verbal information about his problem behavior, the desired alternative behavior, and the associated consequences (e.g., "Kirk, if you finish your work and don't bring it to your teacher, you will not get a treat. If you finish your work and show it to the teacher, you will get a treat."). The verbal explanation alone failed to result in a change in Kirk's behavior; however, when the same verbal information was paired with pictorial depictions of the contingencies, Kirk immediately began to engage in the alternative behavior of showing his work to the teacher, across three classroom routines. From these two reports, it appears that contingency maps, while not yet affirmed as an evidence-based strategy, may enable individuals to understand behavior-consequence relationships and

promote their ability to self-manage and self-regulate their behavior.

CONCLUSION

Despite the availability of numerous types of visual supports, little is known about how to match specific learner or behavioral characteristics to specific strategies; in fact, decisions about the use of specific types of visual supports are often made rather arbitrarily. As noted by Kokina and Kern (2010), the likelihood of obtaining a positive outcome with the use of visual supports is greatly enhanced by first conducting an FBA. In addition to identifying the function and context of problem behavior, an FBA may also help to establish the type of visual support that will be most useful. For example, individuals for whom unpredictability is identified as a setting event or antecedent may benefit from between-activity schedules that enable them to predict upcoming events and then make the transition successfully from one activity/context to the next. Those for whom expectations of independent performance function as an antecedent for problem behavior may require step-by-step, within-activity schedules that enable them to complete specific tasks without assistance. Individuals with poor understanding of social events and expectations might benefit from visually augmented story-based interventions that describe a situation, skill, or concept in terms of relevant social cues, other peoples' perspectives, and appropriate behavior responses. Individuals with special interests might be motivated to engage in appropriate behavior through the use of power cards, while contingency maps may be especially useful as an adjunct to teaching alternative replacement behaviors (including those that are communicative in nature) to replace problem behavior. In addition, most of the research to date has examined the effectiveness of visual supports used in isolation, rather than in the context of multicomponent behavior intervention plans. Future research is needed to identify the relative contribution of various types of visual supports to successful PBS outcomes.

Similarly, little information is available about the prerequisite requirements of strategies such as story-based interventions and power cards, which rely heavily on language and/or literacy skills (Kokina & Kern, 2010). And, as noted by Mirenda and Brown (2009), few researchers have described how they selected the type of symbol used in a visual support intervention (e.g., object, photograph, line drawing), suggesting that a systematic symbol assessment procedure (Beukelman & Mirenda, 2013) was not used to make this decision. Research that explores how to select and individualize visual support strategies systematically is needed to clarify issues such as these so that visual supports can be implemented with maximal benefit.

REFERENCES

Ali, S., & Frederickson, N. (2006). Investigating the evidence base of social stories. *Educational Psychology in Practice, 22*, 355–377.

Association for Positive Behavior Support (2007, March). *Positive Behavior Support standards of practice: Individual level, iteration 1.* Retrieved from http://www.apbs.org/files/apbs_standards_of_practice_2013_format.pdf

Banda, D., & Grimmett, E. (2008). Enhancing social and transition behaviors of persons with autism through activity schedules: A review. *Education and Training in Developmental Disabilities, 43*, 324–333.

Beukelman, D., & Mirenda, P. (2013). *Augmentative and alternative communication: Supporting children and adults with complex communication needs* (4th ed.). Baltimore, MD: Paul H. Brookes Publishing Co.

Brown, K., & Mirenda, P. (2006). Contingency mapping: A novel visual support strategy as an adjunct to functional equivalence training. *Journal of Positive Behavior Interventions, 8*, 155–164.

Brown, K.E. (2004). *Effectiveness of functional equivalence training plus contingency mapping with a child with autism* (Unpublished master's thesis). University of British Columbia, Vancouver, British Columbia, Canada.

Campbell, A., & Tincani, M. (2011). The power card strategy: Strength-based intervention to increase direction following of children with autism spectrum disorder. *Journal of Positive Behavior Interventions, 13*, 240–249.

Cihak, D. (2011). Comparing pictorial and video modeling activity schedules during transitions for students with autism spectrum disorders. *Research in Autism Spectrum Disorders, 5*, 433–441.

Cihak, D.F., Alberto, P.A., Taber-Doughty, T., & Gama, R.I. (2006). A comparison of static picture prompting and video prompting simulation strategies using group instructional procedures. *Focus on Autism and Other Developmental Disabilities, 21*(2), 89–99.

Flannery, K.B., & O'Neill, R.E. (1995). Including predictability in functional assessment and individual program development. *Education and Treatment of Children, 18*, 499–502.

Gagnon, E. (2001). *Power cards: Using special interests to motivate children and youth with Asperger syndrome and autism.* Shawnee Mission, KS: Autism Asperger Publishing.

Gray, A.A. (2010). *The new Social Story book: 10th anniversary edition.* Arlington, TX: Future Horizons.

Gray, C.A. (2000). *Writing Social Stories with Carol Gray* [Video and workbook]. Arlington, TX: Future Horizons.

Keeling, K., Myles, B.S., Gagnon, E., & Simpson, R. (2003). Using the power card strategy to teach sportsmanship skills to a child with autism. *Focus on Autism and Other Developmental Disabilities, 18*, 103–109.

Kokina, A., & Kern, L. (2010). Social Story interventions for students with autism spectrum disorders: A meta-analysis. *Journal of Autism and Developmental Disorders, 40*, 812–826.

Koyama, T., & Wang, H-T. (2011). Use of activity schedules to promote independent performance of individuals with autism and other intellectual disabilities: A review. *Research in Developmental Disabilities, 32*, 2235–2242.

Lequia, J., Machalicek, W., & Rispoli, M. (2012). Effects of activity schedules on challenging behavior exhibited by children with autism spectrum disorders: A systematic review. *Research in Autism Spectrum Disorders, 6*, 480–492.

Lorimer, P.A., Simpson, R.L., Myles, B.S., & Ganz, J.B. (2002). The use of social stories as a preventative behavioral intervention in a home setting with a child with autism. *Journal of Positive Behavior Interventions, 4,* 53–60.

Mechling, L., Gast, D., & Seid, N. (2009). Using a personal digital assistant to increase independent task completion for students with autism spectrum disorder. *Journal of Autism and Developmental Disorders, 39,* 1420–1434.

Mechling, L., & Gustafson, M. (2008). Comparison of static picture and video prompting on the performance of cooking-related tasks by students with autism. *Journal of Special Education Technology, 23*(3), 31–45.

Mesibov, G., Browder, D., & Kirkland, C. (2002). Using individualized schedules as a component of positive behavioral support for students with developmental disabilities. *Journal of Positive Behavior Interventions, 4,* 73–79.

Mirenda, P., & Brown, K. (2009). A picture is worth a thousand words: Using visual supports for augmented input with individuals with autism spectrum disorders. In P. Mirenda & T. Iacono (Eds.), *Autism spectrum disorders and AAC* (pp. 303–332). Baltimore, MD: Paul H. Brookes Publishing Co.

Mitchell, P., & Ropar, D. (2004). Visuo-spatial abilities in autism: A review. *Infant and Child Development, 13,* 185–198.

National Autism Center. (2009). *National Standards Report.* Randolph, MA: Author.

Nichols, S., Hupp, S., Jewell, J., & Zeigler, C. (2006). Review of Social Story interventions for children diagnosed with autism spectrum disorders. *Journal of Evidence-Based Practices for Schools, 6*(1), 90–120.

Reynhout, G., & Carter, M. (2006). Social Stories for children with disabilities. *Journal of Autism and Developmental Disorders, 36,* 445–469.

Reynhout, G., & Carter, M. (2009). The use of social stories by teachers and their perceived effectiveness. *Research in Autism Spectrum Disorders, 3,* 232–251.

Reynhout, G., & Carter, M. (2011). Evaluation of the efficacy of Social Stories using three single subject metrics. *Research in Autism Spectrum Disorders, 5,* 885–900.

Roth, D., Muchnik, C., Shabtai, E., Hildesheimer, M., & Henkin, Y. (2011). Evidence for atypical auditory brainstem responses in young children with suspected autism spectrum disorders. *Developmental Medicine and Child Neurology, 54,* 23–29.

Rowland, C., & Schweigert, P. (2000). *Tangible symbol systems* (2nd ed.). Portland, OR: Oregon Health & Science University.

Rust, J., & Smith, A. (2006). How should the effectiveness of social stories to modify the behaviour of children on the autistic spectrum be tested? *Autism: An International Journal of Research and Practice, 10,* 125–138.

Sansosti, F.J., Powell-Smith, K.A., & Kincaid, D. (2004). A research synthesis of Social Story interventions for children with autism spectrum disorders. *Focus on Autism and Other Development Disabilities, 19,* 194–204.

Schreibman, L., Whalen, C., & Stahmer, A. (2000). The use of video priming to reduce disruptive transition behavior in children with autism. *Journal of Positive Behavior Interventions, 2,* 3–11.

Siegal, M., & Blades, M. (2003). Language and auditory processing in autism. *TRENDS in Cognitive Sciences, 7,* 378–380.

Spencer, V., Simpson, C., Day, M., & Buster, E. (2008). Using the power card strategy to teach social skills to a child with autism. *TEACHING Exceptional Children Plus, 5*(1), article 2. Retrieved August 10, 2012, from http://escholarship.bc.edu/education/tecplus/vol5/iss1/art2

Test, D., Richter, S., Knight, V., & Spooner, F. (2011). A comprehensive review and meta-analysis of the social stories literature. *Focus on Autism and Other Development Disabilities, 26,* 49–62.

Tobin, C., & Simpson, R. (2012). Consequence maps: A novel behavior management tool for educators. *TEACHING Exceptional Children, 44*(5), 68–75.

Waters, M., Lerman, D., & Hovanetz, A. (2009). Separate and combined effects of visual schedules and extinction plus differential reinforcement on problem behavior occasioned by transitions. *Journal of Applied Behavior Analysis, 42,* 309–313.

Curricular Modification, Positive Behavior Support, and Change

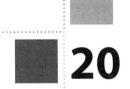

20

Ann Halvorsen and Tom Neary,
with contributions by Deanna Willson-Schafer and Mary Wrenn

Sean

Sean is a tenth grader with a reputation for challenging behavior. He is described as frequently disruptive, disrespectful, and noncompliant and has been ignored, reminded, scolded, confronted, referred, and suspended. Teachers have removed privileges, called his home, devised creative consequences, made accommodations, "caught him being good," nurtured his heart, and counseled him on the long-term benefits of high school achievement. Good people have taken on the challenge of showing him the "error of his ways" and designing reward systems for behaving safely, respectfully, and responsibly. Good people have thrown up their hands and, even though they know better, have talked about his lack of motivation, his apparent need to escape, and his preference for negative attention—and maybe even something medical or beyond their control. Someone said (tentatively and quietly) that this may take referring Sean to someone and maybe even someplace special where people are specially trained to deal with students like this.

If we step back and visualize the likely track Sean is on, we are right to worry that it is heading in the direction of, in the least, underemployment and underachievement and, at the worst, the correctional system. In fact, evidence exists that school systems can identify very early in children's lives which of them are likely to be involved with the correctional system, with an estimated 30% of those juveniles being students with learning disabilities (Children's Defense Fund, 2012). The public school system has an enormous impact on the lives of our citizens. Children are in school, being guided by their teachers for 6 hours a day, 5 days a week, and 10 months a year, from ages 5 to 18. Parents have a major impact on their children in all areas of life, but educators also have a significant opportunity to contribute to the development of the children in their charge.

One of the goals we often acknowledge in education is to encourage lifelong learning (Casner-Lotto & Barrington, 2006). Educators know that schools cannot teach everything and recognize that the critical element is for our students to learn how to learn and want to continue to learn. There may have been a time in the history of our educational systems when some teachers viewed the job as pounding in the facts, whether the child wanted them or not, but in general, almost all teachers want their students to enjoy school and appreciate the things we have to teach. Certainly, that's what we hope for our children. In light of this, it is clear that the learning environment, including what we teach and how we teach as well as the student's active participation in the process, make a difference in whether a student learns how to learn and continues to learn. As Algozzine, Wang, and Violette (2010) pointed out, it is difficult to learn if you are spending more time in discipline-related interactions than those related to learning content.

How do these two variables—what we teach and how we teach—affect student behavior and vice versa? If kindergarten academic variables have been shown to be predictive of problem behavior by the end of elementary school (McIntosh, Horner, Chard, Dickey, & Braun, 2008), and if we can show that preexisting low academic skills lead to problem behavior to escape inappropriate academic tasks, as has been proposed by many (Lee, Sugai, & Horner, 1999; Roberts, Marshall, Nelson, & Albers, 2001), then we cannot escape the implications of our role in this behavioral–instructional dynamic. This relationship was clearly presented as "a coercive cycle of behavioral and educational failure" (McIntosh et al., 2008, p. 132). The teacher presents an academic task; the student engages in problem behavior, the teacher removes the task, the student escapes the task, the student's academic skills do not improve, and the cycle continues with the next presentation. As educators, we have to be engaged in helping our students become more skilled, and when we find ourselves caught in a cycle with a student, we have to look first at our behavior. Our perceptions

and expectations will have an impact on the opportunities we provide.

Despite the rhetoric about what we should be teaching in the schools and how we should be teaching, we do have evidence about effective pedagogy and what enables curriculum to be accessible and engaging for all (e.g., Dean, Hubbell, Pitler, & Stone, 2012; Marzano, 2003). We have research, we have our experience, and our students are continually teaching us what does work to support their learning. The curriculum, the school support structure, the child's readiness, and the family's support are all important variables, but the critical factor is the teacher and what the teacher teaches every day and how it is delivered to each student. There is a measurable difference in student achievement when instruction is taught by highly effective teachers (Dean et al., 2012; Marzano, Pickering, & Pollock, 2001). Sailor (2009) discussed his observations about what makes a successful teacher and described three essential facets:

1. *Science:* The search for sources of evidence to support one's practices

2. *Relationships:* The ability to connect with students, a form of classroom culture-building and understanding of students' lives, which is, in itself, a form of assessment

3. *Inspiration:* As Sailor noted, the "least understood" component, the "I know it when I see it" element—the one we do not yet know how to measure despite our ability to recognize teachers who possess it and inspire their students (p. 263)

We *can* identify the critical components of effective curriculum and instruction that, if implemented consistently and with fidelity, will result in students learning. Evidence-based curriculum and instructional elements constitute the *foundation* for or a key *antecedent* of students' positive behavior and thus meaningful learning for those who, like Sean, have been viewed as having the most challenging behaviors and certainly the most serious reputations. To illustrate these effective strategies and tools, we'll examine the research and, in the process, consider Sean and his fellow students in earlier grades who are experiencing behavior challenges.

DECISION MODEL TO ADDRESS STUDENT NEEDS WITHIN CURRICULUM

Function-Based Intervention

As this chapter will show, by attending to our instruction, ensuring that it is relevant, engaging, and focused, with scaffolds in place to support the learning of individual students that are frequently adjusted based on our formative assessment and provided in a positive climate, we can prevent the large majority of challenging behavior. A small percentage of our students will need more strategic and targeted interventions to support their success in school. It is our belief that addressing challenging behavior through academic support holds the most promise for success.

There are several good, research-based behavior intervention programs available, and selecting and implementing one may seem like a promising solution to challenging behavior in the classroom. However, research has also shown poor effects of these research-based interventions *when they are not based on the assessed function of the behavior* (Filter & Horner, 2009; Ingram, Lewis-Palmer, & Sugai, 2005; Newcomer & Lewis, 2004).

Challenging behavior serves two basic functions: to gain something (attention, tangible or sensory) or to escape or avoid something (Berotti & Durand, 1999, p. 240). When the function is to gain attention, it may be that a behavior plan is the most appropriate intervention, but when escape from academic work is the function, the most appropriate response is academic support (McIntosh et al., 2008). How might education teams identify the function of challenging behavior and

use that information to generate a successful academic intervention?

A FRAMEWORK FOR RESOLVING BEHAVIOR CHALLENGES THAT SERVE THE FUNCTION OF ESCAPE FROM ACADEMIC DEMANDS

Schoolwide Support Structures

Effective schools establish structures of support for both students and teachers so that the resources, expertise, and experience of the school community can be tapped. Early academic and behavioral universal screening and frequent progress monitoring can identify students at risk so that educators can intervene before a cycle of failure begins. Grade-level teams, including special educators, have an opportunity to plan for reteaching or may identify general adaptations a student might need to support their success. The team may adapt materials or consider increasing the level of instruction within the schoolwide response to intervention model. An incentive plan for class participation or task completion can be designed. It is critical that a specific member of the team is designated to create the adaptations, communicate and implement the incentive plan, or make the referral for a more intensive level of instruction. The education team should also set a review date within a month.

Analysis and Intervention

When these initial steps have been implemented with fidelity yet are found to be insufficient, we need to delve more deeply to develop a better understanding of the problem.

Competing Pathways The problem with many behavior intervention plans is that they are designed with a focus on consequences only by providing incentives for demonstrating appropriate behavior and/or providing what we believe is an aversive consequence for demonstrating the behavior of concern. If our plan does not consider the function the behavior serves for the student, it is unlikely our intervention will be successful. When education teams take the time to examine what this behavior might be achieving for the student, they are more likely to build an evidence-based approach that will help the student achieve the same outcome without having to resort to the behavior everyone is concerned about.

One strategy, *competing pathways* (O'Neill et al., 1997), provides a structure for this team discussion. It helps the team develop a testable hypothesis about the function of the problem behavior by identifying the basic pattern of the behavior, including the setting events, triggering antecedents, problem behavior, and maintaining consequences. It represents the team's best guess about what is occurring. The pattern that can be seen in Figure 20.1 suggests that when Sean goes to bed late on school nights and nongraded quizzes are provided on information covered the day before, he protests, slumps, and/or walks out of the room. The result is that Sean does not take the quiz and does not participate in the homework discussion. This, of course, has led to failing quiz grades. Unless we intervene in another way, Sean will be caught in a cycle of educational failure.

Key Conversations When we are attempting to resolve chronic problem behavior, it helps to have people involved who are directly affected by this behavior.

These *key conversations*, if conducted in a structured manner, can provide the insight we need to find a better way for all involved. It's clear that the person most affected by this behavior is the student and, often, we don't consider asking the student to tell us what his or her academic experience is like. This is often the most critical addition to the education team. When the student needs more support, with his or her permission, parents and peers might be invited. Peers have been very helpful in offering insight into the situation because they have a unique perspective less focused on what should be and what is. Using this behavior support team, the next steps would include identifying what we want the student to do and then what alternatives the student might use to achieve that.

When we ask the teacher what he or she wants the student to do instead of protesting, slumping, and leaving the classroom, their teacher might say, "Do the quiz without complaining." If the student did that, he or she could participate in the discussion and likely be more successful (see Figure 20.2).

This may not be sufficient motivation for the student. The other pathway, the one with protests, slumping, and leaving the class, may be a better strategy for the purpose of escaping an unpleasant task. But there may be another pathway that achieves the same outcome for the student (avoiding doing the quiz and the homework discussion). If the student turns in the paper, unfinished, and

Testable hypothesis summary statement

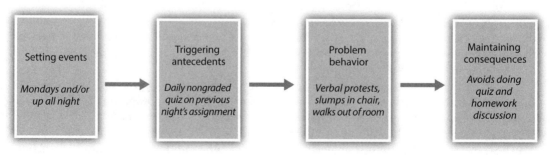

Figure 20.1. Testable hypothesis summary statement.

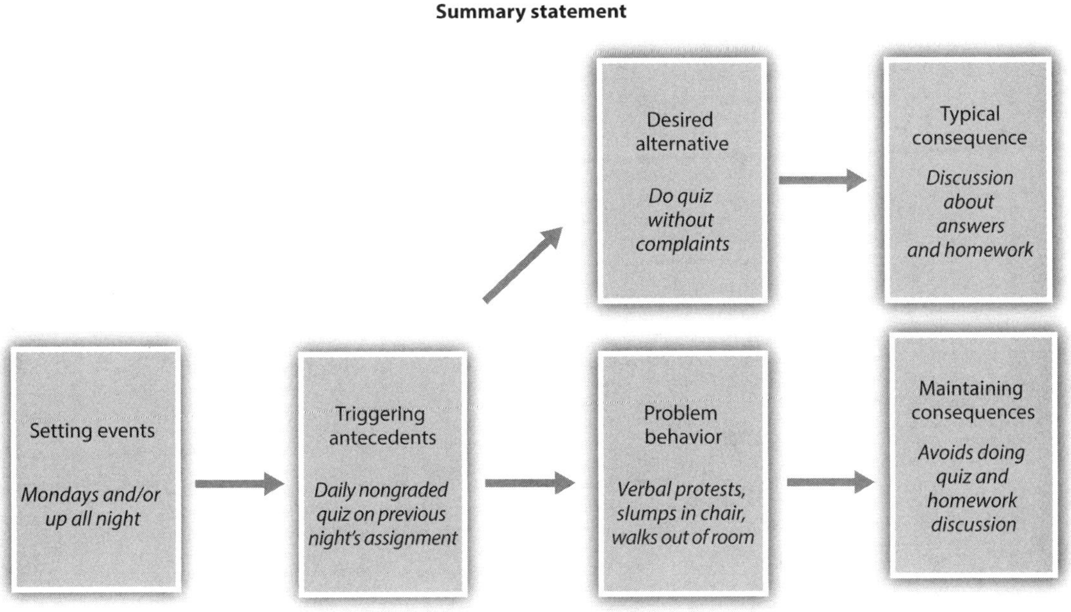

Summary statement

Figure 20.2.   Initial summary statement.

sits quietly without interrupting, he or she could still avoid the quiz and the discussion (see Figure 20.3).

This seems like a counterintuitive strategy, because if we just remove all demands from the student to avoid problem behavior, haven't we just taught the student that this is the way to escape nonpreferred tasks? However, if it actually results in less disruption, it has provided evidence that our hypothesis is correct, and that's a good first step. It's also a less disrupting way to escape, and it may allow the teacher to maintain instruction for the rest of the class without disruption. Allowing and encouraging this pathway (turning in paper and sitting quietly) interrupts the disruptive cycle, giving us an opportunity to begin a preventive and skill-building plan.

Building an Academic Behavior Support Plan

At this point, we have a better understanding of two things: We know the function this disruptive behavior serves for the student (i.e.,

Sean), and we know the student can behave in an appropriate way when the demanding situation is removed. This knowledge allows us to do what we are trained to do—facilitate learning by organizing our learning environment to provide the best chance for learning. For the small percentage of students who require this level of intervention, the work is worth the effort.

The next step involves targeted observations across identified activities, subjects, and settings by team members who know both the student *and* the instructional context. Team members then share that information along with their knowledge of the student, including learning history, learning style, areas of difficulty, intervention history, and (if the student has a disability) how that disability affects his or her learning. Using the competing pathways format, the team can build a plan that might include adaptations, such as bypass strategies that allow students to access or demonstrate mastery in alternative ways, including the use of calculators, spell-checkers, or other compensatory strategies (Friend & Bursuck, 2012). The education team

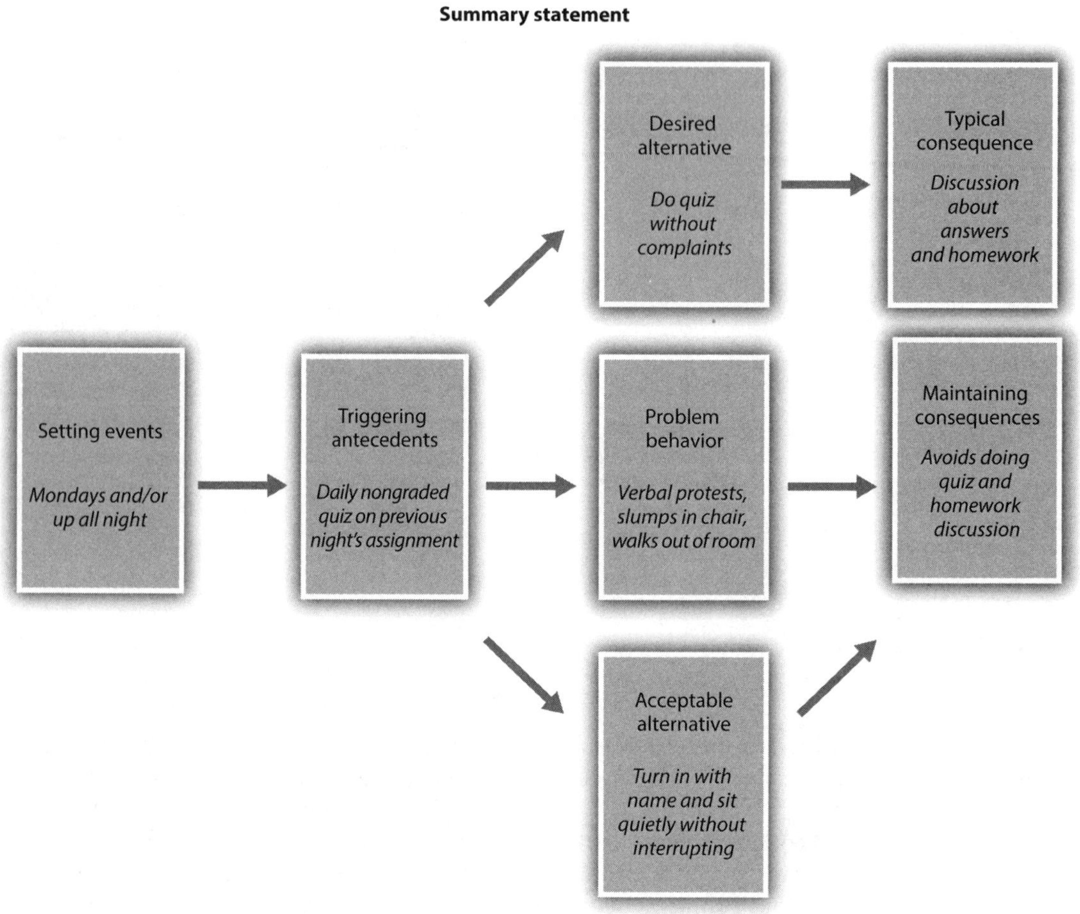

Summary statement

Figure 20.3.   Revised summary statement.

may also make adaptations in materials, classroom organization, or instructional grouping (see Figure 20.4).

Direct Instruction

The team may decide to provide additional instruction, as in reteaching a concept or providing a more intensive instructional program with direct instructional strategies. Direct instruction involves classroom organization and management as well as how curriculum is designed and presented (Rosenshine & Stevens, 1986). In direct instruction, as with scaffolding, academic instruction is enhanced with demonstration, guided practice, and opportunities for independent instruction.

However, direct instruction is often done with small groups or in one-to-one instructional situations, such as in those interventions described earlier, that can be made available through coteaching structures in general education and through the process of defined and supported multitiered support system interventions. Multitiered systems of support (MTSS) will be discussed in more detail later in the chapter. The benefits of direct instruction on behavior were well demonstrated by Nelson, Johnson, and Marchand-Martella (1996), who compared the effects of direct instruction, cooperative learning, and independent practice for students with behavioral disorders. On-task behavior was highest (M = 92.5%) and disruptive behavior was lowest

Setting event changes	Antecedent strategies	Behavior teaching	Consequence modification
Check-in/check-out participation • Review options and expectations. • Establish goals for the day Time to review homework with peer (student choice) Easy warm-up task prior to review	Link topic to Sean's interests. Explain relevance. Provide digital text. Graphic organizer • Highlight big ideas and relationships. Use sentence frame in dyad.	Teach options to problem behavior. Manage conflict with adults. Executive function • Goal setting • Planning and strategy Tech tools • Use of digital text • Internet research strategies	Signal to remind Sean to use options. Acknowledge effort/use of options. Check-in/check-out trading post • Establish point system and chosen privileges.

Figure 20.4.   Behavior support planning for Sean.

(M = 8.7%) in the direct instruction condition. However, Nelson et al. did not look at academic achievement in their study, only at on-task behavior (1996). While it is clear that learning may occur when one is engaged and on task, the complementary addition of the research-based instructional strategies with inclusive service delivery that support small group instruction when needed and the addition of individualized academic goals, expectations, and supports *within* students' behavior plans, are our best combination for both behavioral and academic success.

EVIDENCE-BASED PRACTICES WITHIN GENERAL EDUCATION

Addressing Challenging Behavior Through a Schoolwide Approach

For students who are not academically and/or behaviorally successful at school, we must ask: How can we make curriculum and instruction accessible? Even with a solid educational program, some students will struggle. If a student is found eligible for special education services, that is only the first step. It then becomes the responsibility of the educators to design an effective program of support. Within inclusive schools where the success for every student is the responsibility of every teacher, structures are put into place to ensure success for every

student (Halvorsen & Neary, 2009). One of the most promising structures is establishing a *multitiered system of support* (MTSS), the phrase used by the Kansas Department of Education (2008) initiative to describe its approach to schoolwide problem-solving response to intervention (RTI; Sailor, 2009). MTSS steers schools away from limiting their thinking about intervention to three tiers, followed by an automatic referral for special education eligibility.

An MTSS integrates assessment and intervention within a multilevel prevention system to maximize student achievement and provide strategies to reduce student behavior problems. In this process, schools use evidence-based classroom interventions along with universally applied screening tools to identify students at risk for poor learning outcomes, provide evidence-based interventions, and adjust the intensity and nature of those interventions, depending on a student's responsiveness. Systematic, ongoing progress monitoring occurs, as well as the utilization of these progress data when and if we are assessing students' eligibility for special education services (National Center on Response to Intervention, 2010; Sailor, 2009). As Sailor (2009) noted, a schoolwide problem-solving model has all the essential components to move from a "disability frame" for student challenges to "reframe policy directed to matching resources to identified needs" (p. 33). This team problem-solving focus on prevention, on early intervention targeted to the specific need, with tracking of the results of those interventions and accountability for doing so, is a significant departure from the past. These elements, along with a new focus on sociobehavioral factors that may contribute to learning in addition to potential sensory or cognitive challenges, differentiate MTSS from the old prereferral approaches. The welcome changes engineered through MTSS create a stark contrast to the former child or student study team process, often seen as the paperwork gateway to special education, with ill-defined interventions applied in a haphazard manner and no real resources available to support teachers in systematic application. In 2013, one of the authors reviewed student study team processes in local districts, including some where only 15 minutes of discussion were allotted per child and no student objectives were established to measure student progress on suggested "interventions." Any needed follow-up student study team meetings in one district were used as referrals for special education eligibility assessment.

In contrast, consider the example of a local inclusive middle school, where a schoolwide MTSS academic and behavioral team problem-solving approach has been implemented for years. Located in an urban area near a university, Willard Middle School serves about 560 students in Grades 6–8. It is a diverse school with no dominant ethnicity and students from all socioeconomic backgrounds. About 12% of the students have individualized education programs (IEPs). Most of those students have been identified as having learning disabilities, and about 2% have more significant disabilities.

Over the course of a decade, Willard Middle School has worked to create an inclusive school environment. Central to this effort has been the premise that all supports, whether academic, behavioral, or social, are available for any student who needs them. Special education teachers coteach with general education teachers, following a group of students through their 3 years. These support teachers help address the needs of students with IEPs as well as the needs of any struggling student by working collaboratively with team members to plan and implement curricular supports. Tier-1 interventions such as reteaching, modifying assignments, developing short-term goals with students for academics or improved behavior, or supporting social interactions are emphasized and supported by all team members (see Figure 20.5).

Grade-level teams meet once a week, discussing issues and exchanging strategies for students they have in common. If a student does not respond as hoped to these interventions, additional plans are developed at a school team level. The student needs assessment process (SNAP) team also meets weekly, rotating grade levels. This core team is composed of or involves a variety of general educators, support staff, and administrators meeting with representatives from the grade-level team to discuss these struggling students. The SNAP team looks at a variety of data, reviewing strategies and interventions that have been employed. The grade-level teachers, along with SNAP, develop an action plan, identifying the action, time frame, and those responsible for implementing the different components. Interventions at this level may include further information gathering such as observations; meetings with the family; a daily check-in/check-out with the counselor, teacher, or other team member; a referral for individual or group counseling; or contact with other agencies for support for the student or family. Sometimes the grade-level team just needs encouragement to stay the course or reminders and support to implement some additional Tier-1 supports. Plans are distributed to all members of the student's team and can be reviewed as often as every 3 weeks at the grade-level SNAP meeting.

WILLARD MIDDLE SCHOOL TIER-1 SUPPORTS

Name of student _____ Date _____

Brief description of issues _____
_____
_____

Academic	Behavioral	Socioemotional
Call or e-mail home.	Call or e-mail home or have student call home.	Establish good relationship with student.
Identify and reteach unclear concepts.	Notice and reinforce/reward good behavior.	Call or e-mail home.
Provide tiered, scaffolded, or alternative assignments.	Teach expected behavior.	Find opportunities to praise student.
Use stations to differentiate or reteach.	Have private conversations with the student; establish a good relationship.	Facilitate interactions between student and possible friends.
Develop a plan with students for short-term instructional goals.	Hold team meeting with student to build a sense of community support.	Model desired social skills.
Provide visual supports.	Identify 1–2 behaviors to change, discuss with student, and implement self- or teacher assessment with rewards.	Make sure students know class-mate names.
Modify homework.	Make environmental changes.	Speak to counseling team about the student.
Check for understanding often.	Speak to special education teachers about the student.	
Pair with a highly skilled aca-demic peer.	**Notes**	
Check in with student during independent work time.		
Teach study skills.		
Ensure accountability for all (e.g., use equity sticks).		
Conduct regular binder checks.		
Speak to reading intervention teacher about possible reading assessment.		

Figure 20.5. Willard Middle School Tier-1 supports.

Collaborative efforts to identify and support students who are having difficulty early on have been important to Willard Middle School's success. Another key component was the adoption of schoolwide positive behavior support (SWPBS) as a keystone of their reform. In the early years of this work, Willard Middle School investigated and then implemented SWPBS strategies. These early years were focused on developing the structure: Willard adopted three basic school rules, then taught these rules to all students across settings and rewarded the students for the desired behaviors. The positive behavior support (PBS) team consisted of general and special education teachers, students, administrators, and support staff who continue to meet regularly to review data, monitor goals set by the staff, and plan professional development at staff meetings. Once PBS systems were set, the PBS team put into place an advisory period where students participate in activities and lessons around middle school issues such as bullying, prejudice and hate speech, sexual harassment, and peer pressure, twice weekly. The PBS team manages the development of curriculum for the school advisory period and plans schoolwide activities related to those lessons, which support the development of a more positive school culture. Willard has also developed more social supports for students through, for example, an ambassadors group of mixed grade students who hold ice cream or pizza parties for students new to the school and pair these new students with ambassadors to become familiar with the school culture, including school rules. Ambassadors also seek out and support students at lunch who don't seem to have friends. A weekly game room activity at lunch, by teacher invitation only, provides opportunities for students to enjoy a more organized activity. Ambassadors and focus students may also invite others to attend. Teachers volunteer to supervise the game room and work to support these interactions.

Willard Middle School identifies students who are struggling *before* patterns of failure can be established and provides the academic and behavior support necessary through reteaching and strategic or intensive support. They have achieved positive results from their whole-school approach. Since the adoption of PBS systems and the restructuring of special education support services in 2003, Willard students have gained 125 points in the annual performance index (API) based on the California standards test, reaching a schoolwide score of 811 (out of 1,000 possible points) in 2012, with gains by African American students of 108 points over this same time period. All significant disaggregated groups made similar gains. Discipline data collected by the school reflect similar improvements: Willard Middle School has the lowest rate of suspensions among middle schools in the district. The principal, Robert Ithurburn, credits the collaborative work of all Willard staff, the students, and their families for these outcomes.

A combined model of academic and behavior support through RTI or MTSS has also demonstrated excellent results at King Intermediate School in Kaneohe, Hawaii, with significantly higher reading and behavioral success, compared with the national average. Principal Sheena Alaiasa and her staff have implemented comprehensive MTSS with both academic and behavior support that include frequent and regular classroom observations with feedback to teachers regarding their instruction. Administrative and coaching staff track the instructional environment with a focus on evidence of standards and objectives, use of instructional time, scaffolding, use of academic vocabulary, formative assessment, engagement strategies, relevance, taxonomic level addressed, and classroom climate, using a tool based on *Teach for Success* (Fitterer, Harwood, Lochlear, & Lapid, 2008). Cumulative results are monitored and published each week, with improvement goals established. King has seen a steady improvement in both academic and student behavior. Academic and behavioral data from the

2007–2008 school year showed proficiency in reading on the Hawaii state assessment at 64% and math at 46%. In the 2011–2012 school year, proficiency in reading was at 87% and math at 77% on the Hawaii state assessment. These academic gains have contributed to a remarkable decrease in discipline referrals from 2,900 during the 2007–2008 school year to 175 during the 2011–2012 school year. In terms of the impact on individual students, Principal Alaiasa describes a young man with a history of intensive impulsive behavior and high-frequency discipline referrals for disruption, fighting, and swearing, who had been placed in classes for students with disruptive behavior during his brief school career. At King, he joined a class with high academic and behavioral expectations and experienced a corresponding increase in his math and reading scores, achieving six A grades and reducing his discipline referrals to two for the year. The gains students at King Intermediate can be attributed to the work staff members did to establish good instruction in all classrooms and a schoolwide approach to teaching expected behaviors.

Schools implementing schoolwide, problem-solving MTSS incorporate grade-level planning teams, operate as a professional learning community to develop common assessments, and identify those students who need additional instruction and plan for reteaching and enrichment time. When further support is indicated, problem-solving teams consider, recommend, and may design increased support at more strategic or intensive levels. The key point is that effective schools have put reflective and evidence-based structures in place and are continually reevaluating these structures based on student outcomes. For many students elsewhere, when these schoolwide structures are not in place, it is up to the classroom general or special education teacher to solve academic and behavior challenges on their own, and this is when the best of our intentions break down.

Evidence-Based Instruction that Makes a Difference

Teaching is a challenging job not for the faint hearted. Teachers are responsible for instructing significant amounts of content, demonstrating students' proficiency with the performance of grade-level standards, and preparing them for the high-stakes testing required and the demands of the next grade. Regardless of how diverse the student population is, teachers have a school year to "cover" defined content. A student who exhibits behavior that interrupts learning, who draws the attention and focus of a teacher trying to manage the instruction for 25–30 or more other students, becomes a thorn, and when that thorn is removed, it feels so much better (also known as negative reinforcement). "Disruptions" are one significant source of referrals to the office and, sometimes, referrals to other instructional locations.

When we ask teachers to examine their teaching as a critical first step in resolving behavior challenges, we can be met with resistance, but it is the first step we have to take. And although some may regard curriculum and its adaptation as separate from instruction, we agree with Koga and Hall (2009): "Defining curriculum modification requires us to understand curriculum as a broad concept which involves various educational components and people involved in the educational processes. After all, contents, instruction, input and output inseparably construct daily teaching and learning" (p. 3).

Schools need to question whether evidence-based instructional practices are being implemented and consider whether student data indicate a need to reexamine practices that may better support student access to and participation in the curriculum. Whitehurst (2002) defined *evidence-based research* more broadly than the *scientifically based research* definition provided by the No Child Left Behind Act of 2001 (PL 107-110; § 7801 [37]). In his definition, evidence-based research integrates empirical evidence supported by scientifically based research with other empirical information, professional wisdom, and consensus. This definition acknowledged concerns over the limitations inherent in the exclusive use of randomized experiments as the "gold standard" for all education research, particularly given the constraints of these designs with low-incidence populations and the lack of control over a variety of variables in real school settings (Whitehurst, 2002).

Education teams that work to resolve behavior challenges experience greater success when they begin to examine their teaching practices in comparison to identified evidence-based practices that include, for example, setting and communicating instructional goals with students, employing effective student engagement strategies, providing meaningful feedback, using instructional scaffolding techniques, and utilizing ongoing formative assessment. A group of instructional strategies for improved student achievement was validated by the Mid-Continent Research for Education and Learning (MCREL) organization through two sets of meta-analyses and comprehensive review that occurred over a decade (Beesley & Apthorp, 2010; Dean et al., 2012; Marzano et al., 2001). The impact of these strategies on learning, when implemented with fidelity, has been demonstrated repeatedly across grades and student populations (Dean et al., 2012).

Table 20.1 provides definitions of these strategies as well as other evidence-based instructional practices discussed later.

Universal Design for Learning Differentiates Instruction Universal design in architecture is a simple, elegant set of principles that directs the process of designing structures with *all* people in mind from the start, ensuring accessibility for all types of buildings instead of the sometimes homely and less-than-functional patchwork of "fixes" that need to occur after the fact (Mace, 1985). The development and application of this principle to learning and teaching is a significant

gift to all learners, and its application across behavior planning, curriculum, materials, and assessment—literally all aspects of schooling—has yielded significant positive results (Rose & Meyer, 2006). The universal design for learning (UDL) practice (see Table 20.1) capitalizes on brain research that identifies the roles of three primary brain networks: recognition (the "what" of learning), strategic (the "how" of learning), and affective (the "why" of learning). UDL researchers at the Center for Applied Specialized Technology (CAST) have connected these networks with the range of strategies required to ensure that all students have a variety of means for accessing content (recognition); multiple means of expressing what they have learned (strategic); and are actively engaged in the learning process (affective). From the start, Rose and Meyer (2002) noted that the traditional curriculum itself disables many more than those students who are classified as having disabilities. They and their colleagues set about defining and implementing research-based guidelines to ensure that instruction as well as the curricular materials utilized are differentiated, designed for all students' learning, or simply put, universally designed. We begin with this premise because it is the overarching guide to constructing effective curriculum and instruction.

Differentiated instruction has been defined as instruction designed to "recognize students' varying background knowledge, readiness, language, preferences in learning and interests; and to react responsively" (Hall, Strangman, & Meyer, 2011, p. 3). The differentiation inherent in UDL directs us to design our lessons with *all* our students in mind—that is, in terms of the wide array of backgrounds, skills, and knowledge that each brings to the classroom. UDL has provided a strong research base for the proactive, differentiated design of curriculum and instruction that considers the strengths and needs of all learners, rather than simply "fixing" shortcomings with adaptation or modification

Table 20.1.   Evidence-based practices for curriculum and instruction

Evidence-based classroom practice	Definition
Universal design for learning	This proactive design of inclusive curriculum and instruction eliminates or reduces barriers to academic success for any student, through provision of multiple means of representation, action, expression, and engagement (Rose & Meyer, 2002, 2006).
Setting and communicating objectives	Teachers provide students with information about what they are learning and will be learning; what skills, knowledge, and outcomes are expected; and opportunities to coauthor tailored objectives (Dean, Hubbell, Pitler, & Stone, 2012).
Providing feedback	Teachers provide students with explicit guidance on how they are performing in relation to learning objectives to assist them to refine or improve performance (Hattie, 2012).
Student engagement through cooperative learning structures	These are teacher-structured heterogeneous instructional groupings with five key features: direct instruction of interpersonal and small-group skills, positive interdependence, face-to-face group interaction, individual and group accountability, and group processing (Johnson & Johnson, 2009; Slavin, 1991).
Instructional scaffolding	Teachers provide students with access to known content, skills, or concepts on which to build new concepts, content, or skills (Wood Bruner, & Ross, 1976).
Summarizing and notetaking	Teachers facilitate students' synthesis and organization of information through instruction of notetaking and summarization skills to "capture main ideas and supporting details" (Dean et al., 2012, p. xviii).
Identifying similarities and differences	Students' understanding and use of knowledge is enhanced through instruction in analyzing the ways things are alike and different (Dean et al., 2012).
Homework and practice	Learning is extended through teacher-structured opportunities to practice, review, and apply knowledge/skills (Dean et al., 2012).
Generating and testing hypotheses	Students are taught to ask questions and seek/research answers to questions across content areas (Dean et al., 2012).

Instructional service delivery practice	Definition
Coteaching	At least one general and one special educator share planning and delivery of curriculum and instruction for a heterogeneous group of students that includes 10%–20% students with identified disabilities (Friend & Cook, 2002; Friend & Bursuck, 2012).
Wraparound services	Within the multitiered systems of support (MTSS), intense intervention and support for students who require family and community agency involvement, such as mental health, afterschool providers, mentors, and probation officers through transdisciplinary support plans (Eber et al., 2008).

after the fact (e.g., Coyne, Pisha, Dalton, Zeph, & Smith, 2012; Dalton & Proctor, 2007; Katz, 2013; King-Sears, 2009; Proctor, Dalton, & Grisham, 2007). The UDL framework demonstrates how teachers can accomplish this for students who are struggling as well as those who are working beyond grade-level expectations and supports teachers with the tools to codesign lessons and units with their general education colleagues in a manner that will expand their effectiveness for all. One example noted by Hall et al. (2011) is the array of digital resources, from electronic, more easily adaptable text, to video clips and the importing of graphics/photographs, which provide a myriad of available images to enhance or act as alternatives to traditional text; this lack of such materials provided significant barriers historically to a range of learners (Hall et al., 2011). Digital tools are critical in terms of both students' recognition/access and their expression or actions with content and in engagement or motivation.

When we look at *curricular adaptation* in this context of instruction that has been designed from the start to be accessible to all, what we are able to accomplish is significantly expanded. There will be students who require additional adaptation of content/materials beyond the classwide multiple means; however, the rationale and logic for this becomes clearer to all within a UDL framework. Fisher and Frey (2012b) provided examples of individualized supports and adaptations that demonstrate this. For example, when the teacher is using slides and images to present the African kingdom of Mali, one student has these pictures on her desk, with a peer checking to ensure she has the correct one at hand. Another student with behavior challenges who appears disengaged is offered a choice of several short readings that his group will utilize in the activity that follows. A third student with attention/focusing challenges utilizes a smart pen to record notes while the teacher is presenting the slides.

Curriculum adaptation is a process and a tool to bring subject matter to the student so that he or she may access instruction and learn; it is not an alternate to instruction, nor is it something we do to "occupy" the student while others are engaged in the instruction provided (Cole et al., 2000). It is a powerful tool to increase student progress toward clearly stated goals. In bringing instructional demands within the student's reach, UDL acts as an antecedent behavior intervention as well.

Setting and Communicating Learning Objectives Most of us like to know what we are learning and why we are learning it. Teachers who identify the learning objective and periodically remind students of what the point of instruction is may be better able to maintain student focus and support their understanding of how this relates to other instruction. Students with and without challenging behavior benefit from being prepared for what is about to happen in the

learning activity. So how do we best communicate with students about what we expect them to learn?

The MCREL analysis highlighted the setting of objectives with students themselves and the provision of feedback related to those objectives as having a significant impact on students' achievement (Dean et al., 2012). This process begins with teachers' in-depth understanding of content and performance standards—enough to move fluidly from the standard to which of its elements will be addressed within specific units and lessons, crafting objectives that assist students in understanding what they need to accomplish in terms of knowledge/skills, beyond the activities to be completed. It is a complex dance from the broad standard to objectives that are neither too narrow nor too general and from there to activities. Dean et al. (2012) noted the contrast between learning objectives and learning activities. For example, an *objective* such as "Understand how industrialization in the North impacted the move toward and results of the Civil War" might be coupled with a *learning activity* such as "Read the online excerpt, Chapters 1–3 of Rebecca Harding Davis's *Life in the Iron Mills,* and post a response to at least two of the questions that follow." An activity is a concrete set of actions; the objective is the knowledge or skill we expect students to obtain from their activities of instruction and classroom work.

Connecting objectives with prior learning out loud and in writing *intentionally* is also very important. This assists students to make use of those connections to enhance their performance. Finally, involving students in personalizing objectives or learning contracts has been shown to be an effective student motivator within the differentiated instruction literature (e.g., Tomlinson, 2003, 2007; Tomlinson & Imbeau, 2010), providing students with some control over their learning, building self-regulation or executive function skills (Bransford, Brown, & Cocking, 2000). These are critical areas for students who may experience behavior challenges. Dean et al. (2012) and others suggest teacher supports for students new to objective development, from the use of group or individual KWL (what I know, what I want to know, what I have learned) charts to sentence stems such as "I know that . . . I want to know about . . . or if" (p. 9), accompanied by teacher feedback on the relevance and feasibility of students' objectives within the set time period.

Jeff

Jeff, a fourth grader receiving special education included in general education schooling in a diverse rural California town, needed to understand the intent or goal of each activity, particularly writing activities, which were very challenging for him. Pulling his thoughts together and then either writing or typing them was especially hard. When the prompt was to write about "something your parents do not like you to do" (in his case, playing his Wii), he was more likely to be successful if he had reviewed this prompt on his visual schedule prior to the activity with the particular time it would occur. Next, the activity objective (to practice writing a paragraph about the subject with sentences that support the introductory sentence) needed to be verbally reexplained. His typical writing supports included a word list, a graphic organizer, paper to draw his ideas, and input and support from both his desk partner and an adult, if needed, particularly to assist with connector words (and, with, by) that he often left out of his writing. The elimination of any one of the supports resulted in his throwing himself on the floor, with much yelling and crying. These adaptations supported Jeff's understanding of the lesson's intent or goal and also prevented behavior that would interfere with his learning and the learning of peers in the classroom.

. . . .

Providing Feedback Every special educator learns the importance of providing feedback to students that is specific to or descriptive of the behavior, learning objective, or work presented. Feedback should be timely, occurring as close to the behavior as possible, and give the student information about what she has done correctly and what needs to happen next. In doing so, teachers may first want to engage in "errorless learning" strategies (Terrace, 1963). Errorless learning is a process of setting up students for success by priming their individual performance with, for example, advance visual representations of complex skills, such as how to execute long division, sentence stems, other advance organizers with pictures and text. In her widely adopted work on elements of effective instruction, Hunter (1982) described this as acknowledgment that "practice makes permanent" and stressed the need to circumvent students' practice of errors along the way (p. 34). All feedback processes incorporate the requirement that students understand both the objective they are working toward and the criteria for demonstrating its achievement. Fisher and Frey (2012a) defined the difference between mistakes (accidental, careless) and actual errors related to lack of knowledge. Unlike a simple "careless" mistake, a student's errors may indicate a lack of skills or awareness of what is needed to correct the problem. The process of feedback that helps students correct actual errors should lead to greater understanding and improved performance, as is the case when we use prompts and cue statements or questions that require and enable students to "do the work" and support their doing so. Hattie (2012) reminded us that while we all welcome praise, when it is general and accompanies corrective feedback, the student only hears the praise; thus, it dilutes the substantive part of the message. He suggested providing praise, but not in a way that interferes with other feedback. This recalls Fred Jones's suggestion, "Praise, prompt and leave" (2007), where the teacher may acknowledge the student's having executed a first step and then provide specific direction for the student's *next* step (e.g., "You've got the overview paragraph for your persuasive essay well organized, and the thesis statement is clear, now you need your next paragraph to do what?").

Finally, self-reflection and peer feedback on performance are recommended strategies within certain parameters and can encourage the development of both metacognitive skills and collaboration and, again, may increase motivation by increasing students' sense of control over their learning. Technological tools such as student and small group blogs, wikis, and Google docs with other free applications can enhance these processes, along with graphic organizers and protocols available through resources such as the National School Reform Faculty web site (Dean et al., 2012, p. 18).

Student Engagement Through Cooperative Learning   When cooperative learning structures (CLS) are implemented with fidelity, employing the critical practices listed in Table 20.1, they are positive setting events, facilitating the creation of environments conducive to learning, in which learners will be *actively* engaged (Slavin, 1991). In 1989, Johnson and Johnson selected 754 published cooperative learning studies across content areas and grades, with analyses of effect size data to determine the impact on achievement. Among other outcomes, their findings indicated that students in cooperative learning groups spent significantly more time on task than students in competitive learning situations or students working alone. In addition, students working cooperatively tended to be more involved in activities and tasks, attach greater importance to success, and engage in less apathetic, off-task, disruptive behaviors.

Despite its longevity and research record as a learning tool, cooperative learning remains a misunderstood and therefore oft misapplied practice. Dean et al. (2012) defined CLS as an instructional grouping strategy that enables opportunities for student interaction to "enhance and deepen" learning (p. 37). In the original MCREL meta-analyses 14 years ago (Marzano, 1998a; Marzano et al., 2001), CLS was found to have an effect equivalent to a 27 percentile

point achievement gain (Marzano, 2003, p. 80). The studies conducted in the intervening decade and selected for the next meta-analysis focused on the specific attributes of CLS, including at minimum positive interdependence and individual accountability (Beasley & Apthorp, 2010). A lesser but still impressive positive impact emerged, and Dean et al. (2012) emphasized the importance of all five CLS elements (see Table 20.1) as well as the consistent and systematic utilization of a variety of types of cooperative learning, from informal, ad hoc structures (e.g., think, pair, share), to formal, subject-related timed structures (e.g., unit based for a daily activity period) for different purposes. Referencing Friedman (2006), who noted that "the best companies are the best collaborators" (p. 439), the authors connected the use of cooperative learning with a necessary foundation for future student success, which also depends on collaborative and cooperative skills.

The extent to which students profit from instruction appears directly related to the degree to which they are actively engaged in learning (Algozzine, Ysseldyke, & Elliott, 1997, p. 230). If instruction consists of teachers presenting information and students listening and waiting for their turn, we allow the opportunity for students to lose focus. Research shows that engaged students experience greater satisfaction with school experiences, which may in turn lead to greater school completion and student attendance rates, as well as lower incidences of acting-out behaviors (Voke, 2002, p. 1). As noted, multiple studies have indicated both significant gains in academic success when students were engaged and decreases in challenging behavior accompanying increased engagement (Epstein, Atkins, Cullinan, Kutash, & Weaver, 2008). More frequent and structured cooperative peer interaction across the learning process increases engagement and sets the stage for positive behavior and learning outcomes—for example, initial peer research pairs selecting a topic through joint review, partner reading (Saenz, Fuchs, & Fuchs, 2005) and group service learning projects (Steinberg, Bringle, & Williams, 2010), and low-risk opportunities for practice and sharing information. Effective teachers ensure that all students are involved throughout each lesson, particularly when they are checking for understanding. Sean, our student with challenges from the beginning of this chapter, does not respond to open-ended teacher questions to the whole class. It may be that he is not confident in his ability to respond correctly in front of everyone. His teacher can structure his engagement by providing a sentence frame for all students to check for understanding: "Turn to your partner and complete this sentence: The slope of a line is determined by . . ."; Sean is more likely to participate in this manner.

Connecting Learning to Students' Lives

The perceived relevance of the content and skills we are teaching our students may also affect their engagement and learning. As a student, did you ever try to discern the *point* of some of the curriculum? Educators need to be better at conveying to students the relevance of the content we are addressing, as John Dewey first directed us a century ago (1915). Unless our target student sees the relevance of this instruction to his or her own life, he or she is unlikely to put forth the effort required to learn. Education teams that address challenging behavior will need to find a way to make learning relevant. For example, students may be expected to learn about nutritional food values, referencing this science standard: "All students will demonstrate the ability to access and analyze health information, products, and services." The teacher's learning unit objectives related to this are "Student [will] demonstrate . . . ability to access nutrition information, products, and services and determine the accuracy and validity of nutrition claims" (California Department of Education, 2009). How might we connect this to students' lives?

Learning about nutritional values may sound as compelling as grammar structures to some, but good ideas abound. Secondary-level students working in groups might investigate and identify a nutritional problem of interest to them that has been highlighted in the news. One group that forms around preferences for certain popular soft drinks might choose to explore the reasoning behind the New York City mayor's desire to limit portion size of soda drinks sold in that city. That group's plan could include locating and reviewing online press reports as well as any published criticism on the opposing side of the issue and then investigating for themselves the actual nutritional values of said drinks in relationship to recommended daily needs. They might follow this with a comparison of their own intake of similar and different drink items with recommended nutrition guidelines. Another group whose members have wished for different school snacks might trace back the elimination of "junk" snack foods in California public school vending machines by looking at the nutritional research that informed that decision, the rationale contained within the bill itself, and who its sponsors were, as well as any connections they had to particular food industries. They could then proceed to review the nutritional values within their own food choices, as well as those of ostensibly healthier alternatives. A third group with specific opinions about the school menu might research the history of school lunch programs in terms of what was provided across decades, as well as what we know now about those nutritional values, and make recommendations regarding their school's current offerings.

Alex

Alex is a middle school student who frequently engaged in off-task behaviors during instruction and who consistently failed to turn in writing assignments. When his teacher expressed concerns to Alex's parents, he discovered that Alex was deeply interested in Civil War battles and collected books and memorabilia from this period. One major objective for his grade level was to write arguments and support claims with clear reasons and relevant evidence. By designing a writing prompt related to his interest, Alex's teacher was able to tap into his particular expertise and facilitate a successful writing experience. Often, the challenge in writing for some students is to just get started. This inertia can sometimes be overcome by making the task relevant and engaging.

....

Instructional Scaffolding Instructional scaffolding is a strategy that provides temporary frameworks for students as they learn new concepts and until they can apply acquired skills or strategies independently, as indicated by their learning goals (Rodgers, 2004; Rosenshine & Meister, 1992; Simons & Klein, 2007). Wood, Bruner, and Ross (1976) introduced the practice as a teaching strategy stemming from Vygotsky's zone of proximal development (1978) and generating from the theory that students "construct new knowledge based on what they already know and believe" (Bransford et al., 2000, p. 10). All students, particularly those who struggle academically, can benefit when teachers demonstrate or model a skill ("I do"), practice with the students ("We do"), and then have students demonstrate the skill ("You do"). Some students may require additional demonstration and practice before being required to demonstrate the skill independently. For example, in fourth grade, challenging vocabulary for a story is previewed with Erin, using pictures from the book or additional pictures from other sources. Additional time is provided to allow her to practice reading and writing the words and also practice fitting them into appropriate sentences to help her understand the meaning of the new vocabulary prior to reading the text. These supports make it more likely she will be engaged during classroom instruction, and thus her need to escape the demands of a challenging lesson is removed.

In schools implementing a MTSS, progress monitoring is a key element. Grade-level teams gather and examine student progress on a frequent and consistent basis to quickly identify which students are not mastering key concepts so that they can provide additional and targeted instruction and schedule time each week to reteach those concepts while other students are involved in enrichment in that curriculum area. Reteaching is an instructional scaffold for any student and can be particularly helpful for students with disabilities. Researchers have identified additional instructional strategies that enhance acquisition and mesh well with the concept of scaffolding, including the use of cues, questions, and advance organizers, as well as employing nonlinguistic representations of concepts (Rose & Meyer, 2006).

Summarizing and Notetaking Summarizing and notetaking are well-demonstrated facilitators of higher order thinking skills. The need for these skills occurs through the student's processes of synthesizing and analyzing information as it is presented and engaging in an evaluative process that results in the identification and recording of salient points. The two skills go together and are key components, for example, with the advancement via individual determination (AVID) program adopted by thousands of U.S. middle and high schools over a 30-year period, to improve students' school success and create better pathways to and through postsecondary education (Black, McCoach, Purcell, & Siegle, 2008). These skills must be taught, not assumed, and research has shown that there is not one specific form of notetaking that is best. The MCREL review (Beesley & Apthorp, 2010) suggested explicit teaching of rule-based summarizing strategies, including 1) removing words that repeat information, 2) replacing lists with one word that describes all, and 3) taking out materials not important to understanding (Dean et al., 2012, p. 80). The MCREL review also suggests creating classroom practice opportunities as well as employing a series of frames for summarization depending on the type of text, from narrative to topic restriction, definition, argumentation, and problem solution. The provision of sample notes, teaching a variety of formats (webbing, illustrations, outlines, recorded notes) and creating opportunities for use and revision of notes, enhances practice. In addition, Dean et al. (2012) recommend reciprocal peer teaching through teacher instruction of four comprehension strategies: summarizing, questioning, clarifying, and predicting, taken on gradually by peers working together in each area. Development of these skills will have an impact on individuals' ability to work alone as well as cooperatively and may therefore interact with the whole notion of homework effectiveness and study skill periods at school.

Instruction in Similarities and Differences
"But the greatest thing by far is to have a command of metaphor" (Aristotle, 1932). Understanding similarities and differences significantly affects one's ability to employ higher order thinking skills. The area of identifying and understanding similarities and differences moves us further into critical-thinking skills through comparisons and classifications, as well as use of metaphors, similes, and analogies (Bransford et al., 2000). Dean et al. note that this area is one that helps students make sense of their world (2012). In a study by Fuchs et al., explicit direct instruction with "structured practice, self-assessment and prompting" had a significant impact on students' acquisition of these analytic skills (Dean et al., 2012, p. 120). Dean et al. (2012) supply three rules: Teach students a variety of ways to identify similarities and differences; guide students as they engage in these processes; and provide supporting cues, thus scaffolding their instruction (2012).

Grace

Learning about similarities and differences in early years is often one of the more engaging activities for students, and this interest can be extended up through the grades and across subjects. In a first-grade lesson, groups of students might be provided a variety of objects and asked to classify and organize them by finding their common attributes (e.g., shape, color, length, purpose). The groups would then be guided, through the use of Venn diagrams with overlapping circles, to note which characteristics or attributes two of the items share and which are different.

Grace, a student with moderate disabilities who displays challenging behaviors when curriculum and instruction do not engage her or where the demands of the lesson are too difficult for her, shines in this activity. The math lesson involves making comparisons, finding similarities, and noting differences. As students move across the curriculum and grades, the processes involved in understanding; applying; and developing analogies, similes, and metaphors require both linguistic and nonlinguistic tools. Grace has benefited greatly in this regard throughout her elementary grades. In first grade, she can contribute to a whole-class activity in similarities and differences. In third grade, after several class periods involving research and discussion of family traditions, Grace contributes to the whole-class activity of making books about students' different traditions and indicating similarities. In fifth grade, at the beginning of the school year, she participates with her classmates in a survey designed to help them learn about each other and how they have similar and different likes and dislikes (e.g., movies, musical artists, school subjects, food). Rather than engaging in disruptive escape-related behavior, Grace is able to stay with activities and be an active contributor, because she is engaged in direct instruction of the concept of similarities and differences and how these apply to her daily life.

....

Generating and Testing Hypotheses
When one of the authors was visiting and observing inclusive schools and classrooms across several states, a middle school science teacher asked to talk with her, sharing how much he valued the inclusion of students with any type of learning difficulties in the science curriculum. He described these students as having experienced a great deal of failure before entering middle school science. He described the science curriculum as a last bastion of teaching critical thinking, allowing all students to experiment and

sometimes come up with the wrong conclusions, while testing their hypotheses. As he explained, the value of this lies in the process of gathering data to support a theory and learning what is needed to put that theory to the test. That, as he said, is problem solving, perhaps one of the most essential skills for all students. Kuhn (2007), in a discussion of the content and skills we should teach, concluded that "the two broad sets best serving this purpose are the skills of inquiry and the skills of argument. These skills are education for life, not simply for more school" (p. 111). Teaching these processes does not and must not exist only in science class. Students learn to predict events when reading literature or historical accounts and learn to deduct outcomes from principles within subject matter they have learned to generalize and apply across instances. For 11 studies described as rigorous in their methodology, Dean et al. (2012) found that the effect of this instruction on student learning was greater when teaching the process of generating and testing hypotheses was compared with lectures and teacher-directed activities, in terms of students' understanding of concepts within a problem-solving structure. An example of this might be the lessons we suggested earlier for nutrition studies and making purposeful connections with students' lives.

Formative Assessment   Formative assessments are ongoing assessments or checks for understanding that occur during learning (DeRuvo, 2010, p. 123). If our assessment of student learning is too far removed from day-to-day instruction, we stand a good chance of missing students who need additional instruction, who are practicing errors they are not even aware of. In other words, we would be violating the "rules" of effective feedback that we know from the Dean et al. (2012) analyses—that feedback needs to be *timely*, occurring as close to the performance as possible. We need to provide multiple checks for understanding for all students, especially for our target students with behavior challenges, so that we can adjust

our instruction and provide the scaffolding they need before resorting to their escape strategies. Marzano (2003) recommended the adoption of standards-based quarterly assessments; these are certainly appropriate for overall monitoring and for examining the effects of additional academic interventions through a MTSS approach. However, in conjunction with these, teachers must utilize their toolboxes to ensure understanding is occurring throughout the teaching process, employing tools from choral response and class feedback of quick-written responses using individual think pads or slates/whiteboards, or cell phones to answer multiple choice questions, after which the students' "votes" automatically display through the projector hooked up to the teacher's laptop (Barseghian, 2012). Tomlinson (2007) reminds us that all instruction should embed ongoing assessment of many kinds, including less formal aspects such as conversations with our students and close observations of paired and group work. Using the term "informative assessment" (p. 13), Tomlinson explains that informative assessment is not separate from the curriculum. Tomlinson cites differences among assessment *of* learning, assessment *for* learning, and assessment *as* learning. All assessment should inform our teaching as well as the students' learning (2007). This view of instruction is related to the types of functional, immediate assessment we need to engage in when we are seeking to identify the function of a student's behavior—what is not working for them in the classroom environment or in the demands of curriculum and instruction.

Inclusive Service Delivery Structures
Additional research is emerging on the resources special education can bring to the general education classroom when students are included (Sailor, 2009). Two of these structures, coteaching arrangements (Friend & Cook, 2009; Walsh, 2012) and wraparound services (Eber et al., 2008), defined in Table 20.1, have growing evidence bases, highlighted in the following discussion.

Coteaching Arrangements When special educators spend part or all of the day working in their students' general education classrooms, they are able to design instruction together and be there for its implementation, bringing more flexible means of instruction through strategies such as small groups and parallel activities. First described by Friend and Cook (2002), well-structured coteaching provides for multiple "input" arrangements, and its effectiveness in terms of student outcomes is growing over time (Murawski, Boyer, Melchiorre, & Atwill, 2009; Schwab, 2003; Walsh, 2012; Zigmond & Matta, 2004). Much is available elsewhere on the various approaches to coteaching (e.g., Friend & Cook, 2002; Murawski & Spencer, 2011). Recent research on the outcomes of this service delivery approach to enhance curriculum and instructional arrangements includes Walsh's (2012) 6-year longitudinal examination of a countywide coteaching effort in Maryland, which focused on the effectiveness of coteaching as a systemic strategy to close achievement gaps for students with disabilities. A remarkable 22% increase in statewide reading and math assessment scores occurred among students with disabilities between 2003 and 2009. Concurrently, coteaching was the focus of all professional development, including coaching support and technical assistance provided to facilitate all students' learning in the least restrictive environment, the general education classroom. The achievement gap in reading proficiency decreased from 31% to 9% over this period, and in math, the gap narrowed from a 34% to a 12%. Walsh noted that the strategy is now extended further to address achievement gaps and promote higher achievement for *all* students; coteaching is now a state-recognized tool for continuous improvement.

Renee

A third grader in a rural inclusive school, Renee, had difficulty with whole-class instruction. Regardless of where she sat in class, she would run up to the teacher to examine materials or make an attempt to engage with the teacher during instruction. She often yelled and threw teaching materials on the ground. In observing Renee's behavior across the school day, it became clear that she was less likely to demonstrate these behaviors when she was involved in small groups with frequent opportunities for active engagement with the teacher and her peers. Parallel coteaching was implemented to split the class and provide all students with smaller group instruction, with the general and special educator each teaching half the class. For example, after reading a story about a Japanese family immigrating to the United States, the teachers provided the students with a lesson using realia from Japan (e.g., a silk kimono, a doll, chopsticks, small statues) that represented what they had read about in the story. Each teacher had a selection of materials and a small group of 8 to 10 students surrounding them. Within the smaller group context, when Renee could be close to the teacher and could assist in passing the materials to each student, her behavior changed and she became an active participant, staying with her group. This carried across the coteaching approaches utilized by these two teachers, who could build these conditions into their planning for future lessons.

....

Wraparound Services A final key area of supports that special education can bring to the education of all students, particularly those with very significant behavior challenges, is wraparound services (Eber et al., 2008). Viewed as a more intense tier of intervention in the context of a school-level problem-solving or MTSS approach, wraparound, or integrated, services assume that intervention for some challenging students requires the involvement of family as well as community agencies, such as mental health and afterschool providers, mentor systems, and sometimes probation officers, in developing effective student plans through a transdisciplinary approach. Sailor (2009) reviewed plan development, implementation, and monitoring processes, and recommended specific procedures to increase the likelihood of service effectiveness. A Tier-1 version of wraparound services is seen increasingly in secondary schools that have developed wellness centers, which provide counseling and health supports as well as referrals to community providers to all students, as a preventive, antecedent approach. These interagency agreements can be built on to ensure that the needs of students with individualized behavioral, social, or emotional supports are met on site; this is another tool schools can utilize to increase their capacity to serve all students well.

CONCLUSION

Public schools are a gathering spot for everyone and anyone, regardless of ability, readiness, interests, history, or culture. We as teachers don't have the luxury of selecting certain people to work with, nor would most of us want that dubious "luxury." Students like Sean, Grace, Renee, and Jeff challenge us and challenge the systems where we work. Effective educators and educational systems are flexible and responsive and learn from their experience. As educators, we believe that all people are capable of growth and change. Approaches that simply attempt to manage a student's behavior through rewards and consequences will have limited success in settings that strive to encourage lifelong learning. Instead, we must utilize all the tools we have at hand. As special educators we begin by working to develop and maintain our schools' inclusive, data-based, problem-solving approach for all students; we assist our general education colleagues as they employ the evidence-based instruction, curricular, and intervention strategies outlined previously, and we contribute through coplanning, coteaching, and individualized supports to the construction of classrooms that support all students' learning. In these ways, we focus on success for those whose challenging behavior has led to their widespread, systematic, and unjust exclusion from equal educational opportunities.

REFERENCES

Algozzine, B., Wang, C., & Violette, A.S. (2011). Reexamining the relationship between academic achievement and social behavior. *Journal of Positive Behavioral Interventions, 13*, 3–16.

Algozzine, B., Ysseldyke, J., & Elliot, J, (1997). *Strategies and tactics for effective instruction*. Longmont, CO: Sopris West.

Aristotle. (1932). Poetics. In W.H. Fyfe (Trans.), *Aristotle in 23 Volumes* (Vol. 23). Cambridge, MA: Harvard University Press.

Barseghian, T. (2012). *How teachers make cell phones work in the classroom*. Mind/Shift. San Francisco, CA: KQED. Retrieved from http://blogs.kqed.org/mind shift/2012/05/how-teachers-make-cell-phones-work -in-the-classroom/

Beesley, A.D., & Apthorp, H.S. (Eds.). (2010). *Classroom instruction that works: Research report* (2nd ed.). Denver, CO: Mid-Continent Research for Education and Learning.

Berotti, D., & Durand, V.M. (1999). Communication-based interventions for students with sensory impairments and challenging behavior. In J.R. Scotti & L.H. Meyer (Eds.), *Behavioral intervention: Principles, models and practices* (pp. 237–250). Baltimore, MD: Paul H. Brookes Publishing Co.

Black, A.C., McCoach, D.B., Purcell, J.H., & Siegle, D. (2008). Advancement via individual determination: Method selection in conclusions about program effectiveness (AVID). *Journal of Educational Research, 102*(2), 111–124.

Bransford, J., Brown, A., & Cocking, R. (2000). *How people learn: Brain, mind, experience and school*. Washington, DC: National Academies Press.

California Department of Education. (2009). *Health education content standards for California public schools kindergarten through grade twelve*. Sacramento, CA: Author.

Casner-Lotto, J., & Barrington, L. (2006). *Are they really ready to work? Employers' perspectives on the basic knowledge and applied skills of new entrants to the 21st century USA workforce*. The Conference Board, Corporate Voices for Working Families, the Partnership for 21st Century Skills, and the Society for Human Resource Management. Retrieved from http://www.21stcenturyskills.org/documents/ FINAL_REPORT_PDF09-29-06.pdf

Children's Defense Fund. (2012). *Policy priorities: Juvenile justice*. Retrieved April 27, 2012, from http:// www.childrensdefense.org/policy-priorities/juvenile -justice/

Cole, S., Horvath, B., Chapman, C., Deschenes, C., Eberling, D.G., & Sprague, J. (2000). *Adapting curriculum and instruction in inclusive classrooms: A Teacher's desk reference* (2nd ed.). Bloomington, IN: Indiana Institute on Disability and Community.

Coyne, P., Pisha, B., Dalton, B., Zeph, L.A., & Smith, N.C. (2012). Literacy by design: A universal design for learning approach for students with significant intellectual disabilities. *Remedial and Special Education, 33*(3), 162–172.

Dalton, B., & Proctor, C.P. (2007). Reading as thinking: Integrating strategy instruction in universally designed digital literacy environment. In D.S. McNamara (Ed.),

Reading comprehension strategies: Theories, interventions, and technologies (pp. 423–442). Mahwah, NJ: Erlbaum.

Dean, C.B., Hubbell, E.R., Pitler, H., & Stone, B.J. (2012). *Classroom instruction that works: Research-based strategies for increasing student achievement* (2nd ed.). Alexandria, VA: Association of Supervision and Curriculum Development.

DeRuvo, S.L. (2010). *The essential guide to RTI: An integrated, evidence-based approach.* San Francisco, CA: Jossey-Bass.

Dewey, J. (1915). *The school and society.* Chicago, IL: University of Chicago Press.

Eber, L., Hyde, K., Rose, J., Breen, K., McDonald, D., & Lewandowski, H. (2008). *Completing the continuum of school-wide positive behavior support: Wrap-around as a tertiary level intervention.* In W. Sailor, G. Dunlap, G. Sugai, & R. Horner (Eds.), *Handbook of positive behavior support* (pp. 667–700). New York, NY: Springer.

Epstein, M., Atkins, M., Cullinan, D., Kutash, K., & Weaver, R. (2008). *Reducing behavior problems in the elementary school classroom: An IES practice guide.* Washington, DC: Institute of Education Sciences.

Filter, K.J., & Horner, R.H. (2009). Function-based academic interventions for problem behavior. *Education and Treatment of Children, 32,* 1–19.

Fisher, D., & Frey, N. (2012a). Making time for feedback. *Educational Leadership, 70*(1), 42–47.

Fisher, D., & Frey, N. (2012b). Accommodations and modifications with learning in mind. *Special Edge, 25*(2), i–iv.

Fitterer, H., Harwood, S., Locklear, K., & Lapid, J. (2008). *T4S: Teach for Success.* Phoenix, AZ: WestEd.

Friedman, T. (2006). *The world is flat: A brief history of the 21st century* (2nd ed.). New York, NY: Farrar, Straus, & Giroux.

Friend, M., & Bursuck, W.D. (2012). *Including students with special needs: A practical guide for classroom teachers* (6th ed.). Upper Saddle River, NJ: Pearson.

Friend, M., & Cook, L. (2002). *Interactions: Collaboration skills for school professionals.* Boston, MA: Allyn & Bacon.

Fuchs, L.S., Fuchs, D., Finelli, R., Courey, S., Hamlett, C.L., Sones, E.M., & Hope, S. (2006). Teaching third graders about real life mathematical problem solving: A randomized controlled study. *Elementary School Journal, 106,* 293–312.

Glover, T.A., & Vaughn, S. (2010). *The promise of response to intervention: Evaluating current science and practice.* New York, NY: Guilford Press.

Hall, T., Strangman, N., & Meyer, A. (2003; updated online 2011, January). *Differentiated instruction and implications for UDL implementation: Effective classroom practices report.* Wakefield, MA: National Center on Accessing General Curriculum (NCAC), Center for Applied Specialized Technology. Retrieved from http://aim.cast.org/sites/aim.cast.org/files/DI_UDL.1.14.11.pdf

Halvorsen, A.T., & Neary, T. (2009). *Building inclusive schools: Tools and strategies for success* (2nd ed.). Upper Saddle River, NJ: Pearson.

Harding Davis, R. (1861). Life in the iron mills. *Atlantic Monthly, 7*(42), 430–451.

Hattie, J. (2012). Know thy impact. *Educational Leadership, 70*(1), 18–23.

Hunter, M. (1982). *Mastery teaching.* El Segundo, CA: TIP Publications.

Ingram, K., Lewis-Palmer, T., & Sugai, G. (2005). Function-based intervention planning: Comparing the effectiveness of FBA function-based and non-function-based intervention plans. *Journal of Positive Behavioral Interventions, 7,* 224–236.

Johnson, D.W., & Johnson, R. (1989). *Cooperation and competition: Theory and research.* Edina, MN: Interaction Book Company.

Johnson, D.W., & Johnson, R.T. (2009). An educational psychology success story: Social interdependence theory and cooperative learning. *Educational Researcher, 38*(5), 365–379.

Jones, F.H., Jones, P., Jones, J., & Jones, F. (2007). *Tools for teaching* (2nd ed.). Santa Cruz, CA: Fred H. Jones and Associates.

Kansas Department of Education. (2008). *Kansas multi-tier system of supports.* Topeka, KS: Author. Retrieved June 24, 2013, from http://www.kansasmtss.org/

Katz, J.N. (2013). The three block model of universal design for learning (UDL): Engaging students in inclusive education. *Canadian Journal of Education/ Revue canadienne de l'éducation, 36*(1), 153–194.

King-Sears, M. (2009). Universal design for learning: Technology and pedagogy. *Learning Disability Quarterly, 32,* 199–201.

Koga, N., & Hall, T. (2009). *Curriculum modification.* Wakefield, MA: National Center on Accessing General Curriculum (NCAC), Center for Applied Specialized Technology. Retrieved from http://aim.cast.org/sites/aim.cast.org/files/CurriculumModsNov2.pdf

Kuhn, D. (2007). Is direct instruction an answer to the right question? *Educational Psychologist, 42*(2), 109–113.

Lee, Y., Sugai, G., & Horner, R.H. (1999). Using an instructional intervention to reduce problem and off-task behaviors. *Journal of Positive Behavior Interventions, 1,* 195–204.

Mace, R. (1985). *Universal design: Barrier-free environments for everyone.* Los Angeles, CA: Designers West.

Marzano, R. (2003). *What works in schools: Translating research into action.* Alexandria, VA: Association of Supervision and Curriculum Development.

Marzano, R., Pickering, D., & Pollock, J. (2001). *Classroom instruction that works: Research-based strategies for increasing student achievement.* Alexandria, VA: Association of Supervision and Curriculum Development.

McIntosh, K., Chard, D.J., Boland, J.B., & Horner, R.H. (2006). Demonstration of combined efforts in school-wide academic and behavioral systems and incidence of reading and behavior challenges in early elementary grades. *Journal of Positive Behavior Interventions, 8,* 146–154.

McIntosh, K., Horner, R.H., Chard, D.J., Dickey, C.R., & Braun, D.H. (2008). Reading skills and function of problem behavior in typical school settings. *Journal of Special Education, 42*(3), 131–147.

Murawski, W.W., Boyer, L., Melchiorre, B., & Atwill, K. (2009). *What is happening in co-taught classes? One state knows!* Paper presented at the meeting of the American Education Research Association, San Diego, CA.

Murawski, W.W., & Spencer, S. (2011). *Collaborate, communicate, and differentiate: How to increase student learning in today's diverse schools.* Thousand Oaks, CA: Corwin Press.

National Center on Response to Intervention. (2010). *Essential components of RTI: A closer look at response to intervention.* Washington, DC: U.S. Department of Education, Office of Special Education Programs, National Center on Response to Intervention.

Nelson, R., Johnson, A., & Marchand-Martella, N. (1996). Effects of direct instruction, cooperative learning, and independent learning practices on the classroom behavior of students with behavioral disorders: A comparative analysis. *Journal of Emotional and Behavioral Disorders, 4*(1), 53–62.

Newcomer, L., & Lewis, T.J. (2004). Functional behavioral assessment: An investigation of assessment reliability and effectiveness of function-based interventions. *Journal of Emotional and Behavioral Disorders, 12,* 168–181.

New York City Board of Education. (October 2007). *A guide to the essential elements of instruction.* New York, NY: Author. Retrieved from http://www.thhs .qc.edu/ourpages/auto/2010/10/20/57043719/eei%20 guide.pdf

No Child Left Behind Act of 2001, PL 107-110, 115 Stat. 1425, 20 U.S.C. §§ 6301 *et seq.*

O'Neill, R.E., Horner, R.H., Albin, R.W., Sprague, J.R., Storey, K., & Newton, J.S. (1997). *Functional assessment and program development for problem behavior: A practical handbook* (2nd ed.). Pacific Grove, CA: Brooks/Cole.

Patterson, G.R. (1976). The aggressive child: Victim and architect of a coercive system. In E.J. Mash, L.A. Hamerlynck, & L.C. Handy (Eds.), *Behavior modification and families* (pp. 267–316). New York, NY: Brunner/Mazel.

Patterson, G.R. (1982). *Coercive family process.* Eugene, OR: Castalia.

Patterson, G.R., Reid, J.B., & Dishion, T.J. (1992). *Antisocial boys.* Eugene, OR: Castalia.

Proctor, C.P., Dalton, B., & Grisham, D.L. (2007). Scaffolding English language learners and struggling readers in a universal literacy environment with embedded strategy instruction and vocabulary support. *Journal of Literacy Research, 39*(1), 71–93.

Rodgers, E.M. (2004). Interactions that scaffold reading performance. *Journal of Literacy Research, 36*(4), 501–532.

Rose, D.H., & Meyer, A. (2002). *Teaching every student in the digital age.* Alexandria, VA: Association of Supervision and Curriculum Development.

Rose, D.H., & Meyer, A. (2006). *A practical reader in universal design for learning.* Cambridge, MA: Harvard Education Press.

Rosenshine, B., & Meister, C. (1992). The use of scaffolding for teaching higher-level cognitive strategies. *Educational Leadership, 49*(7), 26–33.

Rosenshine, B., & Stevens, R. (1986). Teaching functions. In M.C. Wittrock (Ed.), *AERA handbook of research on teaching* (3rd ed., pp 376–391). New York, NY: Macmillan.

Saenz, L., Fuchs, L., & Fuchs, D. (2005). Peer-assisted learning strategies for English language learners with learning disabilities. *Exceptional Children, 71*(3), 231–247.

Sailor, W.S. (2009). *Making RTI work: How smart schools are reforming education through school-wide response to intervention.* San Francisco, CA: Jossey-Bass.

Schwab Learning. (2003). Collaboratively speaking: A study on effective ways to teach children with learning differences in the general education classroom. *The Special EDge, 16*(3), 1–4.

Simons, K.D., and Klein, J.D. (2007). The impact of scaffolding and student achievement levels in a problem-based learning environment. *Instructional Science, 35,* 41–72.

Slavin, R.E. (1991). Synthesis of research on cooperative learning. *Educational Leadership, 48*(5), 71–82.

Steinberg, K.S., Bringle, R.G., & Williams, M.J. (2010). *Service learning research primer.* Scotts Valley, CA: National Service-Learning Clearinghouse.

Terrace, H.S. (1963). Discrimination learning with and without "errors." *Journal of the Experimental Analysis of Behavior, 6*(1), 1–27.

Tomlinson, C. (2003). *Fulfilling the promise of the differentiated classroom: Strategies and tools for responsive teaching.* Alexandria, VA: Association of Supervision and Curriculum Development.

Tomlinson, C.A. (2007). Learning to love assessment. *Educational Leadership, 64*(4), 8–13.

Tomlinson, C.A., & Imbeau, M. (2010). *Leading and managing a differentiated classroom.* Alexandria, VA: ASCD.

Voke, H. (2002). *Motivating students to learn.* Association for Supervision and Curriculum Development Infobrief. Retrieved from http://www.ascd.org/ publications/infobrief/issue28.html

Vygotsky, L. (1978). Interaction between learning and development. In M. Cole, V. John-Steiner, S. Scribner, E. Souberman (Eds.), *Mind in society: The development of higher psychological processes* (pp. 79–91). Cambridge, MA: Harvard University Press.

Walsh, J. (2012). Co-teaching as a school system strategy for continuous improvement. *Preventing School Failure, 56*(1), 29–36.

Whitehurst, G. (2002). *Evidence-based education (EBE).* PowerPoint presentation at Student Achievement and School Accountability Conference in October 2002. Retrieved from http://www.ies.ed.gov/director/pdf/ 2002_10.pdf

Wood, D., Bruner, J.S., & Ross, G. (1976). The role of tutoring in problem solving. *Journal of Psychology and Psychiatry, 17*(2), 89–100.

Zigmond, N., & Matta, D. (2004). Value added of the special education teacher on secondary school co-taught classes. In T.E. Scruggs & M.A. Mastropieri (Eds.), *Research in secondary schools: Advances in learning and behavioral disabilities* (Vol. 17, pp. 55–76). Oxford, UK: Elsevier Science.

Strategies for Functional Communication Training

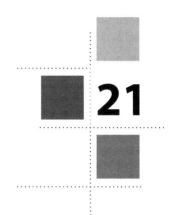

21

V. Mark Durand

Challenging behaviors such as aggression, self-injury, stereotyped behaviors, and tantrums are highly prevalent among children and adults with a variety of developmental disorders. Between 10% and 40% of children with disabilities display frequent and severe challenging behaviors (Einfeld, Tonge, & Rees, 2001; Lowe et al., 2007). Along with frequency, the chronic nature of these behaviors is also of serious concern (Totsika, Toogood, Hastings, & Lewis, 2008). Several studies document that, even with treatment, these behaviors may still be problematic a decade later (Einfeld & Tonge, 1996; Einfeld et al., 2001; Emerson et al., 2001; Green, O'Reilly, Itchon, & Sigafoos, 2005; Jones, 1999).

Challenging behaviors are among the most frequently cited obstacles to placing students in community settings (Eyman & Call, 1977; Jacobson, 1982). Further, their presence is associated with significantly increased recidivism among those individuals referred to crisis-intervention programs from community placements (Shoham-Vardi et al., 1996). Challenging behavior interferes with such essential activities as family life (Cole & Meyer, 1989), educational activities (Koegel & Covert, 1972), and employment (Hayes, 1987). Parental stress is shown to significantly increase when caring for a child with problem behavior (Floyd & Gallagher, 1997; Hastings, 2002; Saloviita, Italinna, & Leinonen, 2003).[1] Mothers of children with disabilities tend to have higher rates of depression, and depressed parents are more likely to have a child with behavior problems (Feldman et al., 2007). In one of the largest studies of its

---

[1] Throughout the chapter I will use the terms *challenging behavior* and *problem behavior* and other variations to indicate those difficulties presented by individuals that interfere with educational, vocational, and family activities.

kind, researchers examining almost 10,000 children found that the single best predictor of early school failure was the presence of behavior problems (Byrd & Weitzman, 1994). In fact, the presence of behavior problems was a better predictor of school difficulties than factors such as poverty, speech and hearing impairments, and low birth weight.

One of the most frequently used approaches to reduce these challenging behaviors involves replacing the problem behavior with an alternative behavior—a technique known as functional communication training (FCT; Carr & Durand, 1985; Durand, 1990). FCT was developed in the early 1980s at the time when controversies erupted over the use of painful or humiliating interventions with people with disabilities. This approach fit with the *Zeitgeist* to offer interventions for even the most severe challenging behaviors that would avoid relying on procedures that might dehumanize the individual (Durand, 1987). The first study documented that a positive approach consistent with today's efforts at positive behavior support (PBS) could effectively treat chronic and severe problem behavior (Carr & Durand, 1985).

FCT entails a multistep process to 1) assess the function of the challenging behavior to be targeted, 2) select an appropriate alternative behavior, and 3) teach the alternative and fade out supports to fit the current environment. There is a wide range of behaviors that have been targeted with FCT, including aggression, self-injury, elopement (Lang et al., 2009), and inappropriate sexual behavior (Fyffe, Kahng, Fittro, & Russell, 2004). FCT is used in homes, schools, and in the community by family members as well as a range of professionals (Dunlap, Ester, Langhans, & Fox, 2006; Durand, 1999; Kemp & Carr, 1995). Research on FCT targets individuals across all ages (from infants/toddlers to older adults), developmental levels (from those with pervasive needs for support to those with average or above average cognitive abilities), language abilities (Mancil, 2006; Petscher, Rey, & Bailey, 2009; Snell, Chen, & Hoover, 2006), and diagnoses such as autism

spectrum disorder (ASD; e.g., Brown et al., 2000), attention-deficit/hyperactivity disorder (ADHD; e.g., Flood & Wilder, 2002), and traumatic brain injury (Gardner, Bird, Maguire, Carreiro, & Abenaim, 2003).

EVIDENCE BASE FOR FUNCTIONAL COMMUNICATION TRAINING

There is an extensive literature on the outcomes of using FCT to treat and reduce challenging behavior. This section selectively reviews the substantial body of research in this area. To date, close to 200 published studies document the successful use of FCT with a range of individuals and their challenging behaviors (Durand, 2012; Kurtz, Boelter, Jarmolowicz, Chin, & Hagopian, 2011; Mancil, 2006; Tiger, Hanley, & Bruzek, 2008). In addition, several parameters necessary for the success of FCT have been individually examined (e.g., schedule thinning) and the research on these aspects of FCT will also be discussed.

A review by Matson and colleagues (2005) evaluates the literature on a number of techniques used to treat aggression and found that FCT was one of the most heavily researched approaches. In their review of research on differential reinforcement of alternative behavior, Petscher and colleagues identified more than 80 studies that used FCT to treat challenging behavior, met specific criteria such as being published in peer-reviewed outlets, and reported behavioral data (Petscher et al., 2009). They used the standards set by the American Psychological Association's Division 12 Task Force on the Promotion and Dissemination of Psychological Procedures to determine if FCT or its variations met the task force's criteria for interventions that are "well established," "probably efficacious," or "experimental" (Chambless et al., 1996; Task Force Promoting Dissemination of Psychological Procedures, 1995). Overall, they found that differential reinforcement of alternative behavior in general and specifically FCT met the criteria for well-established treatments for destructive behavior. This level of evidence was present whether or not extinction for challenging behavior was added as a component of the treatment (Petscher et al., 2009). They also noted that these results were obtained with few unwanted side effects across children and adults with a range of disorders. FCT is frequently cited as one of the few behavior interventions having extensive support from initial efficacy studies (Smith et al., 2007).

Schedule Thinning and Functional Communication Training

An important issue to address when using FCT is the reinforcement for the alternative communication being used to replace challenging behavior. Initially, a rich schedule of reinforcement is recommended to ensure that acquisition occurs quickly (see Chapter 8; Durand, 1990). If reinforcement is delayed too long or is otherwise not sufficient, the individual will return to using challenging behavior to gain access to preferred reinforcers at an acceptable rate (e.g., escape from demands, attention from others; Horner & Day, 1991). However, continued reinforcement of the new communicative response at high rates can be impractical. Too frequent requests for attention, for example, can be annoying to teachers or family members, regardless of the form they take. Requesting escape from work on a continual basis can seriously interfere with educational and vocational goals. In order to address this issue, a number of studies examine if and how the schedule of reinforcement for the appropriate communicative behavior can be reduced or "thinned" from a continuous schedule to a more intermittent one that may be more acceptable in typical settings (Falcomata, Roane, Muething, Stephenson, & Ing, 2012; Hagopian, Kuhn, Long, & Rush, 2005; Hagopian, Toole, Long, Bowman, & Lieving, 2004; Kelley, Lerman, & Van Camp, 2002; Worsdell, Iwata, Hanley, Thompson, & Kahng, 2000).

In one study, for example, researchers gradually increased the time between the appropriate request and the reinforcement (Hagopian, Fisher, Sullivan, Acquisto, &

LeBlanc, 1998). They found that although this attempt at schedule thinning was successful in reducing the amount of effort to respond to appropriate requests for some individuals, it was not successful for all. Similar problems in using delayed schedules have been noted in other studies as well (e.g., Fisher, Thompson, Hagopian, Bowman, & Krug, 2000). One difficulty with using delayed schedules of reinforcement with the alternative response is that the individual may not be able to discriminate when and if the request will be satisfied, resulting in increased requesting—a pattern typically observed with fixed interval (FI) reinforcement schedules. Some researchers have found more success using signals (e.g., red card signaling no response forthcoming, green card signaling a request will receive a response) to indicate the temporal nature of the responses (Hanley, Iwata, & Thompson, 2001).

It is unlikely that one approach to schedule thinning will be effective for all cases when using FCT. For example, the ability of the individual to discriminate reinforcement schedules and the person's history of reinforcement will likely influence efforts to reduce the level of reinforcement for appropriate requests. At the same time, it is important to consider what the prevailing environment can support. Some environments can support relatively high rates of requests (e.g., classrooms with small student-to-teacher ratios) while others cannot (e.g., classrooms with only one teacher and many students). Research on contextual fit with regard to requests for reinforcement and the environment's ability to maintain responses should be an important next step in researching the nature of responses to appropriate requests for reinforcement in FCT (Durand, 2012).

Consequences for Challenging Behavior

A somewhat controversial concern related to FCT use involves the issue of how to respond to the challenging behavior itself. Several studies have examined directly the issue of continuing reinforcement for the challenging behavior. One study looked at whether or not FCT would be an effective approach if the challenging behavior continued to be reinforced while an alternative response was being taught (Shirley, Iwata, Kahng, Mazaleski, & Lerman, 1997). For three individuals who engaged in self-injurious behavior, manual signing was used as the alternative communicative response. The researchers found that self-injury was not initially reduced if it continued to be reinforced concurrently with the new alternative. However, once extinction was initiated for the challenging behaviors, they were reduced and signing increased. Even when extinction was suspended for self-injury, the behavior problems remained at low levels for two of the three individuals (Shirley et al., 1997). On the other hand, one study examined the use of FCT for four students identified as having significant challenging behaviors and diagnosed with severe emotional and behavioral disorders (Davis, Fredrick, Alberto, & Gama, 2012). The students were taught to hand their teacher a card to signal break time (consistent with the function of their behavior problems, which involved escape from task demands). Even though the teachers provided comparable breaks from work for both challenging behavior and appropriate communication, challenging behavior was significantly reduced for all four students. Overall, the collective evidence across many studies suggests that FCT is effective with or without programmed extinction for the challenging behavior (Petscher et al., 2009).

Other studies have shown some difficulty maintaining success with FCT without the use of some form of punishment (e.g., response cost or time-out; Wacker et al., 1990). It is difficult to interpret why some individuals in the previous research did not require negative consequences to reduce their challenging behaviors. One interpretation may be that because these negative consequences are often introduced from the beginning of treatment, this may have affected later behavior. It is possible that if the negative consequences were

never introduced concurrent with FCT, these consequences may not have been required to reduce their challenging behavior. These data suggest that "behavioral contrast" (the tendency to evaluate situations compared with how these situations have been presented previously) may sometimes be at work—with the effectiveness of FCT alone influenced by the removal of the contingencies for challenging behavior (i.e., time-out and graduated guidance; Durand, 2012).

Although there is an extensive body of published research assessing the effectiveness of FCT, the vast majority of these studies employ single-case designs with a small number of participants in each study. Although several larger studies exist (e.g., Durand & Carr, 1992; Hagopian et al., 1998; Kurtz et al., 2003; Wacker et al., 1998), there are to date no formal randomized clinical trials comparing outcomes to no treatment and treatment as usual or to other traditional techniques. This reliance on a single category of research design may limit our understanding of FCT as an intervention.

THEORETICAL BASIS FOR FUNCTIONAL COMMUNICATION TRAINING

It is valuable to understand the theoretical foundation of several aspects of FCT in order to be able to adapt this procedure to diverse individuals and settings. Described next are the concepts behind why challenging behavior is reduced with FCT (functional equivalence) and why the effects of FCT generalize to new people and settings (natural communities of reinforcement).

Functional Equivalence

The mechanism of behavior change that underlies the reduction of problem behavior using FCT is the concept of "functional equivalence" (Carr, 1988; Durand, 1987). The assumption is that problem behaviors are maintained by a particular reinforcer or reinforcers (e.g., attention from others, escape from work). Theoretically, then, these behaviors can be replaced by other behaviors if these new behaviors serve the same function and are more efficient at gaining the desired reinforcers. For example, if a young boy hits himself to get attention from his parent, then teaching him another, more effective way to get this attention (e.g., "Come here, please") should serve the same function for the boy. This then would result in a decrease in the frequency of his self-injury as he becomes successful gaining attention in this new way. FCT is presumed to reduce problem behavior because it involves teaching and reinforcing a replacement behavior that serves the same function.

Natural Communities of Reinforcement

For FCT as an intervention strategy, using communication as the replacement behavior provides an added benefit because of its unique ability to recruit natural communities of desired reinforcers. In other words, if someone learns to ask or otherwise solicit the reinforcers from others, then that person is able to recruit these reinforcers without an interventionist having to specifically train other people how to respond. For example, in one study, my colleagues and I examined whether nonverbal children would be able to recruit reinforcers from community members, thereby resulting in a reduction of their challenging behaviors (Durand, 1999). Five students were identified who 1) exhibited severe and frequent behavior problems and 2) were unable to communicate verbally with others. The teachers of these students were shown how to assess the functions of the students' behaviors and select more appropriate alternatives for them to use. The teachers were then instructed in how to assist their students to use vocal output communication devices to request things such as assistance or attention from others. The teachers were successful in teaching their students to use their devices to gain access to the stimuli previously maintaining their challenging behaviors, and they observed significant reductions in problem behavior in the classroom. Next, the teachers took their students out into typical community settings and observed that the students used their devices to appropriately solicit attention and help from untrained people in settings such as the library and stores at the local shopping mall. Again, challenging behavior was significantly reduced in the community settings once the students were able to recruit reinforcers from others. Importantly, this success was achieved without specifically instructing community members how to respond to the students. The librarians or store clerks responded naturally to the requests made by the students through their devices and this, in turn, resulted in reduced challenging behavior in the community (Durand, 1999).

The concept of "recruiting natural communities of reinforcement" (Stokes, Fowler, & Baer, 1978) is central to the success of FCT outside of structured environments staffed with highly trained individuals (Durand, 1990). This is a particularly important aspect of FCT when comparing the outcomes associated with FCT to other intervention strategies. We conducted an experimental analysis of this bootstrapping aspect of FCT (i.e., the self-sustaining nature of this intervention because of its ability to be maintained by student initiations and without direct training of others) in a study comparing this treatment approach with another, common approach to reacting to challenging behavior—time-out from positive reinforcement (Durand & Carr, 1992). In this study, we selected 12 school-age students, all of whom engaged in a variety of challenging behaviors (e.g., tantrums, self-injury, and aggression). In addition, we screened for students whose challenging behaviors were being maintained by attention from others. The rationale for selecting students who only had attention-maintained problem behavior was to ensure that they would be appropriate for time-out.

Six students were randomly assigned to one of the two treatment conditions—FCT or time-out. Just prior to introducing the treatments, the students were individually placed with teachers who had no knowledge of the study and who were instructed to work with the student on a task. No instructions were given about how to react to behavior problems. Treatment was then introduced by other teachers and was successful in reducing challenging behaviors for each child. Thus the first finding was that both FCT and time-out could successfully reduce challenging behavior. Then the students were placed back with the teachers who were naïve to the treatment program. Students who had received time-out as a treatment quickly found that time-out as a consequence would not occur in this setting, and they resumed their behavior problems. In contrast, the students who received FCT as a treatment used their communicative responses to request attention and the naïve teachers responded appropriately, maintaining the reduction of the challenging behavior. In short, the advantage of FCT was not solely in the initial reduction in challenging behavior—which both treatments could produce—but also in its ability to recruit natural communities of reinforcement (in this case, teacher attention; Shoham-Vardi et al., 1996). The sustainability of treatments outside of special environments (e.g., university clinics) and without highly trained staff is often overlooked in the intervention literature but is essential for the success of these techniques in typical settings.

ASSESSMENT FOR FUNCTIONAL COMMUNICATION TRAINING

Functional behavioral assessment (FBA) is at the core of the process used in FCT (Durand, 1990). The function or functions of challenging behavior are determined, and this information is used to select the alternative communicative behavior that is taught to replace the problem behavior. The primary goal is to identify a socially acceptable behavior that serves the same function as the problem behavior and that therefore can serve as a replacement for the challenging behavior. To assess the function of a problem behavior, the antecedents and consequences of that behavior need to be identified, which can be accomplished in a number of ways.

In order to improve the accuracy of assessment results, it is typically recommended that multiple forms of assessment are used (see Chapters 14 and 15). Functional analysis—manipulating aspects of the environment to assess behavior change—is frequently cited as an effective method of determining the function of a behavior problem (Hanley, Iwata, & McCord, 2003; see Chapter 16). A number of different variations on functional analysis have been developed, including manipulating only antecedents to problem behavior (e.g., removing attention to assess if challenging behavior increases; Durand & Crimmins, 1988) and providing consequences (e.g., talking to a child contingent on misbehavior; Iwata, Dorsey, Slifer, Bauman, & Richman, 1994). However, there are also a number of issues to consider prior to conducting this type of assessment (Durand, 1997; Sturmey, 1994). One issue is accessibility to manipulation. There are certain influences that you cannot or would not manipulate or change in order to perform a functional analysis. Factors such as some illnesses, disrupted family life, and chromosomal aberrations can certainly affect behavior problems, but changing these influences to assess their impact is obviously problematic or impossible.

Another concern involves the ethics of conducting a functional analysis. There are other influences that you could manipulate but may not want to change if they result in an increase in challenging behavior. For example, you may want to know why a child runs out into the road, but it would be inappropriate to set up this situation, given the potential danger. In many instances, deliberately increasing a severe behavior problem in order to assess it can be questioned on ethical grounds. Alternatives to traditional functional analyses are being explored to minimize harm, including using only short probes of behaviors in settings related to their purported function (also called *trial-based functional analysis*; Lambert, Bloom, & Irvin, 2012; Sigafoos & Saggers, 1995). Other problem behaviors can be so severe (e.g., hitting one's head on the floor) that allowing even one instance would be too dangerous. In these cases, assessment that does not involve manipulation (and subsequent increases in challenging behavior) would be recommended.

Because of the issues raised previously, FBA is usually carried out in most settings without the use of experimental manipulations. Typically, the assessment process begins with informal observations and interviews of significant others. Once a broad range of information is collected and hypotheses about the function(s) of the behaviors are developed, more formal assessments are used to validate these hypotheses. A number of assessment instruments are available to provide additional information about the functions of behavior, including the Motivation Assessment Scale (MAS; Durand & Crimmins, 1988; Joosten, Bundy, & Einfeld, 2012), the Motivation Analysis Rating Scale (Wieseler, Hanson, Chamberlain, & Thompson, 1985), the Functional Analysis Interview Form (O'Neill et al., 1997), and the Questions About Behavioral Function (Paclawskyj, Matson, Rush, Smalls, & Vollmer, 2008). These types of instruments can be used to provide additional and convergent information about behavior functions (see Chapter 14). This information is then used to help select the alternative communication to be taught.

Although a full discussion is beyond the scope of this chapter and reviewed elsewhere in this book, there are a number of additional factors that must be considered prior to developing a comprehensive FCT intervention plan, including identifying goals and specific behaviors of concern; selecting the communication skill to be taught, including the appropriate modality (e.g., speech, picture system) and the message or messages that will recruit functionally equivalent responses from others (e.g., asking for help on a difficult task); creating or identifying teaching situations that are triggers for problem behavior; assessing the ability of the environment to maintain a certain level of responsiveness to requests; and identifying any potential obstacles to proper implementation (e.g., parent or teacher who may not believe that student is capable of making changes). To illustrate the assessment process, two cases will be briefly described, and I will return to these cases in the intervention section.

Nathan

Nathan was an 8-year-old boy diagnosed with ASD. He was nonverbal and had limited functional communication skills. His teacher introduced a Picture Exchange Communication System (PECS) to him so that he could make basic requests. Typically he would become extremely upset at school and at home, and this would take the form of slapping his face, hitting his head, and hitting others. After some discussion about the possible reasons behind Nathan's outbursts, we had both his mother and his teacher complete antecedent-behavior-consequence (ABC) charts and the MAS. The results of these assessments differed somewhat between home and school: Nathan's outbursts at home seemed mostly to revolve around asking him to do things he did not want to do (e.g., toothbrushing, sitting at the dinner table, going to bed). At school, he did seem to use his outbursts to avoid or escape unpleasant situations (e.g., particular tasks, going through the cafeteria line, coming inside from the playground) but also to solicit his teacher's attention when she was working with other classmates. Nathan's mother and teacher (with the consultation of his speech-language pathologist) agreed to use the PECS book at home and at school to keep the method of communication consistent. The FCT plan is described later on in this chapter.

Presencia

Presencia was a 2-year-old girl with a preliminary diagnosis of ASD. Presencia did not display "shared attention" (e.g., looking back and forth between a favorite toy and her parents), did not point and look at someone to get something she wanted, and at a year and a half still had no spoken words. Her parents reported that she loved to line things up at home (e.g., toys or silverware) and would become extremely upset if they were touched or put away (Falcomata et al., 2012). Because her tantrums were the most disruptive at home, the assessment revolved around finding the function(s) of these behaviors. Although we tried to get Presencia's parents to fill out ABC charts at home, they never seemed able to complete them. We did have them retrospectively recall the situations surrounding these disruptions and had them complete the MAS with the early intervention team. A major theme that arose was that anytime she was interrupted from a favorite activity, she would scream and fall to the floor. As a result, her parents tried to avoid these situations and ended up rearranging the household (e.g., leaving an area in the living room for her to line up her toys) and their activities (e.g., letting her eat all meals on the floor of the living room so her lining up of items wasn't interrupted) to prevent tantrums. The plan developed for her (and her parents) will be discussed later in the chapter.

INTERVENTION WITH FUNCTIONAL COMMUNICATION TRAINING

The steps to implement FCT include assessing the function of behavior, selecting the communication modality, creating teaching situations, prompting communication, fading the prompts, teaching new communicative responses, making appropriate environmental modifications, and assisting with any cognitive obstacles to using FCT (see Table 21.1). In Nathan's case, we used his PECS book to include a picture of his teacher (so he could give it to her to get her attention), a picture of his favorite nighttime

story (so he could request having it read once to him before bedtime), and a picture of a hand to signify that he needed help on some task. These and others were used so that he would learn to request things he was getting through his tantrums (e.g., teacher attention). The pictures also helped indicate that certain activities were about to occur (e.g., bedtime), so he could learn to adapt to these situations. We also added in other components for a full treatment plan (i.e., restriction of his sleep so he would be tired at bedtime and reduce his bedtime problems, a star chart for good behavior).

Although Nathan's parents were successful at home implementing these procedures and they were reporting much improved behavior, this was not the case at school. In discussing the differences, it became clear that (unlike Nathan's parents), his teacher was doubtful that Nathan would be capable of using PECS to communicate successfully and that this would not help him improve his behavior. When he did not quickly pick up using his pictures at school, she interpreted this as a part of his disability (ASD) and did

Table 21.1. Step-by-step instructions for implementing functional communication training (FCT)

Steps	Description
Assess the function of behavior.	Use two or more functional assessment techniques to determine what variables are maintaining the problem behavior.
Select the communication modality.	Identify how you want the individual to communicate with others (e.g., verbally, through alternative communication strategies).
Create teaching situations.	Identify situations in the environment that are triggers for problem behavior (e.g., difficult tasks), and use these as the settings for teaching the alternative responses.
Prompt communication.	Prompt the alternative communication in the setting where you want it to occur. Use the least intrusive prompt necessary.
Fade prompts.	Quickly fade the prompts, ensuring that no problem behaviors occur during training.
Teach new communicative responses.	When possible, teach a variety of alternative communicative responses that can serve the same function (e.g., "Help me" or "I don't understand").
Modify the environment.	When appropriate, changes in the environment—such as improving student–task match in school—should be implemented.
Assess for and intervene on cognitive obstacles.	Determine if the people implementing functional communication training (FCT) have doubts about their ability to use the technique or the child's ability to change. If so, help them view these issues more optimistically.

From Durand, V.M., & Merges, E. (2008). Functional communication training to treat challenging behavior. In W. O'Donohue & J.E. Fisher (Eds.), *Cognitive behavior therapy: Applying empirically supported techniques in your practice* (2nd ed., pp. 222–229). New York, NY: Wiley; adapted by permission. This material is reproduced by permission of John Wiley & Sons, Inc.

not persist with teaching him PECS. To help his teacher, we pointed out that this type of self-talk (e.g., "See, I knew this wouldn't work") was interfering with her ability to successfully teach him at school. We helped her substitute a more positive view of the situation (e.g., "I know this will be difficult but he is making some progress, and I know how to modify my teaching plan if there is a problem"), which eventually helped her continue prompting him. The cognitive-behavioral approach of Nathan's teacher is based on research showing how pessimistic self-talk can be a significant obstacle in implementing behavior plans; helping teachers overcome these thoughts can improve child outcomes (Steed & Durand, 2013). Eventually, Nathan became more proficient at using PECS in school, and his behaviors improved as well.

In the case of Presencia, we confronted a similar obstacle, but this time it was with her parents. We wanted to set up a system that would warn her when a favorite activity was about to end (using a timer) and giving her the ability to communicate for a little extra time (i.e., pointing to a picture for "5 more minutes"). We also suggested a positive transition activity to reinforce her for moving to the next situation (e.g., allowing her to line up the silverware at the dinner table if she left the living room to have dinner). This way she could have a little more control over the situation but still learn how to transition away from a favorite activity. Unfortunately, both of her parents were extremely reluctant to try to change the routines they had set up at home. Similar to Nathan's teacher, we had Presencia's parents keep a log of what they were thinking in these situations. We found that their thoughts about Presencia and themselves as parents were consistent with a pessimistic attributional style (Durand, 2011). For example, they thought that their daughter would tantrum in all situations—that it was due to her ASD and that she would always have these behavior problems. They also felt that they had absolutely no control of her, and they became extremely anxious when she got upset.

As we had done with Nathan's teacher, we confronted these thoughts through a process called *disputation*, showing them that most of what they were thinking was not fully true (e.g., she did not tantrum all the time, and they were able to intervene with her successfully sometimes) and then helped them with some substitute thoughts (e.g., "We have a plan, and things are getting better"). We also encouraged them to become more mindful when their daughter had a tantrum and, instead of avoiding the tantrums, just become aware of them. This helped them become less anxious about these tantrums. Procedures like these have been demonstrated to help pessimistic parents like Presencia's better implement behavior plans; these procedures lead not only to improved child behavior but also to a better quality of life (Durand, Hieneman, Clarke, Wang, & Rinaldi, 2013). Over the next few weeks, Presencia's parents reported being a little more comfortable asking her to transition away from favorite activities and, although her tantrums were not completely gone, they were much shorter and less intense. They also told us that they were now more optimistic about being able to lead a more typical life at home.

These two cases illustrate how we implanted FCT in the context of more comprehensive plans. The value of FCT is that it allows the person more control over important aspects of his or her environment, and this may account for part of its success as an intervention. In addition, the inclusion of cases where there were attitudinal obstacles to implementing FCT illustrates the hurdles teachers and parents face all too often. Fortunately, we are finding that we can help those who must implement our plans and make them more successful.

FUTURE DIRECTIONS

The extensive body of evidence since we first introduced FCT as an intervention in 1985 (Carr & Durand, 1985) points to its success in reducing challenging behavior. However, we are finding that up to 50% of the families or teachers with whom we work are not able to fully carry out this (or any other) intervention. Evidence is growing that parents and teachers differ in their perceptions of themselves (e.g., feeling out of control or inadequate as a parent or teacher), the child with a disability (e.g., whether or not their child is capable of making behavior improvements), and their degree of optimism about future prospects for change. This can have a negative impact on their ability to implement potentially successful interventions. Our work addresses the needs of these families and teachers by integrating cognitive behavior interventions (optimism training) with PBS (Durand, 2011; Durand et al., 2013; Steed & Durand, 2013). Continuing research in this area promises to broaden the benefits associated with FCT to a larger group of individuals challenged by problem behavior.

In addition to research on those who implement FCT, continuing research is needed in other aspects of FCT itself. For example, the issue of response acceptability (how individuals in the student's environment respond to new communication forms) is a potentially fruitful and important research topic. A related topic is the aspect of FCT referred to as *response milieu* (the nature of the environment in which the student is communicating). Both of these areas lack any systematic study, yet they are essential to the success of this treatment approach. Research on how to assess environments (e.g., How will others respond to a request for assistance?) and if and when to change the communication form or the environment itself (e.g., switching jobs to one that is more accepting of requests for choices) is needed to guide intervention efforts in this area. Answers to these types of questions will likely result in even more successful outcomes for individuals with challenging behavior.

CONCLUSION

There is a large body of evidence showing that challenging behavior can be reduced by replacing it with more acceptable and functionally equivalent communicative responses (FCT). Research shows that this approach can be adapted for use with many different types of problem behaviors (e.g., tantrums, aggression, self-injury, inappropriate verbalizations), across different client populations (e.g., ADHD, ASD, intellectual disability), and in a variety of settings (e.g., home, school, work, community). It is recommended that when designing plans for reducing challenging behavior, teams should consider FCT as an important component in their arsenal of intervention techniques.

REFERENCES

Brown, K.A., Wacker, D.P., Derby, K.M., Peck, S.M., Richman, D.M., Sasso, G.M., ... Harding, J.W. (2000). Evaluating the effects of functional communication training in the presence and absence of establishing operations. *Journal of Applied Behavior Analysis, 33*(1), 53–71.

Byrd, R.S., & Weitzman, M.L. (1994). Predictors of early grade retention among children in the United States. *Pediatrics, 93,* 481–487.

Carr, E.G. (1988). Functional equivalence as a mechanism of response generalization. In R.H. Horner, G. Dunlap, & R.L. Koegel (Eds.), *Generalization and maintenance: Lifestyle changes in applied settings* (pp. 194–219). Baltimore, MD: Paul H. Brookes Publishing Co.

Carr, E.G., & Durand, V.M. (1985). Reducing behavior problems through functional communication training. *Journal of Applied Behavior Analysis, 18*(2), 111–126.

Chambless, D.L., Sanderson, W.C., Shoham, V., Bennett Johnson, S., Pope, K.S., Crits-Christoph, P., ... McCurry, S. (1996). An update on empirically validated therapies. *The Clinical Psychologist, 49,* 5–18.

Cole, D.A., & Meyer, L.H. (1989). Impact of needs and resources on family plans to seek out-of-home placement. *American Journal on Mental Retardation, 93,* 380–387.

Davis, D.H., Fredrick, L.D., Alberto, P.A., & Gama, R. (2012). Functional communication training without extinction using concurrent schedules of differing magnitudes of reinforcement in classrooms. *Journal of Positive Behavior Interventions, 14*(3), 162–172. doi:10.1177/1098300711429597

Dunlap, G., Ester, T., Langhans, S., & Fox, L. (2006). Functional communication training with toddlers in home environments. *Journal of Early Intervention, 28*(2), 81–96.

Durand, V.M. (1987). "Look homeward angel": A call to return to our (functional) roots. *The Behavior Analyst, 10,* 299–302.

Durand, V.M. (1990). *Severe behavior problems: A functional communication training approach.* New York, NY: Guilford Press.

Durand, V.M. (1997). Functional analysis: Should we? *Journal of Special Education, 31,* 105–106.

Durand, V.M. (1999). Functional communication training using assistive devices: Recruiting natural communities of reinforcement. *Journal of Applied Behavior Analysis, 32*(3), 247–267.

Durand, V.M. (2011). *Optimistic parenting: Hope and help for you and your challenging child.* Baltimore, MD: Paul H. Brookes Publishing Co.

Durand, V.M. (2012). Functional communication training to reduce challenging behavior. In P. Prelock & R. McCauley (Eds.), *Treatment of autism spectrum disorders: Evidence-based intervention strategies for communication & social interaction* (pp. 107–138). Baltimore, MD: Paul H. Brookes Publishing Co.

Durand, V.M., & Carr, E.G. (1992). An analysis of maintenance following functional communication training. *Journal of Applied Behavior Analysis, 25*(4), 777–794.

Durand, V.M., & Crimmins, D.B. (1988). Identifying the variables maintaining self-injurious behavior. *Journal of Autism and Developmental Disorders, 18,* 99–117.

Durand, V.M., Hieneman, M., Clarke, S., Wang, M., & Rinaldi, M. (2013). Positive family intervention for severe challenging behavior I: A multi-site randomized clinical trial. *Journal of Positive Behavior Interventions, 15*(3), 133–143.

Einfeld, S.E., & Tonge, B.J. (1996). Population prevalence of psychopathology in children and adolescents with mental retardation: II Epidemiological findings. *Journal of Intellectual Disability Research, 40,* 99–109.

Einfeld, S.E., Tonge, B.J., & Rees, V.W. (2001). Longitudinal course of behavioral and emotional problems in Williams syndrome. *American Journal on Mental Retardation, 106,* 73–81.

Emerson, E., Kiernan, C., Alborz, A., Reeves, D., Mason, H., Swarbrick, R., . . . Hatton, C. (2001). Predicting the persistence of severe self-injurious behavior. *Research in Developmental Disabilities, 22,* 67–75.

Eyman, R.K., & Call, T. (1977). Maladaptive behavior and community placement of mentally retarded persons. *American Journal of Mental Deficiency, 82,* 137–144.

Falcomata, T.S., Roane, H.S., Muething, C.S., Stephenson, K.M., & Ing, A.D. (2012). Functional communication training and chained schedules of reinforcement to treat challenging behavior maintained by terminations of activity interruptions. *Behavior Modification, 36*(5), 630–649. doi:10.1177/0145445511433821

Feldman, M., McDonald, L., Serbin, L., Stack, D., Secco, M.L., & Yu, C.T. (2007). Predictors of depressive symptoms in primary caregivers of young children with or at risk for developmental delay. *Journal of Intellectual Disability Research, 51*(8), 606–619. doi:10.1111/j.1365-2788.2006.00941.x

Fisher, W.W., Thompson, R.H., Hagopian, L.P., Bowman, L.G., & Krug, A. (2000). Facilitating tolerance of delayed reinforcement during functional communication training. *Behavior Modification, 24*(1), 3–29.

Flood, W.A., & Wilder, D.A. (2002). Antecedent assessment and assessment-based treatment of off-task behavior in a child diagnosed with attention deficit-hyperactivity disorder (ADHD). *Education and Treatment of Children, 25*(3), 331–338.

Floyd, F.J., & Gallagher, E.M. (1997). Parental stress, care demands and use of support services for school age children with disabilities and behavior problems. *Family Relations, 46*(4), 359–371.

Fyffe, C.E., Kahng, S., Fittro, E., & Russell, D. (2004). Functional analysis and treatment of inappropriate sexual behavior. *Journal of Applied Behavior Analysis, 37*(3), 401–404.

Gardner, R.M., Bird, F.L., Maguire, H., Carreiro, R., & Abenaim, N. (2003). Intensive positive behavior supports for adolescents with acquired brain injury—Long-term outcomes in community settings. *Journal of Head Trauma Rehabilitation, 18*(1), 52–74.

Green, V.A., O'Reilly, M., Itchon, J., & Sigafoos, J. (2005). Persistence of early emerging aberrant behavior in children with developmental disabilities. *Research in Developmental Disabilities, 26*(1), 47–55.

Hagopian, L.P., Fisher, W.W., Sullivan, M.T., Acquisto, J., & LeBlanc, L.A. (1998). Effectiveness of functional communication training with and without extinction and punishment: A summary of 21 inpatient cases. *Journal of Applied Behavior Analysis, 31*(2), 211–235.

Hagopian, L.P., Kuhn, S.A.C., Long, E.S., & Rush, K.S. (2005). Schedule thinning following communication training using competing stimuli to enhance tolerance to decrements in reinforcer density. *Journal of Applied Behavior Analysis, 38*(2), 177–193.

Hagopian, L.P., Toole, L.M., Long, E.S., Bowman, L.G., & Lieving, G.A. (2004). A comparison of dense-to-lean and fixed lean schedules of alternative reinforcement and extinction. *Journal of Applied Behavior Analysis, 37*(3), 323–338.

Hanley, G.P., Iwata, B.A., & McCord, B.E. (2003). Functional analysis of problem behavior: A review. *Journal of Applied Behavior Analysis, 36,* 147–185.

Hanley, G.P., Iwata, B.A., & Thompson, R.H. (2001). Reinforcement schedule thinning following treatment with functional communication training. *Journal of Applied Behavior Analysis, 34*(1), 17–38.

Hastings, R.P. (2002). Parental stress and behavior problems of children with developmental disability. *Journal of Intellectual and Developmental Disability, 27*(3), 149–160.

Hayes, R.P. (1987). Training for work. In D.C. Cohen & A.M. Donellan (Eds.), *Handbook of autism and pervasive developmental disorders* (pp. 360–370). New York, NY: John Wiley & Sons.

Horner, R.H., & Day, H.M. (1991). The effects of response efficiency on functionally equivalent competing behavior. *Journal of Applied Behavior Analysis, 24*(4), 719–732. doi:10.1901/jaba.1991.24-719

Iwata, B.A., Dorsey, M.F., Slifer, K.J., Bauman, K.E., & Richman, G.S. (1994). Toward a functional analysis of self-injury. *Journal of Applied Behavior Analysis, 27*(2), 197.

Jacobson, J.W. (1982). Problem behavior and psychiatric impairment within a developmentally disabled population I: Behavior frequency. *Applied Research in Mental Retardation, 3,* 121–139.

Jones, R.S.P. (1999). A 10 year follow-up of stereotypic behavior with eight participants. *Behavioral Intervention, 14,* 45–54.

Joosten, A.V., Bundy, A.C., & Einfeld, S.L. (2012). Context influences the motivation for stereotypic and repetitive behaviour in children diagnosed with intellectual disability with and without autism. *Journal of Applied Research in Intellectual Disabilities, 25*(3), 262–271.

Kelley, M.E., Lerman, D.C., & Van Camp, C.M. (2002). The effects of competing reinforcement schedules on the acquisition of functional communication. *Journal of Applied Behavior Analysis, 35*(1), 59–63.

Kemp, D.C., & Carr, E.G. (1995). Reduction of severe problem behavior in community employment using an hypothesis-driven multicomponent intervention approach. *Journal of The Association for Persons with Severe Handicaps, 20*, 229–247.

Koegel, R.L., & Covert, A. (1972). The relationship of self-stimulation to learning in autistic children. *Journal of Applied Behavior Analysis, 5*, 381–387.

Kurtz, P.F., Boelter, E.W., Jarmolowicz, D.P., Chin, M.D., & Hagopian, L.P. (2011). An analysis of functional communication training as an empirically supported treatment for problem behavior displayed by individuals with intellectual disabilities. *Research in Developmental Disabilities, 32*(6), 2935–2942. doi:10.1016/j.ridd.2011.05.009

Kurtz, P.F., Chin, M.D., Huete, J.M., Tarbox, R.S., O'Connor, J.T., Paclawskyj, T.R., & Rush, K.S. (2003). Functional analysis and treatment of self-injurious behavior in young children a summary of 30 cases. *Journal of Applied Behavior Analysis, 36*(2), 205–219. doi:10.1901/jaba.2003.36-205

Lambert, J.M., Bloom, S.E., & Irvin, J. (2012). Trial-based functional analysis and functional communication training in an early childhood setting. *Journal of Applied Behavior Analysis, 45*(3), 579–584. doi:10.1901/jaba.2012.45-579

Lang, R., Rispoli, M., Machalicek, W., White, P.J., Kang, S., Pierce, N., . . . Lancioni, G. (2009). Treatment of elopement in individuals with developmental disabilities: A systematic review. *Research in Developmental Disabilities, 30*(4), 670–681.

Lowe, K., Allen, D., Jones, E., Brophy, S., Moore, K., & James, W. (2007). Challenging behaviours: prevalence and topographies. *Journal of Intellectual Disability Research, 51*(8), 625–636. doi:10.1111/j.1365-2788.2006.00948.x

Mancil, G.R. (2006). Functional communication training: A review of the literature related to children with autism. *Education and Training in Developmental Disabilities, 41*(3), 213–224.

Matson, J.L., Dixon, D.R., & Matson, M.L. (2005). Assessing and treating aggression in children and adolescents with developmental disabilities: A 20-year overview. *Educational Psychology, 25*(2), 151–181.

O'Neill, R.E., Horner, R.H., Albin, R.W., Sprague, J.R., Storey, K., & Newton, J.S. (1997). *Functional assessment and program development for problem behavior: A practical handbook*. Pacific Grove, CA: Brooks/Cole Publishing.

Paclawskyj, T.R., Matson, J.L., Rush, K.S., Smalls, Y., & Vollmer, T.R. (2008). Assessment of the convergent validity of the Questions About Behavioral Function Scale with analogue functional analysis and the Motivation Assessment Scale. *Journal of Intellectual Disability Research, 45*(6), 484–494.

Petscher, E.S., Rey, C., & Bailey, J.S. (2009). A review of empirical support for differential reinforcement of alternative behavior. *Research in Developmental Disabilities, 30*(3), 409–425.

Saloviita, T., Italinna, M., & Leinonen, E. (2003). Explaining the parental stress of fathers and mothers caring for a child with intellectual disability: A double ABCX model. *Journal of Intellectual Disability Research, 47*(4/5), 300–303, 312.

Shirley, M.J., Iwata, B.A., Kahng, S.W., Mazaleski, J.L., & Lerman, D.C. (1997). Does functional communication training compete with ongoing contingencies of reinforcement? An analysis during response acquisition

and maintenance. *Journal of Applied Behavior Analysis, 30*(1), 93–104.

Shoham-Vardi, I., Davidson, P.W., Cain, N.N., Sloane-Reeves, J.E., Giesow, V.E., Quijano, L.E., & Houser, K.D. (1996). Factors predicting re-referral following crisis intervention for community-based persons with developmental disabilities and behavioral and psychiatric disorders. *American Journal on Mental Retardation, 101*, 109–117.

Sigafoos, J., & Saggers, E. (1995). A discrete-trial approach to the functional analysis of aggressive behaviour in two boys with autism. *Journal of Intellectual and Developmental Disability, 20*(4), 287–297.

Smith, T., Scahill, L., Dawson, G., Guthrie, D., Lord, C., Odom, S., . . . Wagner, A. (2007). Designing research studies on psychosocial interventions in autism. *Journal of Autism and Developmental Disorders, 37*(2), 354–366.

Snell, M.E., Chen, L.Y., & Hoover, K. (2006). Teaching augmentative and alternative communication to students with severe disabilities: A review of intervention research 1997–2003. *Research and Practice for Persons with Severe Disabilities, 31*(3), 203–214.

Steed, E.A., & Durand, V.M. (2013). Optimistic teaching: Improving the capacity for teachers to reduce young children's challenging behavior. *School Mental Health, 5*(1), 15–24. doi:10.1007/s12310-012-9084-y

Stokes, T.F., Fowler, S.A., & Baer, D.M. (1978). Training preschool children to recruit natural communities of reinforcement. *Journal of Applied Behavior Analysis, 11*, 285–303.

Task Force Promoting Dissemination of Psychological Procedures. (1995). Training in and dissemination of empirically-validated psychological treatments: Report and recommendations. *Clinical Psychology: Science and Practice, 48*, 3–23.

Tiger, J.H., Hanley, G.P., & Bruzek, J. (2008). Functional communication training: A review and practical guide. *Behavior Analysis in Practice, 1*(1), 16–23.

Totsika, V., Toogood, S., Hastings, R.P., & Lewis, S. (2008). Persistence of challenging behaviours in adults with intellectual disability over a period of 11 years. *Journal of Intellectual Disability Research, 52*(5), 446–457.

Wacker, D.P., Berg, W.K., Harding, J.W., Derby, K.M., Asmus, J.M., & Healy, A. (1998). Evaluation and long-term treatment of aberrant behavior displayed by young children with disabilities. *Journal of Developmental and Behavioral Pediatrics, 19*(4), 260–266.

Wacker, D.P., Steege, M.W., Northup, J., Sasso, G., Berg, W., Reimers, T., . . . Donn, L. (1990). A component analysis of functional communication training across three topographies of severe behavior problems. *Journal of Applied Behavior Analysis, 23*(4), 417–429. doi:10.1901/jaba.1990.23-417

Wieseler, N.A., Hanson, R.H., Chamberlain, T.P., & Thompson, T. (1985). Functional taxonomy of stereotypic and self-injurious behavior. *Mental Retardation, 23*(5), 230–234.

Worsdell, A.S., Iwata, B.A., Hanley, G.P., Thompson, R.H., & Kahng, S.W. (2000). Effects of continuous and intermittent reinforcement for problem behavior during functional communication training. *Journal of Applied Behavior Analysis, 33*(2), 167–179.

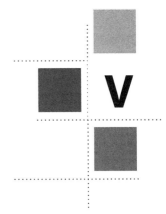

Comprehensive Multielement Positive Behavior Support Plans

STANDARDS ADDRESSED IN THIS SECTION

VI. A. Positive behavior support (PBS) practitioners apply the following considerations/foundations across all elements of a PBS plan:

1. Plans are developed in collaboration with the individual and his or her team.

2. Plans are driven by the results of person-centered and functional behavioral assessments.

3. Plans facilitate the individual's preferred lifestyle.

4. Plans are designed for contextual fit, specifically in relation to (a) values and goals of the team, (b) current and desired routines within the various settings in which the individual participates, (c) skills and buy-in of those who will be implementing the plan, and (d) administrative support.

VI. B. Behavior support plans (BSPs) include interventions to improve/support quality of life in the following areas:

1. Achieving the individual's dreams

2. The individual's health and physiological needs

3. Promoting all aspects of self-determination

4. Improvement in individual's active, successful participation in inclusive school, work, home, and community settings

(continued)

397

5. Promotion of social interactions, relationships, and enhanced social networks
6. Increased fun and success in the individual's life
7. Improved leisure, relaxation, and recreational activities for the individual throughout the day

VI. C. PBS practitioners develop behavior support plans that include antecedent interventions to prevent the need for challenging behavior using the following strategies:
1. Alter or eliminate setting events to preclude the need for challenging behavior.
2. Modify specific antecedent triggers/circumstances based on the functional behavior assessment (FBA).
3. Identify and address behaviors using precursors.
4. Make the individual's environment/routines predictable.
5. Build opportunities for choice/control throughout the day that are age appropriate and contextually appropriate.
6. Create clear expectations.
7. Modify curriculum/job demands so the individual can successfully complete tasks.

VI. D. PBS plans address effective instructional intervention strategies that may include the following:
1. Match instructional strategies to the individual's learning style.
2. Provide instruction in the context in which the challenging behaviors occur and in the use of alternative skills, including communication skills, social skills, self-management/monitoring skills, and other adaptive behaviors as indicated by the FBA and continued evaluation of progress data.
3. Teach replacement behavior(s) based on competing behavior analysis.
4. Select and teach replacement behaviors that can be as or more effective than the challenging behavior.
5. Utilize instructional methods of addressing a challenging behavior proactively.

VI. E. PBS practitioners employ consequence intervention strategies that consider the following:
1. Reinforcement strategies are function based and rely on naturally occurring reinforcers as much as possible.
2. Intervention strategies use the least intrusive behavior reduction strategy.
3. Emergency intervention strategies are used only where safety of the individual or others must be assured.
4. Intervention strategies consider plans for avoiding power struggles and provocation.
5. Intervention strategies consider plans for potential natural consequences. Consider when these should happen and when there should be attempts to avoid them.

VI. F. PBS practitioners develop plans for successful implementation of PBS plans that include the following:
1. Action plans for implementation of all components of the intervention
2. Strategies to address systems change need for implementation of PBS plans

VI. G. PBS practitioners evaluate plan implementation and use data to make needed modifications:
1. Implement plan and evaluate and monitor progress according to time lines.
2. Collect data identified for each component of the PBS plan.
3. Analyze data regularly to determine needed adjustments.
4. Evaluate progress on person-centered plans.
5. Modify each element of the PBS plan as indicated by evaluation data.

The five chapters that make up this section focus specifically on the development and implementation of positive behavior support (PBS) plans. The section begins with Chapter 22, "Building Supportive Environments," and Chapter 23, "Implementing Multi-element Positive Behavior Support Plans." These chapters describe the importance of systems, environments, and contexts when considering the design of supports that are sustainable for an individual who is exhibiting challenging behaviors and the many variables that facilitate or impede implementation of quality behavior support plans. The next three chapters in this section—Chapter 24, "Cultural and Contextual Fit," Chapter 25, "Developing a Multielement Behavior Support Plan for a Middle School Student from a Diverse Background with Significant Behavioral Challenges," and Chapter 26, "Application of a Multielement Positive Behavior Interventions and Supports Plan for Alie , an Elementary Student with Intellectual Disabilities"—present specific plans that were developed for three individuals: a young child with autism, a middle school child with emotional disabilities, and an elementary grade student with intellectual disability. There is great diversity across the individuals described in these chapters—in terms of age, type of abilities and disabilities, and cultural backgrounds. This diversity will demonstrate to the reader the breadth of application of the field of PBS.

Behavior support plans (BSPs) are the culmination of a great deal of well-planned, systematic, and collaborative work, including data collection, functional assessment, environmental analysis, records reviews, and team collaboration—to name just a few. There are a variety of formats that have been suggested for formatting a BSP (e.g., Bambara, 2005; Crimmins, Farrell, Smith, & Bailey, 2007; Horner, Albin, Todd, Newton, & Sprague, 2011), and these vary from school to school, agency to agency, and state to state. However, as with behavior, the form is less important than the function. Important components that are found across most formats include the following:

Name	The target individual's name
Date	Date the behavioral support plan was developed
Behavior definition	An observable and measureable description of the target behavior(s)
Measurement	How the target behavior will be measured (e.g., rate, frequency, duration)
Evaluation	A description of how often the team will review progress and who will be responsible for gathering data
Setting event strategies	What strategies will be implemented to prevent the occurrence of setting events that trigger the behavior (e.g., bus monitor to prevent bullying on the bus on the way to school)
Antecedent strategies	What strategies will be implemented to prevent the occurrence of antecedent events that trigger the behavior and set the occasion for the new response (e.g., visual schedule to make classroom routines more predictable)
Consequence strategies	What strategies will be used to reinforce desired behavior and what strategies will be used when a challenging behavior occurs
Alternative skill instruction	What skill(s) will be taught that provide a positive and functional alternative to the challenging behaviors
Response to challenging behavior	What the response will be when a challenging behavior occurs (e.g., ignore, prompt a communicative alternative)

As you proceed through this section of the book, it is critical to keep in mind the ultimate goal of PBS plans are to improve the quality of the lives of individuals with challenging behaviors and their families. And the foundations and the strategies that are presented here are based on person-centered and respectful visions of a good life.

Fredda Brown

REFERENCES

Bambara, L.M. (2005). Overview of the behavior support process. In L.M. Bambara & L. Kern (Eds.), *Individualized supports for students with problem behaviors: Designing positive behavior plans* (pp. 47–70). New York, NY: Guildford.

Crimmins, D., Farrell, A.F., Smith, P.W., & Bailey, A. (2007). *Positive strategies for students with behavior problems.* Baltimore, MD: Brookes.

Horner, R.H., Albin, R.W., Todd, A.W., Newton, J.S., & Sprague, J.R. (2011). In M.E. Snell & F. Brown (Eds.), *Instruction of students with severe disabilities* (pp. 257–303). Upper Saddle River, NJ: Pearson Education.

Building Supportive Environments

Toward a Technology for Enhancing Fidelity of Implementation

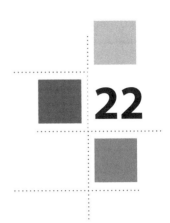

Kent McIntosh, Joseph M. Lucyshyn,
M. Kathleen Strickland-Cohen, and Robert H. Horner

Effective behavior support is achieved through designing supportive environments. When designing behavior support plans (BSPs) for individuals, it is common to examine the proximal (i.e., immediate) environment and how it relates to an individual's problem or adaptive behavior. For example, implementers may identify environmental events and environmental contingencies that evoke or maintain problem or adaptive behavior. Elements of the environment, such as the level of brightness in the room or how a task request is delivered, may be modified to prevent problem behavior from occurring. Likewise, social attention may be withheld for misbehavior and provided contingent on adaptive behavior to help increase the likelihood of adaptive behavior and decrease misbehavior. Such aspects of environmental redesign may be considered manipulation of the proximal environment, because these events serve as immediate triggers or reinforcers for the target behaviors of individuals. As such, effective behavior support involves changes in adult or caregiver behavior (i.e., implementing strategies) to adjust the immediate environment surrounding the individual.

However, it is also common to overlook the distal, or contextual, environment when designing support for individuals. This lack of attention to the broader context (e.g., behavior of peers, school resources, capacity of family members to use recommended strategies) may lead to insufficient behavior change and the ultimate failure of BSPs

The research reported here was supported by the Institute of Education Sciences, U.S. Department of Education, through Grant R324A120278 to the University of Oregon. The opinions expressed are those of the authors and do not represent views of the Institute or the U.S. Department of Education.

(Benazzi, Horner, & Good, 2006). In light of this common error, there has been a contemporary focus on examining the broader context and systems that may support the implementation of effective practices within that broader context (Biglan, 1995; Fixsen, Naoom, Blase, Friedman, & Wallace, 2005; Walker et al., 1996). This chapter focuses on the importance of *context* in individual behavior support and steps to create contexts that support the implementation of effective individual behavior support practices, interventions, and strategies.

SCHOOLS AND COMMUNITIES AS HOST ENVIRONMENTS

Kame'enui, Simmons, and Coyne (2000) used the term *host environments* to describe the broader context of intervention implementation and focus attention on how contextual variables influence implementation. This thinking represents a continuing evolution of service delivery, from earlier notions viewing schools and communities as settings where interventions are delivered, to later notions viewing schools and communities as optimal places to identify individuals needing intervention and contexts that can be manipulated to enhance implementation and delivery of interventions. This shift represents an important frame of reference for interventionists because it exponentially expands the number of malleable variables that can be addressed to enable behavior change for populations of individuals.

From an individual behavior support perspective, the broader environment consists of risk and protective factors that influence individual behavior. Host environments can be viewed as constellations of antecedents and consequences that may either encourage and maintain or discourage the behavior of individuals in these environments. These environmental features may act as setting events in school, home, and the community (Mayer, 1995). Host environments may inadvertently be arranged to support maladaptive behavior for individuals. For example,

the fear of retribution may prevent well-intentioned students from intervening when they observe bullying—in essence creating a school culture in which bullying behavior is tolerated or even reinforced (Whitted & Dupper, 2005). In another example, schools may implement harsh, exclusionary discipline policies intended to curb antisocial behavior, but in reality, the problem behavior may be reinforced by removal from aversive academic tasks or social interactions. Suspensions, often perceived as a powerful deterrent by school personnel, may be perceived by some students as school-sanctioned vacation days (Maag, 2001; Mayer, 1995). This difference in perspectives is troubling, given the research showing detrimental outcomes of suspensions (Hemphill, Toumbourou, Herrenkohl, McMorris, & Catalano, 2006; Skiba & Peterson, 2000).

Likewise, host environments may inadvertently be arranged to support maladaptive behavior of implementers as well. As with students, issuing suspensions in schools may be reinforcing for school personnel because of the momentary relief from aversive student behavior, thereby increasing their likely use in the future (Sugai & Horner, 2002). More generally, the perceived reinforcer for a classroom teacher or interventionist to implement a BSP may be improved student behavior, but implementation may also result in additional work and assignment of more students with challenging behavior to his or her caseload. On the other hand, the contingencies for failing to implement a plan could include additional support, removal of that student from the classroom or caseload, and a special education designation or psychiatric diagnosis, which may provide relief from work and reduce feelings of incompetence. As such, environments may be naturally arranged to discourage effective behavior support without any intent of harm from implementers or their supervisors.

Over time, these interaction patterns can become coercive cycles (Patterson, 1982), wherein problem behavior for the individual is reinforced by the withdrawal of requests from the implementer and withdrawal of requests is reinforced by the cessation of problem behavior from the individual. These patterns of negative reinforcement for the problem behavior of both individuals and implementers can easily become persistent and difficult to remediate because the interactions are effective in removing aversive stimuli and family or classroom harmony can be maintained by avoiding aversive demands (Lucyshyn et al., 2004; McIntosh, Horner, Chard, Dickey, & Braun, 2008). As a result, the home or classroom setting becomes a host environment for maladaptive behavior support strategies.

BUILDING HOST ENVIRONMENTS THAT SUPPORT IMPLEMENTATION OF EFFECTIVE PRACTICES

Fortunately, the same host environments that are arranged to support maladaptive behavior can be redesigned to support adaptive individual and service provider behavior. The context can be changed to support both 1) an entire population of individuals and 2) implementers of BSPs. The next sections describe how host environments can support more effective individual plans through establishing setting events that increase the likelihood of adaptive behavior, enhancing implementer capacity to implement practices, and creating systems to support implementers in their work with individuals.

Establishing Setting Events for Adaptive Behavior

A key component of effective environmental change is to implement conditions to evoke adaptive behavior for whole populations of students or communities (Biglan, 1995; Wandersman & Florin, 2003). The goal is to develop a positive social culture with prosocial norms that signal that adaptive behavior will be reinforced and maladaptive behavior will not. Essentially, the task is to create aspects of the environment that serve as salient setting events for adaptive behavior.

One example of a school approach to shaping the social culture of the student body as a whole is schoolwide positive behavior intervention and support (SWPBIS; Sugai & Horner, 2009). SWPBIS is a systems-level framework for implementing evidence-based practices in schools that focuses on 1) redesigning the physical environment; 2) defining, teaching, and acknowledging prosocial behavior for all students in all settings; 3) using data to measure implementation, outcomes, and the need for additional individual student support; and 4) providing a continuum of interventions for groups and individual students who require more support. The SWPBIS approach, which emphasizes explicit skills instruction to prevent and address maladaptive behavior, has been shown in over 20 studies to effectively produce important outcomes, including reducing levels of problem behavior, reducing the use of exclusionary discipline procedures (e.g., suspensions), reducing bullying behavior, increasing social competence and emotion regulation, increasing academic achievement, and increasing perceived school safety (Bradshaw, Waasdorp, & Leaf, forthcoming; Horner et al., 2009; Luiselli, Putnam, Handler, & Feinberg, 2005; McIntosh, Bennett, & Price, 2011; Nelson, Martella, & Marchand-Martella, 2002; Waasdorp, Bradshaw, & Leaf, 2012).

Although it may seem counterintuitive to focus on all students when attempting to address the behavior of a smaller proportion of students with significant behavior needs, there are a number of compelling reasons for establishing a positive schoolwide culture as a foundation for effective individual student support. First, when the student body as a whole is taught prosocial behavior and acknowledged for using it, the increased rates of prosocial behavior can create norms for behavior that endure. Adaptive behavior becomes the expectation not only from adults but also from peers. Disrespectful behavior is then seen as violating not only school rules but also the social code. New students entering the school then join an environment with setting events for prosocial behavior and peers who model adaptive behavior. Having upper-grade students with high social status teach the expectation can further signal that all students, including those with disabilities, should expect prosocial behavior from one another. This aspect becomes more important as students progress through school, when peers, rather than adults, increasingly gain influence over individual behavior (Dishion & Dodge, 2006). A key challenge in schools is preventing and addressing bullying behavior, because it is more likely to occur in a context without adult supervision and may be reinforced by peer attention (Doll, Song, Champion, & Jones, 2011). Moreover, students with disabilities are more likely to be targets of bullying as well as bully others (Cummings, Pepler, Mishna, & Craig, 2006). With attention to building a positive social culture, school personnel can implement interventions to increase the likelihood that bystanders will intervene to stop bullying behavior (Ross & Horner, 2009). Another beneficial aspect of building a positive culture is that the reduction in problem behavior and improved perceptions of school safety often seen when implementing SWPBIS may reduce fear and anxiety for those affected by threats to personal safety, further supporting students' behavior support needs (McIntosh, Ty, & Miller, forthcoming). Finally, attention to preventive interventions provided to all students can reduce the number of students who require additional support, because a high quality schoolwide intervention can support more students to be successful, which both reduces the number of students who need support and frees resources for the students who truly require individualized behavior support (McIntosh, Chard, Boland, & Horner, 2006).

A number of studies have shown that the schoolwide interventions associated with SWPBIS can be effective for supporting students with significant needs as well. Tobin and colleagues (2012) showed that the effects of SWPBIS on reducing problem

behavior are seen for students both with and without individualized education programs (IEPs). In addition, schools implementing SWPBIS have reduced rates of out-of-school placements for students with severe behavior needs, as well as improved retention of these students when they return to their local schools (Lewis, 2007). Bradshaw, Waasdorp, and Leaf (2013) reported results from a randomized control trial where at-risk students were statistically significantly less likely to receive office discipline referrals and less likely to be referred for special education in schools implementing SWPBIS, compared with control schools.

Creating Systems to Support Implementers

The potential benefits of designing effective host environments extend not only to individuals but also to implementers. One of the most important consequences of attending to host environments has been the focus on building systems that help implementers design and implement effective support plans. Fidelity of implementation (the extent to which implementers use support plans as intended; Gresham, 1989) plays a singularly important role in behavior support. Because this predicts the extent to which interventions are successful (Domitrovich et al., 2008), implementers should set goals regarding the assessment and improvement of fidelity of implementation. As such, it is important to identify how the environment can be altered to improve fidelity. This process is labeled an implementation system, as opposed to an intervention system (Fixsen et al., 2005).

Sugai and colleagues (2010) describe four components of systems for effective implementation of schoolwide behavior support: behavioral expertise, training, coaching, and evaluation. *Behavioral expertise* refers to the capacity to select effective interventions based on scientific evidence and principles of behavior. *Training* involves the systems used to provide new staff with needed skills or existing staff with new skills, whether they are assessment (e.g., functional behavioral assessment [FBA]), intervention (e.g., skills instruction, assistive technologies), or coordination of services (e.g., wraparound and person-centered planning). Training systems consist of a cadre of trainers, a sequenced training curriculum, and assessment procedures to ensure that the recipients can use the required skills. *Coaching* involves a system of ongoing technical assistance to implementers (e.g., assistance in the FBA process, support plan implementation, knowledge of community supports). To be most effective, coaches need to have both implementation and consultation skills, as well as dedicated time to act as coaches. *Evaluation* systems include collection, reporting, and use of data for decision making. Comprehensive evaluation includes assessment of both fidelity of implementation (e.g., percentage of support plan steps implemented) and individual outcomes (e.g., progress toward IEP goals). In addition, effective evaluation systems include regular structures for meeting, making decisions with data, and following up on action plans (Todd et al., 2011). These

systems and their critical features are similar across school and community agencies.

Strategies to Support Implementers

Within these systems, specific strategies can be used to support school personnel and other implementers in implementing support plans. Like plans with students, these strategies, which focus on supporting the plan implementers, can be arranged according to a three-term contingency—that is, antecedent, behavior, and consequence strategies can be arranged for implementers with the goal of increasing fidelity of implementation of individual interventions. A visual depiction of sample strategies is included in Figure 22.1.

Antecedent Strategies Antecedent strategies to support implementer fidelity focus on arranging the implementer's environment to prompt implementation of specific interventions. Examples include making environmental changes (e.g., making intervention materials readily available), providing specific checklists for implementation steps, or providing verbal or visual prompts

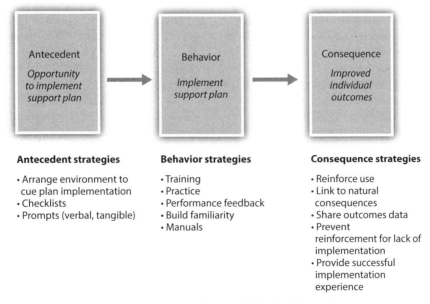

Figure 22.1. Contextual strategies to enhance implementer fidelity of implementation.

to use implementation steps. An example in SWPBIS is a tangible ticket system used to acknowledge prosocial behavior. The tickets themselves have little reinforcing value, as the key mechanism is the developmentally appropriate acknowledgment of students for their success (Biglan, Flay, Embry, & Sandler, 2012). In addition to providing teachers with a way to acknowledge appropriate student behavior, ticket systems also serve as a prompt to school personnel to increase their rates of reinforcement for common expectations being demonstrated in targeted areas. Having tangible discriminative stimuli to prompt acknowledgment of student behavior is therefore an antecedent strategy in the host environment to enhance the fidelity of the intervention (positive reinforcement) for the implementer.

Behavior Teaching Strategies Behavior strategies for supporting implementers involve teaching them needed skills and practices to be successful in implementation (e.g., conducting accurate FBAs, implementing video modeling effectively). As in individual behavior support, effective teaching involves explicit instruction and practice, accompanied by performance feedback. Effective teaching results in implementer fluency with the required skills so they can implement and adapt them across the range of individual needs (e.g., varying levels of communication). Instructional examples and practice can be tailored to the implementer's client population; more examples may be needed for successful response generalization. Familiarity with the intervention will likely decrease the effort required to implement it, increasing its desirability. In addition to instruction, implementation manuals (e.g., Dunlap et al., 2009; Loman & Borgmeier, 2010) may be provided as resources for self-instruction in implementation skills. For example, checklists of critical features for using picture schedules can help implementers use them optimally.

Consequence Strategies Effective host environments also include naturally occurring consequences that maintain the implementing behavior of implementers, and environments can be modified to produce or highlight existing consequences of implementation. One key step is to identify any natural contingencies that may maintain or discourage implementation of the intervention plan. Obvious reinforcers could include observing improved individual performance or lifestyle outcomes and reductions in aversive individual problem behavior. For example, coaches and supervisors can share student outcomes data, overlaid with fidelity of implementation data, to make these consequences more salient for implementers. In situations in which individual behavior change is small or implementation is too inconsistent to show positive results, shaping plans may be needed to reinforce efforts at implementation. For example, it can be useful for supervisors to provide developmentally appropriate praise for consistent implementation, paired with statements that persistence will result in the desired outcomes. In addition, it is helpful to identify and prevent any contingencies that reinforce failure to implement plans. For example, if implementers fail to execute plans effectively, they may receive relief from work responsibilities or be assigned fewer tasks. In these situations, it may be necessary to prevent escape for inaction on behavior plan implementation, while providing the support needed to help the implementer be successful.

It is an encouraging finding that obtaining experience implementing effective strategies can serve to reinforce effective intervention. Research indicates that experience implementing interventions can improve teacher self-efficacy and confidence in the ability to improve student outcomes, which increases the likelihood of sustained implementation, even after withdrawal of coaching (Baker, Gersten, Dimino, & Griffiths, 2004). Such findings have consistently been found in studies of SWPBIS (Kelm & McIntosh, 2012; Ross & Horner, 2006; Ross, Romer, & Horner, 2012). There is also some evidence that implementing particular intervention strategies (e.g., token economies) may increase implementers' use of other behavior support strategies as well (e.g., behavior-specific praise; Elswick & Casey, 2011), although findings in this area are mixed (Lannie & McCurdy, 2007). Finally, implementing effective systems-level interventions may also influence aspects of the workplace. A trial of SWPBIS found improvements not only in student behavior but also in organizational health, the perceived collective effectiveness of the implementers working together to achieve shared goals (Bradshaw, Koth, Bevans, Ialongo, & Leaf, 2008).

ELEMENTS OF HOST ENVIRONMENTS THAT ENHANCE SUSTAINABILITY OF INTERVENTIONS

A critical goal for any organization is to sustain implementation of effective interventions so that more individuals can have improved outcomes (Greenberg, 2004). However, such outcomes are rarely observed (Fixsen et al., 2005; Latham, 1988). An emerging focus of research is on the factors that enhance or inhibit sustainability of interventions (Gersten, Chard, & Baker, 2000), and although elements of the interventions themselves can certainly affect their sustainability, features of the host environment are more predictive of sustainability than intervention effectiveness (Cornell, 2006; McIntosh, MacKay, et al., 2011). As such, it is worthwhile to examine how host environments can be altered to maximize the durability of interventions across all levels of support.

Over the past 15 years, there have been a number of research studies using in-depth interviews or surveys regarding implementer perceptions of contextual factors that support implementation of evidence-based interventions. Regarding school systems, McIntosh and colleagues (2014) summarized studies examining the implementation and sustainability of SWPBIS. These factors included administrator and staff support, effective training systems, access to coaching, efficient teaming, and use of data for decision making. Large-scale quantitative studies have also provided evidence supporting these factors (Coffey & Horner, 2012; McIntosh et al., 2013). Similarly, in relation to individual (Tier 3) supports, Hieneman and Dunlap (2000, 2001) identified factors leading to the effective implementation of community based behavior support, including service provider buy-in, skills of the implementers, and the extent to which the system is responsive to individual needs. Similar to school systems, these factors could be enhanced by attending to characteristics of the host environment.

Based on a long line of experimental research in family systems, Lucyshyn and colleagues (Lucyshyn et al., 2007, 2009) identified a number of strategies for behavior intervention plans that have been shown to lead to a durable implementation of support in the home. This approach can be considered adapting each family environment to make it an effective host environment for positive behavior support. The strategies described include attending to the roles of function and coercive theory in reinforcing maladaptive parent-child interactions, building relationships with parents by establishing trust and involving them in collaborative plan development, building the capacity and willingness of parents to intervene effectively, developing plans (including relapse prevention plans) to build adherence, and planning support deliberately for long-term maintenance (i.e., across the life span). Their research shows that when plans attend to these features, support plans may sustain for years and even decades.

In addition to identifying factors related to sustainability, tools have developed to assess the capacity of environments to implement and sustain effective practices (Fixsen et al., 2005). The two guiding messages are that effective practices are more likely to sustain if 1) they are implemented at a high level of fidelity and, 2) once implemented, they incorporate a continuous regeneration cycle in which the practice is adapted to fit more closely with the changing demands of the context. For both of these messages to be realized, implementers need formal tools for assessing both the level of implementation and the capacity of the setting to support sustain implementation.

Within SWPBIS, there are research-validated external evaluation and school self-assessment tools for assessing implementation fidelity for each tier of support. At Tier 1, the schoolwide evaluation tool (external evaluation) and team implementation checklist, PBIS self-assessment survey, and schoolwide benchmarks of quality (self-assessments) are used to assess fidelity of implementation for universal systems. At Tiers 2 and 3, the individual student school evaluation tool (external evaluation) and benchmarks of advanced tiers and measure of advanced tiers tool (MATT; self-assessments) assess support systems for students requiring additional support. Newer measures, such as the tiered fidelity inventory, blend self-assessment and external evaluation through a process in which an external coach leads the team through evaluation. These measures, all available at www.pbis.org and www.pbisapps.org, assess both the quality of systems for support and the features of individual BSPs. A central feature of both the research and self-assessment tools has been the incorporation of an action planning component, in which school teams are able to use fidelity tool results to define the most useful, specific tasks or actions that they will complete in short time windows (e.g., 2 weeks) to improve implementation. Self-assessments are done frequently (e.g., every fourth meeting) if a school has not implemented to criterion and annually once a minimum criterion is met.

Tobin et al. (2012) emphasized that the durable implementation of SWPBIS at all three tiers of support often requires specific assistance from the host school district. Districts control the funding, policies, data systems, and often the professional development available to a school. The specific role and importance of districts for implementation and sustainability of evidence-based practices is still emerging. One important indicator of this new emphasis is the arrival of the District Capacity Assessment (DCA; Duda et al., 2012). The DCA is a self-assessment fidelity tool for examining if a school district has developed the capacity to complete core functions, such as 1) selecting effective practices; 2) recruiting and hiring skilled personnel; 3) providing essential training to key personnel; 4) coaching trained personnel to implement new practices in their local school; 5) providing feedback on staff performance; 6) collecting, summarizing, and using data for decision-making; and 7) organizing policies and ongoing information loops to assess fidelity, impact, and sustained effectiveness.

The collective messages from emerging tools is that schools improve when groups of people (e.g., faculty, staff, families, students) have common goals, regular opportunities to assess progress, and an active process for investing time/resources in advancing their common goal. Both the fidelity of initial implementation efforts and the sustained performance of those practices implemented to criterion will benefit from ongoing, efficient strategies for monitoring implementation quality.

In family settings, the development of host environments that enhance the sustainability of behavior interventions and supports implemented by family members requires interventionists to view the family as the unit of analysis and the family system as the context in which interventions are embedded and sustained. The family system is composed of 1) family characteristics; 2) parental, marital, sibling, and extended family subsystems; 3) family functions; and 4) family life cycle (Turnbull, Turnbull, Erwin, Soodak, & Shogren, 2011). Any one of these features of the family system can serve to either promote or hinder the implementation and sustainability of behavior interventions, so understanding the strengths and needs of a family from a family systems perspective can contribute to the design of BSPs that are acceptable, feasible, durable, and sustainable across the life cycle of the family. Thus it behooves family interventionists to assess the child and family from an ecological/family systems perspective and to ensure that 1) BSPs are designed to possess a good contextual fit with family life and 2) relevant family-centered supports are identified and put into place to fortify the family system and to increase the likelihood of treatment fidelity and sustainability. Family-centered supports may include, for example, respite care, sibling support, or marital therapy for the parents.

To this end, Lucyshyn and colleagues (Albin, Lucyshyn, Horner, & Flannery, 1996; Lucyshyn & Albin, 1993) developed a family ecology assessment that is based on family ecological theory (Gallimore, 2005; Gallimore, Goldenberg, & Weisner, 1993) and informed by strengths-based assessment and family-centered practices (Dunst, Trivette, & Deal, 1988; Singer & Irvin, 1991; Turnbull & Turnbull, 1991). The family ecology interview is a collaborative, strengths-based assessment of features of family ecology that are relevant to the design of a contextually appropriate BSP. The assessment has two parts: 1) a focused assessment of family activity settings or routines in the home and community with family members and 2) a broader assessment of family ecology, including child and family strengths, formal (e.g., center-based respite care) and informal resources (e.g., respite care by grandparents) used by or available to the family, sources of social support, sources of stress, and family goals for the child and for the family as a whole. The purpose of the assessment is to 1) identify family goals for the child and family as a whole, 2) select and prioritize problematic family routines for intervention and support, 3) generate a family vision of realistic but successful routines, 4) gather information relevant to the design a contextually appropriate BSP, and 5) identify family-centered adjunctive supports that may be necessary to ensure that the plan is feasible and sustainable within the family system. Another purpose of the assessment, available to interventionists who

conduct the interview in a collaborative and collegial manner, is to initiate a therapeutic dialogue with the family that revives hope that may have faded, gains the family's trust, and builds a therapeutic alliance focused on promoting constructive changes in parent and child behavior and in family environments. The family ecology assessment conducted in conjunction with a functional assessment of the child's behavior results in BSPs that promote meaningful and durable improvements in child behavior and family life (Binnendyk & Lucyshyn, 2009; Lucyshyn et al., 2007; Lucyshyn, Albin, & Nixon, 1997; Lucyshyn et al., 2014).

Jacob

Jacob was a fourth grader diagnosed with Asperger syndrome. Jacob's primary instruction occurred in a general education classroom with 22 students and one teacher. Jacob has independently followed a daily visual schedule for the past 2 years. His reading skills were above average, and he spent a considerable amount of time at home on the computer reading about mystical themes (e.g., unicorns, dragons), which were his primary interests. Jacob's 504 plan (accommodation plan) primarily focused on increasing appropriate peer interactions, and he received social skills training with the school psychologist twice per week to improve the quality of his social interactions and his self-advocacy skills. Until midyear, Jacob's academic performance had been only slightly below that of his peers; however, following winter break, Jacob became increasingly off task, particularly during math and writing. When asked to complete his work, Jacob had begun verbally refusing and arguing with his teacher, Mrs. Trocki. As a result, he lost his recess time several times per week for 3 consecutive weeks. With this consequence in place, Jacob's problem behavior appeared to increase rather than decrease. Mrs. Trocki and the school psychologist agreed that an FBA was needed and contacted the district behavior specialist.

The behavior specialist, Ms. Sparks, conducted an FBA interview with Mrs. Trocki and observed Jacob twice during reading and writing classes. Based on the information gathered in the interview and through direct observation, Ms. Sparks concluded that Jacob's problem behavior was maintained by escape from academic tasks that he found difficult and developed a BSP to directly address the function of the problem behavior (i.e., escape from difficult tasks). Ms. Sparks then provided Mrs. Trocki with a list of behavior change strategies to address Jacob's problem behavior, which included 1) teaching Jacob to raise his hand and request help from the teacher or a break from work when he becomes frustrated, 2) reminding him to use these skills at the beginning of independent work time, 3) providing 20 minutes of additional 1:1 instruction in writing and math daily, and 4) checking Jacob's work every 5 minutes and reminding him that for every 20 minutes that he stays on task, he will be allowed to take a 5-minute break from the classroom to go to the sensory-motor lab, a preferred environment.

Two weeks later, Ms. Sparks received a message from Jacob's principal stating that Jacob's problem behavior was escalating. In addition to verbally refusing to work, he had started crying, tearing up his worksheets, and pushing materials off his desk. As a result, his teacher was requesting that a change of placement be considered. When Ms. Sparks contacted Jacob's teacher to discuss why the BSP strategies were not effective, Mrs. Trocki said that she was having considerable difficulty implementing the plan. Mrs. Trocki felt that the BSP was not "reasonable," stating that, "with 21 other students in my classroom, I just do not have time to check Jacob's work every 5 minutes." Mrs. Trocki went on to explain that without additional staff, it was impossible to provide 1:1 instruction and frequent breaks outside of the classroom. She also did not agree that Jacob should be allowed to ask for breaks "instead of completing his work."

The next day, Ms. Sparks met with Mrs. Trocki, the school psychologist, Jacob's parents, and the school principal to develop a new action plan. Together, the team decided that to prevent the problem behavior from occurring, Jacob would be given modified assignments that more closely matched his current skill set. He would also receive small group pull-out math and writing instruction three times per week for 20 minutes. Instead of Mrs. Trocki checking Jacob's work every 5 minutes, the team developed a plan for teaching Jacob to monitor his own behavior and give himself points for staying on task. Ms. Sparks agreed to develop the self-monitoring materials for Jacob, and the school psychologist would meet with Jacob to teach him how to use

the materials. Mrs. Trocki agreed to continue to prompt Jacob to raise his hand at the beginning of independent work and check Jacob's work every 10 minutes during independent work time to provide descriptive praise and help with any questions that Jacob might have. Ms. Trocki would receive a detailed written plan from Ms. Sparks, as well as coaching and feedback from the school psychologist, on how to fade this support as Jacob becomes more successful. In addition, the team agreed that as an alternative to engaging in problem behavior, Jacob would be taught to raise his hand and ask for help or for an easier assignment, and for every 3 points that Jacob earned (i.e., 15 minutes on task), he would earn 5 minutes for reading a book on a preferred topic or drawing at his desk.

In addition to the behavior change strategies, the team developed specific implementation and evaluation plans, detailing 1) who would be responsible for implementing each part of the plan, 2) when each part would be implemented, and 3) how to determine if the BSP was being implemented and if it was having the desired effect. Mrs. Trocki would be provided with a fidelity checklist to rate the extent to which she was implementing the different pieces of the BSP in the classroom. The school psychologist agreed to check in with Mrs. Trocki twice weekly during the first month of implementation to answer any questions or address any issues that might arise. The team members also selected a time that they would all meet again at the end of the first 2 weeks of implementation to evaluate how the plan was progressing and determine if any modifications needed to be made.

At the first plan review meeting, Mrs. Trocki and the school psychologist were happy to report to the school team and Jacob's parents that his problem behavior had improved significantly, with only three incidents of task refusal and no occurrences of tearing up worksheets or pushing materials off his desk for the past 2 weeks. Mrs. Trocki stated that she found the new strategies to be "doable" as part of her typical classroom schedule. She also expressed that she appreciated having the opportunity to check in regularly with the campus-based school psychologist and found the fidelity checklist to be a helpful reminder for keeping track of the different steps of the BSP. Ms. Sparks, the district behavior specialist, agreed to check in with the school psychologist every 2 weeks by e-mail, and to provide future assistance on an as-needed basis, although Mrs. Trocki reported feeling comfortable implementing the revised plan on her own at that point.

....

Amanda

Amanda was an 8-year-old girl who lived at home with her mother, father, and older sister. She attended a general education classroom in her neighborhood public elementary school with the support of an educational assistant and resource room teacher. At the age of six, Amanda was diagnosed with a moderate intellectual disability. Her family was Taiwanese and immigrated to Canada in 1998. The family was referred for family-centered PBS services due to severe problem behavior in the home, including noncompliance and defiance, disruptive and destructive behavior, self-injury, and physical aggression. A family ecology assessment revealed several strengths as well as challenges. Amanda's parents were very caring, willing to make sacrifices for their children, and had a strong marriage characterized by positive reciprocity. Amanda's strengths included her deep affection for her family and strong interest and curiosity in

people. The family, however, was socially isolated, largely due to Amanda's problem behavior, and the parents experienced an inordinate level of chronic stress. Neither parent worked outside the home, with the father choosing to work from his home to protect Amanda's mother from any aggressive behavior. Both parents reported feelings of sadness and frustration. In addition to behavior support, the family expressed an interest in receiving respite care and counseling support.

The functional assessment indicated that the primary function of Amanda's problem behavior was obtaining attention—that is, when Amanda was momentarily alone and her parents were occupied, she engaged in problem behavior to get positive or negative attention. Based on the results of the family ecology assessment and functional assessment, a technically sound and contextually appropriate multicomponent PBS plan was designed in collaboration with her parents for two problematic home routines: 1) child free time in family room while a parent prepared supper in the adjacent kitchen and 2) going to bed in her bedroom. The multicomponent plan included strategies and supports aimed at rendering problem behavior irrelevant, ineffective, and inefficient in regard to the function of problem behavior (see Table 22.1).

Table 22.1. Positive behavior support plan for Amanda

Preventive strategies

1. Use visual supports to increase the predictability of routine expectations and parental attention:
   a. Social Stories about child free time while parent is busy and for bedtime routine
   b. Visual sequence of task steps for child free time, during a parent's busy routine, and bedtime
   c. Countdown timer to predict length of time until parent returned attention
2. Use "first-then" visual positive contingencies to motivate desired behavior (e.g., a picture of Amanda playing independently, followed by a picture of parent playing together with Amanda).
3. Offer choices to encourage cooperation.

Teaching strategies

1. Use safety signals to teach endurance by gradually increasing latency to parent attention.
2. Teach Amanda to ask for attention or help.

Consequence strategies

1. Provide praise and rewards contingent on routine-related desired behavior.
2. Honor appropriate requests for attention or help.
3. Actively ignore and redirect minor problem behavior.
4. Remove adult attention for 30 seconds to 1 minute contingent on major problem behavior.

To empower the family to implement positive behavior supports with Amanda, an implementation plan was also developed that included routine-specific implementation checklists, in vivo coaching, and problem-solving meetings. During implementation support, the interventionist focused on teaching Amanda's parents to use PBS strategies to 1) improve Amanda's behavior and participation in the two target routines, 2) build constructive patterns of parent-child interaction (parent busy → child positive behavior → parent positive attention → child positive behavior), and 3) diminish coercive patterns of interaction (parent busy → child problem behavior → negative attention → child terminates problem behavior). To create a host environment for this transformation, family-centered supports also were put into place. These supports included 1) counseling support, 2) culturally responsive adaptations (e.g., slower pace for training, mother helping to train father), 3) stress management training from the intervention team, and 4) respite care (from a hired care provider).

Plan implementation occurred across a 2- to 4-year period of initial training, maintenance support, and follow-up. Direct observation results across the two routines showed stable decreases in problem behavior to near-zero levels and an increase in Amanda's ability to successfully participate in the routines, with all improvements maintaining at a 1-year follow-up. In addition, over the course of intervention and follow-up, the family reported a cascade of positive collateral effects. Once Amanda's parents were able to successfully support her in the home, they took measured forays into the local community. In doing so, they found that they could successfully support their daughter during walks in the neighborhood, visits to city parks, and shopping trips to grocery and clothing stores. With new-found confidence, the parents began to see a new horizon of possibilities for themselves and Amanda. Both parents sought and secured gainful employment outside the home, greatly improving their family's financial circumstances. These successes then led to the parents attempting and successfully completing day and weekend trips with Amanda and her sister to Seattle, Washington, 116 miles from their home. The ease and success of these trips then fueled summer vacation excursions to the Oregon Coast, Disneyland, and finally a 7-week tour of Asia, including Japan, Thailand, and their native Taiwan. In summarizing her family's experience, Amanda's mother reflected that "through this process of positive behavior support, we were empowered . . . we can go anywhere and do anything with [our daughter] now."

FUTURE DIRECTIONS

In addition to the benefits described here, efforts in building supportive environments have focused on integrating disparate systems to provide a coordinated, integrated services framework for individuals. Although it is becoming more common to consider interventions within host environments, it is still also common for support to be arranged into silos that treat the problems of individuals separately (McIntosh & Goodman, forthcoming). Yet research shows that academic, behavior, and mental health problems may have common origins (Biglan et al., 2012; McIntosh, Sadler, & Brown, 2012), and their effective treatments share common features (Filter & Horner, 2009; Preciado, Horner, & Baker, 2009). In some school systems, academic and behavior support systems have been integrated into multitiered systems of support (Ervin, Schaughency, Goodman, McGlinchey, & Matthews, 2006; Sadler & Sugai, 2009). In community and family support, the concept of systems of care (Stroul & Blau, 2008) describes how different interventions across agencies can be linked to provide coordinated support to individuals and families. The primary goal of redesigning systems into integrated services frameworks is to create a seamless support structure that delivers a range of effective interventions. Such efforts are not easy— they require establishing common vision and goals, often returning to an overarching goal of improving outcomes for individuals. By altering the host environment, the implementation and sustainability of behavior support for individuals can be optimized.

CONCLUSION

With the technologies for behavior support described in this book, implementers have access to evidence-based practices for reducing problem behavior and enhancing quality of life for individuals across a wide range of needs and contexts. However, having effective strategies available is not the same as being able to implement them consistently. The recent focus on host environments is promising because, just as changing the environment is an effective approach for individuals with needs, changing the environment for implementers is an effective approach to implementation of behavior support for individuals and groups.

REFERENCES

Albin, R.W., Lucyshyn, J.M., Horner, R.H., & Flannery, K.B. (1996). Contextual fit for behavioral support plans: A model for "goodness of fit." In L.K. Koegel, R.L. Koegel, & G. Dunlap (Eds.), *Positive behavioral support: Including people with difficult behavior in the community* (pp. 81–98). Baltimore, MD: Paul H. Brookes Publishing Co.

Baker, S., Gersten, R., Dimino, J.A., & Griffiths, R. (2004). The sustained use of research-based instructional practice: A case study of peer-assisted learning strategies in mathematics. *Remedial and Special Education, 25,* 5–24.

Benazzi, L.R., Horner, R.H., & Good, R.H. (2006). Effects of behavior support team composition on the technical adequacy and contextual fit of behavior support plans. *Journal of Special Education, 40,* 160–170.

Biglan, A. (1995). Translating what we know about the context of antisocial behavior into a lower prevalence of such behavior. *Journal of Applied Behavior Analysis, 28,* 479–492.

Biglan, A., Flay, B.R., Embry, D.D., & Sandler, I.N. (2012). The critical role of nurturing environments for promoting human well-being. *American Psychologist, 67,* 257–271.

Binnendyk, L., & Lucyshyn, J.M. (2009). A family-centered positive behavior support approach to the amelioration of food refusal behavior: An empirical case study. *Journal of Positive Behavior Interventions, 11,* 47–62.

Bradshaw, C.P., Koth, K., Bevans, K.B., Ialongo, N., & Leaf, P.J. (2008). The impact of school-wide positive behavioral interventions and supports on the organizational health of elementary schools. *School Psychology Quarterly, 23,* 462–473.

Bradshaw, C.P., Waasdorp, T.E., & Leaf, P.J. (forthcoming). Effects of school-wide positive behavioral interventions and supports on child behavior problems and adjustment. *Pediatrics.*

Bradshaw, C.P., Waasdorp, T.E., & Leaf, P.J. (2013). *Examining variation in the impact of school wide positive behavioral interventions and supports.* Manuscript submitted for publication and reported in House Subcommittee Hearings, February 8, 2013.

Coffey, J., & Horner, R.H. (2012). The sustainability of school-wide positive behavioral interventions and supports. *Exceptional Children, 78,* 407–422.

Cornell, D.G. (2006). *School violence: Fears vs. facts.* Mahwah, NJ: Lawrence Erlbaum.

Cummings, J.G., Pepler, D.J., Mishna, F., & Craig, W.M. (2006). Bullying and victimization among students with exceptionalities. *Exceptionality Education Canada, 16,* 193–222.

Dishion, T.J., & Dodge, K.A. (2006). Deviant peer contagion in interventions and programs: An ecological framework for understanding influence mechanisms. In K.A. Dodge (Ed.), *Deviant peer influences in programs for youth: Problems and solutions* (pp. 14–43). New York, NY: Guilford Press.

Doll, B., Song, S., Champion, A., & Jones, K. (2011). Classroom ecologies that support or discourage bullying. In D.L. Espelage & S.M. Swearer (Eds.), *Bullying in North American schools* (2nd ed., pp. 147–158). New York, NY: Routledge.

Domitrovich, C.E., Bradshaw, C.P., Poduska, J.M., Hoagwood, K., Buckley, J.A., Olin, S., . . . Ialongo, N.S. (2008). Maximizing the implementation quality of evidence-based preventive interventions in schools: A conceptual framework. *Advances in School Mental Health Promotion, 1,* 6–28.

Dunlap, G., Iovannone, R., English, C.L., Kincaid, D., Wilson, K., Christiansen, K., & Strain, P.S. (2009). *Prevent-teach-reinforce: The school-based model of individualized positive behavior support.* Baltimore, MD: Paul H. Brookes Publishing Co.

Dunst, C.J., Trivette, C.M., & Deal, A.G. (1988). *Enabling and empowering families: Principles and guidelines for practice.* New York, NY: Brookline Books.

Elswick, S., & Casey, L.B. (2011). The good behavior game is no longer just an effective intervention for students: An examination of the reciprocal effects on teacher behaviors. *Beyond Behavior, 21*(1), 36–46.

Ervin, R.A., Schaughency, E., Goodman, S.D., McGlinchey, M.T., & Matthews, A. (2006). Merging research and practice agendas to address reading and behavior school-wide. *School Psychology Review, 35,* 198–223.

Filter, K.J., & Horner, R.H. (2009). Function-based academic interventions for problem behavior. *Education and Treatment of Children, 32,* 1–19.

Fixsen, D.L., Naoom, S.F., Blase, K.A., Friedman, R.M., & Wallace, F. (2005). *Implementation research: Synthesis of the literature.* Tampa, FL: University of South Florida, Louis de la Parte Florida Mental Health Institute, The National Implementation Research Network.

Gallimore, R. (2005). Behavior change in the natural environment: Everyday activity settings as a workshop of change. In C.R. O'Donnell & L.A. Yamauchi (Eds.), *Culture and context in human behavior change: Theory, research, and applications* (pp. 207–231). New York, NY: Peter Lang.

Gallimore, R., Goldenberg, C.N., & Weisner, T.S. (1993). The social construction and subjective reality of activity settings: Implications for community psychology. *American Journal of Community Psychology, 21,* 537–560.

Gersten, R., Chard, D.J., & Baker, S. (2000). Factors enhancing sustained use of research-based instructional practices. *Journal of Learning Disabilities, 33,* 445–457.

Greenberg, M.T. (2004). Current and future challenges in school-based prevention: The researcher perspective. *Prevention Science, 5,* 5–13.

Gresham, F.M. (1989). Assessment of treatment integrity in school consultation and prereferral intervention. *School Psychology Review, 18,* 37–50.

Hemphill, S.A., Toumbourou, J.W., Herrenkohl, T.I., McMorris, B.J., & Catalano, R.F. (2006). The effect of school suspensions and arrests on subsequent adolescent antisocial behavior in Australia and the United States. *Journal of Adolescent Health, 39,* 736–744.

Hieneman, M., & Dunlap, G. (2000). Factors affecting the outcomes of community-based behavioral support: I. Identification and description of factor categories. *Journal of Positive Behavior Interventions, 2,* 161–169, 178.

Hieneman, M., & Dunlap, G. (2001). Factors affecting the outcomes of community-based behavioral support: II. Factor category importance. *Journal of Positive Behavior Interventions, 3,* 67–74.

Horner, R.H., Sugai, G., Smolkowski, K., Eber, L., Nakasato, J., Todd, A.W., & Esparanza, J. (2009). A randomized, wait-list controlled effectiveness trial assessing school-wide positive behavior support in elementary schools. *Journal of Positive Behavior Interventions, 11,* 133–144.

Kame'enui, E.J., Simmons, D.C., & Coyne, M.D. (2000). Schools as host environments: Toward a schoolwide reading improvement model. *Annals of Dyslexia, 50,* 31–51.

Kelm, J.L., & McIntosh, K. (2012). Effects of schoolwide positive behavior support on teacher self-efficacy. *Psychology in the Schools, 49,* 137–147.

Lannie, A.L., & McCurdy, B.L. (2007). Preventing disruptive behavior in the urban classroom: Effects of the good behavior game on student and teacher behavior. *Education and Treatment of Children, 30,* 85–98.

Latham, G. (1988). The birth and death cycles of educational innovations. *Principal, 68,* 41–43.

Lewis, T.J. (2007). *Functional assessment and positive behavior support plans.* Paper presented at the Office of Special Education Programs Forum, Washington, DC.

Loman, S., & Borgmeier, C. (2010). *Practical functional behavioral assessment training manual for school-based personnel.* Portland, OR: Portland State University.

Lucyshyn, J.M., Albin, R.A., Horner, R.H., Mann, J.C., Mann, J.A., & Wadsworth, G. (2007). Family implementation of positive behavior support with a child with Autism: A longitudinal, single case experimental and descriptive replication and extension. *Journal of Positive Behavior Interventions, 9,* 131–150.

Lucyshyn, J.M., & Albin, R.W. (1993). Comprehensive support to families of children with disabilities and behavior problems: Keeping it "friendly." In G.H.S.

Singer & L.E. Powers (Eds.), *Families, disability, and empowerment: Active coping skills and strategies for family interventions* (pp. 365–407). Baltimore, MD: Paul H. Brookes Publishing Co.

Lucyshyn, J.M., Albin, R.W., & Nixon, C.D. (1997). Embedding comprehensive behavioral support in family ecology: An experimental, single-case analysis. *Journal of Consulting and Clinical Psychology, 65,* 241–251.

Lucyshyn, J.M., Binnendyk, L., Fossett, B., Cheremshynski, C., Lorhmann, S., Elkinson, L., & Miller, L.D. (2009). Toward an ecological unit of analysis in behavioral assessment and intervention with families of children with developmental disabilities: Conceptual and empirical foundations and implications for assessment and intervention. In W. Sailor, G. Dunlap, G. Sugai, & R.H. Horner (Eds.), *Handbook of positive behavior support,* 73–106. New York, NY: Springer.

Lucyshyn, J.M., Fossett, B., Binnendyk, L., Cheremshynski, C., Lorhmann, S., Miller, L.D., . . . Irvin, L.K. (2014). *Transforming coercive processes in family routines: A longitudinal analysis with 10 families of children with developmental disabilities.* Manuscript in preparation.

Lucyshyn, J.M., Irvin, L.K., Blumberg, E.R., Laverty, R., Horner, R.H., & Sprague, J.R. (2004). Validating the construct of coercion in family routines: Expanding the unit of analysis in behavioral assessment with families of children with developmental disabilities. *Research & Practice for Persons with Severe Disabilities, 29,* 104–121.

Luiselli, J.K., Putnam, R.F., Handler, M.W., & Feinberg, A.B. (2005). Whole-school positive behaviour support: Effects on student discipline problems and academic performance. *Educational Psychology, 25,* 183–198.

Maag, J.W. (2001). Rewarded by punishment: Reflections on the disuse of positive reinforcement in schools. *Exceptional Children, 67,* 173–186.

Mayer, G.R. (1995). Preventing antisocial behavior in the schools. *Journal of Applied Behavior Analysis, 28,* 467–478.

McIntosh, K., Bennett, J.L., & Price, K. (2011). Evaluation of social and academic effects of school-wide positive behaviour support in a Canadian school district. *Exceptionality Education International, 21,* 46–60.

McIntosh, K., Chard, D.J., Boland, J.B., & Horner, R.H. (2006). Demonstration of combined efforts in school-wide academic and behavioral systems and incidence of reading and behavior challenges in early elementary grades. *Journal of Positive Behavior Interventions, 8,* 146–154.

McIntosh, K., & Goodman, S. (forthcoming). *Multitiered systems of support: Integrating academic RTI and school-wide PBIS.* New York, NY: Guilford Press.

McIntosh, K., Horner, R.H., Chard, D.J., Dickey, C.R., & Braun, D.H. (2008). Reading skills and function of problem behavior in typical school settings. *Journal of Special Education, 42,* 131–147.

McIntosh, K., MacKay, L.D., Hume, A.E., Doolittle, J., Vincent, C.G., Horner, R.H., & Ervin, R.A. (2011). Development and initial validation of a measure to assess factors related to sustainability of school-wide positive behavior support. *Journal of Positive Behavior Interventions, 13,* 208–218. doi:10.1177/1098300710385348

McIntosh, K., Mercer, S.H., Hume, A.E., Frank, J.L., Turri, M.G., & Mathews, S. (2013). Factors related to sustained implementation of school-wide positive behavior support. *Exceptional Children, 79,* 293–311.

McIntosh, K., Predy, L.K., Upreti, G., Hume, A.E., Turri, M.G., & Mathews, S. (2014). Perceptions of contextual features related to implementation and sustainability of school-wide positive behavior support. *Journal of Positive Behavior Interventions, 16,* 29–41. doi:10.1177/1098300712470723

McIntosh, K., Sadler, C., & Brown, J.A. (2012). Kindergarten reading skill level and change as risk factors for chronic problem behavior. *Journal of Positive Behavior Interventions, 14,* 17–28. doi:10.1177/1098300711403153

McIntosh, K., Ty, S.V., & Miller, L.D. (forthcoming). Effects of school-wide positive behavior support on internalizing problems: Current evidence and future directions. *Journal of Positive Behavior Interventions.*

Nelson, J.R., Martella, R.M., & Marchand-Martella, N. (2002). Maximizing student learning: The effects of a comprehensive school-based program for preventing problem behaviors. *Journal of Emotional and Behavioral Disorders, 10,* 136–148.

Patterson, G.R. (1982). *Coercive family process.* Eugene, OR: Castalia.

Preciado, J.A., Horner, R.H., & Baker, S.K. (2009). Using a function-based approach to decrease problem behavior and increase reading academic engagement for Latino English language learners. *Journal of Special Education, 42,* 227–240.

Ross, S.W., & Horner, R.H. (2006). Teacher outcomes of school-wide positive behavior support. *Teaching Exceptional Children Plus, 3*(6). Retrieved from http://journals.cec.sped.org/tecplus/vol3/iss6/art6/

Ross, S.W., & Horner, R.H. (2009). Bully prevention in positive behavior support. *Journal of Applied Behavior Analysis, 42,* 747–759.

Ross, S.W., Romer, N., & Horner, R.H. (2012). Teacher well-being and the implementation of school-wide positive behavior interventions and supports. *Journal of Positive Behavior Interventions, 14,* 118–128.

Sadler, C., & Sugai, G. (2009). Effective behavior and instructional support: A district model for early identification and prevention of reading and behavior problems. *Journal of Positive Behavior Interventions, 11,* 35–46.

Singer, G.H.S., & Irvin, L.K. (1991). Supporting families of persons with severe disabilities: Emerging findings, practices, and questions. In L.H. Meyer, C.A. Peck, & L. Brown (Eds.), *Critical issues in the lives of people with severe disabilities* (pp. 271–312). Baltimore, MD: Paul H. Brookes Publishing Co.

Skiba, R.J., & Peterson, R.L. (2000). School discipline at a crossroads: From zero tolerance to early response. *Exceptional Children, 66,* 335–347.

Stroul, B.A., & Blau, G.M. (Eds.). (2008). *The system of care handbook: Transforming mental health services for children, youth, and families.* Baltimore, MD: Paul H. Brookes Publishing Co.

Sugai, G., & Horner, R.H. (2002). The evolution of discipline practices: School-wide positive behavior supports. *Child and Family Behavior Therapy, 24,* 23–50.

Sugai, G., & Horner, R.H. (2009). Defining and describing schoolwide positive behavior support. In W. Sailor, G. Dunlap, G. Sugai, & R.H. Horner (Eds.), *Handbook of positive behavior support* (pp. 307–326). New York, NY: Springer.

Sugai, G., Horner, R.H., Algozzine, R., Barrett, S., Lewis, T., Anderson, C., . . . Simonsen, B. (2010). *School-wide positive behavior support: Implementers' blueprint and self-assessment.* Eugene, OR: University of Oregon. Retrieved from http://pbis.org/pbis_resource_detail_page.aspx?Type=3&PBIS_ResourceID=216, January 24, 2014.

Tobin, T., Horner, R.H., Vincent, C.G., & Swain-Bradway, J. (2012). *If discipline referral rates for the school as a whole are reduced, will rates for students with disabilities also be reduced?* Eugene, OR: Educational and Community Supports.

Tobin, T., Vincent, C.G., Horner, R.H., Dickey, C.R., & May, S.A. (2012) Fidelity measures to improve implementation of positive behavioural support. *International Journal of Positive Behaviour Support, 2*(2), 12–19.

Todd, A.W., Horner, R.H., Newton, J.S., Algozzine, R.F., Algozzine, K.M., & Frank, J.L. (2011). Effects of team initiated problem solving on meeting practices of schoolwide behavior support teams. *Journal of Applied School Psychology, 27,* 42–59.

Turnbull, A.P., & Turnbull, H.R. (1991). Understanding families from a systems perspective. In J.M. Williams & T. Kay (Eds.), *Head injury: A family matter* (pp. 37–63). Baltimore, MD: Paul H. Brookes Publishing Co.

Turnbull, A.P., Turnbull, H.R., Erwin, E.J., Soodak, L.C., & Shogren, K.A. (2011). *Families, professionals and exceptionality: Positive outcomes through partnerships and trust* (6th ed.). New York, NY: Pearson.

Waasdorp, T.E., Bradshaw, C.P., & Leaf, P.J. (2012). The impact of schoolwide positive behavioral interventions and supports on bullying and peer rejection. *Archives of Pediatrics & Adolescent Medicine, 166,* 149–156.

Walker, H.M., Horner, R.H., Sugai, G., Bullis, M., Sprague, J.R., Bricker, D., & Kaufman, M.J. (1996). Integrated approaches to preventing antisocial behavior patterns among school-age children and youth. *Journal of Emotional and Behavioral Disorders, 4,* 194–209.

Wandersman, A., & Florin, P. (2003). Community interventions and effective prevention. *American Psychologist, 58,* 441–448.

Whitted, K.S., & Dupper, D.R. (2005). Best practices for preventing or reducing bullying in schools. *Children and Schools, 27,* 167–173.

Implementing Multielement Positive Behavior Support Plans

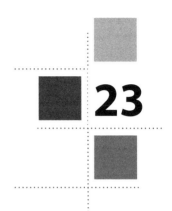

23

Meme Hieneman and Glen Dunlap

The preceding chapters focused on the foundations and principles of positive behavior support (PBS) and considerations in the selection and design of interventions. This chapter is about implementing PBS plans. It provides a discussion of factors related to implementation and outlines and illustrates essential processes for improving the consistency with which strategies are utilized. The primary goal of these strategies is to improve the fidelity with which support strategies are used, as high fidelity is logically associated with desirable outcomes. In the following pages, we will discuss variables related to plan design, implementation, and effectiveness; strategies for translating behavior support plans (BSPs) into practice; mechanisms for tracking fidelity and progress; and data-based decision making in the complex and changing circumstances of a person's life in the community.

The literature on PBS provides an impressive body of evidence on the features,

design, and evaluation of effective, person-centered interventions. In a cursory review, however, it becomes evident that considerably less has been written about the nuts and bolts of implementation. The thesis of this chapter is that practitioners need to put at least as much emphasis on putting plans in place as they do on assessment and plan development.

Effective implementation of PBS can be a complex endeavor. The complexity, however, varies greatly as a function of the characteristics of the focus person, history of problem behavior, interventions (both successful and unsuccessful), and the features of the environments in which support will be provided. An essential component of intervention is assessment of the contexts in which support will be delivered so that all these variables can be understood and addressed, ensuring that the interventions have the social validity, technical adequacy, and practicality to be feasibly implemented.

A major point that needs to be explicit before we proceed is that the comprehensiveness and precision of the design and implementation of an individualized PBS plan must be viewed as a continuum. For some individuals with severe intellectual and communicative disabilities or with other significant risk factors, whose problem behaviors have been present for years and in multiple settings, PBS plans may need to be very detailed and involve extensive planning for all aspects of intervention. For some other individuals, however, plans do not need to be as intensive or comprehensive. The message is that the effort invested in plan development and implementation should be balanced by the needs of the person (and others in their environment affected by the problem behaviors) and the overall goals that need to be addressed by the interventions and supports to be implemented. It would be inappropriate to allocate more time, effort, and resources than are necessary to resolve the presenting problem(s).

This chapter is limited to *individual positive behavior supports;* however, the design of a PBS plan and the probability of favorable outcomes are dependent to a large extent on the prevailing contexts in which the plan will be implemented. The extent to which the pertinent environments are designed to support desirable behavior and discourage problem behavior is a dominant determinant of behavior outcomes (see Chapter 22; Sailor, Dunlap, Sugai, & Horner, 2009). Specifically, when high-quality universal and targeted practices are in place in a particular setting (e.g., classroom, workplace, family home), it is expected that problem behaviors will tend to be less frequent and less intense and the need for an exacting and comprehensive PBS plan will be reduced. Although an individualized PBS plan may still be required, the plan might not need to be as detailed or technically precise. This is the logic of multitiered systems of prevention, as has been articulated compellingly in the writings on schoolwide and programwide PBS (Fox, Dunlap, Hemmeter, Joseph, & Strain, 2003; Sailor et al., 2009; Walker et al., 1996).

In PBS, the primary objective is to improve the quality of individuals' lives within the context of inclusive settings and natural routines. Doing so requires the engagement of parents, teachers, employers, and other typical caregivers so that they may implement support strategies across circumstances and over time. Therefore, a key ingredient of effective implementation is empowering the individuals charged with plan implementation. Such empowerment requires that we design interventions with contextual fit (Albin, Lucyshyn, Horner, & Flannery, 1996), communicate expectations clearly, arrange environments to support implementation, provide effective instruction and reinforcement for the implementers, and gradually fade our assistance while shifting to natural contingencies. This chapter will address these practical elements.

VARIABLES RELATED TO PLAN DESIGN, IMPLEMENTATION, AND EFFECTIVENESS

The implementation of BSPs within typical home, community, and educational or vocational settings is affected by a variety of factors. Possible moderating factors described in the PBS literature include the characteristics of the individual who is the focus of intervention, people supporting the individual, and settings in which the intervention is put in place (Albin et al., 1996). In a two-part study, we asked practitioners, experts, and family members to identify and rate the importance of variables contributing to the success and failure of community-based behavioral interventions (Hieneman & Dunlap, 2000, 2001). Our results were consistent with those suggested by our colleagues—that is, a number of factors were seen as important, and caregiver buy-in was rated as the most essential factor. These factors are addressed in the following sections.

Characteristics and Needs of Individual

A number of factors associated with specific abilities and disabilities of the individuals with challenging behavior may influence the person's responsiveness to intervention. Relevant issues include the individual's cognitive, sensory, motor, social, emotional, and other developmental characteristics, as well as their current skills repertoire (Emerson et al., 2001). The severity, complexity, and history of the individual's behavior and their responsiveness to previous intervention efforts may also contribute to the outcomes. Finally, the individual's motivation and preferences would be anticipated to influence the support process.

Characteristics and Preferences of Implementers

The people implementing the plan and supporting the individual on an ongoing basis also have a critical influence. Considerations include who will be involved in which roles and to what extent and how much time the caregivers have available. The knowledge and capabilities of the caregivers, as well as their physical, intellectual, and emotional characteristics, are relevant. If the caregivers are experiencing considerable stress or depression or they are not fully committed, they may not be able to implement the plan adequately (Hastings, 2002; Head & Abbeduto, 2007).

Characteristics of Environments and Systems

Implementation is also affected by aspects of the surroundings and systems in which the plan will be utilized. These include the structure and resources of the physical settings—specifically their organization, materials available, arrangement, and access to technology. Routines and scheduling are also relevant to a plan's success. This means identifying and integrating strategies within typical activities and events and considering the consistency, predictability, and clarity of these routines (Lucyshyn et al., 2009, Moes & Frea, 2004).

Research in schoolwide and program-wide PBS illustrates the importance of multilevel and proactive systems of support for creating sustainable supports for individuals with behavior challenges (see Chapter 22; Sailor et al., 2009). These concepts can also be applied to the family ecology, recognizing that structural issues (e.g., expectations, routines) impact behavior support in homes (Hieneman, Childs, & Sergay, 2006). In implementing support plans, PBS teams need to ensure that individualized strategies align with the broader practices and that the systems in place support individualization.

To illustrate the importance of these variables in implementing PBS plans, we offer two case examples. Kevin and Jolanda are very different children, participating in unique social and physical environments.

Kevin

Kevin is 3 years old and has been identified as having developmental delays consistent with an autism spectrum diagnosis. He is bright and verbal but has difficulty interpreting social circumstances. He resists new situations and changes in routines by making excuses, whining, and dropping to the floor. Kevin lives with his parents and siblings; both of his parents work outside the home. He attends an inclusive preschool class with a teacher and one instructional aide; neither has training and experience in working with children with autism. However, both are open to new information and are highly motivated. Kevin's home and school environments are highly organized and have consistent routines. There is, however, very little administrative support at the school. The parents use their own fiscal resources to cover the supplemental services and therapies Kevin receives.

Kevin needs a plan that focuses on teaching him how to read social cues and interact positively with his peers and includes a written activity schedule and Social Stories to increase the predictability of his daily life. These strategies can be easily adopted at home and school—in fact, his teacher is finding that all her students appreciate the schedule. For Kevin's team, challenges might be integrating social learning opportunities within existing routines, coordinating support around his family's busy schedule, and keeping the school's administration informed and engaged.

....

Jolanda

Jolanda is 12 years old. She has a severe intellectual disability as well as medical complications (e.g., gastrointestinal problems, sleep disturbance, epilepsy). Jolanda communicates only through gestures and leading others to show them what she needs. She is affectionate but has an extensive history of aggression, self-injury, and property destruction. These behaviors have typically been addressed through reactive strategies such as compliance training, tangible rewards, and manual restraint to manage her aggression. Jolanda's mother is a single parent with no other children and works part time. Jolanda's home is chaotic, with frequent guests, schedule changes, and limited financial resources and access to technology. Jolanda receives intensive services at home, school, and in the community from a variety of trained professionals. However, the agencies supporting Jolanda have rigid procedures, many of which are not consistent with the elements of her proposed PBS plan.

Jolanda requires functional communication training using an augmentative device or gestures to teach her basic replacement skills, coordination among her many service providers, crisis management procedures, and support in developing daily living and self-care skills. The hope is to emphasize more positive and strength-based approaches than those to which she was previously exposed. Implementation methods might include helping her mother access needed resources and negotiating the service system. It may also be beneficial to help her and the school establish routines in which Jolanda can naturally practice her communication and life skills.

....

Both Kevin's and Jolanda's plans need to be aligned with the resources available, fit within natural routines, and be "doable" for the caregivers, given their preferences and competing priorities. In order to be successful, practitioners may have to either make accommodations to the plan to fit within existing circumstances or change some aspects of the environment or patterns of interaction to adapt to the plan. Attaining this "contextual fit" requires a realistic appraisal of potential resources and barriers, working closely with caregivers to ensure the validity of goals and procedures, and continual collection of data on fidelity and outcomes to determine whether the plan is being used and is achieving the desired goals.

TRANSLATING BEHAVIOR SUPPORT PLANS INTO PRACTICE

PBS plans, by definition, should incorporate certain basic features that allow individuals to participate successfully in integrated environments. These features are evident in the literature (Hieneman, Dunlap, & Kincaid, 2005; Horner, Sugai, Todd, & Lewis-Palmer, 1999–2000), in behavior plan templates utilized by school and community programs, and addressed elsewhere in this book. In summary, PBS plans should include relevant information regarding the individual, family, and caregivers; specific behaviors of concern and goals of intervention; assessment-based interventions to prevent, teach, and respond to behavior; strategies focused on improving quality of life; and mechanisms for providing training, monitoring fidelity of implementation, and objectively assessing progress. In addition, it is important to translate the plans into action through effective teaching practices, implementation within natural routines, and making sure the plans work within the settings and systems in which they are utilized.

Effective Teaching Practices

Having clear, comprehensive, and practical written plans facilitates the utilization of the strategies. Since teaching is an essential foundation for promoting durable change, it is particularly important that specific procedures for rearranging the environment and teaching skills be incorporated into the plan. For most caregivers, it is insufficient to simply say "Teach Jolanda skills x, y, and z." The methods need to be explicit. Clear and effective instructional strategies include 1) defining specific skills (e.g., outlining component skills or task analyses); 2) arranging the environment to encourage the use of these skills; 3) prompting, shaping, and chaining procedures; 4) carrying out differential reinforcement and error correction procedures; and 5) using generalization and maintenance strategies. (See Snell & Brown, 2011, Chapter 12 in this book, and Westling & Fox, 2009, for in-depth reviews of systematic instructional strategies.)

The literature offers a variety of evidence-based instructional approaches, each with their own strengths as well as their own limitations. For example, discrete trial training utilizes systematic and intensive methods that involve skill sequencing and repetition to achieve mastery (McEachin, Smith, & Lovaas 1993). Pivotal Response Training targets requisite socially valid responses that lead to greater generalization (Koegel & Koegel, 2006). Verbal behavior training builds on the recognition that language has multiple purposes and teaches skills to meet different functions in a developmental sequence (Sundberg & Partington, 1998). Incidental teaching relies on natural cues and reinforcers, embedding teachable moments in ongoing routines (Charlop-Christy & Carpenter, 2000). Peer-mediated instruction engages friends in the instructional process to promote inclusion and successful interactions (Strain & Kohler, 1998). Finally, functional communication training incorporates functional behavioral assessment (FBA) to identify and teach specific replacement behaviors (Durand, 1990), thereby reducing the individual's need to engage in problem behavior. The methods inherent in these applications should be utilized to efficiently build new skill repertoires.

Implementation within Natural Routines

A defining feature of PBS is that proactive and educational supports are embedded within natural contexts, rather than addressed in separate, structured teaching sessions. Lucyshyn and colleagues (2009) have demonstrated how interventions can be organized and implemented within activity settings. Activity settings can include daily living, chores, homework, outings, leisure activities, and social interactions (O'Donnell, Tharp, & Wilson, 1993). Implementation of plans within natural contexts may be more relevant for the individual and doable for caregivers, making valued routines more successful. For Kevin and Jolanda, we would want to select particular skill targets and instructional practices that would allow them to be most successful in the environments in which they participate. Engaging Kevin's peers and siblings to encourage and reinforce social skills during the natural course of his day may be an effective strategy. Jolanda, however, may require more immediate and systematic methods to gain the skills she needs to request items and refuse unpleasant circumstances, as well as develop skills for independence. Jolanda may also respond more positively if these skills are embedded in community activities that both she and her mother find reinforcing.

Making Positive Behavior Support Plans Work

As mentioned in the introduction, we should expect to have a continuum of precision and comprehensiveness in BSPs. This continuum is based on the needs of the individuals, settings and social environments in which they participate, resources required and available, capability of the people implementing the plan, and monitoring requirements dictated by the agencies or schools supporting them. Plans may range from highly structured and intensive to short and informal.

In order to effectively implement PBS plans, it is beneficial to have appropriate structures and supports within the programs or agencies serving the individual. There may be times that the assistance an individual requires (e.g., professional support, resources needed to implement the plan) outweighs or does not match resources currently available or that policies and procedures of an agency or other group setting do not support effective intervention. In that case, those facilitating the PBS process must choose between changing placements/service providers and collaborating with (or, less preferably, advocating against) the administration to encourage change. Working within systems that embrace PBS principles to help all individuals and establish multitiered and flexible support systems (e.g., schoolwide PBS) is certainly easier.

Since Kevin's preschool has not served children with autism previously, the program may have to be open learning how to more effectively support children with special needs and allow some flexibility in their discipline practices. His plan will likely be relatively simple and fit naturally within existing integrated routines. In Jolanda's case, it may be a challenge to pull all the professionals together to create an integrated and responsive plan, rather than simply continuing status quo. Because of the service requirements and variety of providers involved, Jolanda's plan would probably have to be more specific and comprehensive than Kevin's plan.

· ·

ENGAGING CAREGIVERS IN PLAN IMPLEMENTATION

To facilitate consistent use of behavior strategies, caregivers and professionals who interact with the individual daily and across environments (e.g., family members, teachers) must be fully engaged. Unfortunately, the nonadherence of caregivers—parents in particular—to recommended behavior procedures continues to be a common complaint (Allen & Warzak, 2000). Collaboration has been identified as one of the core ingredients of PBS (Carr et al., 2002). It means that caregivers and professionals supporting the individual work together to achieve mutually agreed-on outcomes. Processes by which parents and service providers are engaged in PBS appear to fall into two broad categories: creating ownership and building capacity. It is necessary to address these elements as well as attend to potential barriers to participation.

Creating Ownership

Ownership is achieved by engaging caregivers in planning and decision making. A number of studies in PBS have engaged parents as partners in plan design and implementation (e.g., Koegel, Streibel, & Koegel, 1998; Lucyshyn et al., 2007; Vaughn, Dunlap, Fox, Clarke, & Bucy, 1997). Other studies have actively involved parents and other caregivers in the FBA, helping to gather information and identify patterns, as well as make decisions about plan components (McNeill, Watson, Henington, & Meeks, 2002; Peterson, Derby, Berg, & Horner, 2002). In school-based intervention, team-based decision making has been identified as a key ingredient to success (Goh & Bambara, 2012). This is a sharp contrast to traditional consultative processes in behavior intervention, encouraging ownership rather than dependence on an expert to resolve problems.

Person-centered planning approaches are commonly incorporated into PBS. These processes are addressed in Chapter 13 of this book and allow individuals, family members, and direct service providers to identify a positive vision for the future and short- and long-term goals for the individual. The teams then map out an action plan, determining how supports will be established and responsibilities are determined. Regardless of how collaborative action planning is accomplished, it is essential that all caregivers are fully engaged, that the goals reflect what is most valued by the people who care most for the individual, and that there is a clear strategy for implementing the action plan.

Building Capacity

Building capacity requires the teaching of skills so that caregivers can implement behavior plans as designed. Parent training programs have been implemented since the field of behavior analysis was established (Shaeffer, Kotchich, Dorsey, & Forehand, 2001). Data have demonstrated improvements in parenting skills but inconsistent results in child outcomes and maintenance

(Maughan, Christiansen, Jenson, Olympia, & Clark, 2005). Johnson and colleagues (Johnson et al., 2007) and Durand and Hieneman (2008) have both evaluated comprehensive parent education curricula for building competency in the PBS process. Preliminary studies of both curricula provide evidence that significant improvements in child behavior can occur when the parents are taught to apply the principles of PBS to resolve their children's behavior challenges. These same practices are being incorporated in curricula for early interventionists and educators (Dunlap, Wilson, Strain, & Lee, 2013).

In PBS, it is not enough to simply provide written plans; we must teach implementers the specific skills needed to implement methods, particularly when working with inexperienced caregivers. In a study conducted by Erbas (2010), the importance of providing parent feedback to improve fidelity and outcomes for children's behavior is clearly illustrated. Sarakoff and Sturmey (2004) demonstrated that utilizing instruction, feedback, rehearsal, and modeling to teach teachers discrete trial training using behavioral techniques produced significantly improved fidelity. Training (and coaching) of practitioners involves the same instructional practices we use with individuals. The overriding goal should be to build the capacity of those implementing the interventions rather than dependence on experts.

Overcoming Barriers to Participation

A common frustration of PBS facilitators is when caregivers do not follow through with plans, even when all the necessary training and support has been provided. We must recognize that caregiver behavior (e.g., cooperation, engagement, nonadherence, or resistance) is mediated by the same variables as the behavior of focus individuals. Social settings may not support implementation, and reinforcers may not be available to encourage follow-through. It is common for caregivers to engage in unproductive

anticipatory responses (e.g., avoiding circumstances, allowing a child to do anything he wants) to avoid problem behavior. They may also escalate and/or concede in response to an individual's behavior, setting up a coercive response cycle (Patterson, 1982). These patterns actively compete with PBS efforts.

An important aspect of PBS is determining whether contingencies are in place to support the caregivers (see Chapter 3). If caregivers are not implementing plans as designed, we might ask whether the strategies are too difficult to implement or the environment somehow does not support intervention. If the consequences of giving in, giving up, or reverting to old patterns of interaction outweigh reinforcement of more long-term consequences for the child because they produce more immediate results, then we must try to adjust these patterns. In this case, a primary role of PBS facilitators would be determining how contingencies of caregiver behavior could be realigned to support implementation (e.g., by providing more encouragement, simplifying strategies to make them more efficient, or presenting data that show improvements over time).

Even when the environment and contingencies appear to be supporting intervention, caregivers sometimes do not buy into plans. A commonly acknowledged but rarely investigated issue pertains to caregiver pessimism (Baker, Blacher, & Olsson, 2005). When caregivers do not believe they or the individuals they are supporting are capable of positive change, they are disinclined to implement interventions. A study by Durand, Hieneman, Clarke, Rinaldi, and Wang (2013) evaluated combining optimism training and parent education in PBS through a highly structured program designed to overcome parental resistance, thereby improving outcomes. Participants received either education in PBS only or the same educational program combined with cognitive-behavior strategies to identify, dispute, and replace beliefs interfering with their follow-through with behavior intervention. All participants demonstrated significant improvements in child behavior and family quality of life, but the group exposed to optimism training had better outcomes and reported greater confidence following the study. Steed and Durand (2012) have replicated this study with teachers and found that educators in the optimistic teaching condition adopted more behavior interventions and reported greater improvements in their students socioemotional functioning. These studies indicate that, in addition to addressing the observable contexts and contingencies surrounding caregiver behavior, it may also be beneficial to address attitudinal issues (e.g., self-talk).

Kevin's parents and teachers are highly motivated and optimistic. However, Jolanda's mother, teacher, and service providers are discouraged and overwhelmed. To assist them, the team will design strategies that produce immediate results and are easy to implement. Using cognitive-behavior strategies, the PBS facilitator can identify sources of resistance and help Jolanda's caregivers become more open to alternative strategies.

....

TRACKING FIDELITY OF IMPLEMENTATION

The primary goal of strategies related to implementation is to improve the fidelity with which interventions are used. A higher level of fidelity means that the PBS plan is being implemented as intended and, assuming that the plan is well designed, favorable effects are more likely to occur (Durlak & DuPre, 2008). So what is meant by *fidelity of implementation?* Simply stated, fidelity refers to the extent to which actual implementation of a PBS plan corresponds to the intent of the plan and the specifics with which the plan's components are described (Billingsley, White, & Munson, 1980). Fidelity is also referred to as *procedural fidelity, implementation fidelity,* and *treatment integrity.* We consider these terms to be equivalent.

Fidelity has been consistently described as having several dimensions. Some of the dimensions to be considered include adherence, quality, consistency, and dosage. *Adherence* refers to whether the basic steps or elements of the plan are being implemented. *Quality* refers to whether the plan is being implemented well (for instance, with precision and enthusiasm), as opposed to just perfunctorily. *Consistency* pertains to whether the plan is being implemented regularly, with elements being implemented at the times indicated by the plan, and *dosage* refers to the amount of intervention applied and whether the plan is being implemented with sufficient frequency, duration, and intensity.

The methods for collecting data on fidelity of implementation are numerous and, of course, they depend on the dimensions that are determined most important for a particular PBS intervention plan.

Kevin is able to tolerate some degree of variability in the consistency with which his interventions are utilized. However, he requires a high level of quality in the implementation of strategies associated with social interaction and perception training. Jolanda's communicative alternatives to problem behavior need to be prompted and reinforced with both consistency and frequency (i.e., dosage) in order to secure those skills as replacements.

....

With many plans, it is essential to assess the extent to which all the steps incorporated in the original plan and associated with high-quality application of the practice are implemented. This assessment of adherence is usually accomplished with a checklist that delineates the steps in the order in which they are to be implemented.

One of Kevin's intervention strategies includes a written activity schedule. The steps for presenting the schedule might include 1) directing his attention to the schedule, 2) prompting with a question (e.g., "Which activity is next?"), 3) waiting at least 10 seconds for a response, and 4) providing verbal acknowledgment of the identified activity and immediately encouraging him to transfer to the activity. The fidelity checklist would include these four steps, along with means of marking whether the step occurred.

....

Checklists are common for measuring fidelity adherence and can be used for most elements of an intervention plan.

Another dimension of fidelity that is often important to measure is dosage.

When learning functional communication skills, Jolanda needs to engage in numerous "practice trials" per day, across settings and situations. The team decided to measure dosage by counting the number of times that her mother, teacher, and behavior specialist prompt her to request attention, items or activities, or breaks throughout the day. A data collection system was designed to keep a tally of such occurrences—for instance, with a golf counter or on an index card. If the plan called for a minimum of 10 trials of each communication target, then the day's tally needs to meet those criteria. If fewer than 20 are recorded, a possible concern with fidelity would be identified.

....

Quality is another dimension that may be relevant when assessing fidelity. For instance, if a team determines that the effectiveness of an intervention will be affected by the enthusiasm with which a reinforcer is delivered, a rating scale could be devised to assess this dimension of fidelity. In a three-point scale, a "3" might indicate that the reinforcer was delivered in a genuine, intensive, and enthusiastic manner, while a "1" would signify that the reinforcer was provided with limited or no eye contact and with a totally dispassionate attitude. Rating scales are useful approaches to fidelity assessment as long as the anchors are described operationally so that observers can achieve reliability.

In addition to the methods described previously, fidelity can be assessed with other measurement strategies. The important features are that 1) the aspect of implementation that is being measured is viewed as the most essential aspect for the procedure to be effective and 2) the measurement strategy is feasible for the intervention team to carry out. And this leads to a key issue about who will be collecting the fidelity data. There are a variety of options, with one possibility being the same person who will be implementing the intervention—that is, self-recording. When the interventionist is self-recording fidelity, the measurement process can serve both as documentation of integrity and as a prompt to help ensure that implementation occurs with high fidelity. But when fidelity is expected or demonstrated to be a concern, then it is important to have a separate observer obtain the data, either in addition to or instead of the interventionist. This can help avoid bias and enhance the validity of the data. The separate observer can be a peer, a coach, a supervisor, or an external consultant.

PROGRESS MONITORING

Prior to implementing BSPs, the following should have occurred: 1) a baseline was established on the behaviors of concern, current status of skills in need of development, and indicators of quality of life being used to evaluate the outcomes; 2) the specific strategies to be used to support the individual's behavior based on the FBA were defined; and 3) the responsibilities for implementation and monitoring were assigned to PBS caregivers. If these things have been accomplished and the data collection methods are clear and reasonable, data-based decision making should be a straightforward process.

An essential element of PBS intervention plans is the collection of data to monitor progress. Progress-monitoring data are the means by which it is determined whether the rate and magnitude of change are satisfactory. The basic methods of defining and measuring behavior were covered in detail in Chapter 10, so this discussion is limited to issues regarding progress monitoring that are vital for implementation.

These issues include identifying priorities among desired outcomes, selecting suitable targets for data collection, and establishing data-collection strategies that are valid, useful, and efficient.

Identifying Priorities

The majority of multielement PBS intervention plans have numerous goals, including primary and secondary outcomes and short- and long-term objectives. However, there are limits to the number of behaviors that can be measured simultaneously and, therefore, the intervention team must distinguish between those urgent behaviors that should be monitored very frequently (e.g., daily) and those behaviors that can be tracked with occasional (e.g., weekly) probes. Levels of urgency are usually easy to determine; however, it is still important for the team to devote deliberate planning to prioritization of goals and behaviors of concern. The most urgent behaviors almost always include the primary reason for the plan being established in the first place, such as violent or dangerous behaviors or behaviors that dramatically disrupt the valued family routines or the learning or working environment (e.g., high-pitched screaming). It is also a good idea to place a high priority on vital or critical skills (e.g., functional communication, tolerance for delays) that are targeted as prosocial replacements for the targeted problem and skills that will allow the individual greater access to his or her community and improve social relationships.

Selecting Targets for Data Collection

When priorities have been established, the most urgent behaviors need to be operationally defined and methods need to be established for monitoring their levels on an ongoing basis. Operational definitions include the context in which the skill is needed, the specific change in behavior expected, and the criteria for success (Cooper, Heron, & Heward, 2007). We usually recommend that frequent data collection be

focused on at least one behavior that is targeted to be reduced and at least one behavior that is targeted to be increased in frequency or established through instruction.

Jolanda's priorities include recording acts of aggression toward herself, others, or property and communicative requests using her augmentative system. In addition, some of Jolanda's other behaviors that are targeted to be reduced (e.g., leaving bedroom at night, inappropriate social interactions) and increased (e.g., independent completion of daily living activities) will also be monitored, although the frequency and intensity of data collection will be less frequent and less formal than the most urgent behavior targets.

....

Finally, it is also essential to monitor data that represent aspects of the person's quality of life (Schalock & Verdugo, 2002). Specifically, teams would use objective information to determine whether the individual's relationships, community participation, independence in daily activities, opportunities for decision making, and overall satisfaction and happiness improve. A good way to track improvements in quality of life is to revisit the individual's person-centered plan at least once per year. For both Kevin and Jolanda, we would be interested in monitoring their levels of participation in daily activities and quality of social interactions with peers. Assessing quality of life can be a complex undertaking, requiring a deeper level of planning (e.g., Kincaid & Fox, 2002), and it ordinarily involves longitudinal, rather than short-term, outcomes (see Chapter 13; Dunlap, Kincaid, & Jackson, forthcoming).

Data Collection Strategies

In deciding how to collect the data needed for progress monitoring, there are several considerations that must be taken into account. A first set of considerations is that the data to be collected must be accurate, reliable, and have face validity—that is, the data that are obtained must truly represent what is actually happening, and they must reflect what is most important in the behavior change process. A second critical consideration is that the data collection strategies must be practical and feasible. The systems of data collection need to be designed with a full awareness of who will be observing and recording the data, how much time it will take, and whether it is possible for the designated observers to collect valid data in the context of their other responsibilities.

One relatively simple method for collecting useful progress monitoring data involves the use of rating scales. This strategy requires only that an observer make a rating of the magnitude of behavior over a period of time, such as an instructional session, a morning, or even a whole day. The ratings are on a perceptual scale, often from 1 to 5, with the anchors operationalized so that there is optimal agreement among observers. These behavior scales (e.g., daily report cards) can correlate well with direct observations, and they can be reliable as long as the anchors are well defined (e.g., Chafouleas, Riley-Tillman, & Sassu, 2006; Dunlap, Wilson, Strain, & Lee, 2013; Iovannone, Greenbaum, Wang, Kincaid, & Dunlap, 2013). Rating scales are convenient and valuable options for progress monitoring, especially when resources for data collection are limited.

Kevin attends an inclusive preschool classroom with 20 children, one teacher, and one instructional aide. The data collection strategy would need to be developed with the understanding that there would be no dedicated observer and that any data recording would have to be conducted within the ongoing responsibilities of the two adults in the classroom. Some data collection techniques that require close and frequent observation, such as interval or duration recording, would be impractical; however, a rating scale to indicate the quality of interactions with his peers each day might be feasible. For Jolanda, on the other hand, data collection would be designed with the recognition that the funding allows for an individual instructional aide at school and a behavior analyst who comes to the house four times per week. Her direct service providers would be able to collect data on individual functional communication training (FCT) probes, performance on the steps of task analyses on daily living skills, and each incident of aggression, possibly using a handheld device to produce immediate graphs. Obviously, the plans for monitoring the effects of Kevin's and Jolanda's interventions would be quite different.

....

DATA-BASED DECISION MAKING

Data collected to monitor fidelity and outcomes of intervention must be synthesized, analyzed, and reviewed to inform ongoing decision making. The formality and frequency of these data reviews will necessarily vary across circumstances. In some cases, it may be necessary to hold regular meetings with all PBS caregivers; in others, these contacts may be organized around typical reporting processes (e.g., grading periods, progress reports) interspersed with periodic e-mails or phone calls, as needed. Agencies, insurance companies, and intensive school programs often require relatively elaborate reports at least quarterly containing data on each individual goal within the individual's plan. Regardless of the nature of these reviews, it is important that they occur regularly, that the data reviewed are objective and relevant, and that the reviews drive data-based decision making.

With every plan, there will be expectations regarding the time lines and magnitude of the anticipated behavior change. It is therefore helpful to create decision rules for gauging a plan's success and making changes based on the data trends. The review period should be based on the frequency of the behaviors of concern and opportunities to practice new skills. For high-rate behaviors, more frequent (e.g., weekly) reviews are indicated. For low rate behaviors, it is more appropriate to evaluate outcomes on a monthly or quarterly basis. For example, a PBS team might decide that the behaviors of concern need to diminish by at least 50% within the first month to continue implementing the plan as designed or that an individual needs to master certain social and communication skills before introducing them to additional settings or challenging situations.

The characteristics of the individual, the history of their behavior, the consistency of the team implementing the strategies, and the specific features of the behavior plan may all affect responsiveness to intervention. For example, longstanding patterns in which problem behavior was intermittently reinforced are usually more resistant to change. High-quality instruction is likely to produce the most rapid improvements. Preventive strategies are often associated with immediate change, whereas learning new skills occurs more gradually. In some cases, behavior escalation can occur temporarily when reinforcers the individual is accustomed to obtaining as a result of their problem behavior are being withheld. As PBS plans are characterized by a combination of these components, it is likely that their overall effectiveness will be enhanced and unwanted results will be minimized.

The primary questions driving data-based decision making in PBS should include the following: Is the plan being implemented as designed and consistently? Are the interventions producing the desired results in terms of changes in behavior and quality of life? If the answers to both of these questions are "yes," then the plan should continue to be utilized and strategies for generalization and maintenance should be planned. If the answer to one or both of the questions is "no," then problem solving is in order.

ENSURING FIDELITY OF PLAN IMPLEMENTATION

As mentioned previously, implementation fidelity may be evaluated via direct observation (e.g., using a fidelity checklist). In addition, it may be assessed indirectly by reviewing documentation and other permanent products or measures. It may also be beneficial to survey caregivers periodically, asking them to assess their perceived level of integrity to components of the BSP. If sufficient fidelity

data have been collected, the interventionists should be able to identify the elements of the plan or the times and contexts in which implementation is superior and those in which it is inadequate in its adherence, frequency (dosage), consistency, or quality.

Variability in data collected on outcome measures for the individual that is not consistent with particular setting events may also indicate inconsistency in plan implementation. Looking for this variability and tracking fidelity data allow PBS caregivers to determine if certain features of the behavior plan are being implemented consistently while other strategies are only adhered to sporadically. The data may indicate that some caregivers are using the plan with greater integrity than others. Fidelity may also diminish over time. All these patterns might indicate that the plan or aspects of the plan have diminished acceptability of the interventions or that additional instruction and reinforcement is warranted.

It is unclear how much deviation in implementation is allowable with regard to affecting outcomes, but if diminished fidelity data correlate with deterioration in the individual's behavior, PBS caregivers need to identify and address specific logistical or motivational barriers leading to this breakdown. For example, observations of plan implementation or discussions with caregivers may help the team identify and resolve a lack of necessary resources, competing priorities, or other issues contributing to fidelity problems. (See preceding sections related to contextual fit and engaging caregivers for other possible explanations.)

Using Data to Track Progress and Resolve Problems

Ongoing data collection and analysis provides tangible evidence of progress but also an opportunity for problem-solving when improvements are insufficient. A question that should be continually asked is whether the data being collected are capturing what is intended and important. It is not uncommon to initiate strategies for tracking progress, only to determine later that they are not useful in evaluating outcomes. For example, teachers could be tracking the percentage of assignments completed when accuracy or rate of completion provides a better indicator of academic performance. In that case, they should be adjusted. Accuracy of data collection is, of course, essential to tracking progress toward desired goals.

Data on behaviors targeted for increase or decrease should be graphed to analyze trends. These graphs may be maintained daily, weekly, or even monthly, depending on the frequency of the behavior of concern. If no progress is being made or changes are occurring in the wrong direction, it is clear that the plan should be discontinued right away and the interventions reevaluated. If there is variability in the data, this may indicate that 1) the data are being collected inconsistently, 2) the plan is not being implemented as designed in all circumstances, or 3) there are setting events affecting the individual's behavior that may need to be addressed. It may be necessary to repeat aspects of the analysis or the entire FBA in order to develop more appropriate strategies.

In examining the graphs of Jolanda's use of FCT skills, it may be evident that she is consistently requesting items and activities with both signs and her augmentative communication device but rarely using either of these to avoid undesirable activities. This would drive the team to reassess how they are teaching her to request a break and, given her progress with requests, might indicate that they can begin introducing brief waiting periods before receiving items or activities.

In Kevin's situation, the team is rating the quality of interactions he has with his peers. If his team finds that high-quality interactions only occur with one or two children or around particular activities, they may want to examine those situations more closely. Reviewing data such as these allows PBS teams to determine whether sufficient progress is occurring, modify aspects of the social or physical environment, tweak instructional practices, or modify reinforcers or their schedule of delivery to improve outcomes.

In addition to reviewing progress related to skill development and reductions in behaviors of concern, teams will want to examine changes in overall quality of life. Asking questions such as these might keep teams focused on the most meaningful outcomes: Is the child going more places or doing more things? Do more peers identify the child as their friend? Has the child become more independent in daily routines? Do the child and family report reduced levels of stress?

Planning in Response to Progress

If an individual is making continual improvements in both behavior and quality of life as a result of consistent plan implementation, it is necessary to determine how to gradually increase the expectations for independence and how to gradually reduce supports. A standard that has been suggested in the Prevent-Teach-Reinforce model is that the plan should remain in place for at least the same duration as the history of the behavior of concern. That does not mean, however, that criteria for performance cannot be increased and that supports must be maintained at the original level. Determining how to maximize natural cues and contingencies through better engagement of typical caregivers should be a basic feature of the data-based decision-making process.

As Jolanda develops more proficiency with her basic functional communication skills, her team considers broadening the goals to include a greater variety of conversational and leisure skills. These skills will be identified based on the data (e.g., where she is most and least successful). The focus for Kevin might shift to self-management and peer-mediated supports, which will lessen the need for service providers and reduce barriers to full integration.

CONCLUSION

The effective implementation of multielement PBS plans is an endeavor worthy of careful planning and diligence. Regardless of the precision and quality with which the plan is designed, it will not be effective unless it is implemented with fidelity, and implementing with fidelity requires attention to a number of contextual variables as well as data collection. In this chapter, we have reviewed those variables that are known to affect implementation and have discussed strategies for enhancing fidelity and the likelihood of favorable outcomes. The greater the care with which we engage in implementation, the more probable the benefits that will result from PBS.

REFERENCES

Albin, R.W., Lucyshyn, J.M., Horner, R.H., & Flannery, K.B. (1996). Contextual fit for behavior support plans: A model for "goodness of fit." In L.K. Koegel, R.L. Koegel, & G. Dunlap (Eds.), *Positive behavioral support: Including people with difficult behavior in the community* (pp. 81–98). Baltimore, MD: Paul H. Brookes Publishing Co.

Allen, K.D., & Warzak, W.J. (2000). The problem of parental nonadherence in clinical behavior analysis: Effective treatment is not enough. *Journal of Applied Behavior Analysis, 33,* 373–391.

Baker, B.L., Blacher, J., & Olsson, M.B. (2005). Preschool children with and without developmental delay: Behaviour problems, parents' optimism and well-being. *Journal of Intellectual Disability Research, 49,* 575–590.

Billingsley, F., White, O.R., & Munson, R. (1980). Procedural reliability: A rationale and example. *Behavioral Assessment, 2,* 229–241.

Carr, E.G., Dunlap, G., Horner, R.H., Koegel, R.L., Turnbull, A.P., Sailor, W., . . . Fox, L. (2002). Positive behavior support: Evolution of an applied science. *Journal of Positive Behavior Interventions, 4,* 4–16.

Chafouleas, S.M., Riley-Tillman, T.C., & Sassu, K.A. (2006). Acceptability and reported use of daily behavior report cards among teachers. *Journal of Positive Behavior Interventions, 8,* 174–182.

Charlop-Christy, M.H., & Carpenter, M.H. (2000). Modified incidental teaching sessions: A procedure for parents to increase spontaneous speech in their children with autism. *Journal of Positive Behavior Interventions, 2,* 98–112.

Cooper, J.O., Heron, T.E., & Heward, W.L. (2007). *Applied behavior analysis* (2nd ed.). Upper Saddle River, NJ: Pearson.

Dunlap, G., Kincaid, D., & Jackson, D. (forthcoming). Positive behavior support: Foundations, systems, and quality of life. In M. Wehmeyer (Ed.), *The Oxford handbook of positive psychology and disability.* New York, NY: Oxford University Press.

Dunlap, G., Wilson, K., Strain, P., & Lee, J.K. (2013). *Prevent-teach-reinforce for young children: The early childhood model of individualized positive behavior support.* Baltimore, MD: Paul H. Brookes Publishing Co.

Durand, V.M. (1990). *Severe behavior problems: A functional communication training approach.* New York, NY: Guilford Press.

Durand, V.M., & Hieneman, M. (2008). *Helping parents with challenging children: Positive family intervention: Facilitator guide/parent workbook.* Oxford, UK: Oxford University Press.

Durand, V.M., Hieneman, M., Clarke, S., Wang, M., & Rinaldi, M.L. (2013). Positive family intervention for severe challenging behavior I: A multisite randomized clinical trial. *Journal of Positive Behavior Interventions , 15*(3), 133–143.

Durlak, J.A., & DuPre, E.P. (2008). Implementation matters: A review of research on the influence of implementation on program outcomes and the factors affecting outcomes. *American Journal of Community Psychology, 41,* 327–350.

Emerson, E., Kiernan, C., Alborz, A., Reeves, D., Mason, H., Swarbrick, R., . . . Hatton, C. (2001). Predicting the persistence of severe self-injurious behavior. *Research in Developmental Disabilities, 22,* 67–75.

Erbas, D. (2010). A collaborative approach to implement positive behavior support plans for children with problem behaviors: A comparison of consultation versus consultation and feedback approach. *Education and Training in Autism and Developmental Disabilities, 45,* 94–106.

Fox, L., Dunlap, G., Hemmeter, M.L., Joseph, G.E., & Strain, P.S. (2003). The teaching pyramid: A model for supporting social competence and preventing challenging behavior in young children. *Young Children, 58,* 48–52.

Goh, A.E., & Bambara, L.M. (2012). Individualized positive behavior support in school settings: A meta-analysis. *Remedial and Special Education, 33,* 271–286.

Hastings, R.P. (2002). Parental stress and behavior problems of children with developmental disability. *Journal of Intellectual and Developmental Disability, 27*(3), 149–160.

Head, L.S., & Abbeduto, L. (2007). Recognizing the role of parents in developmental outcomes: A systems approach to evaluating the child with developmental disabilities. *Mental Retardation and Developmental Disabilities Research Reviews, 13,* 293–301.

Hieneman, M., Childs, K., & Sergay, J. (2006). *Parenting with positive behavior support: A practical guide to resolving your child's difficult behavior.* Baltimore, MD: Paul H. Brookes Publishing Co.

Hieneman, M., & Dunlap, G. (2000). Factors affecting the outcomes of community-based behavioral support: I. Factor category importance. *Journal of Positive Behavior Interventions, 3,* 67–74.

Hieneman, M., & Dunlap, G. (2001). Factors affecting the outcomes of community-based behavioral support: II. Identification and description of factor categories. *Journal of Positive Behavior Interventions, 2*(3), 161–169.

Hieneman, M., Dunlap, G., & Kincaid, D. (2005). Positive support strategies for students with behavior disorders in general education settings. *Psychology in the Schools, 42,* 779–794.

Horner, R., Sugai, G., Todd, A., & Lewis-Palmer, T. (1999–2000). Elements of behavior support plans. *Exceptionality, 8*(3), 205–216.

Iovannone, R., Greenbaum, P., Wang, W., Kincaid, D., & Dunlap, G. (forthcoming). Reliability of an individualized behavior rating scale tool for progress monitoring. *Assessment for Effective Intervention.*

Johnson, C.R., Handen, B.L., Butter, E., et al. (2007). Development of a parent training program for children with pervasive developmental disorders. *Behavioral Interventions, 22,* 201–221.

Kincaid, D., & Fox, L. (2002). Person-centered planning and positive behavior support. In S. Holburn & P.M. Vietze (Eds.), *Person-centered planning: Research, practice, and future directions* (pp. 29–50). Baltimore, MD: Paul H. Brookes Publishing Co.

Koegel, R.L., & Koegel, L.K. (2006). *Pivotal response treatments for autism: Communication, social, and academic development.* Baltimore, MD: Paul H. Brookes Publishing Co.

Koegel, R.L., Streibel, D., & Koegel, L.K. (1998). Reducing aggression in children with autism toward infant or toddler siblings. *Journal of The Association for Persons with Severe Handicaps, 23,* 111–118.

Lucyshyn, J.M., Albin, R.W., Horner, R.H., Mann, J.C., Mann, J.A., & Wadsworth, G. (2007). Family implementation of positive behavior support for a child with autism. *Journal of Positive Behavior Interventions, 9*(3), 131–150.

Lucyshyn, J., Binnendyk, L., Fossett, B., Cheremshynski, C., Lohrmann, S., Elkinson, L., & Miller, L. (2009). Toward and ecological unity of analysis in behavioral assessment and intervention with families of children with developmental disabilities. In W. Sailor, G. Dunlap, G. Sugai, & R. Horner (Eds.), *Handbook of Positive Behavior Support* (pp. 73–100). New York, NY: Springer.

Maughan, D.R., Christiansen, E., Jenson, W.R., Olympia, D., & Clark, E. (2005). Behavioral parent training as a treatment for externalizing behaviors and disruptive behavior disorders. *School Psychology Review, 34,* 267–286.

McEachin, J.J., Smith, T., & Lovaas, O.I. (1993). Long-term outcome for children with autism who received early intensive behavioral treatment. *American Journal of Mental Retardation, 97,* 359–372.

McNeill, S.L., Watson, T.S., Henington, C., & Meeks, C. (2002). The effects of training parents in functional behavior assessment on problem identification, problem analysis, and intervention design. *Behavior Modification, 26,* 499–515.

Moes, D.R., & Frea, W.D. (2002). Contextualized behavioral support in early intervention for children with autism and their families. *Journal of Autism and Developmental Disorders, 32,* 519–533.

O'Donnell, C.R., Tharp, R.G., & Wilson, K. (1993). Activity settings as the unit of analysis: A theoretical basis for community intervention and development. *American Journal of Community Psychology, 21,* 501–520.

Patterson, G.R. (1982). *Coercive family process.* Eugene, OR: Castalia.

Peterson, S.M., Derby, K.M., Berg, W.K., & Horner, R.H. (2002). Collaboration with families in the functional behavioral assessment of and intervention for severe behavior problems. *Education and Treatment of Children, 25,* 5–25.

Sailor, W., Dunlap, G., Sugai, G., & Horner, R.H. (2009). *Handbook of positive behavior support.* New York, NY: Springer.

Sarakoff, R.A., & Sturmey, P. (2004). The effects of behavioral skills training on staff implementation of discrete trial teaching. *Journal of Applied Behavior Analysis, 37,* 535–538.

Schalock, R., & Verdugo, M.A. (2002). *Handbook on quality of life for human service practitioners.* Washington, DC: American Association on Mental Retardation.

Shaeffer, A., Kotchich, B.A., Dorsey, S., & Forehand, R. (2001). The past, present, and future of behavioral parent training: Interventions for child and adolescent problem behavior. *Behavior Analyst Today, 2,* 91–105.

Snell, M.E., & Brown, F. (2011). *Instruction of students with severe disabilities* (7th ed.). Upper Saddle River, NJ: Pearson.

Steed, E.A., & Durand, V.M. (2012). Optimistic teaching: Improving the capacity for teachers to reduce young children's challenging behavior. *School Mental Health, 5*(1), 15–24.

Strain, P.S., & Kohler, F.W. (1998). Peer-mediated social intervention for young children with autism. *Seminars in Speech and Language, 19,* 391–405.

Sundberg, M.L., & Partington, J.W. (1998). *Teaching language to children with autism or other developmental disabilities.* Concord, CA: AVB Press.

Vaughn, B., Dunlap, G., Fox, L., Clarke, S., & Bucy, M. (1997). Parent-professional partnership in behavioral support: A case study of community-based intervention. *Journal of The Association for Persons with Severe Handicaps, 22,* 186–197.

Walker, H.M., Horner, R.H., Sugai, G., Bullis, M., Sprague, J.R., Bricker, D., et al. (1996). Integrated approaches to preventing antisocial behavior patterns among school-age children and youth. *Journal of Emotional and Behavioral Disorders, 4,* 194–209.

Westling, D.L., & Fox, L. (2009). *Teaching students with severe disabilities* (4th ed.). Upper Saddle River, NJ: Pearson.

Cultural and Contextual Fit

Juan's Family as Active Team Members

Bobbie J. Vaughn and Lise K. Fox

24

This chapter provides an illustration of the use of positive behavior support (PBS) with a farm-worker family from Mexico and their child, Juan. The chapter illustrates the necessity for blending cultural competence as a part of contextual fit throughout the PBS process. In many schools, there is a growing population of families from ethnically, linguistically, and culturally diverse backgrounds. This diversity can present challenges to parent and family involvement in traditional school culture and school processes (Chen, Downing, Peckham-Hardin, 2002; Sugai, O'Keeffe, & Fallon, 2012; Wang, McCart, & Turnbull, 2007). Juan's case study provides descriptions of how school personnel can use culturally competent approaches in their collaboration with families to ensure the development of an effective and contextually appropriate behavior support plan (BSP).

As reported in the 2010 Census, a large proportion (37.3%) of the 308.7 million people in the Unites States were from Native American, African American, Hispanic, Asian, and non-European backgrounds (U.S. Census Bureau, 2011). While growth in the total U.S. population was 9.7% between 2000 and 2010, the growth among diverse ethnic groups was much greater, with growth in the Hispanic population by 43% and the Asian population by 43.3%.

In addition, there are large numbers of immigrants in the United States, with one in five people being first- or second-generation U.S. residents. The changing demographics of the nation have critical implications for schools, with increased diversity in the student population and many students coming from homes where English is not the primary language. There has also been growth in the numbers of children living in poverty, with 5.7 million living in poverty in 2010 (Annie E. Casey, 2012). The greatest numbers of children in poverty are children who are Hispanic or Latino (Annie E. Casey, 2012). Changes in the demographics of the school population indicate that schools must reevaluate their approach to parent engagement and support as they strive to collaborate with families to provide effective educational programs.

Research has indicated that higher risks for challenging behavior are associated with families living in poverty (Leventhal & Brooks-Gunn, 2011; Qi & Kaiser, 2003). Providing behavior support to children from diverse families requires an approach that incorporates cultural competence, including understanding and considering family values, beliefs, traditions, and ecology (e.g., socioeconomic status, lifestyle, and family structure) into the behavior support process (Albin, Lucyshyn, Horner, & Flannery 1996; Carr et al., 2002; Lucyshyn, Horner, Dunlap, Albin, & Ben, 2002). The consideration of family factors contributes to the process of establishing contextual fit in the behavior support process. Contextual fit, an essential element of PBS, refers to the use of the PBS process and the development of BSPs that are a "fit" for the individual, family, and unique settings where behavior support will be implemented (Lucyshyn et al., 2002). Attending to contextual fit is particularly critical for the implementation of PBS by families who have complex needs and struggle to support their children with persistent challenging behavior (Vaughn, Wilson, White, & Dunlap, 2002; Vaughn, Dunlap, Clarke, Fox, & Bucy, 1997). When utilized in the behavior support process, contextual fit creates compatibility between the behavior support process and plan and family needs. Contextual fit is addressed through the acceptance of family cultural and linguistic preferences, the development of collaborative partnerships, the consideration of family ecology, the examination of issues related to the feasibility of implementation, and the development of behavior supports that include the improvement of quality of life (McLaughlin, Denney, Snyder, & Welsh, 2012).

In this chapter, Juan's story illustrates the use of cultural competence and contextual fit with a family who came to the United States from Mexico and worked as migrant farm workers. At the time when the BSP was developed, Juan and his family had permanently located in a community in the southeastern United States and no longer moved to follow seasonal work. In the presentation of Juan's BSP, we discuss the manner in which the preschool program staff established a partnership with Juan's family and engaged in collaborative teaming to develop an effective BSP that resolved school issues and supported the family with issues at home.

THE POSITIVE BEHAVIOR SUPPORT PROCESS WITH JUAN AND HIS FAMILY

Juan was a 3-year-old Hispanic boy who experienced developmental delays. His parents initially became concerned about his play skills, challenging behavior, and language development when it seemed he did not meet developmental milestones at the same age as his siblings. Friends at their church gave them a phone number to call and request an evaluation from a Child Find (20 U.S.C. 1412[a][3]; i.e., a mandate from Individuals with Disabilities Education Improvement Act (IDEA) of 2004 (PL 108-446), special education law, that states must identify and evaluate all children with disabilities birth through 21 years) team. The Child Find team included a bilingual psychologist and speech pathologist who conducted the evaluation in both English and Spanish. The evaluation team determined that Juan was eligible for early childhood special education services for autism spectrum disorder. During the evaluation, Juan also demonstrated disruptive behaviors when asked to change activities and during difficult tasks. The behaviors they observed included crying, falling to the floor, refusing to move, pulling away when physically prompted to stand, throwing objects, and running away. Juan's parents indicated that they saw the same behaviors at home. The team recommended enrolling Juan in a blended preschool classroom for children with and without disabilities with English for speakers of other language (ESOL) supports.

Juan's Family

Juan lived with his mother and father, who are vegetable and fruit farmers; his grandmother; and his two older brothers. His mother and father farmed all their lives and attended school sporadically as they were growing up in Mexico. His father spoke and understood English fairly well but did not read well in English or Spanish. Juan's mother spoke and read primarily Spanish. His grandmother did not read and only spoke Spanish. They had a three-bedroom house with an open kitchen and living area. All the children shared one bedroom. Juan's family lived on the land they farmed and rented from the land owner. In previous years, Juan's family traveled the United States from south to north to farm but had recently decided to stay in their community to work year round in one location. Juan's parents wanted their children to receive a stable education, especially with Juan's developmental and behavioral struggles.

Juan's Behavior at Preschool

Juan's parents knew that preschool would be challenging for him. They were anxious about his first day of school, as he experienced severe tantrums when going to new settings. They had experienced this with Juan in going to stores and other community outings. This was very embarrassing for his family. They were concerned that his teacher might not want Juan in her classroom when she saw his disruptive behaviors.

On the first day of school, Juan screamed and cried and threw himself on the ground as he approached the building. Juan's father had to pick him up and carry him into the classroom. He was worried Juan would not be allowed to stay. The teacher encouraged Juan's parents to leave and assured them that he would adjust and settle into the classroom routine. Juan screamed and cried before each

new activity, and during center time, he threw toys at the other children.

Although Juan's teacher was hopeful that he would adjust after a few weeks in the classroom, Juan remained disruptive during transitions and aggressive toward other children. He continued to scream and resist transitions, and without fail, Juan would throw toys during center time and other preschool activities that involved interactions or play with other children.

Juan's preschool teacher called a meeting with the behavior specialist and asked her to come in to observe Juan throughout the day. The behavior specialist wanted to observe activities where he had problems as well as those activities where he was successful. She understood that activities without problems were just as important to analyze as those with problems.

Juan's Behavior at Home

Juan also experienced similar behavior problems at home. He often grabbed toys from his brothers and would interfere with their outside play. When his brothers played ball outside, he would take the ball and run away with it. When they took it back, Juan would throw himself on the ground, screaming and crying. Juan would also tantrum during transitions and became aggressive with his parents and grandmother when they persisted in trying to gain his cooperation.

Step 1: Identifying Goals

The first step of the PBS process involved team building and the identification of team goals. The development of a well-functioning collaborative team is a key to effective PBS. Family members are a critical component of the team since they are regarded as "their child's most powerful, valuable, and durable resource" (Dunlap & Robbins, 1991, p. 188). Including family members in collaborative teams is important and valuable but not necessarily simple. Collaboration requires effort from all team members.

The PBS process for Juan began when his preschool special education teacher and his ESOL teachers contacted the behavior specialist and social worker about Juan's challenging behavior. They felt that Juan's behaviors were serious enough to warrant some additional help from people experienced in supporting students with challenging behavior. They wanted to form a team with Juan's family to help make decisions about how to support Juan over the next year. The ESOL teacher and the bilingual paraprofessional volunteered to call Juan's parents since they are not fluent in English. The paraprofessional explained to them in Spanish that the school was concerned about Juan's behavior and were interested in knowing what they experienced at home but, more important, what they wanted for Juan's future. The school proposed a meeting to plan for his future and asserted to the family that their participation was essential because of their understanding of Juan. The family was pleased that people wanted to help Juan but felt hesitant about the meeting.

Juan's teachers talked with the school principal about Juan's situation and explained that they established a team to help Juan and wanted to encourage his parents' participation on the team. The teachers and other team members wanted the flexibility to hold the meeting at a time and place comfortable for Juan's parents. The principal agreed to allow the staff to meet off campus and offered a small stipend to the team for their "after-hours" effort. The family and school staff met at the neighborhood recreation center close to

the family's house at 7:00 p.m., when both parents could attend. They agreed to only meet for an hour and a half, at the family's request. The recreation center provided a meeting room at no cost, and there were toys and games to entertain Juan's siblings during the meeting.

The team used a person-centered planning (PCP) process (see Chapters 3 and 4), called *personal futures planning,* as the first step in the PBS process. Juan's parents, his grandmother, and the school professionals all participated in the meeting. The school felt that including the grandmother was important because she often took care of Juan and his brothers while the parents worked. The goal of the PCP process was to understand his family's vision for Juan's future, learn more about his life, and gain insight into the family's values and beliefs in relation to Juan's education. PCP results in "maps" that portray aspects and goals of Juan's life. Since the family felt more comfortable speaking Spanish, the ESOL teacher translated orally in English and wrote both in Spanish and in English on the maps. The first piece of chart paper or "map" was titled "Who is Juan?" In response to that map, team members and Juan described Juan's unique interests and personality traits. The ESOL teacher captured the team members' reflections with pictures and words. The next map read "Juan's life," and the additional maps were "Who are the people in Juan's life?," "What works, what doesn't?," "Vision for this school year," and "Where do we start?"(see Table 24.1). By the end of meeting, the family felt

Table 24.1.   Juan's and his family's vision

- Have friends and be invited to parties
- *Tener amigos y ser invitado a fiestas*
- Learn to play with brothers and other friends
- *Aprender jugar con sus hermanos y otros amigos*
- Increase his flexibility with change
- *Aumentar su flexibilidad con cambios*
- Learn to accept going to new places
- *Aprender a aceptar ir a lugares nuevos*

Source: University of South Florida Family Involvement in Functional Assessment Project (2004).

more comfortable about the team process. They left feeling understood and supported by the school. The school team members felt that they had a better understanding of Juan, Juan's family life, the potential for supporting him, and how behavior issues affected his life at home and school.

Step 2: Information Gathering

Juan's family members were important partners in the information gathering or functional assessment process. They were able to bring a unique source of knowledge about Juan's behavior at home and in the community. The information that they brought to the process was key to the development of an effective behavior plan.

In the week following the PCP meeting, the ESOL teacher and behavior specialist called the family to ask whether they could visit them in their home to discuss Juan's behavior at home and in the community. Because the family felt supported at the PCP meeting and had developed rapport with the rest of the team, they felt comfortable with the school team visiting the home. The behavior specialist mailed the family English and Spanish versions of the functional behavioral assessment (FBA) interview for the family to review prior to the meeting. The interview was sent to the family to increase the family's comfort with the questions that would be asked during the FBA process. The ESOL teacher, behavior specialist, and an ESOL assistant (for translation) scheduled a home visit at a time convenient for the family. The school staff assured the family that the information gathered would help everyone better understand Juan's challenging behavior.

The functional assessment included an interview with the family and teachers. When conducting the interview with the family, the staff explained to the family how each section of the interview provided information that would help everyone understand and support Juan both at home and at school. They used a form that asked about the type of challenging behaviors Juan exhibited at home; his physical state (e.g., sleep, eating habits, fatigue, illness, medication); specific events, people or places that upset him (e.g., new places, changes in schedule, play); his communication and social skills; and how people respond to him and what he gets from their response (e.g., time-out, removal from activity, scolding). The school team members explained that this process had a "formal" name (FBA), but the questions really provided a structure for discussing the events associated with Juan's behavior. They explained that this interview process helped the team understand the events that triggered and maintained Juan's challenging behavior. The school team also respectfully included questions during the interview that helped them understand the family's beliefs and values on discipline and child rearing in general. They believed it was important to understand the family's lifestyle and values when thinking about Juan's current challenges.

When the interview was completed, the school team members provided the family with a simple behavior checklist in Spanish. The checklist offered a behavior rating scale that could be completed by the family to provide information on Juan's behaviors across activities that occurred at home. To complete the scale, the family only needed to write a number beside each activity across the week (see Figure 24.1). The school staff explained that keeping track of the difficult activities and the behavior at home provided them with important information that would help in the behavior support process.

The team set a date for the next meeting, which would be held 2 weeks later at the school. They scheduled it at the school on an afternoon before the school-sponsored family barbeque. They wanted to help the family feel comfortable meeting other families and offset travel expenses by providing an evening meal. They told the family that they could bring all family members, including Juan's siblings, in an effort to ensure attendance and create a sense of comfort.

CHILD BEHAVIOR HOME AND SCHOOL ROUTINE CHECKLIST

Insert activities in the left-hand column as they occur throughout the day. Select the number that best describes the behavior, and place it in the box next to the activity by day.

1	2	3	4
Not at all	Seldom	Frequently	Excessively
(Casi nunca)	(Pocas veces)	(Frecuentemente)	(Excesivamente)

Daily routines (Rutinas diarias)	Monday (Lunes) Date (Fecha) _____	Tuesday (Martes) Date (Fecha) _____	Wednesday (Miércoles) Date (Fecha) _____	Thursday (Jueves) Date (Fecha) _____	Friday (Viernes) Date (Fecha) _____
Afterschool play (Juegos después de la escuela)	4	3	3	4	
Bath (Bañarse)	2	1	1	2	
Mealtime (Hora de comer)	1	1	1	1	
Television	1	1	1	1	
Bedtime (Hora de dormir)	3	2	2	3	
Leaving in the car to go out (Montarse en el auto para salir)	4	4	4	4	

Figure 24.1.   Child behavior home and school routine checklist.

Source: University of South Florida Family Involvement in Functional Assessment Project (2004).

In *Individual Positive Behavior Supports: A Standards-Based Guide to Practices in School and Community Settings,* edited by Fredda Brown, Jacki L. Anderson, and Randall L. De Pry. Copyright © 2015 by Paul H. Brookes Publishing Co. All rights reserved.

Step 3: Hypothesis Development

During the meeting at school, the school team and family met to develop hypotheses about Juan's behavior and discuss the design of the BSP. The meeting was held in a large conference room where the school team served some drinks and snacks. They put their hypothesis framework on chart paper on the wall to support the participation of all team members. They wanted this meeting to be casual and interactive. The principal arranged for two paraprofessionals to stay with Juan and his siblings in a classroom where they played and used the computer.

The behavior specialist facilitated the development of the hypotheses by summarizing the functional assessment interviews and observations that had been provided by various team members. The team discussed what things "set off" or triggered the challenging behaviors (i.e., play, transitions), the behaviors associated with the specific triggers (i.e., crying, screaming, throwing things, throwing himself down, hitting others), and finally how the teachers and parents were responding to Juan's behaviors (e.g., move him away from other children, time-out, remove him from the activity). From this information, they hypothesized the function of Juan's behavior. As the behavior specialist led the discussion about the hypotheses, she carefully described the categories on the chart paper and what they meant. The ESOL teacher's paraprofessional wrote and orally translated in Spanish. The behavior specialist said that, from the interviews and the team's feedback, play and transitions seemed to be the contexts where there were triggers for the behaviors. The observations and data from the family and school team gave further insight into the antecedents, the nature of the behavior, and the maintaining consequences that occurred in those contexts.

When the team finished their discussion, the hypotheses provided a starting point for the BSP. In particular, it was clear that Juan wanted to be around other children, but his delayed language contributed to his inability to join in play. At home, the family related a similar situation in how Juan disrupted play with his brothers. The family was afraid his brothers would not want to be around him and that Juan might not have any friends. After some discussion, the team developed two hypotheses related to Juan's behavior at school and two hypotheses related to Juan's behavior at home (see Table 24.2).

Table 24.2. Hypotheses for Juan

Setting (Lugar)	Hypothesis (Hipotesis)
School (Escuela)	When Juan transitions to new places or changes activities, he cries and screams and throws himself down in an effort to avoid activity change. *(Cuando Juan hace una transición a lugares nuevos o cambia actividades, él llora y grita y se tira al piso para evitar el cambio en actividad.)*
School (Escuela)	When Juan wants to play with a group of children during center time play, he throws blocks or disrupts play activities to get attention from peers. *(Cuando Juan quiere jugar con un grupo de niños durante centros o otros tiempos de jugar, él tira bloques o interrumpe las actividades de juego para obtener atención de su compañeros.)*
Home (Casa)	When Juan tries to join his brothers in outside play, he will take their ball and run away. When corrected, Juan screams, cries, and throws himself on the ground. *(Cuando Juan intenta jugar afuera con sus hermanos, él les quita la bola y huye. Cuando se le corrige, Juan grita, llora, y se tira al piso.)*
Home (Casa)	When Juan's family wants to take Juan somewhere in the car (shopping, Laundromat, friends' houses), Juan screams and cries and refuses to go and thus avoids or delays the transition. *(Cuando la familia de Juan quiere llevarlo algún lugar en el auto [ir de compras, a la lavandería, a casas de amigos], Juan grita y llora y se niega ir y por lo tanto evita o retrasa la transición.)*

Source: O'Neill et al. (1997).

Step 4: Behavior Support Plan

Once Juan's team generated hypotheses about his challenging behavior at home and school, they began to develop strategies for a support plan. All strategies would be based on the hypotheses developed from the FBAs. They wanted to identify strategies that would make it unnecessary for Juan to exhibit challenging behavior during center time play and transitions and promote his engagement in learning activities. For each hypothesis, the team agreed to only include strategies that would work for everyone on the team. The plan included ways to change the triggers for his behaviors, teach him new behaviors, and change teacher and family responses. In selecting the strategies, the team considered the resources available to the family and the teachers, ease of implementation, and whether the strategies could be used at home and school.

Hypothesis 1: Transitions at School
Juan's family and the school discussed the first hypothesis related to transitions. To address the triggers of Juan's disruptive behavior during transitions, the teacher created a visual schedule for Juan in addition to their class schedule. The schedule allowed him to predict the transitions. In addition, when Juan made the transition to center and circle time activities, he was allowed to pick a favorite toy or activity. This provided him with an immediate reward for the transition. The teacher also made him a "helper" within activities, to allow him to have a role in the activity. The teacher used cue cards with pictures that depicted sitting, hands down, and quiet voice. She used these with all the children but especially with Juan because of his language challenges. Juan also has a buddy to accompany to activities such as lunch, outside play, and snack time.

Hypothesis 2: Play at School When the team discussed Juan's challenges with play and based on the FBA, they believed that Juan engaged in throwing and other behaviors because he wanted to join his peers in play. It seemed that Juan did not know how to or have the language to ask to play. His limited English proficiency and language delays prevented him from understanding how to gain access to social interaction. If children did not respond to Juan when he walked over to them, Juan threw toys and often took their toys to interrupt their play. The children told the teacher, who then moved Juan to another center for independent play.

His ESOL and preschool teacher taught him the word *play* and the phrase *I sit* and also gave him a picture of the center where he wanted to play. They coached him to go up to his peers and say *play*. They also instructed the peers to allow Juan to join them and acknowledge his attempts at communication. His teacher made sure that he had lots of practice throughout the day, such as during outside play, circle time, lunchtime, and snack time.

Hypothesis 3: Play at Home The team was able to use the teacher's observations of Juan during play with his brothers to help identify strategies with the family to address his challenging behaviors at home. The school team explained that the family needed to change the triggers that caused challenging behavior and help Juan develop the skills needed to play with his brothers and be able to go places in the community as a family.

To address issues related to play, they set up a scheduled time for Juan to play with his brothers using a simple version of ball play, with a ball designed for a toddler that involved turn taking and waiting and had clear beginnings and endings. The game involved rolling the ball on the floor to his brothers and waiting for the ball to be rolled back to him. Previously, Juan tried to join in with his brothers playing softball outside. He didn't understand the game or when it was his turn. He also lacked the physical skills required to throw and catch the ball. Teaching the brothers how to play a simpler version of ball allowed Juan to practice asking for his turn, waiting for others, and offering and receiving high-fives for doing well. He also needed to say *play* and *I sit* at home. All family members, including the grandmother, could join in, which gave Juan more practice. It also provided the family with opportunities to praise him.

Hypothesis 4: Transitions in the Community For transitions to the community, the school team taught Juan's family about using pictures and how they worked to help him make transitions at school. The family did not have a computer, but the teachers asked the family to tell them all the places they go or wanted to go. The teachers created scripted stories for locations the family indicated they wanted to go with Juan using pictures from the Internet and taking digital photos of locations in the family's community. The scripted story provided pictures that illustrated what activities would occur in the setting and what Juan would be expected to do. The family was instructed to share the picture book related to the setting immediately prior to starting the transition and at other times in the day as Juan was interested. They helped the family design a *first–then* board that could be used to present information to Juan about the transition. This included a *first* of getting in the car and *then* of the location where they were going. Juan was provided with a preferred toy once he sat is his car seat. In addition, they helped the family identify some preferred toys from their home to put in a travel bag to use in settings where Juan might get bored (e.g., laundromat, friend's house).

The school team immediately put the four hypotheses and related strategies into a simple two-page BSP in both English and Spanish (see Figures 24.2 and 24.3). The behavior specialist trained the teachers on the use of the support plan strategies. The ESOL teacher and her paraprofessional visited Juan and his family at home and talked through the plan. They wanted to ensure the family still felt comfortable with the implementation at home and in school.

Step 5: Monitoring and Evaluation

Juan's team (school staff and family) reconvened 1 month after the plan's implementation to discuss the BSP. This meeting provided an important opportunity for revisiting, reevaluating, and adjusting the support plan. During this meeting, the behavior specialist and the teacher summarized Juan's progress after 1 month through data gathered from all team members using a child behavior home and school routine checklist and direct observation via videos and pictures. The teacher showed the team, on her laptop, pictures and video of Juan saying "play" and playing with friends during playtime, using his schedule, and saying "I sit" at circle time. The ESOL teacher made a home visit to observe Juan and his brothers playing ball and a transition to the car to go to a family friend's house. Overall, the team and family were happy with the BSP. The changes needed in Juan's support plan were minor. In addition, to discussing what worked and what didn't, the behavior specialist created a simple bar graph with Juan's behavior plotted before and after the support plan implementation. The bars represented the changes in Juan's behavior from baseline to intervention at school and home (see Figure 24.4).

These measures gave the team a general idea of how well the interventions were working for Juan's attention- and escape-maintained behaviors. Reconvening the team provided opportunities for celebrating Juan's successes as well as agreement from the entire team for making the necessary adjustments in the support plan.

CONCLUSION

The support of Juan and his family was successful because the school sought to establish a collaborative partnership with the family in the design and implementation of the BSP. To ensure a collaborative partnership, the school went to great lengths to respect the family's cultural and linguistic preferences,

Triggers (Gatillos de conducta)	Behaviors (Conducta desafiante)	Responses (Respuesta/Su reacción)
School (Escuela) • Center time play (Juegos durante centros)	• Throw toys (Tira juguetes) • Disrupt activity (Interrumpe la actividad)	• Time-out or move to another center by himself (Tomar tiempo solo o ir a otro centro por si mismo)
Home (Casa) • Play with brothers (Jugar con los hermanos)	• Take toys; run away (Quitar los juguetes, huir) Function (Propósito): Get access to peers and play (Obtener acceso a sus compañeros y jugar)	• Scold Juan or take him back in the house (Regañar a Juan y llevarlo de regreso a la casa)

Prevention (Prevención)	New skills (Nueva conducta)	New responses (Nueva respuesta/reacción)
School (Escuela) • Coach Juan to say "sit" or "play" (Entrenar a Juan a decir "sentar" o "jugar") • Coach peers to acknowledge Juan and ask him to play (Entrenar a los compañeros a reconocer a Juan y invitarlo a jugar)	• Say "play" or "I sit" (Decir "jugar" o "me siento") • Use picture of play area (Usar la foto de la zona de jugar)	• Praise Juan and his peers for playing (Alabar a Juan y sus compañeros por jugar)
Home (Casa) • Play simple ball game with brother using the words "play" or "sit" (Jugar un juego sencillo de pelota con su hermano usando las palabras "jugar" o "sentarse") • Coach brothers in how to play with Juan (Entrenar a los hermanos como jugar con Juan)	• Say "play" (Decir "jugar")	• Praise Juan for playing (Alabar a Juan por jugar) • Praise brothers for playing with Juan (Alabar a los hermanos por jugar con Juan) • High-fives from brothers (Choca cincos de sus hermanos)

Figure 24.2. Behavior support plan (BSP) summary for attention. (*Source:* University of South Florida Family Involvement in Functional Assessment Project, 2004.)

understand family ecology, understand the feasibility of plan implementation, and consider the family vision, preferences, and desires (McLaughlin et al., 2012). As schools support an increasing number of students from diverse families, they must develop processes and supports to ensure that strong collaborations with families can be developed and that the behavior support process will be conducted in partnership with the family. This means schools must prepare teachers and other school staff to honor the family's cultural and linguistic preferences within the confines of the classroom and other school areas (Utley, Kozleski, Smith, & Draper, 2002). The first step before a school even begins the PBS process is the development of rapport and trust with the family. At the most fundamental level, this means welcoming the families into the school using their native or preferred language (Waterman & Harry, 2008). This posture sets a tone of respect and comfort for the family and is the first step in establishing rapport.

For schools to be effective with diverse families, they must view the world from the

Triggers (Gatillos de conducta)	Behaviors (Conducta desafiante)	Responses (Respuesta/Su reacción)

School (Escuela)
• Transitions to activities
  (Hacer la transición a actividades)
	• Cries, screams, throws himself on floor
	  (Llora, grita, se tira al piso)
		• Coax, threaten, pick him up
		  (Persuadir, amenazar, recogerlo)

Home (Casa)
• Transition to unfamiliar places
  (Hacer la transición a lugares desconocidos)
	• Cries, screams, throws himself on floor
	  (Llora, grita, se tira al piso)
	
	Function (Propósito):
	Escape/avoid
	(Escapar/evadir)
		• Avoid going places unless necessary
		  (Evitar salir menos que sea necesario)

Prevention (Prevención)	**New skills** (Nueva conducta)	**New responses** (Nueva respuesta/reacción)

School (Escuela)
• Use a visual schedule
  (Usar un horario visual)
• Let Juan choose an activity after he makes transitions
  (Dejar que Juan elija una activad cuando hace la transición)
• Coach peers to acknowledge Juan and ask him to play
  (Entrenar a los compañeros a reconocer a Juan y pedirle jugar)
• Pick a buddy to walk with him
  (Elija un compañero para que camine con él)
	• Use schedule
	  (Usar un horario)
		• Praise Juan for transitions
		  (Alabar a Juan por hacer la transición)
		• Encourage peers to praise him
		  (Fomentar que los compañeros alaben a Juan)

Home (Casa)
• Scripted story about the setting and activities for Juan; first-then board to prompt transition
  (Una historia sobre el escenario y actividades para Juan; un cuadro de primero-después para estimular la transición)
• Travel bag with preferred toys or activities
  (Una bolsa para viajar con juguetes preferidos o actividades)
• Coach brothers to play with him and keep him engaged
  (Entrenar a los hermanos que jueguen con él y que lo mantengan ocupado)
	• Use first-then to make transition to car
	  (Usar primero-después para hacer la transición al auto)
	• Request toy bag
	  (Pedir la bolsa de juguetes)
		• Praise Juan for the transition
		  (Alabar a Juan por hacer la transición)
		• Praise brothers for playing with Juan
		  (Alabar a los hermanos por jugar con Juan)
		• High-fives from brothers
		  (Choca cinco de los hermanos)
		• Preferred treat or toy once in car seat
		  (Convite o juguete preferido cuando este en el asiento del auto)

Figure 24.3. Behavior support plan (BSP) summary for escape/avoidance. (*Source:* University of South Florida Family Involvement in Functional Assessment Project, 2004.)

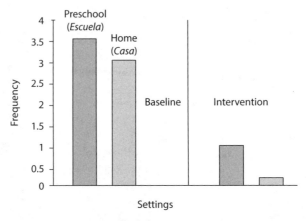

Figure 24.4. Child behavior score for home and school routines (*Puntuacion de conducta para rutinas de la casa y la escuela*). (From University of South Florida Family Involvement in Functional Assessment Project, Louis de la Parte Florida Mental Health Institute, Department of Child and Family Studies. [2004]. *Family involvement in functional assessment: A guide for school professionals.* Tampa, FL: Author.)

family's perspective (Lynch & Hanson, 2004). Reaching out to families in their native language conveys respect and acceptance and acknowledges families' cultural and linguistic differences. Further, meeting with them at a time and location of their choosing extends the welcome and indicates a support of their needs. In the support of Juan and his family, the school provided at all times a bilingual translator and written materials in Spanish for the family. They deferred to the family on where and when the first meeting should occur, rather than insisting that the family come to school. Juan's teachers wanted to gain the family's trust and convey support in the anticipation of creating a collaborative partnership.

Collaborative partnerships are a natural outgrowth of rapport between families and schools. Educators cannot establish collaborative partnerships without family comfort in the context of interactions. Migrant and other complex families might need the encouragement from schools to recognize the importance of their contributions for the education of their child. Collaborative relationships involve reciprocity, which requires give and take but not necessarily equivalent knowledge. Families offer insight into their family system and the cultural values and beliefs of their child, while schools bring

knowledge of their system, academic curricula, and instruction and behavior support. Although families and schools are not experts in each other's systems, both "ways of knowing" are essential elements for partnerships. This mutuality of understanding is especially critical because it has a direct impact on the effectiveness of the behavior support process (Lucyshyn et al., 2002; Turnbull & Turnbull, 2002; Wang et al., 2007).

In this case study, the school was intentional in their development of a collaborative partnership with Juan's family by allowing the family to designate the initial meeting times and locations. The school wanted to gain the trust of Juan's family to fully understand the challenges they faced and how they might provide more comprehensive support to Juan.

Families from diverse backgrounds often lead very complex and difficult lives. In the context of collaborative partnerships, schools must create an atmosphere that allows families the freedom to comfortably discuss their day-to-day family lifestyle, routines and activities, and family priorities (Rao & Kalyanpur, 2002). Gaining this knowledge of their ecology assists school teams in understanding the complexities of the life of the family and provides information that is critical for understanding and supporting the family capacity for implementing interventions within the PBS process. Schools might find it necessary to assist families in meeting their basic needs—something that for many precedes engagement in the behavior support process. Further, these family challenges might have a direct impact on the child's behavior in school.

Although Juan's family did not reveal their income or legal status, the school understood that they lived in a crowded home earning farm-worker wages. The school also realized that the family worked long hours with little energy left to cope with Juan's challenging behavior. As revealed in the person-centered plan, their priority was for Juan to learn to play with children and to respond to changes in his schedule. This provided the school with insight into the family's aspirations for their children and how those directly relate to their day-to-day needs—something school teams must consider when determining the feasibility of implementation.

The feasibility of implementation comprises acceptability, effectiveness, sustainability, and satisfaction (McLaughlin et al., 2012). Through considering contextual fit, schools can create effective interventions that resonate with families and maintain over time. If schools consider cultural and linguistic preferences and family ecology, then families are more likely to view interventions as acceptable and sustainable. For families, interventions must fit with their cultural values and achieve socially validity—that is, interventions should be designed so that families can comfortably implement the interventions across contexts, including the community, and willingly teach other family members how to use interventions within home and community routines (Sprague & Horner, 1992).

To ensure that interventions were feasible, the school worked diligently to understand the ecology of the family and the likelihood that the proposed interventions would be implemented by Juan's family. They began the process of understanding the family values through PCP. Here, the

school learned about their journey from Mexico and their education. Their greatest aspiration for Juan was to have friends and play with his brothers. They also felt hampered by his inability to go different places and wanted the family to participate in family outings. The school team gained more knowledge during the FBA process, where they discussed the family's overall understanding of Juan's challenging behavior and the family's overall perspectives about discipline. These revelations provided a window into the potential barriers to implementation and the support the family needed to partner in the PBS process.

PCP provides a family-centered mechanism for an open discussion to ascertain what the family wants for their child as an outcome associated with improved behavior. PCP walks the family through a process that offers the family an opportunity to speak to different aspects of their child's life and what the child needs to obtain the vision the family and child have for their lives (Kincaid & Fox, 2002). For Juan's family, the person-centered process opened the door to a strong alliance with the school and the development of a collaborative partnership. For the school, understanding the family's vision for Juan was a critical step in the process and provided the school professionals with a deeper understanding of how to best support Juan within the family ecology and how to guide the development of Juan's behavior supports in a manner that fit with the family and would result in outcomes related to their desired quality of life.

REFERENCES

Albin, R.W., Lucyshyn, J.M., Horner, R.H., & Flannery, K.B. (1996). Contextual fit for behavioral support plans: A model for "goodness of fit." In L.K. Koegel, R.L. Koegel, & G. Dunlap (Eds.), *Positive behavior support: Including people with difficult behavior in the community* (pp. 81–98). Baltimore, MD: Paul H. Brookes Publishing Co.

Annie E. Casey Foundation. (2012). *Kids count data book*. Retrieved from http://datacenter.kidscount.org/DataBook/2012/

Carr, E.G., Dunlap, G., Horner, R.H., Koegel, R.L., Turnbull, A.P., Sailor, W., . . . Fox, L. (2002). Positive behavior support: Evolution of an applied science. *Journal of Positive Behavior Intervention, 4,* 4–16.

Chen, D., Downing, J.E., & Peckham-Hardin, K.D. (2002). Working with families of diverse cultural and linguistic backgrounds: Considerations for culturally responsive positive behavior support. In J.M. Lucyshyn, G. Dunlap, & R.W. Albin (Eds.), *Families and positive behavior support: Addressing problem behavior in family contexts* (pp. 133–151). Baltimore, MD: Paul H. Brookes Publishing Co.

Dunlap, G., & Robbins, F.R. (1991). Current perspectives in service delivery for young children with autism. *Comprehensive Mental Health Care, 1,* 177–194.

Kincaid, D., & Fox, L. (2002). Person-centered planning and positive behavior support. In S. Holburn & P.M. Vietze (Eds.), *Person-centered planning. research, practice, and future directions* (pp. 29–50). Baltimore, MD: Paul H. Brookes Publishing Co.

Leventhal, T., & Brooks-Gunn, J. (2011). Changes in neighborhood poverty from 1990 to 2000 and youth's problem behaviors. *Developmental Psychology, 47*(6), 1680–1698.

Lucyshyn, J.M., Horner, R.H., Dunlap, G., Albin, R.W., & Ben, K.R. (2002). Positive behavior support with families. In J.M. Lucyshyn, G. Dunlap, & R.W. Albin (Eds.), *Families and positive behavior support: Addressing problem behavior in family contexts* (pp. 3–44). Baltimore, MD: Paul H. Brookes Publishing Co.

Lynch, E.W., & Hanson, M.J. (2002). *Developing cross-cultural competence: A guide for working with young children and their families.* Baltimore, MD: Paul H. Brookes Publishing Co.

McLaughlin, T.W., Denney, M.K., Snyder, P.A., & Welsh, J.L. (2012). Behavior support interventions implemented by families of young children: Examination of contextual fit. *Journal of Positive Behavior Interventions, 14,* 87–97.

National Center for Cultural Competence. *A guide to infusing cultural and linguistic competence in health promotion training.* Washington, DC: Georgetown University Center for Child and Human Development.

O'Neill, R.E., Horner, R.H., Albin, R.W., Sprague, J.R., Storey, K., & Newton, J.S. (1997). *Functional assessment and program development for problem behavior: A practical handbook.* Pacific Grove, CA: Cengage Learning.

Qi, C., & Kaiser, A. (2003). Behavior problems of preschool children from low-income families: Review of the literature. *Topics in Early Childhood Special Education, 23,* 188–216.

Rao, S., & Kalyanpur, M. (2002). Promoting home-school collaboration in positive behavior support. In J.M. Lucyshyn, G. Dunlap, & R.W. Albin (Eds.), *Families and positive behavior support: Addressing problem behavior in family contexts* (pp. 219–239). Baltimore, MD: Paul H. Brookes Publishing Co.

Sprague, J.R., & Horner, R.H. (1992). Determining the acceptability of behavioral interventions. In M. Wang, H. Walbert, & M. Reynolds (Eds.), *Handbook of special education* (Vol. 4). Oxford, UK: Pergamon Press.

Sugai, G., O'Keeffe, B.V., & Fallon, L.M. (2012). A contextual consideration of culture and school-wide positive behavior support. *Journal of Positive Behavior Interventions, 14,* 197–208.

Turnbull, A.P., & Turnbull, H.R. (2002). Comprehensive lifestyle support: From rhetoric to reality. In J.M. Lucyshyn, G. Dunlap, & R.W. Albin (Eds.), *Families and positive behavior support: Addressing problem behavior in family contexts* (pp. 349–370). Baltimore, MD: Paul H. Brookes Publishing Co.

U.S. Census Bureau. (2011). *Overview of race and Hispanic origin: 2010.* Retrieved from http://www.census.gov/prod/cen2010/briefs/c2010br-02.pdf

Utley, C.A., Kozleski, E., Smith, A., & Draper, I.L. (2002). Positive behavior support: A proactive strategy for minimizing behavior problems in urban multicultural youth. *Journal of Positive Behavior Interventions, 4,* 196–207.

Vaughn, B.J., Dunlap, G., Fox, L., Clarke, S., & Bucy, M. (1997). Parent professional partnership in behavioral support: A case study of community based intervention. *Journal of The Association for Persons with Severe Handicaps, 22,* 186–197.

Vaughn, B.J., Wilson, D., White, R., & Dunlap, G. (2002). Family-centered intervention to resolve problem behaviors in a fast-food restaurant. *Journal of Positive Behavior Interventions, 4,* 38–45.

Wang, M., McCart, A., & Turnbull, A.P. (2007). Implementing positive behavior support with Chinese American families: Enhancing cultural competence. *Journal of Positive Behavior Interventions, 9,* 38–51.

Waterman, R., & Harry, B. (2008). *Building collaboration between schools and parents of English language learners: Transcending barriers, creating opportunities.* Tempe, AZ: National Center for Culturally Responsive Educational Systems.

Developing a Multielement Behavior Support Plan for a Middle School Student from a Diverse Background with Significant Behavioral Challenges

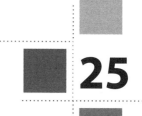

25

Randall L. De Pry and Julie Esparza Brown

Students with chronic or persistent problem behaviors benefit academically and socially when their environments are predictable, proactive, preventive, and positive (Sailor, Dunlap, Sugai, & Horner, 2009; Sugai et al., 2000). Schools that match this profile engage in instructional and behavioral support practices that are differentiated across learners and embedded within existing systems of support (De Pry & Cheesman, 2010; McIntosh, Horner, & Sugai, 2009; Scott, 2007). These practices are referred to as *schoolwide positive behavior intervention and support* (SWPBIS; Sugai et al., 2000) and *response to intervention* (RTI; Fuchs & Fuchs, 2006). When combined, they are often referred to as multitiered systems of support (MTSS; Sugai & Horner, 2009). Schools that use MTSS provide adults with a framework for the application of instructional and behavioral supports that are implemented with fidelity and result in the ongoing use of data-based practices for supporting all learners (Sailor, Doolittle, Bradley, & Danielson, 2009; Tillery, Varjas, Meyers & Collins, 2009).

At the individual level, these outcomes can best be achieved when multielement behavior support planning is in place. Multielement plans of behavior support focus first on improving the quality of life of the individual, with a secondary purpose of reducing the problem behavior (Carr et al., 2002). This interrelationship between improving quality of life through skill development and systemic change, which then results in reductions in problem behavior, is a defining characteristic of positive behavior support (PBS). Multielement plans of behavior support are based on functional assessment data and shared common values, such as a focus on quality of life, contextual fit, person-centered thinking, and environmental or systemic supports. This chapter illustrates the development of a multielement plan of support for a student from a diverse background with significant behavioral challenges. The student characterized in this case study, "Mario," is a combination of several students that the authors have encountered over their careers; Mario's story illustrates an approach for including the student in the planning process. The chapter is divided into three sections: background, context, and process. The background section explores Mario's strengths and areas of concern. The context section describes critical features of the school, home, and community in which Mario lives. Finally, the process section examines the problem-solving and behavior implementation planning processes, including an example of Mario's student-directed functional assessment summary form.

BACKGROUND

Student

Mario is an 11-year-old boy at Sotomayor Middle School. His working-class neighborhood borders the school and consists of apartments, duplexes, and single-family homes. There is a mix of Latino and Anglo-American families residing in the area. Mario has lived with his maternal aunt and uncle along with their two young children for the past 3 years. Three years ago, his father was deported back to Mexico and has been unable to return to the United States. At that same time, his mother had to move to another state to find employment. Mario's aunt and uncle have reported that they are concerned with Mario's lack of respect toward them, their children, and other extended family members, as well as other problem behaviors he is displaying at school.

Although Mario was born in the United States, he is still acquiring standard English since his parents' and aunt and uncle's first and most commonly used language is Spanish. Therefore, he continues to receive services from the English learner program (ELP) that began in kindergarten, and he is identified as an English learner.

Strengths

On a continuum of 1 to 5 (1 being low and 5 being high) on an English language proficiency test, he scores at a level of 3. This means he continues to qualify for services to improve his academic English skills through the ELP and receives one class period per day of English language development (ELD). English learners are expected to progress one level per year in their acquisition of English, and Mario's progress is slower than expected. Although Mario sounds verbally fluent in English, he lacks the breadth and depth of vocabulary and language skills, or "academic language," needed to be successful in a curriculum taught in English. Further, as is typical of his language community, he frequently includes English and Spanish phrases within his speech (i.e., code switches) and has difficulty understanding common English idioms and metaphors.

Mario is physically active and seems to enjoy hands-on learning. School peers like Mario when he is social and seem to want to be his friend. He is able to verbally communicate his wants and needs appropriately, but when he is upset, he tends to use more Spanish phrases interspersed with English. This makes it difficult for teachers to understand him when he is upset. Mario has bonded with the school's Latino counselor, because during stressful times, Mario can communicate with him in both English and Spanish. The counselor also serves as a positive Latino role model for Mario. Mario participates in his own individualized education program (IEP) meetings with careful planning and support (Agran & Hughes, 2008; Martin, Marshall, Maxson, & Jerman, 1996). He works well with teachers on a one-to-one basis and seems to benefit from instructional methods that provide high levels of positive reinforcement and explicit instruction in needed skills and academic language (Archer & Hughes, 2011).

Problem Behaviors

Mario's problem behaviors include yelling, threatening, pushing, being out of his seat, not following teacher directions, and sometimes crying. The highest intensity problem behaviors are yelling and threatening, often directed at both teachers and peers, particularly during content area instruction. This has resulted in fewer opportunities to fully include Mario in general education classes where content instruction occurs with his same-age peers.

Teachers have learned to never ask Mario to read aloud in front of his peers, since this is the most likely scenario to elicit the problem behaviors. These types of problem behaviors have resulted in eight suspensions for the current academic year, and his IEP team has met to discuss possible next steps. The suspensions have been particularly difficult for Mario's aunt and uncle since they have no time-off provisions at their employment and must leave Mario at home alone when he is suspended. Although they leave firm rules about not allowing friends to visit on these days, they have no way of monitoring this and suspect he violates the rule in the afternoons.

Mario's special education teacher has learned that a few of his general teachers want him removed and placed in a more restrictive environment due to the threatening and uncooperative nature that he exhibits during his outbursts. Overall, the intensity and frequency of problem behavior increase during high-demand academic activities—particularly activities that involve reading and math. Problem behaviors are virtually nonexistent during electives and ELD class, which includes some friends from his neighborhood and language supports.

During the last IEP meeting, it was noted that problem behaviors are more likely when Mario is late for school. School data indicate that this occurs at least five times per month. During these periods, Mario arrives at school up to 45 minutes late and often complains of arguments with his aunt and uncle that morning. Usually, he asks for a carton of milk after calming down, since he doesn't seem to get breakfast on days he has trouble at home. On these days, he is generally unkempt in appearance and seems on edge for most, if not all of the instructional day.

Direct observation data suggest that some peers seem to be rejecting Mario by not including him in groups during free periods and lunch. This is most notable on difficult days or days when Mario is late. Moreover, the adults in the building have put Mario on a "watch list" and seem to be responding to his problem behavior in a more punitive and harsh manner, given his history of problem behavior. His special education teacher indicates that, given these conditions, they are having some difficulty finding a solution that supports his needs and the needs of his peers and teachers.

CONTEXT

Sotomayor Middle School has been implementing SWPBIS for the past 4 years. The school reached 80/80 on the School-Wide Evaluation Tool (SET; Sugai, Lewis-Palmer, Todd, & Horner, 2005) at the completion of year 2 of implementation and has recently begun to focus on how to fully support students who need targeted and individualized levels of behavior support. The SET is an evaluation instrument that measures implementation features associated with SWPBIS. Sotomayor Middle School has a total enrollment of 925 students, with Latino students representing 48% of the student body and English learners totaling 30% of all students. On last year's state testing, only 52% of the students scored proficient or above average in literacy, compared with the regional average of 63%. They fared better in math, with 54% of students scoring proficient or above average, compared with the county's average of 56%. The school is a Title-I school, with 91% of students qualifying for free and reduced lunch. The school has worked to integrate their RTI and SWPBIS implementation efforts, due to similarities in the problem-solving, data-based decision-making, and communication processes involved with each (Sailor et al., 2009). The administrative team is now using the term MTSS to characterize the integrated model (Sugai & Horner, 2009).

A vision for an integrated approach was promoted by the school's principal. She has provided strong support for these efforts and attends meetings held by the school leadership team whenever she can. Moreover, she has incorporated instructional and behavioral supports into the school improvement plan as one of her top-three school goals. She has articulated to her faculty, staff, and parents that, by using an integrated approach, the faculty and staff can better serve the whole child in general education settings. In other words, students who are experiencing behavior difficulties in the classroom are likely to need additional instructional or academic supports due to the impact that their social behavior is having on learning and peer/teacher relationships. Each student is viewed individually, and data are used to make determinations related to differentiated instructional and behavioral supports (De Pry & Cheesman, 2010). The faculty, staff, and parents have widely endorsed this model.

In retrospect, this broad support occurred because of the way the principal sought buy-in from all groups. For example, she held meetings with each stakeholder group, including parent groups from each of the school's cultural communities to elicit their feedback and support. To build trust with parents, she held dinner meetings and ensured that there were interpreters available; child care was also provided at the meetings, in which children and their siblings were involved in fun educational activities taught by some of the school's teachers. All parents received invitations in their native language whenever possible, which was followed up by phone calls by the school's cultural liaison. At Sotomayor, the cultural liaisons were primarily instructional assistants from the local community who work closely to facilitate partnerships with non–English-speaking families.

Sotomayor Middle School has made a number of significant and systemic changes since beginning implementation 4 years ago. The school attended both awareness and implementation trainings related to SWPBIS and RTI and brought back materials to share with the rest of the faculty and staff. These materials have been supplemented with new materials on MTSS that provide guidance on the integration of tiered support models (see Swift Schools, 2013). Material related to culture and language have also been shared and discussed during faculty meetings so that all staff have the opportunity to examine their own socialized biases, fears, and assumptions. This was considered to be a first step in dispelling stereotypes about Latino and other minority students and increasing expectations regarding their school performance and behavior (Bal, Thorius, & Kozleski, 2012; Noguera, 2012). In fact, the faculty decided that, during the coming term, they would invite a local community group to facilitate a discussion on overcoming racism. Since it is offered afterschool, this opportunity is voluntary, but to date 80% of the faculty have committed to it. During faculty and grade-level team meetings, these materials have been used to guide discussion and planning.

As a result of building trust with her faculty, the principal requested that a team facilitator and a representative sample of faculty and staff (e.g., general education teachers, special education teachers, support staff, educational assistants) be brought together to form what is known as the school leadership team. The team agreed that focusing on proactive, preventive, and culturally responsive strategies is an important change from the way that the school had been operating previously. Formerly, the school staff used reactive, consequence-based methods to try to change academic and social problem behaviors. Consequence-based methods resulted in an excessive use of office discipline referrals (ODR), in-school suspensions, and in some cases, out-of-school suspensions. As part of a retrospective analysis of these methods, the leadership team found a number of culturally based misunderstandings. For example, during the prior year, one of their newly arrived students who only spoke Spanish refused to make eye contact with teachers. The staff interpreted her behavior as a sign of disrespect. Upon investigation, the staff learned that making eye contact with people in respected positions is disrespectful in her culture. This incident taught the faculty the importance of making sure that someone fluent in the student's language and who is knowledgeable about their culture is part of all meetings whenever possible.

An analysis of ODR data 2 years prior to implementation indicated that the school averaged 546 ODRs per year. The majority of the referrals (63%) came from the classroom, with remaining referrals being given in non-classroom settings such as hallways and the cafeteria. Recent data indicate a 58% reduction in referrals, given the focus on providing comprehensive instructional and behavioral supports for all learners. Faculty report that this reduction in the use of referrals has resulted in a more positive school climate and more time to engage in instructional activities.

As part of the implementation, Sotomayor Middle School identified common, schoolwide behavior expectations and has agreements to teach these directly and explicitly to their students at the beginning of the school year. Faculty and staff use "booster sessions" when data indicate that reteaching may be necessary. ELD teachers begin the year by explicitly teaching the schoolwide behavior expectations to ensure that all students understand them. To further support the diverse school community, the behavior expectations are translated into the school's most common non-English languages, Spanish and Vietnamese. Posters are located around the school and the translated expectations are sent to parents at the beginning of each year.

Sotomayor Middle School also engaged in meaningful conversations about the problem behaviors occurring most frequently. The staff noted that it was difficult to understand their data without engaging in a conversation about what each of the behaviors meant on the ODR form (e.g., "disrespect," "bullying"). The school leadership team facilitated a number of meetings where faculty and staff worked together to operationally define these terms and incorporated those definitions into their faculty handbook. Data suggest that a standardization of commonly used terms has led to greater consistency for faculty and staff.

Having clearer definitions of what constitutes problem behavior allowed the faculty and staff to have meaningful discussions about which behaviors would be managed in the classroom and which behaviors require administrative support. These discussions led to decisions about how consequences were given at the classroom and office levels and resulted in the identification of more consistent and instructionally focused ways of handling problem behavior. Some faculty and staff changed their approach to these types of problem behaviors and now view them as a "learning error," as opposed to more common within explanations for "why" the student engaged in problem behavior (e.g., "hyper," "bad," "disabled"). This change in attribution lead to meaningful discussions about how to set up the classroom environment to ensure success for all learners, the identification of meaningful data sources that can be used to guide instructional decisions, a focus on the design and delivery of lessons using strategies that provide differentiated instructional supports, and the increased use of evidence-based methods to establish important academic and social behaviors.

As part of supporting an integrated approach to instructional and behavioral supports, the school identified software that allowed for the collection and dissemination of data related to academic and social/behavioral performance (AIMSweb, 2013; SWIS, 2013). These data are used at every meeting, to monitor student progress and performance and guide decision making. Faculty and staff noted that having access to data increased the likelihood that they would make accurate instructional decisions. This was particularly true when trying to make sense of behavioral data at the schoolwide, classroom, nonclassroom, and individual levels. Staff were able to better support students by accessing data from their computers and viewing it in a graphed format. This process allowed the staff to disaggregate the data by student subgroups to ensure that no one group was receiving a disproportionate number of referrals, since both local and national data indicated disproportionate discipline outcomes in many schools across the country (De Pry & Cheesman, 2010; Skiba, Michael, Nardo, & Peterson, 2002; Vincent, Randall, Cartledge, Tobin, & Swain-Bradway, 2013).

Sotomayor Middle School also held conversations about the merits of acknowledging students who engaged in the schoolwide behavior expectations. A system was developed where students in classroom and common school areas could receive a "Caught You Being Good" card that was given when a student was noticed engaging in a behavior that aligns with the schoolwide behavior expectations. When the students received the "Caught You Being Good" card, faculty and staff made an effort to verbally state why they were being acknowledged in a genuine and meaningful way. As part of increasing efforts to become culturally responsive, "Caught You Caught You Being Good" was translated in the three major languages spoken at the school: English, Spanish, and Vietnamese. Data suggested that when the cards were used as intended, students had a tendency to engage in the behavior expectation again. It was also noted that faculty who showed genuine enthusiasm, as well as behavioral specificity as part of their verbal acknowledgment, seemed to have better results.

Sotomayor Middle School made significant changes in the school climate by focusing on proactive and preventive strategies. The changes made by the school are primarily focused on adult behaviors (teachers and staff), as opposed to more typically addressing student problem behavior after it occurs. In other words, the school was focusing on proactive and preventive strategies, as opposed to reactive measures only. Students, faculty, and staff report that the school is a better place for learning, and data seem to support this assertion. Math and reading scores on the state assessment have been trending upward across grades levels. The team believes that this is a result of faculty having more time to teach and support the wide variety of learners in their classrooms. In fact, the school leadership team calculated

the amount of time saved through the reduction of ODRs alone and concluded that they collectively saved approximately ten 6-hour schools days of time by teaching positive alternatives instead of reacting to problem behavior and excluding students.

While the school has embraced differentiated instructional and behavioral support for all learners, a number of challenges still existed. Mario's progress remained a challenge from both an academic and social/behavioral perspective. Mario and other students who are learning English can suffer academically from teachers who have low expectations, limited knowledge of the academic language necessary to succeed in an all English curriculum, and limited afterschool options. With this in mind, the following section examines the process that was used to understand Mario's current levels of performance, expectations of teachers and family, and processes for providing support using a multielement behavior intervention planning method.

PROCESS

Given the frequency and duration of Mario's problem behavior and its impact on academic performance, his teacher initiated the school's problem-solving process. The process has five major steps: 1) defining the problem, 2) analyzing the data, 3) developing a plan, 4) implementing the plan, and 5) evaluating performance.

Step 1: Define the Problem

Teacher Interviews   The PBIS coach scheduled meetings with Mario's teachers. During these meetings, discussions were held about Mario's strengths and areas of concern (see Table 25.1). The teachers provided examples of academic work and discussed areas where Mario was meeting benchmarks. In addition, a discussion was held about significant areas of concern and interventions that were currently in place to provide targeted or individualized support. The PBIS coach asked formal questions using a structured interview format called the Functional Assessment

Table 25.1.   Strengths and areas of concern for Mario

Strengths	Areas of concern
1. Home/community • Strong extended family support • Strong community support	1. Home/community • Argumentative • Disrespectful • Misses parents
2. Communication • Speaks both English and Spanish • Adequate communication and auditory processing in both languages	2. Communication • Difficulty expressing anger verbally, especially in English • Difficulty interpreting the nonverbal actions/intentions of others
3. Health • Physically active	3. Health • None
4. School • Works well one on one • Responds well to positive reinforcement • Has friends from his neighborhood	4. School • Difficulty following teacher directions • Engages in yelling, threatening, and hitting and leaves desk during content instruction • Decreased opportunities for inclusion due to problem behaviors • Reluctance to engage in large group academic tasks such as reading aloud

Interview (FAI; O'Neill et al., 1997). The FAI provides useful data for the team by bringing greater clarity to the problem behavior, including data on what precedes the behavior (characterized as setting events and predictors) and what happens directly after the program behavior occurs (characterized as consequences or maintaining function). Questions related to communication, when the problem behavior is most likely and least likely to occur, how the student prefers to be acknowledged (reinforcement inventory), and what programs have been tried in the past and their effect were particularly useful. Following the meeting, the teachers and coach reviewed the data and began to develop hypotheses for why the problem behavior was occurring. These hypotheses, often referred to as *summary statements,* included listing any setting events, antecedents, or predictors; the problem behavior; and the possible function related to the problem behaviors. Table 25.2 lists the summary statements that were created based on the FAI for Mario.

Family Interview   Mario's aunt and uncle were invited to be interviewed. Mr. Ortega, a Latino counselor, informed the team that it was important to invite either the uncle only or the uncle and aunt, out of respect. While it is always preferable to have multiple respondents, scheduling the interview was difficult. To accommodate the scheduling difficulties, the PBIS coach and Mr. Ortega met Mario's uncle and aunt at a restaurant in the family's neighborhood for about 40 minutes. Since that was not enough time to complete the interview, the counselor asked follow-up questions as part of a phone interview. Both interviews provided important information and a context for building a multielement behavior intervention plan that has strong "contextual fit" (Albin, Lucyshyn, Horner, & Flannery, 1996) as well as cultural congruence (Au, 2009). The summary statement, collaboratively created with the aunt and uncle, is included in Table 25.2.

Student Observation   Mario was observed in a variety of settings at his school. The PBIS coach used the Functional Assessment Observation (FAO) form to collect data across settings (O'Neill et al., 1997). He used the FAO in settings where the problem behavior occurred, and also in settings where it did not occur, to bring greater

Table 25.2.   Summary statements

Setting event	Antecedent/predictor	Behavior	Consequence/function	Probable function
When Mario arrives to school late due to a conflict at home	And is asked to read aloud	He yells and makes threatening comments in English and Spanish	And he is sent out of the room.	Escape/avoidance
When Mario arrives to school late due to a conflict at home	And is asked to work with peers to collaboratively solve a math problem	He walks away from the instructional group	And is eventually sent to a desk in the back with a study carrel.	Escape/avoidance
When Mario is not invited to join a peer group during breaks	And is subsequently asked to work with same peers during content instruction	He argues and occasionally threatens peers	And is sent to time-out or the office.	Escape/avoidance
Uncle and aunt interview				
When Mario gets up late for school and is disrespectful by refusing to acknowledge his aunt and/or follow her directions	And is given a verbal time limit to be ready to be out the door	He yells and refuses to follow her directions	Because he doesn't want to go to school.	Escape/avoidance

understanding to Mario's entire school day. Data were collected during each class period over 10 consecutive days. The PBIS coach would position himself in a nonintrusive place in each setting to collect data—ideally where the student could be seen and heard without creating any type of interruption. Observation data that were collected included identification of the specific problem behavior, any antecedent or predictors that occurred just prior to the behavior of concern, and the hypothesized function of the behavior. The PBIS coach would record each behavioral event on the FAO form. To assist in trying to understand why an incident occurred (particularly for incidents where it was not obvious), the observer silently asked the following questions about the problem behavior: What was Mario trying to get or receive? What was Mario trying to escape or avoid? The direct observation data were combined with the interview data to provide a basis for the development of the behavior intervention plan.

Mario Interview Mario was interviewed using the Student-Directed Functional Assessment Interview (SDFAI; O'Neill et al., 1997). This instrument allowed Mario to provide his personal perspective on what problem behaviors were occurring and why. The PBIS coach, along with Mr. Ortega, found a low-demand time when Mario was not experiencing any difficulties to conduct the interview. The interview started with Mario listing behaviors that he felt may be a concern. This portion of the interview was followed by Mario being able to review his schedule and rate how he feels he's doing. For example, at 9 a.m. Mario has his math class. On the schedule analysis, he listed math class as a setting where he feels he has significant problem behavior. On the other hand, he listed art class as a setting that was not problematic for him. Occasionally the PBIS coach and counselor asked follow-up questions such as, "What makes this setting difficult for you?" or "What do you like about this class?" These types of questions resulted in a variety of responses, related to difficulty with the content (e.g., reading aloud) or not liking the teacher, class, or activities. To record this data, the PBIS coach simply turned the SDFAI form over and wrote down Mario's answers on the back for later review. Upon completion of the interview, Mr. Ortega asked Mario if he would like to meet again with his teachers to talk about what they learned and collaboratively plan for next steps (Martin, Marshall, & De Pry, 2008). He agreed, and a meeting was scheduled. The involvement of a Latino counselor helped Mario feel comfortable enough to provide honest and reflective answers. Also, although Mario has good oral English skills, he is not yet a fluent English speaker and, at times, particularly discussing topics that are stressful, he prefers to answer in Spanish.

Step 2: Analyze the Data

The PBIS coach called a meeting where critical stakeholders (e.g., a grade-level team representative, Latino counselor, family member) were able to meet late one afternoon, after the aunt's workday, and discuss the data that were collected. The counselor asked that the number of school personnel be limited since families are often overwhelmed when meetings are too large. The PBIS coach facilitated the meeting and used a process for seeking input from those in attendance. While Mario's aunt spoke some English, Mr. Ortega provided interpretation to ensure clear communication. The primary purpose of this meeting was to review the data, draw initial conclusions, and determine next steps. A separate meeting was scheduled for later that week that included Mario, a general education teacher who represented the grade-level team, his special education teacher, and a counselor. The PBIS coach reviewed the data collected from the interviews and direct observation and a consensus was reached that Mario has a more difficult time at school on days where he has arrived late as a result of a conflict at home. Under these conditions, problem behavior increased when high-demand academic tasks were presented to him, such as reading aloud. Typical responses included yelling, threatening, pushing, or leaving his desk, which served as a method for Mario to avoid these tasks, even when it

resulted in him being sent down to the office or home. The team agreed that for Mario to meet academic and social benchmarks at school and avoid getting further behind, a plan of support was needed.

Step 3: Develop a Plan

The data derived from Step 2 were summarized and used for the next step—plan development. Sotomayor Middle School was piloting an innovative strategy for increasing student buy-in and relevance associated with the behavior intervention planning and implementation process. The model that the school used is based on research literature focusing on person-centered planning and self-determination, where the student becomes an active participant in the development of their behavior intervention planning meeting (Kern, Dunlap, Clarke, & Childs; Martin, Marshall, & De Pry, 2008; O'Neill et al., 1997; Reed, Thomas, Sprague, & Horner, 1997; Wehmeyer, Baker, Blumberg, & Harrison, 2004). Those in attendance included Mario, a general education representative from his grade-level team, his special education teacher, and Mr. Ortega. The meeting was scheduled for an hour and the intended outcome was to provide a process where Mario could contribute to his behavior intervention planning and implementation. Figure 25.1 provides an example of Mario's completed plan. The following is a brief description of the process that was used and meeting protocols.

MEETING PROTOCOLS AND GUIDELINES: HOW TO COMPLETE THE STUDENT-DIRECTED FUNCTIONAL ASSESSMENT SUMMARY FORM

Team Members, Date, Sources of Information

The facilitator of the meeting (often the special education teacher, given his or her familiarity with the student) starts by initially welcoming everyone. The facilitator lists the student's name first and then the names of other team members who are in attendance. Next, the facilitator writes down

Student-Directed Functional Assessment Summary Form

Team members: Mario, Mr. Dean, Mr. Ortega, and Mrs. Valenzuela

Meeting date: February 12

Sources of information: Functional assessment interview (teachers and aunt), functional assessment observation (10 days), student functional assessment interview (Mario)

Step 1: Gathering information

	My information	My classroom teacher's information	My special education teacher's information	Agreements (A)
What I'm doing well	1. *Science is my favorite subject.* 2. *I like working with certain groups on projects (A2).* 3. *I like most of my teachers, Mr. Ortega, my counselor, and helping (A1).*	1. *You can be very cooperative and friendly (A1).* 2. *You seem to enjoy work where you can create things, such as project-based learning (A2).* 3. *I really appreciate how you help me with students who are learning English.*	1. *I appreciate how you help me and your peers in the resource room (A1).* 2. *I've seen lots of growth in your reading.* 3. *You seem to enjoy cooperative learning experiences (A2).*	A1. *I like to help and can be friendly.* A2. *I like working in groups on projects and stuff.*
What I need to work on	1. *Reading is hard for me (A2).* 2. *Yelling and arguing with certain teachers and kids (A3)* 3. *Leaving when I get pissed off (A1)*	1. *Not following my directions and getting angry (A3)* 2. *Walking out of the room when you're mad or being sent to the office (A1)* 3. *Focusing more on your academics and work completion (A2)*	1. *Social/problem-solving skills that will help you when you're angry or frustrated (A3)* 2. *Getting to school on time and staying in class even when you're upset (A1)* 3. *Fully participating in your reading group, including completing and turning in your assignments (A2)*	A1. *Staying in class/groups even when I feel upset* A2. *Working harder on my reading, math, and stuff* A3. *Getting mad at teachers and kids*

Step 2: Why I do what I do

My summary statement (Sources: Student functional assessment interview and discussion)

Setting event	Predictor	Behavior (A)	Consequence/function
When I get in an argument at home and end up coming in late	*Mrs. Smith asks me to read or to turn in my work.*	*I yell at her and sometimes I leave the room because I don't like to read out loud.*	*She gets mad at me and calls the office. Sometimes I get sent home. (escape/avoidance)*

Step 3: Identifying my new behavior(s)

Thinking about a new behavior. (Directions: Circle new behavior.)

What I need to work on (A)	My new behavior (B)
A1. *Staying in class/groups even when I feel upset* A2. *Working harder on my reading, math, and stuff* A3. *Getting mad at teachers and kids*	1. *Picking my own time to read out loud or asking if I can wait for a while when I'm upset* 2. *Asking if I can wait for a while* 3. *Chillin' out in the back of the room for a few minutes until I calm down*

Figure 25.1. Mario's student-directed functional assessment summary form (From De Pry, R.L., & Hanson, A. [2009]. *Student-directed functional assessment summary sheet.* Unpublished assessment, University of Colorado at Colorado Springs; adapted by permission. As cited in Hanson, A. [2009]. *Using a student-directed functional behavior assessment to improve behavior of a student with emotional and behavioral disorder in an inclusive classroom.* Unpublished manuscript, University of Colorado at Colorado Springs.).

Step 4: Creating our plan

Our strategies for success (Sources: Team discussion)

Way before (setting event)	Just before (antecedent/predictor)	New behavior (B) (replacement response)	Just after (maintaining consequence)
If I'm late, I'll call on my cell so you know. My aunt can also call you if I can't. (Mario) If you missed breakfast and we know you're coming in, we can have something for you. (Mrs. V) You can have 10–15 minutes to chill out in the resource room before going to your first class. This is a time to eat or calm down. (Mr. D) If you're on time, you can put a check mark on your data collection sheet for each class so we can review it at the end of the week. (Mr. O)	I will talk with you the day before and show you what section I will be asking you to read. If you want, we can practice it together before you leave for the day. (Mrs. V) I will check in with you each day to see if you need any help with work that has been assigned. (Mr. D) You can also stop by our rooms when you have questions. (Mrs. V, Mr. O, and Mr. D) I will check with you in the morning to remind you that I'm going to ask you to read and see how you're doing. (Mrs. V) If you're looking upset, I will privately prompt you to use your strategies. (Mrs. V)	If I'm doing okay, I'll try to read. (Mario) If I'm upset, I will try to let you know ahead of time or ask you if I can "pass" for a while. If I pass, I will try to raise my hand and let you know when I'm ready to give it a try. (Mario) You can also use these red and green cards to let me know how you're doing. Red means upset and green means you're fine. Either using the cards or saying pass is fine with me. (Mrs. V) If I'm really upset, I can put out the red card or go to the back of the room and quietly sit in the empty desk over by the long table with the computers until I'm ready to return to my desk. (Mario) If that doesn't work, you can come over to my room for 10 minutes and settle down or request a few minutes with Mr. Ortega. (Mr. D)	Each class when you're on time and in your seat results in one "Caught You Being Good" card. (Mrs. V) Trying or attempting to read will result in you receiving a "Caught You Being Good" card, which I can give you right then or directly after class. (Mrs. V) Using any of the other strategies successfully will earn you a "Caught You Being Good" card, which I will give to you after class. (Mrs. V and Mr. D) If you yell (once), I will ask you to sit quietly in the back of the room. Any other outbursts will result in time in the office. (Mrs. V) Leaving the room without permission will result in time in the office. (Mrs. V)

Step 5: Reviewing our plan

Will this really work?

I don't think so (1)	Maybe (2)	Probably (3)	I really think so (4)
		X, X	X

For scores of 1 or 2, what adjustments are needed?
No adjustments are needed at this time.

Final steps: Practice, classroom implementation, and evaluation methods

Practicing the new behavior(s)	Who	When
1. Ways of communicating with my teacher (pass, red/green cards)	1. Mrs. V and Mario	1. Next Monday
2. Identifying my "second desk" and practicing quietly, moving to the back of the room	2. Mrs. V and Mario	2. Next Monday

(continued)

Figure 25.1. *(continued)*

Classroom implementation	Who	When
1. *Start plan Immediately following practice of ways to communicate with my teacher*	1. *Mario, Mrs. V., Mr. D*	1. *Next Tuesday*
2. *Start plan immediately following practice of moving quietly to my second desk*	2. *Mario, Mrs. V., Mr. D*	2. *Next Tuesday*

Evaluation methods	Who	When
1. *Counting the number of times on my data collection sheet that I'm on time to class*	1. *Mario, Mrs. V., Mr. D*	1. *Review each week*
2. *Counting the number of times I used my strategies and received "Caught You Being Good" cards*	2. *Mario, Mrs. V, Mr. D*	2. *Review each week*

Signatures (and titles)

_____

_____ (title)

_____

_____ (title)

_____

_____ (title)

_____

_____ (title)

Copies needed

_____   _____   _____

Me   **My teachers**   **My parent(s)**

all sources of information that will be used for this meeting, such as the FAI, SDFAI, and FAO. It is essential that the focus be on the student, emphasizing that the plan will be cocreated and coimplemented by those around the table and others as appropriate. Ultimately, the plan is about improving the student's school experience in such a way that has a positive impact on academic and social benchmarks—in other words, his or her quality of life (Carr, 2007; Carr et al., 2002).

Our Information

The facilitator coordinates with the student and completes the "What Am I Doing Well?" section. The student is prompted to focus on academic, social, or others areas that he or she wants to highlight and share. The facilitator records any student responses directly on the form, trying to use the student's words as much as possible. Following the completion of this section, the general education and special education teachers have opportunities to share what they feel the student is doing well based on the assessments that were previously conducted. The adults are encouraged to operationally define terms in a manner that make them easily understood by the student. For example, the term *academically engaged* is less meaningful than *on task* from the perspective of the student. Then, coordinating with the student, the facilitator completes the

"What Do I Need to Work On?" section. The student self-identifies areas that need attention or that he or she considers problematic. If the student appears to have a difficult time with the question, referring to his or her response on the SDFAI (O'Neill et al., 1997) can be useful. The teachers follow the same process described previously, purposefully relying on relying on data collected and any personal experiences that they have they have had with the student. It is critical that the teachers name the behavior without judgment or accusation. Upon completion of each section, the team looks for areas of agreement and circles where they occur in at least two areas. A final discussion around proposed areas of agreement follows, and agreed-on responses are written on the form in the section titled "Agreements."

My Summary Statements

The summary statement from the SDFAI (O'Neill et al., 1997) is reviewed, and verified with the student regarding the listed setting events, predictors, problem behavior, and maintaining consequences/functions. On occasion, we have noted that students gain new insights into their own behavior by engaging in a simple "behavior analysis" using their own summary statement. For example, a student may not be aware that they are more susceptible to verbal outbursts in class after having a difficult time at lunch due to a disagreement with a peer. Therefore plan development can be a "teachable moment" as team members develop a new understanding of when, where, and why problem behavior occurs. In traditional models, adults often engage in this conversation as they seek to understand problem behavior without the student present.

If the behavior identified matches the agreements listed previously, the student is asked if the summary statement matches his or her understanding of the problem behavior. If the student is interested in focusing on a different behavior, then the team will work collaboratively to create a new summary statement and check for agreement. Using phrases such as "way before" (to identify the setting event), "just before" (to identify the antecedent or predictor), and "just after" (to identify the consequence) helps the student have a better understanding of what is being asked. As noted previously, whenever possible, the team should try to use the student's language or exact words to emphasize that this is *his or her* plan of support.

Thinking About a New Behavior

The next step is to write down the information collected from the "Agreements" section in the box titled "What Do I Need to Work On?" Review the list and ask the student to identify a new behavior that he or she can learn to "replace" the problem behavior. Brainstorming positive responses is encouraged before creating the final list. The facilitator should encourage responses that are likely to make the problem behavior less relevant, effective, or efficient (O'Neill et al., 1997) and, if possible, identify a response that is functionally equivalent. Deference should be given to student preferences that provide a positive alternative to the behavior of concern (see Figure 25.1). Identification of 2 to 5 alternative behaviors will give the team enough choices to discuss and eventually choose the alternative behavior they want to focus on specifically.

Our Strategies for Success

Step 4 replicates the competing behavior path model (O'Neill et al., 1997) and actively includes the student in a discussion of strategies and interventions using data from the collaborative teaming processes described previously. The team's objective is to identify at least two instructional or environmental strategies per category. Putting a team member's name or initials in parenthesis after the strategy increases ownership and is useful later on when the behavior intervention plan is being implemented. The strategies should be clear, detailed enough for full understanding, and focused on the following: 1) changing adult behavior, including instructional strategies; 2) detailing environments and contexts where the problem behavior occurs; and 3) teaching or implementing new responses for the student. Implementers should be mindful of O'Neill and colleagues' statement that "behavior support plans are designed to alter patterns of problem behavior. The process by which this is done, however, involves change in the behavior of family, teachers, staff, or managers in various settings. Plans of behavior support define what *we* will do differently" (1997, p. 65).

This step acknowledges the importance of contextual fit not only for the adults who will be asked to implement the plan but also for the student (Albin et al., 1996). Put less formally, we have observed that many students reject plans of support for a variety of reasons but, when given a choice, will self-identify strategies that are as rigorous and relevant as those that adults would have selected in the absence of the student. The facilitator should seek agreements and mutual understanding before moving to the next category.

Will This Really Work?

The next step involves having a member of the team review the plan aloud and indicate after each entry whether the student and other team members agree or disagree with the idea. In some cases, it makes sense to have the student complete this step (e.g., "Let's read the list and check to see if you agree with each of the items we've come up with"). Team members evaluate the plan by providing a score of 1, 2, 3, or 4. A score of 1 indicates that the rater does not think the plan will work. A score of 2 indicates that "maybe" the plan will work. If anyone on the team rates a plan as a 1 or 2, discuss what adjustments are necessary and update the plan. A rating of 3 indicates the plan will "probably" work, and a rating of 4 indicates the plan will work. Repeat this evaluation following any updates to the plan and be sure that consensus has been reached before moving on.

Final Steps: Practice, Classroom Implementation, and Evaluation Methods

The final steps serve as an action plan for implementation and evaluation of the plan. If there are any considerations or action steps for implementation in the classroom, list those directly on the form. Finally, identify how the plan will be evaluated, who will be involved in the evaluation of the plan (encouraging student participation, including self-monitoring and self-graphing as appropriate), and when the evaluations will occur.

Copies and Signatures

At the conclusion of the meeting, team members are asked to sign the form, starting with the student. The facilitator should indicate who should receive a copy of the completed plan and distribute it to all parties.

MARIO'S PLAN

Mario's plan (see Figure 25.1) was developed following the steps highlighted previously. The plan emphasizes reaching an understanding of the behaviors of concern and possible reasons they were occurring. The final plan includes data from a wide variety of stakeholders, with an emphasis on active student participation. The strategies listed, in many cases, match those that the teachers may have suggested, had they developed the plan in isolation; however, since they were Mario's ideas, there is some evidence to suggest that they will be taken more seriously by the student and his teachers (Shogren, Faggella-Luby, Bae, & Wehmeyer, 2004).

Steps 4 and 5: Implement and Evaluate the Plan

O'Neill et al (1997) define functional assessment as "a process for gathering information that can be used to maximize the effectiveness and efficiency of behavioral support" (p. 3). The challenge from our perspective is to collect the highest quality information (data) and use that information to create contextually and culturally relevant behavior support plans that are implemented with fidelity across stakeholders. In Mario's case, the members of the team practiced new behaviors, such as when and how to say "pass" and how to use the red and green cards (see Figure 25.1) on the date indicated on the summary sheet. Mrs. V. worked with Mario to get his "second desk" cleaned up just in case he decided to move to the back of the room (as opposed to leaving the classroom). She also worked with his special education teacher to reevaluate the reading intervention program that was used with Mario. After additional assessment, the special education teacher changed the reading intervention program, increased the times she met with Mario, and lowered his instructional group size to two students in order to intensify his reading instruction. The goal was to provide a short-term targeted intervention so that Mario could increase his reading skills and be more successful in content classes. Finally, Mr. Ortega (the counselor) met with Mario and created a space where he could sit and work quietly if he needed to come over to his office. The space included a timer that Mario could set for 10 minutes as indicated on his plan.

Mario also had an opportunity to learn how to record his own data on his self-monitoring data collection sheet. Included on the sheet was a space for Mario to also record the number of "Caught You Being Good" cards he has received each day. Mario indicated that he wanted to mail copies of the "Caught You Being Good" cards he received each week to his mother and father, which increased his motivation to improve his behavior. This also created consistent communication with his parents. In addition, his aunt and uncle promised to enroll him in a local soccer league if he was able to improve his behavior at a level recommended by the school team. This was particularly motivating to Mario, since his father had taught him how to play soccer.

CONCLUSION

Data from initial studies that have used this method, in conjunction with established functional behavioral assessment processes, indicate positive student benefits associated with participation in the functional behavioral assessment and behavior intervention plan (Hanson, 2009; Pastor-Clark, 2010). Research on the importance of contextual fit as part of the development and implementation of multielement behavior support plans indicates that "school-based teams made up of team members who are knowledgeable about the student, the setting, and behavioral theory are able to develop technically strong behavior support plans that are also reflective of the team's skills, knowledge, resources, and beliefs" (Benazzi, Horner, & Good, 2006, p. 168). Mario's case study illustrates the importance of including multiple stakeholders in the functional behavioral assessment and behavior intervention plan and extends the discussion by intentionally including the student as a member of the team. O'Neill et al. (1997) writes that functional assessment "requires the collaborative participation of the person with disabilities, those who know that person best, and often a person with significant competence in the theory and procedures of behavior analysis" (p. 2).

Mario's case study also illustrates a planning process that is nested within a school engaged in systemic change efforts specifically addressing academic, social/behavioral, and culturally responsive supports for all learners and their community. This model underscores that academic, behavioral, and cultural beliefs are not easily separated and should be analyzed together as opposed to separately (De Pry & Cheesman, 2010). In doing so, we're hopeful that PBS practitioners in school settings can incorporate innovative strategies for increasing student participation in behavior support planning.

REFERENCES

Agran, M., & Hughes, C. (2008). Students' opinions regarding their individualized education program involvement. *Career Development for Exceptional Individuals, 31,* 69–76.

AIMSweb. (2013). *AIMSweb.* Retrieved November 17, 2013, from http://www.aimsweb.com/

Albin, R.W., Lucyshyn, J.M., Horner, R.H., & Flannery, K.B. (1996). Contextual fit for behavioral support plans: A model for "Goodness of fit." In L.K. Koegel, R.L. Koegel, & G. Dunlap (Eds.), *Positive behavioral support: Including people with difficult behavior in the community* (pp. 81–98). Baltimore, MD: Paul H. Brookes Publishing Co.

Archer, A.L., & Hughes, C.A. (2011). *Explicit instruction: Effective and efficient teaching.* New York, NY: Guilford Press.

Au, K. (2009). Isn't culturally responsive instruction just good teaching? *Social Education, 73,* 179–183.

Bal, A., Thorius, K.K., & Kozleski, E.B. (2012). *Culturally responsive positive behavioral support matters.* Tempe, AZ: Equity Alliance. Retrieved from http://www.equityallianceatasu.org/sites/default/files/CRPBIS_Matters.pdf

Benazzi, L., Horner, R.H., Good, R.H. (2006). Effects of behavior support team composition on the technical adequacy and contextual fit of behavior support plans. *Journal of Special Education, 40,* 160–170.

Carr, E.G. (2007). The expanding vision of positive behavior support: Research perspectives on happiness, helpfulness, and hopefulness. *Journal of Positive Behavior Interventions, 9,* 3–14.

Carr, E.G., Dunlap, G., Horner, R.H., Koegel, R.L., Turnbull, A.P., Sailor, W., . . . Fox, L. (2002). Positive behavior support: Evolution of an applied science. *Journal of Positive Behavior Interventions, 4,* 4–16, 20.

De Pry, R.L., & Cheesman, E.A. (2010). Reflections on culturally responsive teaching: Embedding theory into practices of instructional and behavioral support. *Journal of Praxis in Multicultural Education, 5,* 36–51.

De Pry, R.L., & Hanson, A. (2009). *Student-directed functional assessment summary sheet.* Unpublished assessment, University of Colorado at Colorado Springs, Colorado Springs, CO.

Fuchs, D., & Fuchs, L.S. (2006). Introduction to response to intervention: What, why, and how valid is it? *Reading Research Quarterly, 41,* 93–99.

Hanson, A. (2009). *Using a student-directed functional behavior assessment to improve behavior of a student with emotional and behavioral disorder in an inclusive classroom.* Unpublished manuscript, University of Colorado at Colorado Springs, Colorado Springs, CO.

Kern, L., Dunlap, G., Clarke, S., & Childs, K. (1995). Student-assisted functional assessment interview. *Diagnostique, 19,* 29–39.

Martin, J.E., Marshall, L.H., & De Pry, R.L. (2008). Participatory decision-making: Innovative practices that increase student self-determination. In R.W. Flexer, T.J. Simmons, P. Luft, & R. Baer (Eds.), *Transition planning for secondary students with disabilities* (3rd ed., pp. 340–366). Columbus, OH: Merrill.

Martin, J.E., Marshall, L.H., Maxson, L., & Jerman, P. (1996). *Self-directed IEP: Teacher's manual.* Longmont, CO: Sopris West.

McIntosh, K., Horner, R.H., & Sugai, G. (2009). Sustainability of systems-level evidence-based practices in schools: Current knowledge and future directions. In W. Sailor, G., Dunlap, G. Sugai, & R. Horner (Eds.), *Handbook of positive behavior support* (pp. 327–352). New York, NY: Springer.

Noguera, P.A. (2012). Saving black and Latino boys: What schools can do to make a difference. *Kappan, 93*(5), 9–12.

O'Neill, R.E., Horner, R.H., Albin, R.W., Sprague, J.R., Storey, K., & Newton, J.S. (1997). *Functional assessment and program development for problem behavior: A practical handbook* (2nd ed.). Pacific Grove, CA: Brooks/Cole.

Pastor-Clark, G. (2010). *Facilitating inclusion of a primary student with significant identifiable emotional disabilities and learning disabilities using student-directed functional behavior assessment.* Unpublished manuscript, University of Colorado at Colorado Springs, Colorado Springs, CO.

Reed, H., Thomas, E., Sprague, J.R., & Horner, R.H. (1997). The student guided functional assessment interview: An analysis of student and teacher agreement. *Journal of Behavioral Education, 7,* 33–49.

Sailor, W., Doolittle, J., Bradley, R., & Danielson, L. (2009). Response to intervention and positive behavior support. In W. Sailor, G., Dunlap, G. Sugai, & R. Horner (eds.), *Handbook of positive behavior support* (pp. 729–753). New York, NY: Springer.

Sailor, W., Dunlap, G., Sugai, G., & Horner, R. (Eds.). (2009). *Handbook of positive behavior support.* New York, NY: Springer.

Scott, T.M. (2007). Issues of personal dignity and social validity in schoolwide systems of positive behavior support. *Journal of Positive Behavior Interventions, 9,* 102–112.

Shogren, K.A., Faggella-Luby, M.N., Bae, S.J., & Wehmeyer, M.L. (2004). The effect of choice-making as an intervention for problem behavior: A meta-analysis. *Journal of Positive Behavior Interventions, 6,* 228–237.

Skiba, R.J., Michael, R.S., Nardo, A.C., & Peterson, R. (2002). The color of discipline: Sources of racial and gender disproportionality in school punishment. *Urban Review, 34,* 317–342.

Sugai, G., & Horner, R.H. (2009). Responsiveness-to-intervention and school-wide positive behavior supports: Integration of multi-tiered system approaches. *Exceptionality, 17,* 223–237.

Sugai, G., Horner, R.H., Dunlap, G., Hieneman, M., Lewis, T.J., Nelson, C.M., . . . Ruef, M. (2000). Applying positive behavior support and functional behavioral assessment in schools. *Journal of Positive Behavior Interventions, 2,* 131–143.

Sugai, G., Lewis-Palmer, T., Todd, A., & Horner, R.H. (2005). *School-wide evaluation tool* (v. 2.1). Eugene, OR: Educational and Community Supports, University of Oregon.

Swift Schools. (2013). Retrieved November 17, 2013, from http://www.swiftschools.org/

School Wide Information System (SWIS). (2013). Retrieved November 17, 2013, from https://www.pbisapps.org/

Tillery, A.D., Varjas, K., Meyers, J., & Collins, A.S. (2009). General education teachers' perception of behavior management and intervention strategies. *Journal of Positive Behavior Interventions, 12,* 86–102.

Vincent, C.G., Randall, C., Cartledge, G., Tobin, T.J., & Swain-Bradway, J. (2013). Toward a conceptual integration of cultural responsiveness and schoolwide positive behavior support. *Journal of Positive Behavior Interventions, 13,* 219–229.

Wehmeyer, M.L., Baker, D.J., Blumberg, R., & Harrison, R. (2004). Self-determination and student involvement in functional assessment: Innovative practices. *Journal of Positive Behavior Interventions, 6,* 29–35.

Application of a Multielement Positive Behavior Interventions and Supports Plan for Alie, an Elementary Student with Intellectual Disabilities

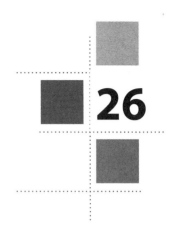

26

Richard W. Albin and Anne W. Todd

This chapter is about Alie, a 9-year-old third grader with intellectual disabilities and social behavioral needs who lives with her parents and her 5-year-old brother. Alie's story is set within the context of a team of educators at West Hill Elementary School dedicated to providing Alie with the academic and social supports she needs to succeed within an inclusive school setting. We describe the processes and activities used by the school's administrators, faculty, and staff, in collaboration with Alie's parents, to design, implement, and monitor the effects of an individualized multielement positive behavior intervention and support (PBIS) plan for Alie. There are two main goals for this chapter. The first is to use Alie's story as an example to illustrate how a school-based team, grounded in positive behavior support, can implement intensive behavior, academic, and other supports within the context of implementing school-wide positive behavior intervention and support (SWPBIS) for all students in the school. Our second goal is to use Alie's story to illustrate key features of the delivery of comprehensive, intensive support within the context of a multitiered system of support (e.g., SWPBIS; Horner, Sugai, Todd, & Lewis-Palmer, 2005; Sugai & Horner, 2009; Walker et al., 1996). (See Sugai and Horner [2009], Sugai et al. [2000], and http://www.pbis.org for a further description of the three-tiered prevention approach to academic and behavior support that characterizes SWPBIS.)

ALIE AND HER SUPPORT TEAM

Alie is a 9-year-old third grader at West Hill Elementary School. She enjoys listening to music, participating in the children's choir, drawing, handwriting, using clocks and numbers, helping with classroom tasks such as passing out and collecting papers and materials, playing soccer, taking care of her pet cat, and helping to prepare meals and snacks. She lives with her parents and her 5-year-old brother. Alie thrives on predictability and does very well with routines. Alie has intellectual disabilities and sociobehavioral needs and receives specially designed instruction as defined by her individualized education program (IEP), which includes personal care, life skills, academic, and sociobehavioral goals. She has been attending West Hill Elementary School since first grade and knows several other students. She receives much of her instruction in the special education classroom but attends part of the day in the third-grade classroom down the hall.

Alie's support team is composed of key support and instructional staff and includes her special education teacher, Ms. Jocelyn Beckman; an instructional assistant, Ms. Amy Suarez; a district liaison who is trained in positive behavior support and serves as Alie's behavior specialist, Dr. Bert Bonner; and Alie's mother, Ms. Cassi Yin, as core team members. Other school and related services personnel, as well as other members of Alie's family and friends, participate in Alie's support process and meetings as needed or when interested. Alie's core team meets every 2 weeks at West Hill and communicates daily via the daily/weekly record, a communication tool that is part of West Hill's SWPBIS process.

Assessments of Alie's skills indicate that she requires varying levels of instruction and support to meet her IEP goals. She receives Tier-1 supports (i.e., general supports for all students) for some tasks that she performs at school (e.g., using a calculator, listening to music, making transitions between school activities) and at home (e.g., getting dressed, helping in the kitchen, feeding her cat). Tier-2 supports (i.e., specialized group interventions) are provided in the areas of personal hygiene, computer use, keyboarding, articulation of speech, and staying on school grounds during outside activities. Areas in which Alie requires Tier-3 supports (i.e., intensive, individualized interventions) include academics (e.g., reading, time-telling, money use, and handwriting) and interactions with peers. (See http://www.pbis.org for a more thorough

description of the multitiered continuum of schoolwide positive behavior and academic support.)

Alie's teachers describe her problem behaviors as engaging in inappropriate language (e.g., teasing comments, profanity, repeated name calling), asking inappropriate questions (e.g., "Can I hug/kiss you?"), hugging peers, touching peers, and standing too close to peers. These behaviors occur during activities where adults are not in close proximity (e.g., at recess, in the hall, in the cafeteria) and potentially lead to instances of Alie's teasing, taunting, and verbal or physical harassment of others as defined by the school's discipline code. Because of these behaviors, Alie's peers often avoid or stay away from her, further limiting her social interactions. Unfortunately, a few of her peers also may tease and provoke Alie when adults are not around, which serves as reinforcement for Alie, with implications that her problem behaviors will increase and may escalate in severity.

To understand the process underlying Alie's behavior support plan (BSP), it is important to understand how the whole school context affects the delivery of intensive individualized behavior support. We believe strongly that investing in whole school PBIS systems both 1) reduces the need for individualized student supports by reducing the number of students who need them and 2) makes it more likely that behavior changes resulting from individualized support will be maintained (Horner, Albin, Todd, Newton, & Sprague, 2011). The next section of this chapter describes the schoolwide systems and practices in place at West Hill that have an impact on behavior support for all students in the school, including those receiving individualized behavior support.

DELIVERING INDIVIDUALIZED BEHAVIOR SUPPORT IN A WHOLE-SCHOOL CONTEXT

Alie's school has an enrollment of 450 students in kindergarten through fifth grades.

West Hill Elementary has been implementing primary-level (Tier 1) SWPBIS for the past 7 years and meets appropriate quality assurance standards on the School-Wide Evaluation Tool (SET; Horner et al., 2004) and Team Implementation Checklist (TIC; Sugai, Horner, Lewis-Palmer, & Rossetto Dickey, 2012). Behavior expectations for all students are clearly defined; taught at the beginning of the school year, with booster trainings occurring throughout the year; and acknowledged. A system for promoting, recognizing, and rewarding appropriate social and academic behaviors is present and regularly used (e.g., students receive "West Hill stars" in recognition of meeting "I'm a West Hill star" expectations). A continuum of behavior support strategies, including primary-level (Tier 1) support, secondary-level (Tier 2) support options, and tertiary-level (Tier 3) individualized interventions is present, with policies and procedures in place for systematic implementation. Finally, consequences for inappropriate behavior for all students are clearly defined and documented through the School-Wide Information System (SWIS). A bullying prevention program (Ross, Horner, & Stiller, 2009; Sugai, Horner, & Algozzine, 2011) has been embedded into West Hill's SWPBIS program. This program teaches social responsibility skills that include a "stop/talk/walk" routine. A key component of the stop/walk/talk routine teaches *all* students and *all* staff the appropriate responses and actions to take when someone is either the victim, the teaser (bully), or a bystander.

West Hill implements a Check In–Check Out (CICO) Tier-2 intervention (Crone, Hawken, & Horner, 2010; Hawken, Adolphson, MacLeod, & Schumann, 2009) for students needing more targeted sociobehavioral support than the SWPBIS Tier-1 program provides. CICO provides students with numerous structured opportunities for contact with adults throughout the school day. Students check in with an adult after arriving at school, receive periodic ratings on their behavior from their teacher(s) throughout the day (as many as 10 times), and check out with an adult to review their behavior ratings at the end of the day. Students in CICO may also bring their daily rating card home to receive feedback and reinforcement from their parents and family. In each of these instances, students receive adult attention, feedback, and praise related to their behavior and reinforcement in the form of rating points that can be used for tangible reinforcers (Crone et al., 2010). Research indicates that CICO is particularly effective for students who engage in problem behaviors maintained by adult attention (March & Horner, 2002).

West Hill uses a web site (http://www.pbisapps.org) for progress monitoring and for monitoring the fidelity of implementation of SWPBIS. West Hill's PBIS Assessment data indicate that SWPBIS is being implemented with high fidelity. This means that 1) all schoolwide procedures are defined, taught, acknowledged, and corrected; 2) data are used for problem solving and decision making; 3) the team has active administrative and district support; and 4) procedures are systematic and documented. (Visit http://www.pbisapps.org for more information on the available evaluation and progress-monitoring tools.)

West Hill also uses the SWIS suite of PBIS applications for monitoring patterns of students' problem behaviors resulting in an office discipline referral (ODR) and for progress monitoring of students receiving CICO (CICO-SWIS) and individual student BSPs (Individualized Student Intervention System [ISIS-SWIS]). CICO-SWIS allows PBIS teams to monitor the progress of each student in CICO and the overall effectiveness of CICO in the school. ISIS-SWIS allows teams to define data-collection measures specific to the goals of each student receiving an individualized BSP, as well as measures to monitor overall fidelity of plan implementation; upload and store all BSP-related documentation such as a functional behavioral assessment (FBA) and other assessment documents, written BSPs, and implementation and evaluation plans;

and enter and summarize data for decision making and progress monitoring, including generating graphs.

With these data systems in place, as well as clearly defined and documented systems for gathering, entering, and reporting those data, the West Hill PBIS team has relevant and timely data available for decision making regarding positive behavior support across the continuum of three tiers. The rates of problem behavior at West Hill are within the national median of elementary schools using SWIS for the full previous school year. However, patterns of problems are reported during lunch, during hallway transitions, and on the playground.

A team-based approach is used at West Hill for implementing and monitoring SWP-BIS as well as Tier-2 and Tier-3 support options (Todd, Horner, Sugai, & Colvin, 1999). The school PBIS team meets monthly to 1) review SWIS data on ODRs, 2) identify students at risk or experiencing a level of problem behavior indicating the need for more intensive Tier-2 or Tier-3 supports, 3) monitor CICO-SWIS and ISIS-SWIS data for students currently receiving more intensive supports, and 4) discuss and respond to any teacher requests for assistance the team received since the previous meeting. Tier-2 targeted group support options (e.g., CICO, remedial reading groups) are available and regularly used to meet the academic and behavioral needs of students requiring additional supports. The capacity for designing, implementing, and monitoring Tier-3 individualized PBIS support plans is present within the team and school. If a Tier-3 individualized plan is needed, an action team specific to the focus student, consisting of teachers, behavior specialists, parents and advocates, and other relevant school and related services staff, is identified to design, implement, and monitor the individualized PBIS plan. The team follows the time line for getting individualized support plans in place as recommended by McIntosh, Frank, and Spaulding (2010), which suggests using student ODR patterns for individual students

during the first 8 weeks of the school year as *one* of the team's "markers" for potential problem solving. The West Hill team's guideline defined that they would begin tracking any student who received two ODRs and begin a review/assessment process for students when they received a third ODR.

Using a team-driven support model means that team meetings and group meetings are a critical element of the process. For meetings to be perceived as functional, productive, and efficient, all meeting participants should participate. Unfortunately, such meetings are not always common. To build and sustain PBIS across all three tiers, meetings need to be predictable, meaningful, efficient, and effective, with outcomes benefitting students. There also is a need to prevent meeting cancellations when the primary facilitator, data analyst, or minute taker are absent. Having effective meetings should not depend on the presence of any one individual team member. West Hill's administration invested in training and coaching to build a systematic meeting structure for developing, implementing, and evaluating all three tiers of support for all West Hill teams. The training targeted team-based problem solving and decision making using accurate and current data. The Team-Initiated Problem Solving (TIPS) model (Newton, Horner, Algozzine, Todd, & Algozzine, 2009) adopted by West Hill builds on and uses the problem-solving model of Deno (1989, 2005) that was specifically designed for school-based problem solvers. The TIPS model applies Deno's model to problem solving and decision making by school PBIS teams. The model involves five steps:

1. *Problem identification:* Measure student performance; decide whether a problem exists.

2. *Problem definition:* Measure degree of discrepancy between desired student performance and actual student performance; decide whether problem is important enough to address.

3. *Design intervention plan:* Generate alternative hypotheses and solutions

regarding the problem; decide which hypothesis/solution appears to be best.

4. *Implement intervention:* Initiate selected solution, measure fidelity of implementation, and collect student performance data; decide whether solution is being implemented as intended and is beginning to reduce discrepancy.

5. *Problem solution:* Use collected data to continue measuring possible discrepancy; decide whether the solution has solved the problem.

TIPS training focuses on two components for elements of effective meetings: meeting foundations and problem solving. Meeting foundations include 1) procedures conducted prior to a meeting (e.g., define agenda; establish meeting roles, such as facilitator, notetaker, timekeeper; review data in advance; define the meeting time frame); 2) procedures for conducting the meeting (e.g., use agenda; review old business; review current data on outcomes and implementation fidelity for interventions in place; identify and define problems; use data to identify intervention options; select solutions/interventions with proven effect, feasibility, and contextual fit; build action plan for implementation); and 3) procedures following meetings (e.g., distribute minutes, share data and decisions with all staff, perform activities/actions noted in action plan). Problem solving is the heart of TIPS and teaches teams the concept of using data to define problems with precision (what, where, when, who, why) before defining an implementation plan and evaluation plan (Todd et al., 2011). The TIPS training process involves not only the presentation of content and materials but also extensive coaching during actual team meetings at the school. Research indicates PBIS teams that receive TIPS training and coaching show improvements in implementing effective meeting foundations and use their data with more thoroughness (Todd et al., 2011, 2012). An effective team management process is an important element in the long-term sustainability of

SWPBIS within school environments that are characterized by regular changes in staff, resources, and student-related problems. Furthermore, team use of data has been identified as a significant school-level factor in the sustained implementation of SWPBIS (McIntosh et al., 2013).

DEVELOPING AND IMPLEMENTING AN INDIVIDUALIZED SUPPORT PLAN FOR ALIE

West Hill Elementary School's PBIS team had the capacity to provide individualized function-based behavior support to students requiring Tier-3 intervention and support within the context of its SWPBIS systems. In Alie's case, when the PBIS team reviewed Alie's SWIS data, they determined that an individualized intervention was the appropriate next step for Alie. Alie's action team was identified to conduct the activities needed to design, implement, and monitor Alie's BSP. Alie's action team's focus was on the sociobehavioral component of Alie's IEP and followed a sequence of steps and activities for designing and implementing a function-based BSP delineated by O'Neill, Albin, Storey, Horner, & Sprague (2015) and Horner et al. (2011). These steps are 1) define the problem, 2) conduct assessment for behavior support planning, 3) design a function-based BSP and a plan for its implementation, 4) implement the BSP with fidelity, and 5) monitor the effects of the plan. The activities conducted by Alie's team and results thereof are presented in the following sections.

Define the Problem

The PBIS team at West Hill Elementary routinely tracked the school's ODR incidents in SWIS, and Alie's social behavior had been on their "radar" as a potential problem since she was in the first grade. Alie had received three referrals for two behaviors—minor physical contact and minor inappropriate language—during first grade. Receiving the third referral met the threshold for review at the next PBIS team meeting for West Hill students. The office referral form used by West Hill staff is compatible with SWIS data entry requirements and identifies not only the student and staff member making the referral but also the behavior, location where it occurred, time that it occurred, perceived motivation for the behavior, action taken, and others involved in the incident. Data suggested that Alie's behaviors had occurred in less structured settings (hallway and cafeteria) clustered around lunchtime, involved other students, and resulted in parent contacts to discuss Alie's behavior. The incidents were viewed by the referring teachers as attempts by Alie to get peer attention. At that time, Alie's teacher and parents did not see a need for a formal behavior plan. The PBIS team agreed to continue their "watch," and Alie was added to the PBIS team's list of students for regular monitoring. At the end of Alie's first-grade year, it was determined to keep her on the school's regularly monitored student list, which monitored the number of ODRs per student.

When Alie entered second grade, her teacher and the PBIS team were already on alert and tracking her data. After Alie received her second ODR within the first 8 weeks of school, the PBIS team decided that Alie needed additional social behavior support. A decision was made to add Alie to the students participating in West Hill's CICO program. PBIS team members knew from the data available to them that a number of West Hill students were benefiting and showing social behavior improvements from participating in CICO. The West Hill CICO coordinator and Alie's special education teacher and classroom assistant agreed to provide any added support that Alie needed to be in the CICO program.

As noted earlier in this chapter, CICO is a Tier-2 targeted group intervention that has been shown to be effective in reducing problem behaviors and ODRs of elementary and middle school students (Filter et al., 2007; Hawken et al., 2009; Simonsen, Myers, & Briere, 2011), including students with learning disabilities (Fairbanks, Sugai, Guardino, & Lathrop, 2007; Hawken, MacLeod, & Rawlings, 2007), very low academic performance

(Todd, Campbell, Meyer, & Horner, 2008), and IEPs (Simonsen et al., 2011). Through the remainder of second grade, Alie's teacher (or her classroom assistant) rated Alie's behavior during the previous period in relation to safety (staying on school grounds), respect (keeping her hands to herself and using nice words), and responsibility (following the daily schedule) 10 times daily. These ratings were done on a 3-point scale (with 2 indicating "good," 1 indicating "okay," and 0 indicating "need for improvement") and were recorded on Alie's daily progress report (DPR) card that listed the three school expectations ("Be Safe, Be Respectful, Be Responsible"), arranged by 10 time periods. Alie picked up a new DPR card each morning when she checked in with the CICO coordinator and returned her completed card to the coordinator at the end of the day when she checked out. Alie and the coordinator reviewed her points earned during check out and determined whether Alie had met her daily goal of receiving 80% of points available. Alie practiced her basic math skills to manage her points and use them at the school's trading post (a place to exchange earned points for desired items). At checkout, Alie received a copy of her card to take home and have signed by her mother, who also provided Alie with praise and reinforcement when she met her goal and encouragement to try hard the next day when she did not. Alie returned the signed card to the coordinator when she checked in the next morning. Using CICO facilitated Alie's success at meeting her daily goal for 9 out of 10 school days for the last 6 months of the school year. Alie had no additional ODRs for the remainder of second grade.

However, when Alie entered the third grade, the CICO data showed a steadily decreasing trend in meeting the daily goal, and instances of inappropriate touch became a pattern with an increasing trend by the sixth week of the school year, when Alie received her third ODR. As a result of her third ODR, West Hill's PBIS team called for an action team to be activated for creating, monitoring, and evaluating an individualized support plan, providing Alie with Tier-3 supports for explicit instruction in skills and a self-management system that provided more feedback and reinforcement that was better targeted to Alie's needs than the CICO program. Although West Hill's office referral form provided some good information regarding why Alie's problem behaviors may have been occurring, the first step for Alie's action team was to conduct a more formal FBA in order to better understand the contexts and function for Alie's problem behaviors.

Conduct Comprehensive Assessment for Behavior Support Planning

FBA is the foundation for a BSP that is technically sound (O'Neill et al., 2015). Academic assessment and person-centered planning provide additional information for developing an individualized plan that both is technically sound and has good contextual fit (Albin, Lucyshyn, Horner, & Flannery, 1996; Horner et al., 2011). Effective assessment examines the settings and contexts in which behavior occurs and sets the stage for developing a BSP that makes problem behavior irrelevant, inefficient, or ineffective. The primary goal of an FBA is to improve the effectiveness of a BSP. Meta-analyses of behavior intervention research indicate that conducting an FBA and using it to plan and select interventions increases intervention effectiveness (Didden, Duker, & Korzilius, 1997; Marquis et al., 2000). Research has also shown that intervention strategies that were logically linked to FBA information (i.e., FBA indicated interventions) were more effective than interventions that were either contraindicated by FBA or not linked to an FBA hypothesis (Ingram, Lewis-Palmer, & Sugai, 2005; Newcomer & Lewis, 2004).

Alie's team created a plan for conducting a functional assessment that included Alie's behavioral specialist, Dr. Bonner, completing interviews with Alie's teacher and classroom assistant using the FACTS (Functional Assessment Checklist for Teachers and Staff; March et al., 2000). Research has shown that the FACTS has strong technical adequacy

and social validity as an FBA interview measure (McIntosh et al., 2008). Dr. Bonner also conducted direct observations of Alie in the settings where her problem behaviors were most likely to occur, and the action team reviewed Alie's SWIS and CICO-SWIS data. To address the contextual fit of Alie's BSP, Alie's mother was informally interviewed by the special education teacher, Ms. Beckman, to gather information on the family's goals and expectations for Alie and their wishes and values regarding intervention strategies. The FACTS (Part A) gathered information on Alie's strengths; her problem behaviors; and where, when, and with whom problem behaviors were most likely. To identify when and where problem behaviors occur, the FACTS (Part A) lists the student's daily schedule of routines, activities, and classes and asks the respondent(s) to rate the likelihood of problem behavior in each context on a 1 (low) to 6 (high) scale. The information collected from Alie's FACTS (Part A) confirmed the information gathered from her office referral forms about her behaviors and where and when they occurred. Alie's problem behaviors were inappropriate language and inappropriate touching, and these behaviors were most likely to occur at lunch, midday recess, and during transitions. The likelihood of problem behaviors in these three contexts or routines was rated as 5 or 6 on the FACTS 6-point scale. According to FACTS instructions, routines rated as 4, 5, or 6 are selected as the focus for completing the FACTS (Part B).

The FACTS (Part B) collects more detailed information on the routines where problems are most likely to occur. Because Alie's problem behaviors were similar in all three of the contexts/routines identified, one FACTS (Part B) was completed for the three settings combined. For Alie, the frequency of problem behaviors was increasing, as was the level of danger, because some of Alie's peers were responding in ways that could escalate the situation. Part B asks respondents to identify predictors of the problem behaviors, setting events that may increase likelihood of problem behaviors, and the consequences that appear likely to maintain problem behaviors. For Alie, predictors were peers present in unstructured settings (lunch, recess, transitions) with low levels of adult supervision (higher than 10:1 student-to-adult ratio). Setting events potentially influencing the likelihood of problem behaviors that were identified were illness, lack of sleep, and lack of peer interactions. There was strong agreement between the two respondents that Alie engaged in problem behaviors to get peer attention and that they worked for her. Both respondents were very confident (with the highest confidence rating of 6 on the Part B confidence scale) of the summary statement resulting from the FACTS (Part B): *During lunch, midday recess, and transitions when peers are present and adult supervision is low, Alie engages in inappropriate language and touching to get peer attention. These behaviors are more likely if Alie is ill, lacks sleep, or has had little peer interaction.*

In the informal interview, Alie's mother, Cassi Yin, expressed her desire to see Alie learn better social and communication skills. She also noted that having Alie self-manage her own behavior would be wonderful. She recalled that Alie had enjoyed having the CICO card during the second grade and thought that teaching Alie self-management skills was an excellent goal.

To follow up on the FACTS interview information, Dr. Bonner conducted 12 direct observations of Alie at lunch (four times), recess (four times), and during transitions (four times) in the hallway. He used a variation of the Functional Assessment Observation Form from O'Neill et al. (2015). This event-driven recording form provides information on targeted behaviors, predictors and antecedents, actual consequences, and perceived functions of problem behaviors. Dr. Bonner observed six incidents where Alie engaged in inappropriate touch (two) or stood very close but did not actually touch a peer (four), and three incidents of inappropriate language. In each incident, Dr. Bonner perceived that Alie's behavior served to elicit peer attention. Although the number of incidents

was small, Dr. Bonner was confident that his direct observations confirmed the summary statements from the FACTS interview.

Using the TIPS model, the team used the assessment data to create the following precision problem statement: *Alie engages in inappropriate language and inappropriate touch during lunch, the midday recess period, and when transitioning from one activity to another, when the student to teacher ratio was 10:1 or greater, to gain peer attention. These behaviors are likely to be more frequent when Alie is ill, low on sleep, and/or lacks peer attention.* The team agreed that this problem statement was accurate and that they had sufficient assessment information to begin developing a BSP.

Design an Individualized Function-Based Support Plan and an Implementation Plan

To develop a plan for Alie, the action team used the precision problem statement (summary statement from the functional assessment) to build a competing behavior model for Alie's problem behaviors and appropriate desired and alternative behaviors (Horner et al., 2011; O'Neill et al., 2015; see Chapters 22, 23, and 24). The logic behind the competing behavior model is that problem behavior competes with desired appropriate behaviors, making it essential to understand both how the problem behavior is reinforced and meets Alie's needs and how to organize (or reorganize) the environment to promote the effectiveness and success of desired appropriate behaviors and minimize the need for, and effectiveness of, problem behaviors. The problem statement summarizes the context for Alie's problem behavior. The competing behavior model adds the *desired behavior* expected of Alie in the context and an acceptable *alternative* replacement behavior that would produce the same consequence as problem behavior. The desired behaviors for all students at West Hill include the use of appropriate language and keeping hands to self. The consequences aimed at maintaining these desired behaviors are points earned through the West Hill Star program and peer and adult attention and praise. The alternative replacement behavior identified by Alie's team was use of a self-management routine. Alie's competing behaviors model is presented in the top half of Figure 26.1.

The next step in completing the competing behaviors model is for the team to identify intervention strategies that will make problem behaviors irrelevant, ineffective, and inefficient. A comprehensive individualized PBIS support plan typically will include multiple components, addressing the various elements of the context in which problem behaviors are occurring—setting events, immediate antecedents and predictors, response instruction, and consequences for both appropriate and problem behaviors. Alie's IEP team decided to create a social-communication goal that emphasized the use of a self-management routine for using appropriate language ("nice words") and keeping her hands to herself during interactions with peers. In addition, the team identified several additional antecedent strategies (e.g., setting event and predictor strategies), aimed at preventing problem behaviors and making them irrelevant, and several consequence strategies designed to increase effectiveness and reinforcement for appropriate behaviors and decrease effectiveness of problem behaviors. The bottom section of Figure 26.1 presents the team's strategies for Alie. The competing behavior model form also notes Alie's sociobehavioral goal: Alie will use a daily self-management routine to monitor appropriate interactions with peers by using appropriate language, keeping hands to self, and responding appropriately when asked to stop, with no more than two incidents of inappropriate language or touching per week. When Alie meets her daily goal, she will have an opportunity to spend additional time with peers.

The behavior specialist, Dr. Bonner, served as a coach to the team in developing and implementing an individualized BSP for Alie that met criteria defined by Horner et al. (2011). These criteria require that the plan be technically sound (e.g., consistent with FBA,

using a competing behavior model to develop a plan), contextually appropriate (e.g., consistent with the values, skills, resources, and administrative support of those who will implement the support), comprehensive (e.g., produce a functional change across the range of situations, times, and contexts needed to meet lifestyle goals), and sustainable (e.g., can be implemented for as long as support is needed).

To be technically sound, Alie's plan was based on the functional assessment results and used the competing behavior model to move from assessment to support. To be contextually appropriate, Alie's team included her mother, and the planning process was built on Alie's strengths, preferences, and needs. Designing Alie's support as a self-management system created opportunities to be comprehensive, using skills in all content areas and settings across the school day. It also served as a nonverbal communication tool between school staff and Alie's parents. The team kept Alie's big picture in mind, noting that her problem behaviors increased slowly during her first 3 years of school. The team agreed to meet twice a month to monitor and adjust Alie's plan as needed. At the same time, Alie's IEP team inserted her self-management goal, which facilitated the sustainability of the plan over time.

Alie's teacher began each school day with a "Prepare for Your Day" activity. Students spent the first 15 minutes of the day filling out their daily schedule, which was written on the board with the time the activity starts and the name of the activity. Participating in "Prepare for Your Day" was a tier-1 intervention in the special education classroom. All students participated. "Prepare for Your Day" provided students a time to get oriented for each day's schedule and incorporated opportunities for students to practice mastered academic skills in time-telling, handwriting, addition, and basic communication. Alie used a picture schedule with a 3-point rating scale, similar to the West Hill CICO point card. Alie's card had specific expectations that aligned with being safe, respectful, and responsible (West Hill's

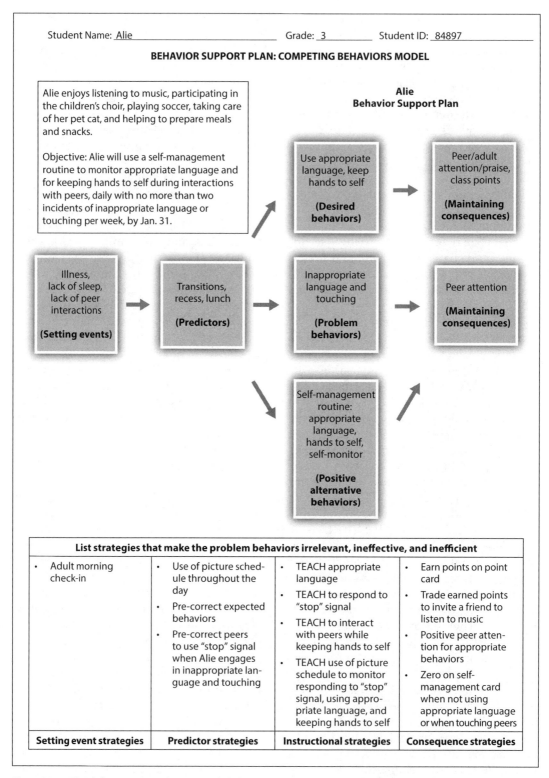

Student Name: Alie_____   Grade: _3_____   Student ID: _84897_____

BEHAVIOR SUPPORT PLAN: COMPETING BEHAVIORS MODEL

Alie enjoys listening to music, participating in the children's choir, playing soccer, taking care of her pet cat, and helping to prepare meals and snacks.

Objective: Alie will use a self-management routine to monitor appropriate language and for keeping hands to self during interactions with peers, daily with no more than two incidents of inappropriate language or touching per week, by Jan. 31.

**Alie
Behavior Support Plan**

Use appropriate language, keep hands to self

(Desired behaviors)

→

Peer/adult attention/praise, class points

(Maintaining consequences)

Illness, lack of sleep, lack of peer interactions

(Setting events)

→

Transitions, recess, lunch

(Predictors)

→

Inappropriate language and touching

(Problem behaviors)

→

Peer attention

(Maintaining consequences)

Self-management routine: appropriate language, hands to self, self-monitor

(Positive alternative behaviors)

List strategies that make the problem behaviors irrelevant, ineffective, and inefficient			
• Adult morning check-in	• Use of picture schedule throughout the day • Pre-correct expected behaviors • Pre-correct peers to use "stop" signal when Alie engages in inappropriate language and touching	• TEACH appropriate language • TEACH to respond to "stop" signal • TEACH to interact with peers while keeping hands to self • TEACH use of picture schedule to monitor responding to "stop" signal, using appropriate language, and keeping hands to self	• Earn points on point card • Trade earned points to invite a friend to listen to music • Positive peer attention for appropriate behaviors • Zero on self-management card when not using appropriate language or when touching peers
Setting event strategies	**Predictor strategies**	**Instructional strategies**	**Consequence strategies**

Figure 26.1. Alie's behavior support plan: competing behaviors model. (From O'Neill/Horner/Albin/Sprague/Storey. *Functional Assessment and Program Development for Problem Behavior,* 3E. © 2015 South-Western, a part of Cengage Learning, Inc. Reproduced by permission. www.cengage.com/permissions)

behavior expectations for all students), and she had 15 check-in times throughout the day to facilitate her use of her self-management card. Prior to implementing use of the self-management card and intervention, Alie received explicit individualized instruction for using appropriate language, keeping hands to self, responding to the schoolwide stop signal (that was a component of the tier-1 bully prevention practices), and using her self-management point card. Once Alie

met mastery on these skills, she used her self-management routine throughout the school day. Figure 26.2 presents a sample of Alie's self-management card for 8:15–10:45 a.m.

Alie used this card to prepare for her day by copying the day of the week, the current date (in two different formats), and the schedule for the day, and the times for each activity. Since one of Alie's IEP objectives was to read digital time, read analog time, and match digital to analog times, Alie's self-management

		Be respectful		Be responsible	Be safe	
Check-in time	Activity	I kept my hands to myself.	I used nice words.	I used a clear voice.	I stayed on school property/ in class.	Total points earned
🕐 8:15	Prepare for day	② 1 0	② 1 0	② 1 0	② 1 0	8
🕐 8:35	Reading	2 ① 0	2 ① 0	② 1 0	② 1 0	6
🕐 9:00	Computer	2 ① 0	② 1 0	② 1 0	2 ① 0	6
🕐 9:25	Math	② 1 0	2 1 ⓪	2 ① 0	② 1 0	5
🕐 10:00	Recess	2 ① 0	2 ① 0	2 ① 0	2 ① 0	4
🕐 10:20	Snack	② 1 0	② 1 0	2 ① 0	② 1 0	7
🕐 10:45	Third-grade class	2 ① 0	② 1 0	2 ① 0	② 1 0	6
Totals		10/14	10/14	10/14	12/14	42/56

Today is Friday   Today's date is November 9, 2012

Comments

Figure 26.2. Alie's morning self-management card.

card had blank clock faces (open circles) for Alie so that she could draw clock hands to match each digital time. With Alie's love of drawing, making the clock faces was a highly preferred activity and served as a motivator to prepare for her day. At the end of each period, Alie rated each of the four expected behaviors (i.e., hands to self, using nice words, using a clear voice, and staying on school property) with a 3-point rating scale. When Alie thought she did a good job, she circled the 2; if her perception was that she did okay, she circled the 1; and if she had a difficult time, she circled the 0. Alie added up her points and wrote the total in the far right column. At the end of each day, Alie used a calculator to add up total points for the day. She then recorded her daily total points in her self-management ledger (a bank ledger for checkbooks). She could then either save her points or trade her points at the school's CICO trading post. Alie typically traded twice a week to spend time with a friend listening to music and looking at books about cats, thereby getting the peer attention she wanted in addition to preferred activities. If Alie used inappropriate language or touched peers, she received a zero on her card, and an incident report was documented for the SWIS system.

As Alie used her self-management card through the day, she essentially took her own data. Instructional staff helped her with her ratings and addition and used those data to drive feedback—both acknowledgment for doing well and corrections when errors were made (e.g., Alie not using nice words during math on November 9, 2012 [see Figure 26.2]). Alie's self-management card was printed back to back so that she could use one side for the morning and one side for the afternoon. This strategy helped to scaffold support and feedback through the day, which facilitated Alie's success. With the data in Figure 26.2, Alie's team could calculate the percentage of possible points earned across the day for each specific behavior. As noted in Figure 26.2, on November 9, 2012, Alie earned 10 out of a possible 14 points (71% of possible points) for keeping her hands to

herself, using a clear voice, and using nice words in the morning. She earned 86% of possible points for staying on school property and in class (12 of 14) for the morning. She earned 75% of possible points across the morning. Alie's team chose to enter the percentage of *total* daily points earned to monitor Alie's progress toward meeting her self-manager goal of 80% of points earned daily. Alie's data were entered into her ISIS-SWIS file daily. As noted on Alie's ISIS-SWIS dashboard (see Figure 26.3), Ms. Beckman was appointed to enter the data.

Figure 26.4 presents a sample of Alie's report showing the percentage of possible points she earned compared with the fidelity of implementation weekly rating by staff. As noted, Alie's early success in implementation seemed related to implementation fidelity. Later, Alie's percentage of points appeared to level off around the 80% criterion that was her daily goal for points earned. Instructional staff reviewed these data weekly, and the action team conducted data reviews at its biweekly team meetings. Alie's file was set up to calculate a percentage score for the day by adjusting the possible point total per day, as appropriate. This feature allowed the team to compare days, even if Alie had a half day of school (7 of possible 15 rating periods) or left early (14 of possible 15 rating periods). The data in Figure 26.4 indicates that the program was working for Alie and her team. At the team meeting, when these data were reviewed, the team decided to continue with the plan as currently defined. Over time and with continued progress, the team planned to slowly decrease the number of rating periods and total points per day, reducing the staff time needed to sustain Alie's self-management program.

Implement the Behavior Support Plan with Fidelity

Developing a BSP that is technically sound, has good contextual fit, is comprehensive, and is sustainable is an essential element for effective support, but it is not sufficient by

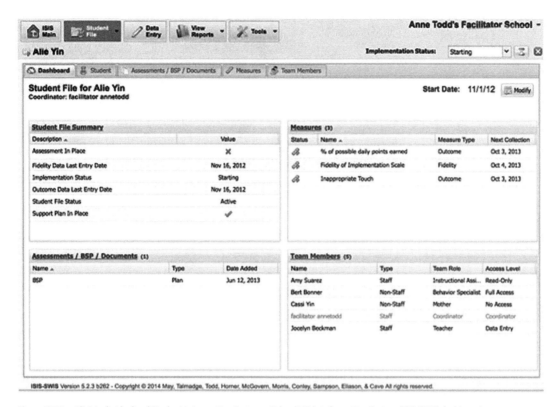

Figure 26.3. Alie's Individualized Student Intervention System—School-Wide Information System (ISIS-SWIS) dashboard.

itself. To be effective, a BSP must be implemented with adequate fidelity. There are two stages in implementing a support plan—particularly a multicomponent plan—with fidelity. The first stage involves those activities necessary for the initial implementation of the BSP itself. There may be materials to prepare, purchase, or develop; training for plan implementers; schedules to develop; and/or preparatory activities involving the focus student/individual. Once implemented, the second stage involves ensuring that BSP interventions are in fact implemented as planned and described in the BSP. In other words, are we doing what we said we would do? Behavior plans are written for the plan implementers. They describe what plan implementers should be doing in order to successfully change the behavior of the focus student. We have found it useful

and strongly recommend producing a separate implementation plan for implementing the BSP. An implementation plan identifies responsibilities and time lines for activities required to get a BSP in place and responsibilities and procedures for ensuring that the BSP is implemented with fidelity (Horner et al., 2011).

Alie's action team developed an implementation plan for components of Alie's BSP (see Figure 26.5). All instruction for new skills (appropriate language, hands to self, responding to the stop signal) was delivered by Alie's classroom teacher within a week of developing the plan. Alie received 30 minutes of instruction daily (three 10-minute sessions distributed throughout the day in natural contexts) on these skills until she met mastery as determined by the instructional goals. Once Alie met mastery, she built

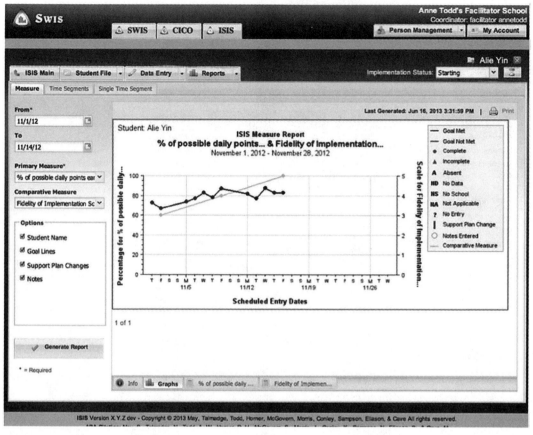

Figure 26.4. Individualized Student Intervention System—School-Wide Information System (ISIS-SWIS) screenshot of Alie's percentage of daily points and fidelity of implementation rating.

fluency as she used her self-management system throughout the day. Responsibilities for intervention strategies related to antecedents (prevention), consequences, and a safety component were specified in the implementation plan.

To monitor the fidelity of implementation of the BSP, Alie's instructional assistant and teacher rated their perceptions of how well they implemented the plan. This fidelity of implementation check was set up in Alie's ISIS-SWIS student file as a weekly rating on a 5-point scale. When the team met at its biweekly meeting, they reviewed the ISIS-SWIS data that included the frequency of inappropriate language and inappropriate touch, percentage of daily points earned, and fidelity of implementation data.

Monitor the Effects of the Behavior Support Plan on Alie's Behavior

Use of an efficient data/information system provides timely information for decision making. West Hill uses the SWIS suite for gathering, entering, and summarizing problem behavior. During third grade, Alie's action team was developed and an individual student file within the ISIS-SWIS module of the SWIS suite was set up for Alie. Figure 26.3 shows Alie's ISIS-SWIS dashboard. As illustrated in the student file summary quadrant, Alie's file was active, with a support plan downloaded and in place, ready for implementation. It also shows that Alie's assessment files have not been downloaded, since there is an X for assessment in place. In

Tasks	Person responsible	By when	Review date	Evaluation decision • Monitor • Modify • Discontinue
Prevention: Make problem behavior irrelevant (environmental redesign). *Adult will meet Alie to greet and prompt/guide through daily schedule.*	Jocelyn and Amy	Daily	11/1	Fade prompting and physical presence when Alie is successful 8/10 days.
Teaching: Make problem behavior inefficient (teach new skills). *Teach Alie appropriate language and no touch point card routine:* *1. Teach appropriate language.* *2. Teach to interact with peers while keeping hands to self.* *3. Teach to respond to "stop" signal.* *4. Teach use of picture schedule to self-monitor.* *Points earned for* *a. Using appropriate language* *b. Keeping hands to self* *c. Responding to "stop" signal*	J.B., A.S., and B.B.	11/12	11/17	Extend self-monitoring intervals when Alie is successful 8/10 days. Adjust or discontinue if unsuccessful 2 consecutive days.
Extinction: Make problem behavior ineffective (i.e., minimize reward for problem behavior). *Teach staff and students to use the Tier-1 "stop" signal when Alie uses inappropriate language and/or touches peers.*	B.B. and J.B.	Daily	11/17	Modify if behavior becomes unsafe.
Reinforcement: Make desired behavior more rewarding. *Count daily points and trade points for extra social time with peers to listen to music or other activity of choice.*	All staff	Daily	11/17	Transition to more natural rewards when Alie is successful 8/10 days.
Safety: Ensure safety of all (i.e., explain what to do in dangerous situations, if needed). *Peers taught to use the reporting to an adult routine ("talk") when Alie does not respond to "stop" signal.*	PBIS team	–	–	Review quarterly.

Figure 26.5. Implementation plan for Alie's behavior support plan (BSP). (From SNELL, MARTHA E.; BROWN, FREDDA, *INSTRUCTION OF STUDENTS WITH SEVERE DISABILITIES,* 7th Edition, © 2011. Reprinted by permission of Pearson Education, Inc., Upper Saddle River, NJ.)

the lower right quadrant, we see that Alie's BSP was added to her file on June 12, 2013. The SWIS facilitator set up three measures with data entry schedules for each. As noted in the upper right quadrant, these included a staff fidelity of implementation measure, a measure to track instances of inappropriate touch for three daily 5-minute observation periods, and a measure for Alie's self-perception rating of the day. Finally, in

the lower right quadrant is the list of Alie's action team members and their role and access level to Alie's ISIS-SWIS file. (For more information regarding ISIS-SWIS, go to http://www.pbisapps.org and click on the ISIS-SWIS link.)

In general, once a BSP is in place, it is important to adapt the plan and its implementation as needed, based on the ongoing monitoring of plan effects and reassessment of support needs. The cycle of assessment, plan development, and implementation often continues and needs adjustment as a student develops. Ideally, plans may shift in focus to increased self-management and reduced external support. The need for support or for specific types of support may change as a student acquires skills, experiences redesigned settings and contexts (e.g., revised curriculum or instructional procedures), or is exposed to new settings or contexts in which support is needed because a successful plan has eliminated barriers to new opportunities. In Alie's case, as social and academic demands increased from first grade to third grade, Alie required varying levels of support across all three tiers.

Outcomes for Alie

Alie's team produced an evaluation plan focused around her sociobehavioral goal that identified a long-term objective and short-term objectives for Alie (see Figure 26.6). The evaluation plan also identified measurement procedures for monitoring implementation of Alie's BSP and for measuring her progress. Overall, Alie met her sociobehavioral goal, as well as her other IEP goals. Although she did display some problem behaviors after implementation of her BSP, she did not receive any further ODRs and did use her self-management system throughout the remainder of third grade. The West Hill PBIS team met Alie's mom at end of the school year and collected information from the family that indicated their high level of satisfaction with the self-management strategy and the outcomes of the BSP. The PBIS team and Alie's family agreed that Alie would remain on the list of students to be tracked for the next school year. The team set a planning meeting for first week of the school year to adapt Alie's BSP for a successful transition to fourth grade.

CONCLUSION

The main purpose of this chapter was to tell Alie's story and to use it as a means to illustrate key features of the delivery of individualized

PBIS within the context of a multitiered system of support in school. There are several messages that we hope readers take away from this chapter. The first message is that individualized behavior support is only one part of a comprehensive three-tiered system of support. SWPBIS provides three levels of support that affect all students—not just those students requiring the most intensive supports. Tier-3 behavior supports should occur within a schoolwide context that will reinforce and sustain individual student gains. A second systems-level message is that data-based decision making is an essential feature of effective support for academic and social behavior. Collecting and using appropriate data to guide decisions on support at an individual student, school, or larger level are important elements of effective systems.

This chapter also provides several messages more directly related to Alie and effective tier-3 behavior support. First, behavior support is not just about reducing problem behavior but also about assisting students to be more successful in achieving their educational, social, and personal goals. Alie's sociobehavioral goal focused on learning to use a self-management system and having appropriate interactions with peers. Second, behavior support should be based on a clear understanding of the precise nature of the problem (what, where, when, who), including the function (why) of problem behavior. Functional assessment information provides a basis for decisions leading to effective BSPs.

Last, although support strategies may be organized and labeled into tiered levels of support, individual students should not be. There are Tier-1, Tier-2, and Tier-3 strategies, but not Tier-1, Tier-2, or Tier-3 kids. Any student may require varied levels of support across different domains and aspects of life. Multitiered systems of support fit everyone's needs.

REFERENCES

Albin, R.W., Lucyshyn, J.M., Horner, R.H., & Flannery, K.B. (1996). Contextual fit for behavior support plans: A model for "goodness-of-fit." In L.K. Koegel, R.L. Koegel, & G. Dunlap (Eds.), *Positive behavioral support: Including people with difficult behavior in*

Social behavioral goal

Alie will use a self-management routine to monitor appropriate interactions with peers by using appropriate language, keeping hands to self, and responding appropriately when asked to stop, daily, with no more than two incidents of inappropriate language or touching per week, by January 31.

What is the long-term objective?

Alie will keep her hands to herself and use appropriate language when interacting with peers, with no more than two incidences of inappropriate language and touch per week.

What are the short-term objectives?

Alie will use appropriate language when interacting with peers, with no more than 2 instances of inappropriate language per day for 8 out of 10 days.

Alie will keep hands to self when interacting with peers, with no more than 2 instances of inappropriate touch per day for 8 out of 10 days.

Alie will stop touching peers or using inappropriate language when peers use the "stop" signal, resulting in no more than 2 instances per week.

Alie will use a picture schedule to self-monitor her use of appropriate language and keep hands to self throughout the day and will earn 2 points per period, as defined by her daily schedule, 8 out of 10 days.

Expected date: 8 weeks

Evaluation procedures

The individual student intervention system module within the schoolwide information system suite (ISIS-SWIS) will be used for data entry and progress report generation. A fidelity of implementation measure, direct observations, and self-ratings will be used to monitor implementation of the plan and measure student progress.

Data to be collected	Procedures for data collection	Person responsible	Time line
Is plan being implemented?	Self-rating scale	April	Weekly
Is plan making a difference?	Rate of inappropriate language, touch (5-minute probes)	Bert/Amy	Twice weekly, 5-minute probes, during lunch and recess
	Self-rating	Alie/Bert	Daily

Plan review date

Team will meet every week to review student progress data and fidelity of implementation data.

Figure 26.6. Evaluation plan for Alie's BSP. (From SNELL, MARTHA E.; BROWN, FREDDA, *INSTRUCTION OF STUDENTS WITH SEVERE DISABILITIES,* 7th Edition, © 2011. Reprinted by permission of Pearson Education, Inc., Upper Saddle River, NJ.)

the community (pp. 81–98). Baltimore, MD: Paul H. Brookes Publishing Co.

Carr, E.G., Dunlap, G., Horner, R.H., Koegel, R.L., Turnbull, A.P., Sailor, W., . . . Fox, L. (2002). Positive behavior support: Evolution of an applied science. *Journal of Positive Behavior Interventions, 4,* 4–16, 20.

Crone, D.A., Hawken, L.S., & Horner, R.H. (2010). *Responding to problem behavior in schools: The behavior education program* (2nd ed.). New York, NY: Guilford Press.

Deno, S.L. (1989). Curriculum-based measurement and alternative special education services: A fundamental and direct relationship. In M.R. Shinn (Ed.), *Advanced applications of curriculum-based measurement* (pp. 1–17). New York, NY: Guilford Press.

Deno, S.L. (2005). Problem-solving assessment. In R. Brown-Chidsey (Ed.), *Assessment for intervention: A problem-solving approach* (pp. 10–40). New York, NY: Guilford Press.

Didden, R., Duker, P.C., & Korzilius, H. (1997). Meta-analytic study on treatment effectiveness for problem behaviors with individuals who have mental retardation. *American Journal on Mental Retardation, 101,* 387–399.

Fairbanks, S., Sugai, G., Guardino, D., & Lathrop, M. (2007). Response to intervention: Examining classroom behavior support in the second grade. *Exceptional Children, 73,* 288–310.

Filter, K.J., McKenna, M.K., Benedict, E.A., Horner, R.H., Todd, A.W., & Watson, J. (2007). Check in/check out: A post-hoc evaluation of an efficient, secondary-level targeted intervention for reducing problem behavior in schools. *Education and Treatment of Children, 30,* 69–84.

Hawken, L.S., Adolphson, S.L., MacLeod, K.S., & Schumann, J. (2009). Secondary-tier interventions and supports. In W. Sailor, G. Dunlap, G. Sugai, & R. Horner (Eds.), *Handbook of positive behavior support* (pp. 395–420). New York, NY: Springer.

Hawken, L.S., MacLeod, K.S., & Rawlings, L. (2007). Effects of the Behavior Education Program (BEP) on office discipline referrals of elementary school students. *Journal of Positive Behavior Interventions,* 9, 94–101.

Horner, R.H., Albin, R.W., Todd, A.W., Newton, J.S., & Sprague, J.R. (2011). Designing and implementing individualized positive behavior support. In M.E. Snell & F. Brown (Eds.), *Instruction of students with severe disabilities* (7th ed., pp. 257–303). Upper Saddle River, NJ: Pearson.

Horner, R.H., Sugai, G., Todd, A.W., & Lewis-Palmer, T. (2005). School-wide positive behavior support. In L. Bambara & L. Kern (Eds.), *Individualized supports of students with problem behavior plans* (pp. 359–390). New York, NY: Guilford Press.

Horner, R.H., Todd, A.W., Lewis-Palmer, T., Irvin, L.K., Sugai, G., & Boland, J. (2004). The School-Wide Evaluation Tool (SET): A research instrument for assessing school-wide positive behavior supports. *Journal of Positive Behavior Interventions,* 6, 3–12.

Ingram, K., Lewis-Palmer, T., & Sugai, G. (2005). Function-based intervention planning: Comparing the effectiveness of FBA indicated and contraindicated interventions plans. *Journal of Positive Behavior Interventions,* 7, 224–236.

March, R., Horner, R.H., Lewis-Palmer, T., Brown, D., Crone, D., Todd, A.W., & Carr, E. (2000). *Functional Assessment Checklist for Teachers and Staff (FACTS).* Eugene, OR: University of Oregon, Educational and Community Supports.

March, R.E., & Horner, R.H. (2002). Feasibility and contributions of functional behavioral assessment in schools. *Journal of Emotional and Behavioral Disorders,* 10, 158–170.

Marquis, J.G., Horner, R.H., Carr, E.G., Turnbull, A.P., Thompson, M., Behrens, G.A., . . . Doolabh, A. (2000). A meta-analysis of positive behavior support. In R.M. Gerston & E.P. Schiller (Eds.), *Contemporary special education research: Syntheses of the knowledge base on critical instructional issues* (pp. 137–178). Mahwah, NJ: Lawrence Erlbaum Associates.

McIntosh, K., Borgmeier, C., Anderson, C.M., Horner, R.H., Rodriguez, B.J., & Tobin, T.J. (2008). Technical adequacy of the Functional Assessment Checklist: Teachers and Staff (FACTS) FBA interview measure. *Journal of Positive Behavior Interventions,* 10, 33–45.

McIntosh, K., Frank, J.L., & Spaulding, S.A. (2010). Establishing research-based trajectories of office discipline referrals for individual students. *School Psychology Review,* 39, 380–394.

McIntosh, K., Mercer, S.H., Hume, A.E., Frank, J.L., Turri, M.G., & Mathews, S. (2013). Factors related to sustained implementation of schoolwide positive behavior support. *Exceptional Children,* 79, 293–311.

Newcomer, L.L., & Lewis, T.J. (2004). Functional behavioral assessment: An investigation of assessment reliability and effectiveness of function-based interventions. *Journal of Emotional and Behavioral Disorders,* 12, 168–181.

Newton, J.S., Horner, R.H., Algozzine, R.F., Todd, A.W., & Algozzine, K.M. (2009). Using a problem-solving model to enhance decision making in schools. In W. Sailor, G. Dunlap, G. Sugai, & R. Horner (Eds.), *Handbook of positive behavior support* (pp. 551–580). New York, NY: Springer.

O'Neill, R.E., Albin, R.W., Storey, K., Horner, R.H., & Sprague, J.R. (2015). *Functional assessment and program development for problem behavior: A practical handbook* (3rd ed.). Belmont, CA: Cengage Learning.

Ross, S., Horner, R., & Stiller, B. (2009). *Bully prevention in positive behavior support.* Retrieved from http://www.pbis.org/

Simonsen, B., Myers, D., & Briere, D.E., III. (2011). Comparing a behavioral check-in/check-out (CICO) intervention to standard practice in an urban middle school setting using an experimental group design. *Journal of Positive Behavior Interventions,* 13, 31–48.

Sugai, G., & Horner, R.H. (2009). Defining and describing schoolwide positive behavior support. In W. Sailor, G. Dunlap, G. Sugai, & R. Horner (Eds.), *Handbook of positive behavior support* (pp. 307–326). New York, NY: Springer.

Sugai, G., Horner, R., & Algozzine, B. (2011). *Reducing the effectiveness of bully behavior in schools.* Retrieved from http://www.pbis.org/

Sugai, G., Horner, R., Lewis-Palmer, T., & Rossetto Dickey, C. (2012) *Team implementation checklist* (version 3.1). Retrieved from http://www.pbis.org/

Todd, A.W., Campbell, A.L., Meyer, G.G., & Horner, R.H. (2008). The effects of a targeted intervention to reduce problem behaviors: Elementary school implementation of check in-check out. *Journal of Positive Behavior Interventions,* 10, 46–55.

Todd, A.W., Horner, R.H., Berry, D., Sanders, C., Bugni, M., Currier, A., Potts, N., Newton, J. S., Algozzine, B., & Algozzine, K. (2012). A case study of team-initiated problem solving addressing student behavior in one elementary school. *Journal of Special Education Leadership,* 25(2), 81–89.

Todd, A.W., Horner, R.H., Newton, J.S., Algozzine, R.F., Algozzine, K.M., & Frank, J.L. (2011). Effects of team-initiated problem solving on decision-making by schoolwide behavior support teams. *Journal of Applied School Psychology,* 27(1), 42–59.

Todd, A.W., Horner, R.H., Sugai, G., & Colvin, G. (1999). Individualizing school-wide discipline for students with chronic problem behaviors: A team approach. *Effective School Practices,* 17(4), 72–82.

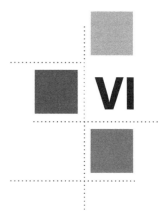

VI

Future Directions

STANDARDS ADDRESSED IN THIS SECTION

II. A. Practitioners of positive behavior support (PBS) understand the importance of and use strategies to work collaboratively with other professionals, individuals with disabilities, and their families. Practitioners do the following:

1. Understand and respect the importance of collaboration in providing effective PBS services
2. Use skills needed for successful collaboration, including the ability to do the following:
   a. Communicate clearly
   b. Establish rapport
   c. Be flexible and open
   d. Support the viewpoints of others
   e. Learn from others
   f. Incorporate new ideas within personal framework
   g. Manage conflict

V. A Practitioners understand the importance of multielement assessments, including the following:

1. Person-centered planning
2. Quality of life

(continued)

481

3. Environmental/ecology
4. Setting events
5. Antecedents and consequences
6. Social skills/communication/social networks
7. Curricular/instructional needs (e.g., learning style)
8. Health/biophysical

V. B. Comprehensive assessments result in information about the focus individual in at least the following areas:
1. Lifestyle
2. Preferences and interests
3. Communication/social abilities and needs
4. Ecology
5. Health and safety
6. Problem routines
7. Variables promoting and reinforcing challenging behavior:
   a. Preferences/reinforcers
   b. Antecedents
   c. Setting events
8. Function(s) of behavior
9. Potential replacement behaviors

V. C. Practitioners who apply PBS conduct person-centered assessments that provide a picture of the life of the individual, including the following:
1. Indicators of quality of life comparable to same-age individuals without disabilities (e.g., self-determination, inclusion, friends, fun, variety, access to belongings)
2. The strengths and gifts of the individual
3. The variety and roles of people with whom they interact (e.g., family, friends, neighbors, support providers) and the nature, frequency, and duration of such interactions
4. The environments and activities in which they spend time, including the level of acceptance and meaningful participation; problematic and successful routines; preferred settings/activities; the rate of reinforcement and/or corrective feedback; and the age appropriateness of settings, activities, and materials
5. The level of independence and support needs of the individual including workplace, curricular and instructional modifications, augmentative communication and other assistive technology supports, and assistance with personal management and hygiene
6. The health and medical/biophysical needs of the individual
7. The dreams and goals of the individual and his or her circle of support
8. The barriers to achieving the dreams and goals
9. The influence of this information on challenging behavior

VI. A. PBS practitioners apply the following considerations/foundations across all elements of a PBS plan:
1. Behavior support plans are developed in collaboration with the individual and his or her team.
2. Behavior support plans are driven by the results of person-centered and functional behavioral assessments.
3. Behavior support plans facilitate the individual's preferred lifestyle.
4. Behavior support plans are designed for contextual fit, specifically in relation to the following:
   a. The values and goals of the team
   b. The current and desired routines within the various settings in which the individual participates

    c.   The skills and buy-in of those who will be implementing the plan
    d.   Administrative support
  5. Behavior support plans include strategies for evaluating each component of the plan.

VI. B. Behavior support plans include interventions to improve/support quality of life in at least the following areas:
  1. Achieving the individual's dreams
  2. The individual's health and physiological needs
  3. Promoting all aspects of self-determination
  4. Improvement in individual's active, successful participation in inclusive school, work, home, and community settings
  5. Promotion of social interactions, relationships, and enhanced social networks
  6. Increased fun and success in the individual's life
  7. Improved leisure, relaxation, and recreational activities for the individual throughout the day

The final section of this book addresses future applications and research directions for positive behavior support (PBS). Chapter 27, "Positive Behavior Supports and Quality of Life," and Chapter 28, "Ronda's Story," describe the desired outcomes of PBS practices via the lives of individuals whose PBS supports have resulted in quality lives. Although improvement in quality of life has been acknowledged as the outcome of primary importance for well over a decade (Carr, 2007; Carr et al., 2002), it continues to be a challenge. These first two chapters in this section describe the lives of five individuals that are experiencing quality lives based on their own interests, talents, and personalities. This we believe is the future for more and more individuals with challenging behaviors. Chapter 27 is written by the three mothers of four adult sons. They describe the processes and challenges of struggling to find the supports needed for their sons, along with the joys, outcomes, and lessons learned through their combined experiences. Each young man is different from the others in terms of interests, talents, and the geographical environments in which they live. Their stories provide examples of how the critical components of PBS can be successfully applied across lifestyles.

Chapter 28 describes Ronda, a fiercely independent elderly woman who lives in her own apartment, loves working, and never intends to retire. Ronda is supported by a supported living agency imbued with the values, assumptions, practices, and desired outcomes of PBS since the agency's inception in 1997. As aging accompanied by Alzheimer's and dementia increase the need for more intensive support, Ronda and her staff struggle together to find strategies that provide the needed support while maintaining her need for retaining her independence and control over her own life. This chapter provides a picture of supports for adults that are what we hope will soon become available to all individuals whose disabilities include challenging behavior.

As the field of PBS evolves, the contexts of its relevant and successful implementation have expanded greatly. Evidence of successful applications is now available across multiple contexts and populations, some of which include early childhood, individuals with mental health support needs, juvenile justice systems, and school or systems-wide PBS. Chapter 29, "Taking Positive Behavior Interventions and Supports into the Future," provides a comprehensive overview of emerging practices and thoughtful recommendations and a vision for future steps based on current and emerging research.

The final section of the book provides both suggestions for and evidence of future directions for the field of PBS. Evidence of valued outcomes from respectful and effective interventions that adhere to the values and assumptions of PBS practices found in the first section of this book is demonstrated repeatedly in the first two chapters. These will provide practical strategies and inspiration as to what is possible for families and services providers. The final chapter provides data-based evidence of PBS applications across many contexts and suggestions for both future research and future directions for PBS applications.

Jacki L. Anderson

REFERENCES

Carr, E.G., Dunlap, G., Horner, R.H., Koegel, R.L., Turnbull, A.P., Sailor, W., Anderson, J.L., Albin, R.W., Kern Koegel, L., & Fox, L. (2002). Positive behavior support: Evolution of an applied science. *Journal of Positive Behavior Interventions, 4*, 4-16.

Carr, E.G. (2007). The expanding vision of positive behavior support: Research perspectives on happiness, helpfulness, and hopefulness. *Journal of Positive Behavior Interventions, 9*, 3–14.

Positive Behavior Supports and Quality of Life

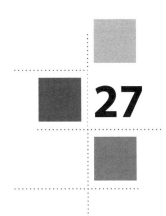

27

Lisa S. Fleisher, Sharon Ann Ballard-Krishnan, and Nila F. Benito

The sine qua non of PBS is its focus on assisting individuals to achieve comprehensive lifestyle change with a view to improving quality of life, not only for persons with disabilities but also for those who support them.

(Carr et al., 2002, p. 7)

When a child is born, parents, family members, and close friends each have their own visions for the future. As is the case with most parents, their hopes for the future are endless, with a common denominator: "I want them to have a fulfilling life. I want them to be healthy, happy, and successful." When that same child exhibits significant behavioral challenges, those dreams are often set aside—even shattered. Individuals with challenging behaviors are often not welcome in community schools, camps, stores, restaurants, theaters, at friends' homes, or even in faith-based communities and settings. The host of behavioral challenges can have a significant impact on opportunities in education, employment, and the community, and the health and social well-being of the child and his or her family (Koegel, Koegel, & Dunlap, 1996), as exemplified throughout this book and later in this chapter. In these instances, it is critical to have systems in place that honor the family's values, are driven by science and standards, and lead to the provision of person-centered individualized supports, with revived hopes, dreams, and opportunities for a quality of life (QOL).

This chapter is unique, as we are three authors bringing multiple perspectives. We are each professionals, advocates in the field of positive behavior support (PBS), and most important, parents of sons, ages 21–35, each with histories of significant behavioral challenges. Throughout the chapter, each of us has included examples from our respective sons to elucidate our lessons learned and the concepts related to the value and science of PBS.

We are personally aware of the impact that such challenging behavior has on the QOL of individuals and their families. We share our visceral fears, raw frustrations, real nightmares, and triumphs that have fiercely compelled us to fully embrace the values of PBS. These experiences demonstrate the need to provide nonstop planning and never-ending implementation of PBS processes, 24 hours a day, 7 days a week, 365 days a year. While the four men and three families represented in this chapter are very different from one another, what we have in common is the good fortune to have discovered and embraced the science and values of PBS. We have experienced firsthand the critical life-altering impact that PBS has on the QOL of our sons and our families. We bring perspectives and experiences that span our sons' lifetimes—at home, at school, at work, and in the community. We demonstrate how real lives have been achieved through the application of the values and science of PBS. Our four sons have systems of support, characterized by dignity, that have ultimately led to their attainment of "enviable lives" (Turnbull & Turnbull, 1999).

MEET STEVE, NICHOLAS, VINCENT, AND JOSEPH

Our sons, Steve, Nicholas, Vincent, and Joseph, are four wonderfully engaging men. Our families and their histories vary. Their skills and interests are fascinating, yet different. What they have in common is a history and repertoire of challenging behaviors that, *without the appropriate supports*, could have led to segregation, exclusion, isolation, difficulties with the law, and even worse, horrific abuse.

Steve

Steve Fleisher is currently 35 years old and lives in his own apartment on Long Island in New York. He commutes 2 hours each way to his part-time job at the law offices of Neal Rosenberg in lower Manhattan, where he does assorted office work and serves as a messenger to deliver documents (via subway), engages in banking activities, and runs other local errands. He is a valued member of his office and clearly welcome at the businesses he frequents.

Steve is an active member of the Self-Advocacy Association of New York State (SANYS), participates in planning regional activities, and attends the annual statewide conference. He helped lead the establishment of a local

self-advocacy chapter for individuals who are not supported by agencies but rather have pursued self-determination as their option. Steve is thrilled to have been elected their first copresident. One year he was the top solicitor of donations to support the annual fund-raising efforts of the self advocacy organization. Steve is a paid speaker and does PowerPoint presentations at local colleges, conferences, and state agency training sessions about his life before and after self-determination. He is repeatedly invited back because of what he has to share, as well as his enthusiasm for public speaking.

Steve is a loving, generous member of his immediate and extended families, and most recently, he was honored and overjoyed to be deemed "best bro" at his brother's wedding.

Nicholas

Nicholas Krishnan is 22 years old and has always been a busy guy. When he was a toddler, he learned to ski, play the violin, perform gymnastic routines, and swim. In his youth, he rode horses and became a disabilities activist, making regular trips to Washington, D.C. Before exiting elementary school, Nicholas was accepted to play percussion in the school band and at a prestigious fine arts camp, which he attended for 3 consecutive years. In middle school, Nicholas started singing in the choir and running on the track team. While in high school, Nicholas played percussion in the marching and concert bands, sang in the men's glee club, ran track, and swam on the men's varsity swim team, earning varsity letters in band, choir, track, and swimming.

Today, Nicholas focuses his attention on learning all he can in the areas of audio production and video editing. He enjoys his work as a volunteer at a local television station, sings in his church choir, and belongs to a world percussion performance group. Nicholas enjoys taking online music courses through the Berklee College of Music.

Nicholas's greatest outcomes were realized thanks to his own determination and the tireless efforts of his family and a close circle of friends and professionals who wanted him to be successful. And what do people remember most about Nicholas? "Nicky is always happy."

Vincent

Vincent Benito has a kind and loving heart. At 22 years old, he became the new owner of his own healthy vending snacks business, with all the supports required to be successful. This was a dream that was 4 years in the making, and with the effort of many, it is now a reality. Vincent's idea for a healthy vending business grew out of his enjoyment of Doritos and pepperoni pizza, with an eventual shift to eating healthier, paired with his love of dancing, swimming, and fitness, including his college conditioning class and workouts at the local gym.

Vincent likes people around him to be happy. As a result, he may do some things just to please others, rather than because he wants to. He has a silly sense of humor that is infectious. Vincent is very thoughtful and patient with his younger brother Joseph, who also has autism. Vincent cares so much for Joseph that he will even give Joseph one of his favorite pillows when Joseph is upset.

Vincent enjoys going to the beach as much as possible, reading books (including the phonebook and dictionaries), listening to music, and online shopping. His best friend since preschool joined the Navy last year and Vincent misses him tremendously.

Joseph

Within 3 weeks of being diagnosed with autism at age 2, Joseph Benito began attending a community preschool program and has continued to be included in general classes from elementary to high school. Joseph is a "cool dude." He often finessed his female classmates to carry his lunchbox for him in elementary school. His personality and smile light up a room. Today, at age 21, Joseph is attending classes at the local community college and participating in a government office internship with the personal supports he needs.

Although he prefers to be on his computer or on vacation, Joseph is planning for his career as an administrative assistant and artist. At age 19, Joseph began enjoying creating art by painting his own take on classic masterpieces, such DaVinci's *Mona Lisa* and Van Gogh's *Starry Night*. Joseph is curious about the world, and his favorite activities involve a focus on traveling and planning vacations to new places as often as possible.

Visual supports are essential for Joseph, with the most important being his calendar, where he records all activities and any changes to his schedule. Thanks to school and community inclusion, Joseph has some close friends who support and believe in him. Joseph enjoys hanging out with his friends, including his brother Vincent, who also has autism.

⋯⋯⋯⋯⋯⋯⋯⋯⋯⋯⋯⋯⋯⋯⋯⋯⋯⋯⋯⋯⋯⋯⋯⋯

The purpose of this chapter is to reflect on the PBS standards of practice at the individual level (APBS, 2007) by sharing how the values and the scientific-based methodologies of PBS, our insights, our fears, and common sense have enabled us to help create and support our sons to have "enviable lives." This chapter is written for multiple audiences. We hope that parents will garner some fresh insights regarding new approaches to behavioral concerns and renewed strength not to give up on providing an enviable life for their sons and daughters. We hope that the dreams, skills, and fears of parents, as the one constant across all life domains and settings, can be viewed with respect, treated with value, and supported through action. We hope that professionals, practitioners, and others will continue to believe in the immense potential for a quality life for those children and adults who present the most challenging of behaviors. We hope this quest not only changes problematic behaviors but also inspires comprehensive dignified lifestyle changes in the home, in the community, at school, at work, and everywhere else it matters for that person.

WHAT DOES POSITIVE BEHAVIOR SUPPORT HAVE TO DO WITH QUALITY OF LIFE?

The dependent variable that best exemplifies the field of PBS is Quality of Life, specifically QOL for people with challenging behaviors and problems adapting.

(Carr, 2007, p. 4)

A focus on QOL was not always a reality, particularly for people with significant developmental disabilities. Emblazoned in our memory are those horrific images from the 1970s of neglect, abuse, and hopelessness from Willowbrook and other institutions and "state schools" and the individuals with developmental disabilities whose lives were forever affected. These nightmarish images were captured most vividly in historical documents, such as the photographic essay "Christmas in Purgatory" (Blatt & Kaplan, 1974), the video "Unforgotten: Twenty-Five Years after Willowbrook" (Fisher & Fisher, 2008), and books such as *The Willowbrook Wars* (Rothman & Rothman, 1984).

Through his involvement with SANYS, Steve Fleisher (one of the focus men in this chapter) has come to know many people who spent the majority of their formative years in Willowbrook and other state-run institutions. He spent a year, himself, in a residential school and was subject to seclusion and aversive interventions. These horrific images haunt him regularly, leaving a vision that helps him value the preferred lifestyle he now enjoys and propels his work in self-advocacy.

The 1970s and 1980s ushered in not only the Education of All Handicapped Children Act of 1975 (PL 94-142, now codified as IDEA, the Individuals with Disabilities Education Act) but also changes in attitudes and higher expectations for people with disabilities pertaining to capacity, self-determination, equity, and inclusion of people with significant disabilities across typical settings. Institutional care was being challenged with the principle of normalization (Wolfensberger, 1972), with the principle that "people with disabilities have available to them patterns and conditions of everyday life which are as close as possible to the norms and patterns of the mainstream society" (Nirje, 1969, p. 181). This shift in focus promoted supports and services that were individualized and person centered, opening the door for a fresh assumption to emerge. In other words, if adequate and appropriate supports were available, opportunities and possibilities for rich lives within the community were limitless.

Further fueled by the human rights movement and the consequent disability rights movement, the world underwent a profound transition regarding how people with disabilities were viewed. The expectation of QOL emerged as a human rights value.

Progress has occurred during the past several decades, as this vision for richer and more meaningful lives for people with even the most significant intellectual disabilities continued to grow. Sadly, despite these changes affecting attitudes and the education of individuals with intellectual disabilities, QOL outcomes continued to remain out of reach for many individuals with significant communication and behavioral challenges. Those people were often excluded from everyday social arenas and routinely subject to inhumane methods of behavior management. We continue to fight these ghosts, not because they are history, but because the indignities and hopelessness—as well as many of the aversive interventions, such as seclusion, restraint, contingent electric shock, capital punishment, as well as the overuse of medication—continue today.

Thankfully, in the mid-1980s, PBS was emerging as an alternative theoretical framework and methodology for understanding behavioral challenges and working with the people exhibiting them. With a strong foundation of applied behavior analysis, PBS pioneers introduced a broader understanding of the communicative functions that behaviors served for the individual (Carr & Durand, 1985), the role that context and appropriate supports play, and how individualized supports can positively transform problematic behaviors. The most important commitments, messages, and practices instilled individuals with person-centered values and enhanced the quality of their lives in the process. They noted that it was not enough to simply decrease problematic behaviors without otherwise improving a person's life and condition. Rather, improving the quality of individual lives, as the outcome of all interventions, was the goal (Carr et al., 2002; Horner et al., 1990; Koegel et al., 1996).

Although no single definition or framework for QOL exists, it is universally agreed that QOL is a complex concept, which has been viewed from many perspectives and has strongly influenced health care delivery and social services (Lyons, 2010; Rapley 2003). From a research perspective, the growing emphasis on QOL for people with intellectual disabilities generated the formation of a special interest research group within the International Association for the Scientific Study of Intellectual Disability. An outcome of this group's work involved presenting an empirically derived taxonomy consisting of eight QOL domains. These eight QOL domains included 1) emotional well-being, 2) interpersonal relations, 3) material well-being, 4) personal development, 5) physical well-being, 6) self-determination, 7) social inclusion, and 8) rights (Schalock, 2000, 2004, 2011). The domains were relevant to all people, including individuals with the most significant intellectual, communication, and behavioral challenges, as emphasized in the seminal paper, "Positive behavior support: Evolution of an applied science" (Carr et al., 2002).

Self-advocates learned about and embraced these concepts and began demanding and putting pressure on the systems that support them as they strive for a quality life. For example, self-advocates in New York joined forces with artist and advocate Beth Mount, countless state-level administrators, and families and advocates to design what a group of self-advocates named "Wheel Power: We have choices" (O'Brien & Mount, 2010). Wheel Power illustrated the multiple "spokes" by which each individual could be supported to attain personal satisfaction (and QOL) through choice and person-centered community inclusion. Their vision included the dimensions of neighborhood and community membership, creative expression, family and friends, homelife, spiritual and religious life, work, and learning and teaching. The Wheel provides a framework that enables self-advocates to share existing and hoped for stories of valued social roles and support each other in giving voice to their personal vision.

In summary, QOL might simply be defined as a life steeped in happiness, contentment, and personal satisfaction (Carr, 2007; Taylor & Bogdan, 1990), with the end product, "an enviable life" (Turnbull & Turnbull, 1999).

Clearly, Steve, Nicholas, Vincent, and Joseph and their families and communities enjoy aspects of life that could be considered "enviable." Their lives represent a wealth of examples involving social relationships, personal satisfaction, employment, self-determination, recreation, community adjustment and community/school inclusion, emotional and physical well-being, and exertion of rights (Carr et al., 2002; Schalock, 2000, 2004, 2011). Yet, undeniably, the picture is more complex. These joys and opportunities have not come easily and continue to be day-by-day, moment-to-moment challenges. Although all four men are extremely different from one another in age, preferences, skills, talents, strengths, needs, joys, and fears, each has been identified as being on the autism spectrum. They each continue to present complex, ongoing challenging behaviors and related challenges to those who support them. It is frightening to imagine what their lives and futures might have been like if they had lacked their extraordinary and relentless families and intelligent advocacy for appropriate systems of support, all rooted in the science and values of PBS.

The remainder of this chapter focuses on what we have learned, applying as family members the values and science of PBS. We also share other "lessons learned," always challenged and informed by the quest for QOL for our sons. Each lesson learned is illustrated by one or more vignettes, focusing on Steve Fleisher, Nicholas Krishnan, Vincent Benito, or Joseph Benito, written by their respective mothers Lisa Fleisher, Sharon Ann Ballard-Krishnan, or Nila Benito.

WHAT HAVE WE LEARNED? THE VALUES OF POSITIVE BEHAVIOR SUPPORT

It is good to have an end to journey toward; but it is the journey that matters, in the end.

(Ursula K. Le Guin, 2000, p. 220)[1]

Attempts at assisting a person to alter their challenging behaviors must be person centered:

> PBS involves a conceptual shift in our approach to addressing difficult behavior associated with disabilities away from a simple reduction of the occurrence of such behavior (e.g., punishment) to a comprehensive strengths-based teaching approach that considers the person and his or her total life span or ecology. (Sailor, 2009, p. vi)

A PBS mind-set involves setting goals and using methodologies that reflect the person's hopes, desires, preferences, and needs. It is a mind-set filled with respect for the individual, utilizing interventions that clearly convey respect for the person and honoring that person's preferences.

QOL planning cannot simply point to the *outcomes* of what we are striving for with an individual, because the *processes,* the means and journey by which we get there, are equally critical, particularly for people with developmental disabilities and behavioral challenges. Interventions that are meaningless, unfulfilling, and even worse, dehumanizing and restrictive, have no place. Thus these four men, our families, and their circles of support have insisted on one nonnegotiable: Not only will QOL be a critical outcome for their futures; it will be a goal and characteristics of every activity, interaction, and intervention in every moment of their daily lives.

Dare to Dream?

Families, schools, employers, and communities will only reach for the stars if they dare to believe that the stars are reachable. So often,

particularly in regard to people with significant disabilities, parents are admonished to be "realistic" about what their son or daughter can achieve. In these instances, people with disabilities are often steered into stereotypic and limited school, work, and life options. Individuals are stripped of their dreams, and they dare not dream for bigger outcomes. Person-centered planning (PCP), a critical component of PBS, helps start the journey.

Person-Centered Planning

PCP is a process that helps individuals achieve a quality lifestyle based on their choices, rather than a deficit model. It is often an emotionally powerful and uplifting process through which a group of people, known as the person's "circle of support," help the individual articulate his or her dreams, sometimes also referred to as their "vision for the future" or "North Star," as well as their nightmares. The intent is to enable the circle, consisting of family members, friends, and others who care deeply about the person, plan for the positive outcomes, with careful consideration of the obstacles (the nightmares) that could potentially get in the way. At facilitated meetings, the group helps identify the person's strengths, capacities, preferences, joys, and fears, along with what works and what doesn't. Their intensive knowledge of the individual, paired with each of the participants' unique abilities to reliably listen to verbal input and interpret nonverbal input and contributions make their attendance at the meetings essential. Ultimately, the PCP process results in an action plan, or road map. The PCP describes how a team of people will help the individual work toward achieving his or her dreams of a life with relationships and meaningful activities all pointing toward a positive future.

There are many types of PCP facilitation processes, as outlined earlier in Chapters 3, 4, and 13. Some of the more familiar ones include Personal Futures Planning (Mount,

---

[1] From *The left hand of darkness* by Ursula K. Le Guin, copyright (c) 1969 by Ursula K. Le Guin. Used by permission of Ace Books, an imprint of The Berkley Publishing Group, a division of Penguin Group

2000), the McGill Action Planning System (MAPS; O'Brien, Pearpoint, & Kahn, 2010), and Planning Alternative Tomorrows with Hope (PATH; O'Brien, Pearpoint, & Kahn, 2010). It is not unusual for a group to utilize several of the processes as they meet the needs of the individual. PCP is an ongoing process that is frequently revisited for the purpose of updating the plan and keeping it relevant to a specific time in the person's life. The following sections are written by family members; the first describes the life-changing experience that PCP can have for families as they plan for their children's futures.

Person-Centered Planning: A Life-Changing Experience for Vincent, Joseph, and Their Family[2]

When Vincent and Joseph were 2 and 3 years old, I was fortunate to meet Glen Dunlap and Lise Fox, two of the foremost leaders in the area of PBS and their work with young children and their families. They asked me a question that no one else had: "What are your dreams for your sons' lives?" I thought about my dreams for them, and some of the dreams I had for their lives when they were first born that no longer seemed possible were painful to face. However, being guided through the PCP process gave us the hope we were looking for. At first, I was afraid to share my dreams. It was just too painful. It was very hard to dream about QOL for my children that I love so much. All the "experts" I had spoken to up to that point told me to be "realistic." They encouraged me to give up the dream that my sons would have any kind of "typical" life experiences and told me my sons would both probably never realize that I was their mother.

Through the PCP process, there were questions that compelled us to overcome our fears and build a vision of an enviable QOL. It all started when we drew up person-centered plans for Vincent, age 3, and Joseph, age 2. The "North Star" dreams we started striving for included being toilet trained, having friends, riding a bike, being included in school, never living in a group home, be invited to birthday parties, and making

choices. While Vincent and Joseph far surpassed those first dreams, some took longer to achieve. It took 26 months for Vincent and Joseph to learn how to ride a bike independently, and today they are working on owning their own homes. They love their lives and make more choices than most young adults their age and are truly living the enviable lives we could only dream about so many years ago.

Steve and Nicholas also have lives guided by dreams; the types of dreams that others might have only scoffed at.

Steve's Person-Centered Planning Experience[3]

After a 1-year horrendous, scarring experience in a residential school, at age 20, Steve engaged in his first PCP experience. For several Saturdays, in the comfort of our family home, Steve, our family, and his circle of support gathered to begin planning his journey to a better future. Beginning with MAPS, with Steve as the center of the process, all were asked to share our nightmares, as well as our "no holds barred" visions for his future.

Steve's nightmares were very vivid, since Steve had been living the nightmare for the past year. Focusing largely on impairments and problematic behaviors, schools and professionals throughout his previous few years also projected a bleak trajectory for Steve's future, contributing to the family's nightmares. The group PCP process of articulating the nightmares, along with the visions, enabled Steve's circle to effectively plan for a positive future while guarding against the obstacles that may stand in the way of achieving Steve's dreams.

Given the opportunity through PCP, Steve's own vision included a home of his own, a well-paying job, and a Lamborghini "with two *Baywatch* babes!" After a misdirected detour through traditional adult services, Steve's circle of support rallied together. They assisted him and our family to enlist state support through self-determination, with self-directed supports and services, to help put Steve's dreams into place.

[2]This and all other text about Vincent and Joseph written by Nila S. Benito.

[3]This and all other text about Steve written by Lisa S. Fleisher.

Look at him now! Although he doesn't have the *Baywatch* babes or the Lamborghini, Steve has an apartment of his own, a self-respecting job, opportunities to engage in all social activities of his choice, and the necessary transportation and supports needed to enable him to live a life of his choosing![4]

Dare to Dream: The Quest for a Faith-Based Community for Nicholas[5]

Nicholas's quest to find an accepting faith-based setting was challenging. This was mostly due to Nicholas's autism-related behaviors. His loud vocalizations were not permitted at most places of worship, where being silent was expected. As Nicholas's parents, we refused to give up the dream that someday Nicholas would be fully accepted at a place to worship in his community. We felt that this was important to Nicholas's QOL, especially in the future, when Nicholas's father and I are dead.

It took almost 2 decades for Nicholas to find a warm and embracing church community. It was well worth the wait. Nicholas's congregation not only accepted him; they embraced him, just as he was. Ultimately, Nicholas learned the expected rituals, including the portions of the service where silence was expected! It just took time. Because Nicholas could sing, the music director invited Nicholas to be a member of their volunteer choir, which performs every weekend.

Little did Nicholas's father and I realize the profound impact that the church had on Nicholas's thinking and actions. It became most apparent as he watched his beloved grandmother dying before his eyes. Nicholas gently reached through all the breathing tubes and intravenous equipment, placed his beloved grandmother's cool hand in his, and recited the entire Lord's prayer. He glanced up, giving his cue for all to join him in prayer, as he did his best to provide comfort to someone he dearly loved.

Nicholas was simply amazing! We all had tears rolling down our faces. Prior to that moment, we would have never expected that Nicholas,

a young man with extremely limited expressive language, would have ever led the family in prayer. His demonstration of love, compassion, and a desire to bring comfort to his grandmother and all of us present was exactly what she would have wanted.

Nicholas was the first and last person to pray with his grandmother in her final hours of life on this Earth. He begged to stay by her side. Nicholas seemed to know that he was able to share something important, intimate, and contextually significant with his grandmother: his newly found faith.

....

Nicholas's family learned, from that experience forward, that it is never too late to dream. Daring to dream and having the courage to do so is empowering for any individual. Steve had his own dreams.

Steve's Dreams

When Steve was 12, he approached my husband and me, and asked us, "What are we going to do about my Bar Mitzvah?" It was a question that took us both by surprise: Steve had difficulty participating in group learning activities, exhibited very limited frustration tolerance, and had a repertoire of challenging and avoidance behaviors at school, at home, and in community activities. Consequently, as a family, we were not active in a local synagogue and had not enrolled Steve in religious afterschool programs, as we might have, had he been a typically developing child without these challenges. Sadly, we had accepted that a significant milestone in his heritage, a Bar Mitzvah, would not be something that Steve would be engaged in. As Steve's parents, we had "given up the dream."

Taken by surprise with his request, I continued a crucial conversation with Steve. It went something like this:

Mom: Your Bar Mitzvah?

Steve: Jewish boys have a Bar Mitzvah when they are 13 years old, right?

[4]Steve's self-directed life is featured in the documentary *We Have Choices* (Smith, 2010), which highlights several people in New York State, including Steve, who have pursued "self-determination" (or consolidated supports and services) to pursue individualized, self-directed supports and services.
[5]This and all other text about Nicholas written by Sharon Ann Ballard-Krishnan.

Mom: Right.

Steve: I am going to be 13 years old next year, right?

Mom: Right.

Steve: I am a Jewish boy, right?

Mom: Right.

Steve: So what are we going to do about my Bar Mitzvah?

Unbeknownst to my husband and me, a Bar Mitzvah was still part of Steve's dream for himself! It was time to plan for a Bar Mitzvah!

We thoughtfully planned to help make Steve's dream come true. We found an overwhelming supportive Rabbi, who suggested that Steve would do what he could, without a preset formula for what he had to perform for his Bar Mitzvah. We all agreed that if Steve chose to memorize and chant no more than the short introductory blessing, then it would be fine. Steve and his father, together, would coparticipate in the religious service, followed by a party, which we thought was Steve's real motivation behind his request for a Bar Mitzvah.

The Rabbi helped arrange for a private tutor, who engaged Steve in songs and history. After Steve was comfortable and enjoying the activities, the tutor introduced the blessings, which Steve learned to sing with amazing ease. Finally, the cantor, who had never met Steve, called the house to arrange for a series of weekly sessions where Steve would meet with a group of three youngsters who were also preparing for their Bar Mitzvahs. I explained to the cantor that Steve did not read Hebrew, did not read much English, had low frustration tolerance, had limited sustained attention, and was not successful in working in groups. The cantor responded, "We will see. We will begin next Monday at 4 o'clock."

During the months that ensued, it was amazing to watch not only Steve's unexpected progress in learning the material but even more surprising his engagement, along with the other students. There were no displays of avoidance or disruptive behaviors.

At Steve's Bar Mitzvah, much to the surprise of all, Steve had memorized and chanted the multiple lengthy Hebrew blessings. He proudly read from the Torah, which is the ancient Hebrew scroll. He sang songs during the service. Last, Steve delivered an extremely moving speech that

he had personally prepared and practiced, to a roomful of teary-eyed family, friends, congregants, and religious leaders.

....

Steve's accomplishments, with the resulting absence of challenging behaviors, were a poignant reminder of what someone could achieve when allowed to pursue his dreams and when given the right context and the right people to support him. Guided by the values of PBS, these men and our families were given the opportunity to dream and follow their dreams. Choice and methodologies designed around emphasizing strengths, preferences, and natural consequences enabled them to achieve well beyond all others' expectations. Equally as important, engagement helped decrease otherwise problematic behavioral challenges.

WHAT WE HAVE LEARNED: THE SCIENCE OF POSITIVE BEHAVIOR SUPPORT

The values of PBS provide a foundation for creating a life of quality and purpose for *all* people. However, dreams are shattered unless there are tools available to help individuals and their families reach their North Star. The key to PBS is prevention. While it is the frequency or intensity of the problem behaviors that poses the greatest obstacles, it is the PBS focus on learning new skills and replacement behaviors and modification of the environment that yield the greatest promises for the meaningful enhancement of life opportunities.

From our perspective, the following four principles are critical understandings that have emerged from the science of PBS—principles that have enabled dreams to be realized.

Principle 1: Focus on the Critical Problem Behaviors that Interfere with Quality of Life

Each of the four men brings different behavioral, emotional, cognitive, and physical responses to the world around them, with concomitant hosts of atypical and often baffling behaviors. Some of their behaviors appear bizarre (e.g., an often paralyzing fascination with the serial numbers on American currency, an insatiable drive to collect advertising circulars, seemingly unprovoked loud vocalizations.). Other behaviors could seriously affect their or someone else's health or safety (e.g., pica, elopement, or an overwhelming interest in picking the cuticles of others). Still others could get them into trouble with those in authority positions (e.g., employers, school administrators, or community establishments), such as impulsive reactions to changes in routines under unexpected circumstances (e.g., fire drills, closed streets or buildings, airport security, or when given instructions from security enforcement officers). Each one of the individuals has also, at times, engaged in problematic physical interactions with others, including peers, teachers, family members, community members, support staff, security, or other public officials. Some have engaged in other activities (e.g., phone calls, messages through social media networks, or impulsive behaviors in stores or other community establishments) that, if not interpreted with their disability-related behaviors in mind, could have put them in jeopardy with the law.

Each of us has heard the innumerable excuses about why a given child or adult can't have opportunities or participate in inclusive or preferred activities—always with the adamant rationale that his or her behavior will get in the way or that he or she doesn't have either the necessary skills to act appropriately or the skills to engage in the task. It is not hard to imagine the knee-jerk conclusion offered by some people that "perhaps community inclusion wasn't a realistic possibility," dismissing any comprehensive problem solving on ways to address the challenges while maintaining access to inclusive life opportunities.

Sometimes dreams and realities present themselves with extreme challenges. As parents, we have to take a deep breath and be dream makers with our children. In the

following scenarios, we describe dreams that Steve and Nicholas had. Equally important, we focus on the critical behaviors and skill impairments that could easily serve as impossible obstacles to their quest for those dreams and QOL. In the sections that will follow, we address how principles of PBS were employed to address the challenges, design learning and support strategies, and enable them to successfully participate and thrive.

Steve

Steve had wanted a respectful, paying job for years, but the list of barriers was lengthy. Avoidance, perseverative behaviors, anxiety about his performance, and reactions to numerous stressful situations affected his successful participation throughout his schooling and early adulthood. He had difficulty communicating his anxiety and preferences, which impeded his ability to effectively utilize the supports he had available to him. Although he has strong cognitive abilities, severe learning disabilities, marked by dyslexia, math disabilities, a severe articulation disorder, and fine motor and perceptual motor difficulties (and anxiety and concomitant behavioral challenges) are evident. These difficulties made finding a rewarding job very challenging.

Perhaps the greatest barrier to employment was that Steve often didn't get up when he was supposed to and frequently spent entire days in bed. For Steve, the repeated response from the support agency was, "We can't [won't] look for a job until he shows that he can get up every day on time."

Staying in bed was not limited to employment. Steve loved theater, music, attending sporting events, riding trains, and multiple other activities with his family. Yet he frequently stayed in bed when activities were planned with recreation groups through his adult service providers and sometimes even with his family, even when he had agreed the night before that this was an activity he wanted to do.

Steve loves to ride trains. He grew up riding the subway but loves riding all sorts of transportation: subways, railroads, trolleys, monorails, and buses. In fact, when he visits cities, the top of his agenda is typically to ride each mode of public transportation within the city, even if the goal of the outing is nothing other than to ride the transportation. However, Steve also hates crowds—which doesn't mesh well with NYC subways! When the trains would get too crowded, Steve had a history of exhibiting a host of challenging behaviors, including yelling into the crowd, putting his belongings on adjacent seats so others won't crowd him, and other agitated behaviors that could elicit significant negative responses from other riders, particularly in a crowded urban setting. It jeopardized his ability to use public transportation for enjoyment, as well as for his employment.

Nicholas and the Marching Band

Nicholas dreamed of joining the marching band. Nicholas has played the marimba for many years, takes private music lessons, and has absolute pitch—a rare and precious musical gift. When Nicholas wanted to join the high school marching band, our family wanted to support Nicholas's dream of doing so. Yet we didn't want Nicholas's autism-related behaviors to jeopardize his relationships with the other band members or the entire band's ability to win awards at high-stakes competitions.

Nicholas displayed the following autism-related behaviors that could have potentially interfered with his success as a member of the marching band:

- He vocalized loudly, at seemingly unpredictable times.
- His arms would wind up in the air, like a spinning top, and he would increase the volume of his vocalizations as his arms went higher.
- He would run, with little to no warning, toward venues offering his favorite foods, like hotdogs, pizza, and ice cream, at times when he should have been standing at attention or playing his music.
- Because of his other medical issues, he would slump, almost like melting, making it difficult when required to stand at attention for prolonged periods of time.
- Nicholas had a one-to-one adult assistant with him for support and to help prevent elopement. We wondered how that would look on the marching band field and to the judges at competition.

The good news is that we knew Nicholas would be able to play the music. However, we needed to work with Nicholas to address these other issues that could adversely affect his success in making friends and helping the marching band succeed at competitions.

Principle 2: Understanding that Behaviors Serve a Function for the Individual

The premise that behavior serves a function for the individual has changed the fundamental way challenging behaviors are perceived. For the Fleishers (Steve's family), exposure to the literature on PBS was the "aha!" after years of fruitless attempts to decrease the frequency of problem behaviors, with countless number of behavioral programs tried by multiple schools and agencies that used reinforcers, withholding of reinforcers, and punishers, to no avail. It has become clear that simple manipulations of consequences are not sufficient to change many challenging behaviors, just as a simple review of immediate antecedents in an antecedent-behavior-consequence (ABC) analysis is not sufficient to understand the function of those problem behaviors. In contrast, functional behavior assessment (FBA), a process of gathering information from multiple sources, often including an ABC analysis, assists the team in understanding what reliably predicts and maintains a person's challenging behavior. (See Chapters 14 and 15 for a more detailed review of FBA.) Done in tandem with PCP, FBA provides the data to enable teams to take a holistic view of an individual's life, examining what might be contributing to the challenging behaviors and thus how to best create a support plan. Medical, psychological, physiological, or neurological conditions are considered in regard to how they might affect the behavior. For behaviors that appear to have "no apparent antecedent," setting events or triggers that might be contributing to behaviors under a variety of contexts are examined. This might include information about routines and other activities associated with positive and problematic behavior, the amount of opportunity the individual has to make choices and express individuality, the person's preferences (and dislikes), strengths, and what works and what doesn't work in a variety of contexts; these data are all collected and contribute to the bigger picture.

Principle 3: Teaching New Skills ("Told Is Not Taught!")

Understanding the premise that behaviors serve a function for the individual, it is absolutely clear that any attempt to reduce the problem behaviors, without providing more appropriate alternatives that are valued by the individual and serve the same function, will likely be fruitless. How unfortunate it is that the primary intervention suggested in so many settings continues to be, "He has to learn there are consequences!" We recognize, instead, that often those problem behaviors are exhibited because of skill impairments—the individual doesn't have within his or her repertoire more appropriate behavior responses to serve that function. What we have learned is that, with the use of effective instructional strategies, based on operant and cognitive learning models, we can "select and teach replacement behaviors that can be as or more effective than the problem behavior" (APBS, 2007, VI D4). Clearly, this means that the replacement behaviors selected and taught must be tailored to the individual and serve the function of the previous challenging behavior, thereby providing greater reinforcement. We have also learned, unequivocally, that "told is not taught"—if there are behaviors that are important, we cannot assume that the individual will learn them incidentally. If they could have, they would have—but they did not! These skills need to be taught.

Nicholas's family was fully aware of the need to identify replacement behaviors that would help Nicholas "blend in" with others in the marching band.

Nicholas and the Marching Band

Nicholas, his one-to-one assistant and I addressed the marching band concerns by thinking about what Nicholas really "should be doing" at every moment during a marching band performance. The goal was set to help Nicholas look like a natural marimba player on the marching band field. It would have to be clear to the judges in the competition stands that Nicholas was playing the music alone and that the one-to-one staff person was only there to help with equipment and to keep Nicholas's focus on playing the marimba. A one-to-one staff person with musical performance skills was able to help Nicholas. We all worked as a team to build newly taught marching band behavior skills into Nicholas's performance routines.

The first task was to help Nicholas keep from spinning his arms in the air, which also increased the volume of his vocalizations. It had to look natural. As a marimba player, Nicholas should have a mallet or two in each hand, his arms down, and be ready to play. So, to keep his arms down, Nicholas was taught to always "plant his mallets," keeping the marimba mallets (one in each hand) touching the next two upcoming notes when he was not playing. This way, Nicholas's hands and arms were busy doing something that he learned, and he looked fine from the audience's seats and judge's perspective. No more hands spinning in the air!

....

These interventions kept Nicholas focused on what he should be doing. He was always prepared to start playing at the precise time in his next section of music. He could focus on the conductor. Nicholas learned that his hands and arms had to stay down with his mallets on the keyboard to play well—not just because someone simply demanded he put them down.

For Steve, it became apparent that anxiety was the primary contributor to his challenging behaviors, with avoidance or escape being his most frequent response.

Steve

Sleep was the safest of those avoidance responses. His most challenging behaviors occurred when escape or avoidance was not possible or was prevented by someone or something out of his control. In relation to crowded subways, it became evident that he disliked when people got too physically close to him, and he feared that crowds would impede his ability to get to the door when he needed to exit.

Steve was taught to identify his level of stress and rate it on a 1–10 scale. With his self-rating system, he has come to recognize that when his stress is under five, he might be able to handle unexpected or other stressful events, with appropriate supports and modifications to the environment. Steve and his support staff recognize that his ability to problem-solve or accept support is greatly diminished once his stress level reaches a seven, putting him at greatest risk for engaging in challenging behaviors, which he later regrets.

He has learned a variety of prevention strategies or routines to enable him to control his environment or accept support and thus maintain levels under five. For example, he has learned that time is his greatest ally. It enables him to handle difficult or unexpected events when he is not being hurried to respond. He also recognizes that, due to his math disabilities, estimating time and space are very challenging for him. Thus he will often allow those who support him to help him "plan backward," so that he allots sufficient time for an event or activity. Having sufficient time enables him to let a crowded train pass or excuse himself from a stressful situation to "calm down" and then return. He is using this method with increasing frequency. He is also learning to communicate that his stress level is rising to the person supporting him at the time. This understanding about the impact of his rising stress has increased his motivation to use learned strategies and support to keep that level of stress under seven. He is also learning to use more appropriate escape or avoidance strategies, including verbally expressing his need for a "break," in order to keep the stress level within the "under seven" range.

....

Principle 4: Strategies that Modify the Environment

In addition to teaching new skills, a key to addressing behavioral challenges is to modify the environment so as to make the behavior irrelevant, inefficient, and ineffective. While replacement behaviors may be identified and taught and many of these challenging behaviors may be reduced with appropriate intervention, it is likely that some of these behaviors will never be fully extinguished, given the characteristics of the individuals and the unpredictability of the world in which we live. Therefore, one challenge to those trying to provide support is to identify ways to not only decrease behavior and teach more effective replacement skills or behaviors but also create school, work, and community environments that can support the individual in living the enviable life, despite the probability that those problem behaviors may never be ameliorated.

We have learned that, with appropriate supports that include prevention through environmental modification, we can enable people who have a history of engaging in challenging behaviors to successfully participate and thrive. Failure to provide this support is what Carr (2007) describes "dysfunctional systems"—a major barrier to QOL. The term *environmental modification,* however, is far broader than the words suggest. It is the context that encompasses everything in the physical and emotional space around the person. The physical space might be too large or small, too crowded, too loud or too quiet, too bright, too cold, moving too quickly, or too unpredictable. The cognitive, language, motor, or social demands of the task may be too challenging at the moment (even if achievable under other conditions). In addition, while often overlooked as a setting event, the style of interactions and level of rapport between the people providing the support and the individual are variables that can greatly affect the individual's behavior responses (McLaughlin & Carr, 2005). The challenge is to develop person-centered support plans and find the schools, workplaces, service agencies, and communities who will share the vision and embrace the science of PBS:

Support makes it possible to accept and live with problems that we cannot completely resolve. We may not be able to cure every condition or to prevent every disorder, but we can offer support that improves lives even if we are unable to perfect lives . . . the special mission of PBS, our major contribution to the field, involves the detailed analysis and development of support mechanisms that improve QOL, engendering personal satisfaction and happiness for legions of people and their families who need help now and cannot wait for a cure. (Carr, 2007, p. 6)

Nicholas's vocalizations appeared to be inherently a part of him as an individual, as were his spinning arms and untimely elopement to access his favorite foods. There were so many autism-related issues going on with Nicholas, his family chose to "take a number" and prioritize those behaviors that were most important to work on first. Much of what may have seemed annoying to others in the community did not really bother anyone at home. Yet Nicholas's parents realized that his behaviors could interfere with his dream of playing in the band. What brought the most value to Nicholas was working on expected behavior in a real band setting—something that would have been impossible to teach him at home. Engagement in the natural context was critical to Nicholas's ability to learn and utilize these new replacement behaviors.

Steve

To date, Steve has had three rewarding and respectful part-time jobs. Steve's first job was in the café of an independent arts movie theater, where he had a range of responsibilities, including café setup, serving customers, and working the cash register. That job lasted for 3 years. For the past 4 years, he has been working in an attorney's office, engaging in assorted clerical responsibilities and as a messenger, traveling through New York City. His third part-time job has also been ongoing for the past 9 years; in this job he is employed by SANYS, where he does presentations, as needed, typically using PowerPoint, in a variety of settings, including

university classes, government and agency training sessions, and conferences.

Success at these jobs, despite the numerous barriers that Steve presented, has been made possible for several reasons, most of which relate to the prevention of challenging behaviors by modifying the environment.

Steve has had the most extraordinary employers at each of the jobs. They were bosses who believed that fair is not necessarily "the same for everyone," accepting Steve for who he was. This enabled Steve's team, which included a job developer, to craft a job description and related supports, reflective of what was learned about Steve through his ongoing PCP and behavioral assessment procedures.

There were hopes that his job-related performance and behaviors would grow but not an expectation or demand that they must. For example, each employer recognized that there would be days that Steve would be unable to face the world and drag himself out of bed. This was part of understanding and accepting who Steve was. He was not in jeopardy of losing his job if he called in to indicate he was unable to come in that day. He would not, however, get paid. While pay is a very strong, natural consequence, as always throughout his life, there was never a reinforcer or punisher strong enough to modify his behavior, if there were other setting events that were having an impact on the behavior. While at the jobs, there were always safe places that Steve could escape, if he needed to (the rear door of the café or down the elevator of the law office). When stress overwhelmed him, he could dash out to calm himself down, regroup, and come back to work.

Steve's employers slowly increased their expectations as Steve made progress. At the same time, there was an understanding that variability in performance and behavior was inevitable and that, on any given day, he might not be able to complete a task or demonstrate behavioral modulation that he had demonstrated on previous days. Whether on the trains, at work, or in the community, his one-to-one support staff person (now serving the role of job coach) was there to provide whatever support was needed to enable him to be successful. Although most days Steve engaged in most job tasks on his own, with minimal support, there were other times that the job coach worked side by side with him, as coparticipant, ensuring successful completion of the job requirements. Finally, there were times at work, on the trains, and in the community that the coach's role was to be a buffer between Steve and the world.

Not surprising, given the enormous support but not demand to progress, Steve showed enormous growth. He rarely misses workdays due to avoidance. He increasingly uses proactive planning to try to avoid stressful situations. And he is a valued worker who feels great about himself.

....

Nicholas and the Marching Band

As Nicholas's mother, I am convinced that the personality, attitude, and vision of the high school band director were key to Nicholas's success in the band program and the related environment.

The band director's acceptance of Nicholas and his ability to appear undistracted by Nicholas's vocalizations while continuing to teach the class made everyone around Nicholas accepting and willing to try whatever it took to make the marching band experience work for Nicholas. Nicholas's band peers soon embodied those virtues exhibited by the band director. The warm daily greetings, smiles, and laughter offered by all deescalated Nicholas's inherent and everpresent anxiety. Nicholas felt at home in band class, all thanks to the band director's calming leadership.

The band director allowed Nicholas to use whatever was needed to make the marching band experience work. For example, he allowed Nicholas to chew gum during rehearsals and performances to prevent spontaneous vocalizations. He understood that Nicholas didn't make noises while chewing gum. Nicholas was permitted to use a tall director's type chair while playing on the marching band field. The chair helped Nicholas maintain his posture, without melting at the knees, and the arms of the chair were the physical prompt for Nicholas not to run toward the food stand while performing. This was paired with the consistent routine of taking Nicholas directly to the concession stand to have his favorite food to celebrate, once the performance was over.

The most fascinating transformation I remember was that whenever Nicholas changed into the same marching band uniform that everyone else was wearing, his behavior suddenly became more uniform! He became something more than just himself while wearing that uniform. He seemed

to understand that proper band behavior came along with wearing the uniform and that all members in the band were expected to exhibit those behaviors. Nicholas was not the only one who had to be quiet and stand at attention. Everyone in the uniform did, so he did.

When Nicholas was utilizing his new behavioral instruction to "plant the mallets," Nicholas's flailing arms soon became musical hands. Because Nicholas was permitted to chew gum, his loud and unexpected vocalizations disappeared. All the audience could hear was music. All that the audience could see was a musician, who eventually was selected to play critical solos on the marching band field. Common sense allowed Nicholas to participate in the marching band, perform at every competition, and attend band camp for his entire high school career. Nicholas earned a varsity letter and numerous other awards, including his favorite "best friend award," given to him by his marching band peers.

....

Support Staff Need to Learn New Skills Too!

What is equally notable is the recognition that new skills or replacement behaviors are necessary not only for the individual who engages in "problematic behaviors" but also for the people providing support to that individual, even when the skills or behaviors are counterintuitive. When situations get difficult, people tend to rely on "common sense" solutions—not necessarily the supports or reactions that will best support the individual, as documented in their FBAs and behavior support plans. For successful behavior support to occur, families, teachers, and support staff need to learn the skills needed to employ strategies consistent with the individually designed support plan.

Steve

It had been evident for quite a while that Steve often stayed in bed to avoid a variety of things: He avoided potentially stressful situations, he avoided unpredictable situations, and he slept due to fatigue after being awake all night worrying about those (or other) situations. He also stayed in bed when he saw no value in waking up. It was recognized that Steve needed to be taught to better identify and communicate his preferences and fears. Various strategies had been tried countless times in his past, to no avail.

However, behavior change ultimately occurred when his support network (family and staff) learned to better read his verbal and nonverbal cues, to enable him to "avoid or escape" when he verbalized he was at "stress level six" or was "having a panic attack." It was critical to refrain from even the mildest forms of coercion and mostly to earn his trust that when he communicated verbally or nonverbally; we would respect his preferences, whether we agreed or not.

....

WHAT ELSE HAVE WE LEARNED?

The remainder of this chapter includes the wisdom and adages that we, as parents, have learned. They keep our compasses due north, even in crisis situations. All are founded on the principles of PBS, yet have been enhanced by our roles as parents and advocates throughout our sons' entire lives while looking toward their futures.

"Getting Ready" Actually Means "Never"!

If we spend our lives "getting reading to live," we may never enjoy the act of living.

Steve

Steve lives in his own apartment, not with his family or in a group residence. He did not need to wait until he could manage his budget, cook and clean independently, or manage his social emotional reactions to the world around him. Instead, he has 24/6 support staff (he spends one day a week at home with family) who he and our family hire (using state dollars) and train to provide the intensive supports he needs in his home, job, and community. As a result of PCP and a job developer who identified the "right job," with the "right boss" and the "right supports," he wakes up and gets ready every day for work—and he did not need to first prove he would get up every day at a specific time.

He rides public transportation, with his support staff serving to buffer the everchanging bombardment of challenging events in NYC. He receives support on the job, as necessary, for the job tasks that are too challenging. He is a valued worker and friend and loves going to work. The behavioral challenges that plagued his very existence when he lived in a group residence with inappropriate supports are now infrequent and most importantly do not prevent him from living a quality community based life.

....

If Vincent needed to wait until he had all the skills to run a vending business; or if Nicholas needed to first demonstrate "hands down" or "no vocalizations" before he could practice with the band; or if Steve, whose first job was in the café of a local independent theater, had to first demonstrate that he could arrive on time every day or had all the skills to work as a server in a café or not flee when the demands behind the serving counter got too stressful, they would never have met the "entry" criterion. They would all still be "getting ready." With the right supports, they all thrived in their jobs. Just as Nicholas learned to play with the marching band by participating with the marching band, job-related skills and behavioral modulation for Vincent and Steve were learned in the most meaningful context—the context of the real jobs they wanted.

Nila's Experience, as a Parent

Having my two sons, Vincent (age 3) and Joseph (age 2), diagnosed with an intellectual disability and autism in 1994, I wanted to learn what I needed to do to support them in having the best QOL possible. I searched and searched. I looked for experts and was told about this doctor and that doctor. I took my sons to these doctors only to walk out with a number of prescriptions that I was told might help them. One doctor told me that my sons would never realize that I was their mother. At first, I was stuck in a medical model. How do we fix this? Is there a cure? How do you stop this from getting worse? Seeking answers to these questions was daunting and overall just created more questions.

After talking with several families, I realized that most were willing to try anything. Many families were very involved with special diets and a therapy that took at least 40 hours a week, with their child learning skills, sitting at a table. I asked one mom who had a 6-year-old daughter, "When does your daughter get time to play?" She said, "Oh there is no time for that right now. She has got to learn these skills before it's too late."

Another family told me they did not take their 12-year-son out to dinner, the movies, the mall, or on vacation because he wasn't ready. No time to play? Not ready? It just didn't make any sense to me. I thought about my life and the times when I had to make decisions. If I had waited until I was sure I was ready, then I would have *never* moved forward. Being "ready" took on a whole new meaning to me; we are quite often as ready as we are ever going to be.

....

Value the Person

Nicholas is a member of a world percussion performance group. He is included as a regular performer, not because people have altruistically agreed to include a person with disabilities, but because he is an excellent drummer. His drumming brings something valuable to the ensemble. They value Nicholas, the drummer and performer, for the expertise he brings to the group. They treat him with respect, with friendship, and as a community member. In turn, Nicholas exhibits few problem behaviors when he is fully engaged in performing.

The degree to which others "value the person" is highly related to the assumptions they hold about what that person can achieve. In 1984, Anne Donnellan wrote that "the criterion of least dangerous assumption holds that, in the absence of conclusive data, educational decisions ought to be based on assumptions that, if incorrect, will have the least dangerous effect on the likelihood that students will be able to function independently as adults," concluding that "we should assume that poor performance is due to instructional inadequacy rather than to

student deficits" (p. 142). Thus, for us, as with Donnellan, the least-dangerous assumption is to assume that individuals, even those with significant challenges, will be able to achieve their dreams with the appropriate instruction and supports.

Joseph

Many in Joseph's circle of support who were asked to help identify the kinds of jobs that would be based on his strengths and interests and provide him with satisfaction and joy held the opinion that it was unrealistic to consider that he would one day have a job. One team member stated that "Joseph's parents must be in denial if they think he can work after high school." His school team and state funding agency staff concurred, often emphasizing his lack of verbal communication as an obstacle, "He can only express his needs and wants." It was Joseph's same-age peers without disabilities who were the most creative and positive about his options as an adult. One peer shared, "I think Joseph can do anything he wants to do. He is better on the computer than I will ever be." Getting the peers and the few adults, who believed in Joseph, to share their perspective with those who didn't was a transformation experience that changed perspectives on not only Joseph's potential but the potential of other individuals similar to him.

....

Relationships, Relationships, Relationships: Relationships Are to Positive Behavior Support as Location Is to Real Estate

Quality lives for all people are built around relationships. Relationships affect how we perceive each other, including what quirks we might accept or overlook. We turn to relationships for friendship and support, as well as social connectedness; this in turn often creates connections with other people and other life opportunities, a concept frequently referred to as social capital (Condeluci, 2002). It is those social connections that enable us to network to meet new friends, find jobs and meaningful social outlets, engage in community, assist with transportation needs, and arrange for preferred housing and living choices.

When one has the characteristics that are likely to result in challenging, unwanted, undesirable, or unattractive behaviors, quality relationships become all the more important. In Joseph's example, it was the long-established relationship that Joseph had developed with peers that affected their perceptions of him and consequently the perceptions of the nonbelieving school team and agency providers that have a positive impact on Joseph's ultimate life potential. In the example provided earlier, it took Nicholas's family almost 2 decades to find Nicholas a place to worship in which he not only was welcome but ultimately became a full, valued member of the choir. What did it take? As with all things that work best for Nicholas, it took the right people and Nicholas's own learned skills. The people who invited Nicholas into the church knew him from his years in the high school band and choir. The choir director was a student in the high school band with Nicholas many years before they became adults and would rediscover each other again. The organist was his accompanist for the high school choir and realized that Nicholas could sing, even though he rarely spoke a word. They appreciated Nicholas's musical gifts and intellectually understood his autism-related vocalizations. To them, Nicholas's musical skills and happy personality outweighed the occasional inconvenience of a random vocalization. At Nicholas's newly found church, the congregation soon learned that his loud laughter stemmed from his pure joy of being there. And that made others smile too. Nicholas's initial acceptance and, ultimately, his fully valued participation in his church choir and the congregation were made possible because of the relationships he had developed though his entire life of meaningful skill cultivation and relationship building.

Relationships affect everyday experiences in the community as well, particularly when someone has what others might perceive as peculiar behaviors that may be reflected in seemingly odd requests or unusual behavior responses. There are a host of reasons these behaviors and requests may be triggered. It is the development and nurturing of sincere and often simple (but important) relationships that can prevent disastrous outcomes that might otherwise be seriously life altering or potentially lead to trouble with law enforcement. It is the critical everyday relationships that enable others to learn to see beyond the quirkiness of one's actions or words.

Steve

Steve has an intense, at times immobilizing, fascination with the serial numbers on American currency, as well as the condition of the bills (e.g., bills free from writing or smudges, new bills in color, old bills with the older designs, serial numbers beginning with B2 or A1 or F6). He has specific requests for bills when he cashes his paycheck or when he gets change after shopping. He will often stop at supermarket service desks to ask to exchange bills. There was great concern by Steve's family and support staff that this would create a severe problem in the community, with the expectation that there would be little tolerance for his seemingly ridiculous requests. However, the relationships that Steve has developed with these community people have astounded all the skeptics. Tellers and supermarket clerks each spend considerable amounts of time searching through their stacks for the "right" bills. They patiently explain to their uninitiated and new coworkers what Steve is looking for with his currency request. Further, rather than the recoil, as one might have anticipated, there is always a warm, "Hello," whenever Steve walks to their windows and a warm waving of good-bye as he leaves the store.

....

Relationships with support staff are critically important for all individuals who rely on others for support. Respect and the true ability to see, enjoy, and positively engage with the person behind the disabilities and their related behaviors are essential to their QOL, day in and day out. McLaughlin and

Carr (2005) demonstrated that the quality of rapport between individuals with developmental disabilities and their direct support was a setting event for either problem or desired behavior. The staff members who understand and accept the person for who he or she is aptly embrace the values and science of PBS.

As families, we have witnessed incredibly powerful reciprocal relationships, where our sons have positively influenced the lives of staff members, as well. One such person is Anthony, Nicholas's staff member. Recently, Anthony commented to the newspaper reporter from *The Oakland Press,* "I thought that he was going to have to have all this special attention, but he didn't." Anthony continued, "When I met Nick, I knew everything was going to be a piece of cake. He was a lot of fun to be with . . . We formed a very, very, very good friendship." As a result of their friendship, Anthony chose to return back to school to study media arts production, an interest that came to Anthony through his work supporting Nicholas with his studies in video editing and Nicholas's related volunteer work at two local community television stations.

Their collective joys of engaging in their favorite common interest, audiovisual production, infused with Anthony's fun-loving personality that uplifted Nicholas's spirits along the way, clearly led to a sense of well-being for both Nicholas and Anthony. Their relationship developed into one that is now deeply rooted in mutual respect, for their natural relationships, the skills they share, and the manner in which they interact with one another. Anthony demonstrated, through his work with Nicholas, what true support leading to QOL outcomes can resemble.

Respect, Respect, Respect

The key is to never forget that, regardless of the intensity of the behavioral challenges or other disabilities, the person exhibiting those problem behaviors is a human being, who has something valuable to contribute. This was clearly the case with Anthony and Nicholas's mutual respect for one another, resulting in a relationship that benefited both individuals. Yet there are people who continue to think it is okay to dehumanize people who aren't behaving well. Rather than valuing the person, they see only a "problematic person" that needs to be fixed, as if the person is a thing or object to be somehow manipulated. Using that mind-set, they are likely to propose equally simplistic, disrespectful interventions to address the behaviors; this leads to unhealthy relationships defined by power and control. Nicholas, who has extremely limited verbal language and has been a victim of abuse by someone trying to control his behavior in the past, once shared some of his brief thoughts with an auditorium full of professionals. Near the end of his self-produced video presentation (which he uses instead of verbal presentations), Nicholas emphatically stated, "What you see is not who I am!" (Krishnan, 2012). Nicholas's plea underscores huge ethical considerations to think about when working with people while looking for solutions to resolve troubling behaviors.

When Steve discovered we were writing this chapter, he expressed that he wanted to be interviewed to share his perspective not just as a person with great support needs but also as a representative of "self-advocates." The message that he wanted to be shared more than anything is the desire to be respected. He shared, "We want to be treated as human beings, not like second-class citizens. We hate when someone is bossy or treats us like they are our parents. We want people to make suggestions for us, but we want it to be our choice." And Steve concluded with his intent to advocate for those who were less able to advocate for themselves about the right to privacy, respect, and self-direction in their own lives.

These are critical admonitions about how people often underestimate what individuals with disabilities are capable of, solely based on obvious quirky characteristics or annoying behaviors. Nicholas and Steve refer to the unacceptable practice of infantilizing or disrespecting people with disabilities, speaking *about them* rather than *to them* (even while they are standing right there); sharing their personal information without obtaining consent; making decisions for them without ascertaining their preferences, choices, and decisions about issues; and most egregious, using intervention strategies that are humiliating, dehumanizing, and affect the very core of who that person is. Legislation is not robust enough to curtail all the cruelty they have witnessed and endured in their own lives. Thankfully for them, there are some good guys who come along, lift them up, and help them start seeking the quality they have looked for, all over again.

Nicholas concluded his presentation saying, "Helping facilitate a life worth living is what it is really all about." His words serve as a great reminder to value the person by honoring their own sense of purpose, personal fulfillment, and what makes them most happy, even during the most trying times. And please be kind.

Learn to Listen:
Whose Goal Is It, Anyway?

While the benefits are obvious, the enthusiastic and positive inclination to set ambitious goals can easily be a double-edged sword. Parents and professionals often believe they have the responsibility, knowledge, and the hindsight to know "what is best" for a child (with or without disabilities) or an adult with developmental disabilities. Individuals typically won't select goals or activities or foods that they have never been exposed to, and parental responsibility involves providing those experiences in supportive manners. While that may often be the case regarding raising children, where does that stop? We can all think of examples where parents, thinking they know best, tried to plan their adolescent or adult child's future; we recall well one father who was insistent that his college-bound son was going to be a doctor. He relentlessly pressured his son to begin the premed curriculum. The father

persisted until the son earned a D– in his first chemistry class. The function of the son's behavior was pretty obvious. The son ultimately pursued a Ph.D. in political science and a successful university career.

The tendency for others to try to determine what is best for the individual and how to best achieve those goals is even stronger when the individual has developmental disabilities. Living with someone who has expressive language difficulties can be extremely challenging. Without the give and take of reciprocal dialogue, relationships are often based on the most educated guesses we can make about someone. Thus how do you assist the person to discover what they might enjoy, appreciate, and gain satisfaction and QOL from, while at the same time refraining (or preventing others) from imposing their views on appropriate goals or activities? And how do you sensitize support teams into recognizing that even subtle coercion can be the setting event for challenging behaviors? Like the future political scientist, individuals coerced (even subtly) into lifestyles not of their choosing will communicate using whatever means necessary. Using behavior as one's best means to communicate starts young.

Nicholas's family had him participate in many different types of activities, starting when he was very young. These included academics, the fine arts, athletics, and travel. The hope was to help Nicholas become an interesting person while he became interested in what the world around him had to offer. In the following section, Nicholas's mother explains how she learned to understand his preferences.

Nicholas's Preferences

Being busy always seemed to positively fuel Nicholas's well-being. As new interests emerged and Nicholas's schedule started looking too ambitious, I observed Nicholas closely to figure out signs of Nicholas's pleasure or displeasure with his activities. It didn't take long for me to figure out which activities Nicholas was relieved to drop. When Nicholas didn't like an activity, he would consistently request to use the restroom, even after he had just gone. This seemed to be Nicholas's personally designed "escape and avoidance" behavior. Nicholas would increasingly spend more time in the bathroom, singing and dancing in front of the mirror, than with the intended activity itself. It seemed that Nicholas was on a quest to find his own fun. Yet when Nicholas sincerely enjoyed participating in an activity, he would only use the restroom before and after, preferring to spend most his time at the setting of the activity.

Nicholas's behavior has always been the most reliable means of communication, so much that Nicholas's father and I can "read" Nicholas, simply by paying close attention to his behaviors.

....

For Nicholas's family, behavior is Nicholas's unspoken language.

Power and Control: Support and Control Are Not the Same

Attempts at controlling someone's behavior and dominating the person are vastly different from supporting an individual's needs, especially when behaviors reflect one's attempts at communicating those needs. When control becomes more dominant than support, the relationships between the individuals suffer tremendously, adding another layer of complexity to the resolution of the true behaviors that must be ameliorated. Caution must be used if attempting to eliminate one's behaviors, since they may be the only means of communicating at that time. Behaviors carry meaning for the person. Hence, when addressing problematic behaviors, it is crucial for support providers to step back and avoid interventions that even remotely resemble control and dominance over the person. It is crucial to step back and attempt to be objective and separate out which support decisions are consistent with the person's values, likes, preferences, and support needs and which are simply imposed on the person in response to the discomfort level of the support provider. It is irrelevant whether the support staff feel uncomfortable as Steve goes from bank to bank exchanging currency to obtain the bills that he prefers.

It isn't uncommon for people to collect certain currency. In any instances of attempts to steer Steve away from the comfort that exchanging currency brings him, one might ask, "Who is truly receiving the support?"

If It Isn't Dangerous or Destructive, Get over It

An interesting rhetorical question to ask oneself is, "If there is nobody to witness someone's behavioral challenges, and if it isn't dangerous or destructive to the person or others, is the behavior problematic at all?" What is a problematic behavior? Who decides? Have you ever stood at the freezer door and eaten ice cream with a spoon directly from the container? Or took a swig from the milk container? Or forgot something as you were jumping into the shower or tub and had to go get it with no clothing on? Or watched movies that were of questionable taste? Or "told off your boss" while staring at yourself in the mirror? Or had countless other private thoughts or personal interactions that you were happy were not recorded, documented, or observed?

Imagine how it would feel to have someone in your home or in the community with you all the time, documenting and assessing your every move, in the name of "support": judging whether you should take another donut or two; deciding which of your benign habits and much-needed coping behaviors should be modified; looking to change who you are as a person; telling you that, finally, when you are out and about, you cannot have that one bottle of cola that you have been so badly craving; tattling to others, every day of your life, for the rest of your life; having the completion of data forms become a more important priority than engaging with you; not being able to find the meaning of "support" in the support staff.

As families of sons with disabilities, we learned early on that we could be unintentionally "picking" on our sons, day in and day out, in our quest to teach proper behavior. We didn't want to do that, since we needed time to enjoy our guys, too. Hence we learned to "pick our fights" by using the adage, "If it isn't dangerous or destructive, or have the clear potential for adverse QOL consequences, just get over it!"

Three Magic Words: "It's Your Choice"

Resist the temptation to make people earn what they really need most; what makes them capable of regrouping, and those things which bring comfort and peace.

(Krishnan, 2012)

Steve

The worst affront to Steve is when he perceives that someone is trying to control him. Even when that person thinks they are being subtle and only making "suggestions," he predictability reacts with even greater degrees of rigidity; deliberateness; and when sufficiently frustrated (from being pressured), aggression. Is it that, given his speed of processing information, that often the world is moving too fast and his responses of rigidity or what appears to be defiance is really his attempt to slow it down? Is it a reaction to years of things being done to him, with a poor contextual match between what he preferred or needed and what those in control imposed? Is it years of time-out and punishments, including isolation and aversive consequences, for situations that he didn't understand or were beyond his ability to control at the moment? Have these interventions to control, designed by multiple psychologists and behavior specialists, created such trauma that the perception of external control has in fact become the trigger for defensive behavior?

Whatever the reason, the magic words for Steve are, "It's your choice." The people supporting Steve know to preface any remarks to him with those three words. They understand that less is more, and they must retreat to enable him to think through the strategies that he knows and uses when he is not under stress. They can ask if he wants their help in problem solving but only continue to speak if he indicates he would like their input. They know that time is Steve's best ally, because when not under pressure, Steve does make the right decision on the things that could jeopardize the life he enjoys. Steve's support providers know that once they say, "It is your choice," they must honor their commitment. They can't really intend "as long as you choose what I think is right." When that trust is established, Steve frequently will ask for or accept offered assistance or, on his own, he will make the right choice. And everyone sighs a breath of relief.

The most common application of behavior principles is the use of positive consequences to try to increase positive behaviors and negative consequences to decrease the frequency of undesirable behaviors. However, we argue that preferred activities should not be used to manipulate individuals by withholding those items or activities that all other people, treated with dignity, do not have to earn. Natural consequences work as well, if not better, and are respectful. If someone doesn't go to work one day, he will lose his pay for the day. He might lose his job. But he should not be losing his opportunity to play basketball on the weekend. Some care providers, intentionally or not, ultimately impede rather than support the growth of positive behavior and, most important, the opportunities to achieve QOL, through threats, coercion, punishment, or other means to control behavior, totally void of supporting the person.

Steve and the Beach Boys

Steve, a great Beach Boys fan, saw the advertisement for a concert and asked my husband and me to purchase tickets and go with him. He paid for his ticket, we paid for ours, and he gleefully entered the concert on his calendar, counting the days. One week before the concert, a number of unpredictable events collided in Steve's life, and he had a meltdown, which resulted in some very problematic behaviors. His support staff and others thought that he should be prevented from going to the concert as a "consequence." How, they reasoned, could we justify taking him to such an event that was so special to him and was sure to bring him joy, just days after he had engaged in what they considered such egregious behavior? As his parent, we chose not to pair the two events—they were totally unrelated to one another. There were indeed natural consequences that resulted as a function of his behavior, and those he had to live with.

We went to the concert. It was a spectacular star-filled night in an outdoor theater overlooking the ocean. The music was invigorating and the air was charged with energy. Listening to Steve sing along and dance to the music along with scores of other concertgoers was watching him enjoy life to the fullest. His joy, evident at that concert, was what allowed him to pick up the pieces, recoup, and get back on track. Observing his joy also served as much needed reinforcement for us as his parents. Life is very hard for someone who is challenged by everyday events that everyone else takes for granted and equally hard for the families who work so diligently to keep the support system in gear. Nights like that night remind us why we do what we do and give us the energy to keep on doing it!

....

The Right Support
Isn't Too Much Support

Often service providers believe that the need for more and more intensive supports results, by definition, in a more restricted lifestyle. Or worse, providers recommend types of support guided by dollars rather than human values and the knowledge about what a particular person needs to promote a valued life.

Steve commutes to NYC and works in a law office. Vincent runs his own business. Nicholas plays the marimba in the marching band and enrolls in college courses. They have lives and relationships that are bringing joy to them and those they engage with. When siblings, cousins, friends, or neighbors talk about their jobs, Steve and Vincent can proudly enter the conversations with a description of where they work or what they do. When others talk about their postsecondary school experiences, Nicholas can share his college or music school experiences and Joseph can share his experiences at the local community college and participating in his government office internship. They are each able to engage in those proud life experiences because they have the support they need. Could some perceive it as a lot of support or extraordinary support? Perhaps. Yet each of them, for various reasons, requires

intensive one-to-one support for meaningful outcomes; this is the right level of support.

This need does not change across settings. Interestingly, neither does the cost of providing that support! In fact, Steve's individualized supports in his home, work, and community cost New York State significantly less than supports provided in traditional adult services. What is the difference? They are the right supports, just like prescription lenses for someone with a visual impairment, and in each situation, the outcome is QOL—engaging in preferred, valued activities of one's choosing.

The issue of intensity (and appropriateness) of supports parallels the conceptual reframing of intellectual disability that began in the 1990s. An intellectual disability is now regarded less as an inherent limitation within the individual than as an outcome of the interaction between the person's capacities and the intensity of supports he or she needs, within the context in which the person wants to function (Luckasson et al., 2002; World Health Organization, 2001). The same concept is reflected within the PBS framework: "By support, we mean all those educational methods that can be used to teach, strengthen, and expand positive behavior, and all those systems change methods that can be used to increase opportunities for the display of positive behavior" (Carr et al., 2002, p. 4).

Vincent

When Vincent's school team members were interviewed about the vision for his life after high school, two of them stated that he needed (what they believed is) "too much support to have a real job." Others shared that his "e-e-e" sound and pacing would be too distracting for any workplace and his vulnerability a barrier to integrated employment. The key here is that these team members were focusing on their preconceived ideas of what employment should be and that support is something that should be quantified and measured on a scale of not too much to too much. Theses notions were actually the biggest barriers in moving Vincent toward achieving employment goals.

....

We have also heard the argument that suggests that the levels of support are unfounded since the goals are unrealistic: "Despite all the supports, it is unlikely that the person will make much progress. After all, they will likely never learn to do the task by themselves." "They might always need a person to buffer their impulsive reactions in the community to unexpected, unpredictable events." "Medicaid (the funding source) is supposed to be funding 'habilitation.'" "There need to be goals and demonstration that the individual is making progress toward those goals." Once again, we will argue that sometimes, getting up every day, going to work, enjoying the community and dignity of work *is* enough, even if there has been limited demonstration of new skills or little prospects of reductions of levels of support.

Supports Are Reflective and Responsive: Where to Look When Positive Behavior Support Strategies Do Not Seem to Be Working

Sometimes, even with the best efforts, strategies may not work. When this happens and people involved have good intentions, celebrate everyone's best efforts and don't give up. Someone's life depends on it. Resist the inclination to blame the individual. Behavior is very complex. It may be necessary to revisit the FBA. We must all take responsibility to try another way.

Humbly accept the powerful role of setting events that could be serving to "set the stage" for challenging behavior. While observers may figure out some of these setting events, the individual may be the only one who knows some of the others. Pain and other medical or psychological issues, such as stress, could serve as a setting event, and this may not be obvious to outsider observers (Carr & Owen-DeSchryver, 2007). Particularly with individuals with limited communication skills, a thorough physical exam, including dental, may be in order before anything else, recognizing that desensitization interventions might be necessary to enable the person to receive the medical diagnostic or treatment procedures (Carr & Herbert, 2008). It is possible that many of the responses we call "behavioral issues" might actually be manifestations of trauma-based responses (Harvey, 2012, p. 2). The most disconcerting situation is when the team of specialists blames the individual, perhaps labeling them with a destructive psychiatric label, because there were "no apparent antecedents."

Steve

Steve was enrolled in a residential school program, with the hope of understanding and addressing some of the challenging behaviors he was experiencing. This was prior to his identification as a person with autism spectrum disorder. On the second day of school, he refused to get out of bed. When the resident counselor tried to physically remove him from his bed, he resisted physically. Upon investigation, the clinical staff concluded that he had no reported difficulties earlier that morning or on the residence the previous night. There were "no apparent antecedents." The psychiatrist on staff proposed that although there were no clinical signs of psychosis, there was no other explanation, and perhaps his unexplained behavior responses were due to psychosis. An antipsychotic medication was recommended.

It wasn't until the following week, when my husband and I came to visit, that Steve shared that an assignment was distributed in one of his classes. With his learning disabilities and math disabilities, he was unable to complete it in class but was embarrassed to tell the teacher. He believed, as would have happened in his former school, that the teacher expected that anyone who hadn't finished their work would finish it overnight and bring it in completed the next day. However, at the residence, the understanding was that there was no homework and so there was no provision for anyone to see that he had an "assignment" that he was unable to complete. In the morning, he was afraid to go back to school without his homework and felt inadequate. There *was* a setting event, but Steve was the only person who knew what it was.

....

A Little Knowledge Can Be Dangerous: Positive Behavior Support without Fidelity

The values and science of PBS has changed lives. It has saved our sons' lives. The danger is when people begin using the name of PBS without the adherence to the values, science, and standards. It is frightening when years of development of theory and evidence-based methodology becomes rhetoric. How often do we hear a school or a service provider agency say, "But, of course, everything we do is positive"? We laughed as yet another novice psychologist told us "everything we do is positive" while presenting a "behavior support plan" designed to address very complex behavior: The primary intervention proposed was the opportunity to earn a can of cola, followed by an explanation for why a "crisis plan" was needed in case the behavior occurred, despite the "positive support plan."

PBS, which must reflect both the value and science, cannot simply be taught in a short staff development workshop. PCP is not a meeting, a form, or a completed support plan. And simple interventions or support plans that ignore the complexity of human behavior are inadequate.

Similarly, data-based decision making is a fundamental element of PBS. Data-based decision making is critical during the assessment, program development, and evaluation stages of behavior support. Practitioners of PBS understand the importance of multi-element FBAs that are person centered, with a focus on pinpointing behaviors and creating interventions that improve or support QOL. Data-based decision making, however, can only be as good as the data that are collected. Who is defining the target behavior(s) to be pinpointed and the tools for the assessment? How reliable are the recorders? How free from bias is the interpretation? How deep is their understanding of the values and science of PBS? Too often, the mandate to collect data, without the understanding or commitment to multidimensional assessment and intervention, reduces the focus and

interventions to trivial goals and objectives, because those are data that can be easily collected.

Good assessment data form the basis of quality support plans and access to QOL. Irrelevant data, hiding behind the rhetoric label of PBS (without fidelity), can be harmful, with adverse lifelong consequences, as it is used to label, blame, and exclude, all in the name of PBS.

PBS without fidelity may perpetuate so-inclined schools and agencies to blame the individual and deny them the very outcome that the field of PBS is committed to—QOL. PBS without fidelity will contribute to be dream takers, not dream makers. As a field, it is critical that we enhance training and advocacy so that those who are empowered to act in the role of behavior specialists, team members, and family advocates hold the vision and demonstrate the skills of the science of PBS.

POSITIVE BEHAVIOR SUPPORT IS A WAY OF LIFE

Dreams, dreams shattered, dreams changed, dreams fulfilled, and dreams yet to come—we all have dreams for the people we care for. We also have dreams for those who support them.

We dream of the day when QOL for all, including people with behavioral challenges, is no longer debatable but understood and when opportunities and supports are available to all—not just those individuals whose families have the education, resources, and tenacity that were available to the four men described in this chapter. We hope that someday soon, there can be adequate numbers of PBS professionals in the community and in schools, who can be available to provide affordable services to individuals and their family members who need help across their life span. We dream of the day when parents' looming fears are alleviated: "What will happen when we die? Who will carry on when we can't?"

We dream that legislation and funding agencies will embrace these values and provide the leadership, caring expertise, and funding to enable people to live dignified lifestyles, through individualized comprehensive supports. Steve is fortunate to live in New York State, which has offered individuals (with their circles of support) the opportunity to self-direct their supports and services by controlling their own individualized, portable budget. This has provided Steve (with his family's support) significant control over his life, including the freedom to live where and with whom he chooses; hire (and fire), train, and supervise his own support staff; and engage in his home, work, and community, all guided with dignity by his choices, preferences, and support needs. We hope that this opportunity for control of one's supports becomes the norm and not the exception. Finally, we hope that those designing funding formulas will understand the power of appropriate supports in relation to the frequency of behavioral challenges and QOL and resist the temptation to reduce support dollars when the frequency of behavioral challenges has reduced—we understand too well that problem behaviors have been reduced because the person is receiving the right supports!

CONCLUSION

This chapter focuses on the quest for quality lives for individuals with challenging behaviors. It highlights the lives of four men, our sons, to model the kinds of life opportunities that are possible with the application of PBS with fidelity. It has provided a window into how the value and science of PBS has been applied to help mitigate the impact of challenging behaviors on QOL.

PBS has enhanced our lives, as we see the dreams we dared to dream become reality. What should be absolutely clear, however, that PBS is not an easy fix. PBS is not an intervention, a program, or a treatment. We learned that it has to become a way of thinking, living, and acting. It permeates every aspect of our sons' lives—lives driven by person-centered values of choice, relationships, meaningful

participation, and dignity. We have learned to think about and implement PBS strategies, practically every minute of every day and in every setting. As so eloquently stated by Ann and Rudd Turnbull, whose work on behalf of their son, Jay, served as the model for PBS and comprehensive lifestyle support (Turnbull & Turnbull, 1999) and, at times, served as our beacon in the fog, "PBS should not be conceptualized as being superimposed on one's living condition but rather it should permeate all aspects of a custom-designed lifestyle characterized by personal control, independence, integration, and productivity" (Turnbull & Turnbull, 2011, p. 69).

However, we never said it was easy. When crises arise, they may come without warning anywhere, at any time—on weekends and weekdays, in the early morning or late at night, and even on holidays. Challenging behaviors exhibited by our loved ones can take us to our knees in grief and leave us walking on pins and needles with concerns, day in and day out. As families, we cannot always wait until a respected expert accepts our case, or some type of sporadically scheduled help arrives, or an agency assigned shares our vision, values, and knowledge about the science of PBS.

Our expertise in PBS was nurtured by love and necessity. Embracing the values, science, and standards of PBS enhanced our learning. Our lives were changed for the better, thanks to great people who cared, knew what they are doing, and were determined to improve the quality of our sons' lives with each and every encounter, never giving up.

We hope that with this chapter, we were able to share some of that experience with you to humanize a science, help you understand the joys and fears through family perspectives, share our celebrations, and share ideas to help ramp up some of your successes.

Ultimately, we hope that you have been able to read how the use, value, and science of PBS improves the quality of peoples' lives and that you will feel ready to apply the principles of PBS in your lives, families, and professional practice.

REFERENCES

Association for Positive Behavior Support (APBS). (2007). *Positive behavior support standards of practice: Individual level.* Retrieved from http://www.apbs.org/files/apbs_standards_of_practice_2013_format.pdf

Blatt, B., & Kaplan, F. (1974). *Christmas in purgatory: A photographic essay on mental retardation.* Syracuse, NY: Human Policy Press.

Carr, E.G. (2007). The expanding vision of positive behavior support research perspectives on happiness, helpfulness, hopefulness. *Journal of Positive Behavior Interventions, 9,* 3–14. doi:10.1177/1098300 7070090010201

Carr, E.G., Dunlap, G., Horner, R.H., Koegel, R.L., Turnbull, A.P., Sailor, W., . . . Fox, L. (2002). Positive behavior support: Evolution of an applied science. *Journal of Positive Behavior Interventions, 4,* 4–16.

Carr, E.G., & Durand, V.M. (1985). Reducing behavior problems through functional communication training. *Journal of Applied Behavior Analysis, 18*(2), 111–126. doi:10.1901/jaba.1985.18-111

Carr, E.G., & Herbert, M.R. (2008). Integrating behavioral and biomedical approaches: A marriage made in heaven. *Autism Advocate, 50*(1), 46–52.

Carr, E.G., & Owen-DeSchryver, J.S. (2007). Physical illness, pain, and problem behavior in minimally verbal people with developmental disabilities. *Journal of Autism and Developmental Disorders, 37,* 413–424. doi:10.1007/s10803-006-0176-0

Condeluci, A. (2002). *Cultural shifting.* St. Augustine, FL: Training Resource Network Press.

Donnellan, A. (1984). The criterion of the least dangerous assumption. *Behavioral Disorders, 9,* 141–150.

Fisher, D. (Producer), & Fisher, J. (Director). (2008). *Unforgotten: Twenty-five years after Willowbrook* [Video]. New York, NY: City Lights Home Entertainment.

Harvey, K. (2012). *Trauma-informed behavioral interventions: What works and what doesn't.* Washington, DC: American Association on Intellectual and Developmental Disabilities.

Horner, R.H., Dunlap, G., Koegel, R.L., Carr, E.G., Sailor, W., Anderson, J.A., . . . O'Neill, R.E. (1990). Toward a technology of "nonaversive" behavioral support. *Journal of The Association for Persons with Severe Handicaps, 15,* 125–132.

Koegel, L.K., Koegel, R.L., & Dunlap, G. (1996). *Positive behavioral support.* Baltimore, MD: Paul H. Brookes Publishing Co.

Krishnan, N. (2012). *PBS in the community: Challenges, strategies & successes.* Paper presented as part of a panel at the 9th Annual International Conference on Positive Behavior Supports, Atlanta, GA, March 15, 2012.

Le Guin, U.K. (2000, c1969). *The left hand of darkness.* New York, NY: Ace Books.

Luckasson, R., Borthwick-Duffy, S., Buntinx, W.H.E., Coulter, D.L., Craig, E.M., Reeve, A., . . . Tassé, M.J. (2002). *Mental retardation: Definition, classification, and systems of supports* (10th ed.). Washington, DC: American Association on Mental Retardation.

Lyons, G. (2010). Quality of life for persons with intellectual disabilities: A review of the literature. *Enhancing the Quality of Life of People with Intellectual Disabilities, Social Indicators Research Series, 41,* 73–126. doi:10.1007/978-90-481-9650-0_6

McLaughlin, D.M., & Carr, E.G. (2005). Quality of rapport as a setting event for problem behavior: Assessment and intervention. *Journal of Positive Behavior Interventions, 7,* 68–91. doi:10.1177/10983007050070 020401

Mount, B. (2000). *Person-centered planning: Finding directions for change using personal futures planning.* Amenia, NY: Capacity Works.

Nirje, B. (1969). The normalization principle and its human management implications. In R. Kugel & W. Wolfensberger (Eds.), *Changing patterns in residential services for the mentally retarded* (pp. 179–195). Washington, DC: President's Committee on Mental Retardation.

O'Brien, J., & Mount, B. (2010). *Wheel-power: We have choices!* Adapted from O'Brien, J. (2010). *SSR: Supporting social roles/|A second bottom line for services to people with developmental disabilities.* Toronto, ON: Inclusion Press.

O'Brien, J., Pearpoint, J., & Kahn, L. (2010.) *The PATH and MAPS handbook: Person-centered ways to build community.* Toronto, ON: Inclusion Press.

Rapley, M. (2003). *Quality of life research: A critical introduction.* London, UK: Sage.

Rothman, D.J., & Rothman, S.M. (1984). *The Willowbrook wars.* New York, NY: Harper & Row.

Sailor, W., Dunlap, G., Sugai, G., & Horner, R. (Eds.). (2009). *Handbook of positive behavior support.* New York, NY: Springer. doi:10.1007/978-0-387 -09632-2

Schalock, R.L. (2000). Three decades of quality of life: Mental retardation in the 21st century. In M.L. Wehmeyer & J.R. Patton (Eds.), *Mental retardation in the year 2000* (pp. 335–355). Austin, TX: PRO-ED.

Schalock, R.L. (2004). The concept of quality of life: what we know and do not know. *Journal of Intellectual Disability Research, 48*(3), 203–216.

Schalock, R.L. (2011, May 5). *Quality of life: A conversation with Dr. Robert Schalock.* Retrieved from http://www.youtube.com/watch?v=1PorQtVq1Bo

Smith, J. (Director). (2010). *We have choices* [Motion Picture]. Research and Training Center on Community Living (RTC), Institute on Community Integration. Retrieved http://rtc.umn.edu/rtcmedia/wehavechoices/

Taylor, S., & Bogdan, R. (1990). Quality of life and the individual's perspective. In R. Schalock (Ed.), *Perspectives and issues* (pp. 27–40). Washington, DC: American Association on Mental Retardation.

Turnbull, A., & Turnbull, R. (2011). Right science and right results: Lifestyle change, PBS, and human dignity. *Journal of Positive Behavior Interventions, 13*(2), 69–77. doi:10.1177/1098300710385347

Turnbull, A.P., & Turnbull, H.R. (1999). Comprehensive lifestyle support for adults with challenging behavior: From rhetoric to reality. *Education and Training in Mental Retardation and Developmental Disabilities, 34*(4), 373–394.

Wolfensberger, W. (1972). *The principle of Normalization in human services.* Toronto: National Institute on Mental Retardation.

World Health Organization. (2001). *International classification of functioning, disability, and health (ICF).* Geneva, Switzerland: Author.

Ronda's Story

Living a Quality Life

28

Scott Shepard and Ronda Michaelson

Throughout her 70 plus years, Ronda has persevered, sometimes in spite of all the support professionals with good intentions. Ronda's story is similar to that of many senior adults labeled with intellectual and developmental disability; however, her drive to be independent, along with the evolution of positive behavior support (PBS), self-determination, and person-centered services, have helped create opportunities for her that were unavailable to many other adults and seniors with developmental disabilities. Ronda and I want to share her story. We want to show what PBS really means—what a life based on PBS can look like. Although we do include some examples of the more concrete elements of the PBS technology, our intent is to show what a life can look like when PBS becomes a way of looking at the world and a way of supporting people.

Ronda was born in the late 1930s to a loving family, which soon included a younger brother. She attended special schools in the Los Angeles area, including Widney High School, which Ronda attended in the late 1950s until 1961. Widney High School started as Los Angeles's "Crippled Children's High School" in 1939 and later changed its name to J.P. Widney Special Education Center. Special education centers were set up to serve students with special needs in the Los Angeles area before free appropriate public education for students with disabilities in the 1975 Education for All Handicapped Children Act (PL 94-142, later to be amended in 1991 as the Individuals with Disabilities Education Act, or IDEA, PL 102-119). As recent as 1970, schools in America educated only one in five students with disabilities (United States Department of Education, 2007). While increasing numbers of students with intellectual disabilities now attend the same school campuses as their typical peers, there are still special education centers open in the Los Angeles area today (including Widney High School) that continue to be completely segregated, serving only students with disabilities.

Following Ronda's leaving Widney High School, her parents joined a group of families who founded LARC Ranch (Los Angeles Retarded Children's Ranch, later changed to "Los Angeles Retarded Citizen's Ranch") in the Santa Clarita Valley of North Los Angeles County in 1961. There were not many community living options at the time for adults with developmental disabilities, other than state institutions. This group of parents had the best of intentions and wanted a safe place for their sons and daughters to live. Ronda was placed at LARC Ranch when it opened in 1961 and lived at the 90-person facility for 30 years. In 1990, when Ronda moved out of LARC Ranch, the average age of people residing there was 44 years old. After living in a transition home from 1990 to 1992, which focused on teaching her independent living skills, Ronda moved into her own apartment in 1992, when she was 54 years old. Ronda continues to live on her own in a one-bedroom apartment, benefiting from a housing certificate, and receives supported living services through our agency (Avenues Supported Living Services), which is funded by the North Los Angeles County Regional Center in Southern California. Ronda also receives supported employment services, which provide a job coach who sees her weekly at her jobsite. Ronda has lived in her own apartment for more than 20 years and continues to be passionate about working and being as independent as she can. Like many seniors, Ronda has experienced a variety of medical challenges as she has gotten older, including short-term memory loss associated with Alzheimer's disease, carpal tunnel surgeries, a pacemaker, and loss of mobility that has necessitated the use of a walker.

Instead of describing how we as professionals have taught Ronda new skills and behaviors, Ronda and I are going to share some of the significant lessons that Ronda has taught us and how we have learned to listen to her in the process of providing supported living services and assisting her

through some behavior difficulties. We are hopeful that these lessons will be beneficial to others who are also trying to listen to and address the needs of adults and seniors they are supporting.

RONDA'S STORY

The following quotes are taken from interviews and simply spending time with Ronda over the past 20 years. Together, Ronda and I have put together a PowerPoint presentation that she shares at conferences and with students in university settings. Ronda considers herself to be a lifelong learner and enjoys sitting in on university courses and conferences and participating as a presenter. She prefers to be asked questions that she can answer, as opposed to trying to recite her presentation by herself. The following are excerpts taken from some of her presentations:

Q: If your parents were still alive, do you think they would have helped you to move out of LARC Ranch like you did?

Ronda: I don't think so. Barbara helped me move out. She used to work at the Ranch. (Barbara Stamper was the owner/operator of the residential group home that Ronda moved into from LARC Ranch. Barbara had worked at LARC Ranch, teaching home economics, cooking, and sewing, prior to opening her transition group home for women with intellectual and developmental disabilities in 1982. This is how Ronda first met Barbara.)

Q: Where did Barbara help you to move in 1990?

Ronda: To a group home—the *best* group home!

Q: What did Barbara help you and the other women with?

Ronda: To take the bus, cook, banking, and things. To be independent.

Q: Who else did you meet at Barbara's home?

Ronda: Marcella. My best friend!

Q: How long did you stay at Barbara's home?

Ronda: Three years. I wanted to stay, but Barbara said it was time.

Q: Where did she help you to move?

Ronda: To my apartment of course. I'm in a different one now.

Q: Who else helped you?

Ronda: My supported living agency.

Q: What happened to them after 9 months living in your apartment?

Ronda: I fired them! (Giggle)

Q: Why did you fire them?

Ronda: I didn't like them.

Q: What supported living service agency did you and your brother hire after the first one?

Ronda: Avenues.

Q: How long have you been with Avenues?

Ronda: Since 1993. I haven't fired you yet! (Loud giggle)

Q: If you ever want to fire us, whom can you call?

Ronda: The Regional Center. (The Regional Center is the funding source for the agencies that provide services to children and adults with intellectual and developmental disabilities in the state of California.)

Q: Who pays your bills?

Ronda: I do!

Q: Do you get any discounts on your bills?

Ronda: I have Section 8 (a housing voucher program that pays a percentage of her rent based on her income).

Q: What other bills do you pay?

Ronda: Gas, electricity, cable . . . you know.

Q: How about the beauty shop?

Ronda: Yes, for my permanent!

Q: How did your friend Marcella end up living at your apartment complex 10 years ago?

Ronda: I talked to Michael (Ronda's apartment manager) and told him to find her an apartment.

Q: Now that you have lived in your own place, do you think you would you ever choose to move back to the Ranch?

Ronda: No way! Only to visit.

The care home that Ronda spent 3 years in after LARC Ranch was a fairly unique living situation. Directed by Barbara Stamper, a former employee of LARC Ranch, the home was intentionally set up as a transition home and not as a place where people were expected to live out their lives. The purpose of this home was to assist a small group of up to six women with intellectual and developmental disabilities to gain the skills they needed to make the transition to live more independently in homes of their own in the community. Since its inception in 1982, Barbara's home helped more than 50 women with disabilities learn independent living skills and transition into their own homes. A few women who made the transition from her home got married and had children; most, like Ronda, simply got the opportunity to begin a life of their own in their own place.

REFLECTIONS

Reflections on Community Living

Similar to the supported work movement started by Marc Gold, Lou Brown, and others in the 1970s, which demonstrated that adults with intellectual disabilities could learn the skills needed to engage in meaningful, productive work and become valued members of the work force, publicly funded supported living services began in the late 1970s as an alternative to institutional and restrictive residential placement (O'Brien, 1993). The first move toward integrated community living were residential facilities (including smaller institutions, intermediate care facilities, and group homes), which were seen as providing a more desirable (and normalized) living option than large institutional placement. Although "smaller" numbers of people with intellectual and developmental disabilities living together is generally seen as better as far as service quality, even small group homes can be "institutional." If adults with disabilities do not have a say over who they live with, do not have a say in the rules where they live, or do not have control of their finances or choices in the hiring and firing of the staff that support them, it is still an institution—just a smaller one.

John O'Brien (1993) has described supported living as a situation where "a person with a disability who requires long term, publicly funded, organized assistance allies with an agency whose role is to arrange or provide whatever assistance is necessary for the person to live in a decent and secure home of the person's own." (p. 1)

There are many implications of supported living. What makes a house someone's home? Who has the key? Whose name is on the mailbox, the lease, rental agreement, or mortgage? Who is "the boss," and who makes the rules? The philosophies of PBS, self-determination, and person-centered thinking should be the foundation of all supports. Supported living is a wonderful match for adults who need significant levels of support (including individuals who require support 24 hours a day, 7 days a week, 365 days a year) and for those who have developed severe reputations and may display significant behavior challenges. Supported living is

meant to be person-centered and should be individualized based on the unique needs of the person. For people who have not developed traditional forms of communication (i.e., people who are labeled nonverbal), the values of PBS come into play as we strive to actively "listen" to what the person's behaviors are saying to us.

Often it is stereotypes that lead us to believe that a person's behaviors or lack of independent living skills preclude them from living in their own home in the community. These beliefs are the barriers to making supported living a reality. Table 28.1 lists myths and facts of supported living services.

Reflections on Interdependence

Ronda helped teach an important concept to her staff—something that we try to get across to all our staff when supporting people in the community and in their own homes. This is the concept of *supporting,* rather than *care providing. Supporting* means doing things *with* people and involving them in all aspects of their lives. Decisions about what support is needed and how it is provided is framed within the notion of *self-determination*—that is, the person being supported is included in all decision making as much as possible. Conversely, *care providing* means doing things *for* people, with or without their involvement. When the focus is on care providing, decisions are generally made by professionals (and sometimes family members) about what is best for the person and do not generally include the opinion or preferences of the person(s) being supported.

When Ronda and her brother hired Avenues to support her in 1993, we wanted to figure out how we could do a better job of listening to her than the previous agency so that we would not repeat the mistakes of the previous agency that she fired. So before the paperwork to transfer services to our agency was complete, we coordinated a meeting with the previous supported living services agency to learn more about Ronda and her

Table 28.1. Myths and facts of supported living

Myth	Fact
Only people who are "independent" can live in their own homes.	All needed support services can be provided to someone in his or her own home and the community.
People who need 24-hour care are not eligible.	People can receive 24-hour care, 365 days a year, as needed, to be safe in their own homes.
People with medical challenges can't receive necessary services and life supports in their own homes through supported living services.	People who need the use of respirators and other intensive medical support needs can receive these necessary supports in their own home.
People who display problem behaviors won't be successful living in their own place.	It is generally easier and more successful to support individuals with behavior challenges to live in their own homes. Many behavior issues actually arise in facilities because the person is living with other people who also display behavior challenges.
If you do not communicate traditionally and/or you do not have a communication system in place, then you cannot *choose* to live in your own place.	Even if you do not communicate traditionally, are "nonverbal," and/or do not currently have a communication system in place, your family and support team can help you by advocating for supported living. Your family and support team can also assist you by inferring meaning and documenting the communicative intent of your behaviors.
You will need to live with another person with a disability.	Regardless of the amount of support you need, you should not be required to live with another person with a disability unless you want to. If you want or need to live with someone else, you should be able to choose your roommate(s). (Sometimes you might not be able to afford the rent without splitting it with someone and/or you may choose to live with a roommate who can provide some of the support you need.)

relationship and experiences with them. We were greeted by the agency's supported living coordinator. She let us know that Ronda just did not understand or accept that her agency knew which types of services were best for Ronda—not Ronda herself. (At that time, Ronda was 55 years old, with twice the life experience of the young supported living services coordinator.) This professional informed us that on one recent occasion, Ronda actually refused to let a staff member come into her apartment. (Ronda lived in a secure apartment complex and needed to "buzz" visitors in with a button; otherwise they would not be able to enter.) We asked for more information about the incident when Ronda refused to let staff in and found out that her regular support staff member was sick that day, so the supported living services agency sent over a male replacement staff member whom Ronda had never met. Ronda declined to let the stranger in. Ronda was a single woman in her 50s and about 5-feet tall.

We shared that we would have been worried if Ronda *had* let a strange male into her complex that she had never met before. Ronda later told us that her parents had always instructed her, "Don't let a stranger in. It's not safe!"

When asked what other information she could relate about Ronda, Ronda's former supported living services coordinator shared that Ronda would page her "about 50 times a day!" We later learned that since Ronda didn't have any phone numbers and only a pager number, she would simply page the coordinator nonstop until she called. When we asked what kind of things Ronda paged her about, she shared the following stories:

> Here are two examples of Ronda paging me this past month. Ronda paged to ask me if I could go grocery shopping with her. I asked her if she knew which bus to take to the grocery store, and Ronda said, "Yes." I asked her if she had her list of groceries that she needed to buy, and Ronda again said, "Yes."

I asked her if she had money in her checking account, and could she write a check for her groceries, and she again said, "Yes." So I asked her, "Do you really need me to help you?" Ronda replied, "No." The second example is when Ronda called to ask me if I could take her to the bank. I asked Ronda, "Do you know which bus to take to get to the bank?" Ronda replied, "Yes." I asked her, "Do you know how to deposit your check?" She again said, "Yes, I do!" So I said, "Do you really need me to go with you and help you?" She replied, "No, I don't." These are the kind of calls you will get from Ronda every day!

These examples provided by the supported living services coordinator helped us understand that Ronda did not need their help or our help in these situations; she was simply lonely and wanted company. One of the important things that Ronda has taught us is that we cannot fade ourselves out of someone's life as a paid support simply because we have taught him or her a set of skills. We can only fade our paid support once there are more people in that person's life—more people who are friends, neighbors, family, and unpaid, natural supports.

Teaching people to be "independent" is not necessarily the primary goal when supporting people in community living. When we look at our lives, most of us will realize that we are not independent; further, most of us do not have a goal of being independent in all aspects of our lives. We all have varying levels of "interdependence" on and with others. We rely on family, friends, coworkers, neighbors, and others daily, and in many areas of our lives. It is more natural and rewarding to develop relationships that allow us to do things with people as opposed to doing things strictly on our own. When Avenues supported living services first began to support Ronda after she hired us in 1993, we typically spent time supporting her after her workday, Monday through Saturday. Sundays, however, she was "busy" with her friends at church and didn't want or need to see us. Our goal was to help Ronda develop

additional relationships and social connections, thus requiring less time with paid supports. Eventually Ronda was connected with a Saturday "social group" with other women, attending a variety of community events, such as Dodger baseball games, the zoo, museums, and so forth. She also joined a bowling league and joined in activities and developed social relationships within the context of her various jobs. A critical focus of PBS is developing quality of life enhancement changes (APBS, 2007, Section VI, A and B). The importance of thoughtful planning to improve a person's quality of life, including the promotion of social relationships and enhanced social networks, leisure, and recreational activities, cannot be overstated when talking about the success of multielement behavior support plans in the life of Ronda and other adults with intellectual and developmental disabilities.

After hearing the prior supported living services agency's descriptions and perceptions of their interactions with Ronda, we had a much better idea of how we might be able to begin trying to do a better job of listening to and supporting Ronda. However, Ronda still needed to teach us a few lessons about how we should listen to her better:

> After talking to Ronda's former group home provider, Barbara, I found out that Ronda really enjoyed making a hamburger hot dish recipe called "PTA special." This gave me the idea to call Ronda and "tell" her that I would pick her up on an upcoming Friday at 3:00 so we could go shopping for the ingredients for her PTA special and then fix it together at her house. When I showed up at Ronda's place at 3:00 that Friday, there was no Ronda to be found. I waited for an hour and left a couple of messages on her phone, then left. She called me back a bit after 6:00 to let me know that she already had eaten dinner and didn't need my "help," but that I could come over and visit now if I liked. (From Scott Shepard's staff progress notes, 1993)

I learned a few things from Ronda being a "no show" when I came to visit. First, my time with Ronda is *her* time. Second, while she hates it when someone asks her if she needs help, we can still spend time together that involves learning and doing things that are helpful to Ronda—they just need to be set up and agreed on on her terms. Once we got this straightened out, we established an incredible relationship of (mostly) mutual respect and learning together that has continued for the past 20 years.

POSITIVE BEHAVIOR SUPPORT AND RONDA

There are considerations regarding the implementation of PBS that differ for adults and children (minors). For youth, it is typical for parents to make the rules and decisions in the lives of their children; even when the child participates in the process and choices are respected, it is the parents who are ultimately in control, with educators and other professionals (and hopefully the youth him or herself) contributing to the decision making. However, once these youth become adults, regardless of any disability labels, they have the right to refuse supports and services (which includes behavior support) and make their own rules in their homes. If PBS is to be successful, we must work *with* people, not "on them."

Reflections on Choosing Target Behaviors

Determining which behaviors to target for change in a person's life must be a team-based process, and it is critical that the individual themselves, especially as adults, be a key part of this team and process. Ronda's self-advocacy helps remind us that when we have "ideas" about how to support her, we should always remember the motto, "Nothing about us without us!" (Charlton, 1998). A primary criterion for determining what behaviors to target for change is whether or not that change will make a significant difference in the quality of that person's life. If the behavior change is not anticipated to have a positive impact on the person's

quality of life, then it is hard to justify the need for behavioral intervention. Changing a person's behavior may make *our* lives easier or make the person easier to manage for us, but these are not appropriate criteria to use to justify behavioral intrusion into someone's life.

Behavioral Concerns for Ronda

From our perspective as supporters, Ronda's biggest behavioral challenge is her refusal to accept supports that have an impact on her health and safety. For example, when Ronda had her hip replaced, postoperative instructions were for her not to do laundry, mopping, cleaning, or other physical chores on her own. This was a huge challenge for Ronda, as she does not like to accept support from others but wants to do routines of daily living her way, in the order and manner she wants without any assistance. The consequences of doing too much physical activity were significant, however. If Ronda didn't allow the support recommended by her doctor, she ran the risk that her new hip would not completely heal and she might not regain her full strength or mobility. Once Ronda was able to listen to her doctor and agree to additional *temporary* support, she was able to direct her support staff while they did her chores so that they did them in the manner and the order in which she approved. This approach differs greatly from the more traditional behavioral approach of arranging consequences to reinforce targeted behavior and extinguish interfering behaviors, yet is very consistent with PBS and the values that drive supported living practices.

It has been an ongoing challenge trying to convince Ronda to be safe by engaging in new suggested routines and behaviors designed to keep her healthy and safe. For example, there were complaints from Ronda's manager that she was leaving her shades open in the morning when she was taking a shower and walking through her apartment without any clothes on. It took many efforts to support Ronda to change her behavior. Ronda will not allow staff to move items, put groceries away for her, hang up or put away clothes, or close the shades in her apartment, as she wants to do all these things by herself. If staff try to do any of these things, Ronda will scream and rush over to put things back or redo them herself. Staff who persist in trying to make changes in Ronda's home without her permission end up being "fired" by Ronda. We had team meetings with Ronda and her support staff where we tried to encourage Ronda to draw her shades the night before but with marginal success. (She would follow through with the new behavior routine for a few days and then go back to her old routine.) We set up a support plan to have staff come over and remind her the night before to draw her shades, embedding this new step into her evening routine, but Ronda would refuse to listen to the staff or would draw the shades until they left and then open them again. We had more success when we decided to have her apartment manager speak to Ronda directly about the issue. Ronda respects him as the landlord who makes the rules for the tenants in the complex. As a result of this respect, she agreed to keep her blinds closed at night until she completed her morning routine the next day. Ronda still needs occasional reminders, but for the most part, that issue is resolved. We learned that Ronda will respect the authority of her apartment manager in issues related to housing. Closing her apartment door when she goes to get her mail or do her laundry in the laundry room has also been an issue that took years to resolve. Unfortunately, Ronda learned the hard way when her purse was stolen from her apartment several years ago. We still use this real-life event to remind her of the natural consequences of leaving her door open while she leaves her apartment to do laundry or to get her mail.

In previous years, when doctors and physical therapists prescribed specific procedures for Ronda to follow and specific equipment for her to use, Ronda's behaviors escalated to screaming, throwing objects, and refusing to change any of her routines to accommodate her doctors' requests. Her support team has always worked with medical professionals to find compromises between health and safety and Ronda's wishes. However, more recently, as Ronda has aged, it has become more imperative that she comply with her doctor's recommendations.

We have always tried to include Ronda's numerous doctors and medical professionals (dentist, ophthalmologist, neurologist, physical therapist, podiatrist, foot specialist, and her regular doctor) by proactively contacting them about Ronda's behaviors and resistance prior to her appointments so that they can be clear and direct with her. We often "fax" a note to Ronda's doctors prior to her appointments to give them an update on how Ronda is following (or not following) their recommendations. This way, the doctor has a heads up and can bring up these issues more discretely than if we try to bring it up or "tattle" on her in front of her. It is important for Ronda to hear directions directly from her doctor, as she respects directions when they come from the authority at "the top." However, it is still challenging at times for Ronda to follow through without staff reminders and support. Putting things in writing for her to read also helps her process the information better than if people just "tell her" verbally.

Ronda's employers have also expressed concerns about her behavior at work. The two most critical issues involve missing her ride to work and refusing to stop work on time, which leads to her clocking out 15 minutes or more late and missing her scheduled ride home. Our behavior support strategies at work, similar to other areas of her life, involve Ronda's supervisor, who we have encouraged to be the one to directly tell her what she needs to work on. When her supervisor informs her about the rules or what she needs to do, this has the biggest positive impact on her work behaviors. When her job coach or supported living services staff try to give her feedback on her work behaviors or try to intervene on the job, Ronda simply ignores them and/or uses profanity or harsh words while telling them to leave her alone. Now we simply remind Ronda of what her supervisor told her.

Identifying Triggers

As we look at developing community, work, and in-home supports for adults, we utilize a variety of functional behavioral assessment (FBA) and person-centered planning (PCP) strategies to assist us with this process. When we looked at behavioral "triggers" for Ronda (i.e., stimuli that tend to promote or exacerbate challenging behavior), it was helpful to observe and find out answers to two questions: *"What works?"* and *"What doesn't work?"* (adapted from Smull & Sanderson, 2009). Information obtained about "What doesn't work?" was included in our functional assessment, as these are the variables that are associated with and/or trigger her problem behaviors. Information obtained about "What works?" was included in our behavior support plan, which represents proactive strategies that promote positive behavior change. In getting to know Ronda better through our observations and by interviewing people who knew Ronda, we found out the following information about what works and doesn't work when supporting Ronda.

What Doesn't Work: Triggers to Challenging Behaviors

The following discussion focuses on those variables that we identified as triggers for Ronda. It is important to note that these triggers were discovered within the context of her daily routine, and all the naturally occurring stimuli within those contexts and did not involve a formal FBA.

Rushing, Hurrying, or Interrupting Ronda While She Is Engaged in a Routine (at Work or at Home) We found that whenever we (support staff) try make Ronda go faster, try to stop her from doing something, or interrupt her once she has started a routine, such as a work task, hanging clothes, doing her laundry, putting things away, or organizing things, her behaviors are likely to escalate to screaming and refusing.

Holding Any Type of "Official" Meeting with Large Numbers of Professionals Where Ronda Is the Focus Formal meetings such as individualized program plan meetings, in-home support services, annual review meetings, or other types of team meetings where the focus relates to Ronda are triggers for Ronda. Attempting to hold meetings in her apartment with more than two professionals has led to her pulling her hair, screaming, and refusing to participate.

Attempting to "Help" or Do Things for Ronda When staff offer too much assistance, Ronda screams, uses profanities, pushes, hits, and basically refuses to listen or accept support. Her typical response to people asking if they can "help" her is to yell or shriek "I can do it!" at the top of her lungs, while pushing the people aside.

When Ronda Is Not Working and/or Has Little to Do When Ronda is idle (e.g., not working, not engaged in any activities), she is more likely to feel sad and lonely; she increases her calls to friends and support staff at these times to where it becomes excessive (making 10 calls or more to each person on her phone list in a given evening where she is not actively engaged in something). Problem behaviors are associated with those times when Ronda is not working or not engaged in any number of social events and routines in her life.

When People Try to Change Ronda's Routines or Behaviors by Prompting Her or Giving Her Directions When a staff member attempts to take charge or give her directives, Ronda reacts by either "firing" that person or refusing to work with that person for an extended period of time. The exception is that Ronda is more willing to accept

some direction and requests to change existing routines if these requests come from
people she knows to be in charge (e.g., her
supervisor at work) or staff who have developed long-term relationships with her that
are based on dignity and respect (such as Jill
Martin and myself who have known her for
20 years).

*Using Physical Support or Assistance
that Is Not Requested or Initiated by Ronda*
When anyone attempts to provide physical support (touching her) or to provide
more help than is needed, Ronda will typically engage in aggression (pushing, hitting), screaming, and/or refusal to listen
to anything that person says. People who
have inadvertently been guilty of this have
included nurses and other medical professionals, which has led to Ronda ignoring
their instructions during a medical examination or procedure. We always have vet-
eran support people with Ronda when she
attends doctor appointments to teach and
guide the medical professionals through the
process of interacting directly with Ronda
(as opposed to talking to us) and letting
them know not to touch Ronda without first
telling her what they are doing and why so
that she understands what is going on.

What Works: Ronda's Positive Support Plan and Antecedent Change Strategies

The following strategies are included in Ronda's PBS plan. These strategies are based on
observations of Ronda's triggers, setting
events, personal preferences, and maintaining consequences of her behaviors and
routines. Antecedent-behavior-consequence
(ABC) information (details of antecedents,
behaviors, and consequences) obtained
from staff observations and interviews with
coworkers and community members was
helpful, as it helped us identify patterns in
antecedents and consequences to her behaviors that told us where, when, during what
activities, and with whom her behaviors
were most and least likely to occur.

*Giving Ronda the Time that She Needs
to Get Through Her Routine(s) without
Interrupting or Prompting Her Once She Has
Started* We help Ronda find bank tellers
and cashiers that know her and then get into
their lines at the bank/grocery store to do her
business. The people who know her are more
patient with her and understand that she
needs a little more time to do her business.
Staff have also learned some helpful strategies, such as placing themselves in front of
Ronda's grocery cart while in line so that
Ronda doesn't (purposefully) push her cart
into the person in front of her so that she can
start putting her items on the conveyor belt.

*Proactively Talking with Ronda About
Ideas and Strategies to Assist Her with
Lengthy Routines Before These Routines Are
Started* Speaking to Ronda about assisting
with routines the day before they occur will
usually prevent her from getting upset and
refusing to accept support during the actual
routine. For example, staff may have the following conversation with her: "Ronda, you
were late and missed the bus to get to work
today; should I stop by earlier tomorrow so
you can start your routine earlier? If not,
can we make a checklist together for your
morning routine that might help you to stay
on track?" We have learned that it helps to
sit down with Ronda on a one-to-one basis
a day or more in advance to review and
rehearse any proposed changes in her routine or supports. These informal discussions
take place at a time when Ronda is calm and
receptive to talking about possible changes.
If we try to talk to her about changes at
the time when these changes are about to
occur, Ronda escalates to the point where
she is unable to listen to or process what we
are trying to say, and she refuses any support or redirection that involves a change
in routine. With Ronda's short-term memory challenges that have been brought on
by Alzheimer's disease, it is also important
to assist Ronda to write down the things we
discuss on her calendar and in written form
(as checklists or notes).

Doing Things with Ronda, as Opposed to Attempting to Do Things for Ronda   As with many of the examples already provided, we try to teach staff and team members to include Ronda in all aspects of her support as opposed to doing things for her and without her participation or choice. We can do this by simply asking her which parts of the floor she wants us to mop first or which items of laundry she wants us to wash first. If we need to assist her to put away or to carry her heavy grocery items due to doctor's orders, we still give her something lighter to carry, and we ask where she wants us to put them, as Ronda always has a specific counter, cupboard, or place where she wants things. If Ronda balks at support we are providing, we remind her of which person (doctor, work supervisor, apartment manager, etc.) told her it was important that she allow us to help her. This usually helps her to be more accepting of any support.

Holding Team and Annual Planning Meetings at Ronda's Place of Employment or at a Restaurant, While Minimizing the Number of People in Attendance   Ronda has been attending individual planning meetings focusing on her behaviors and skills since before most of us were born, and her behaviors and affect begin to change whenever she finds herself in a "meeting" about her where she is outnumbered by professionals. At this point, Ronda has experienced over 65 years of various program-planning meetings of some type, where people have set goals for her and talked about her impairments, needs, and challenges. Historically, Ronda has not fared well at these meetings and generally has been uncooperative (displaying her discomfort by pulling hair, screaming, and spitting at meetings in which groups of people are talking about her "goals and objectives"). When we look at the nature of these meetings over the years, it is easy to see why Ronda would be uncomfortable, as most of these meetings involved a number of professionals talking about what Ronda's problems were and what they felt she needed to be working on.

It has been difficult to remove the stigma and other negative feelings that Ronda associates with these types of meetings. Our strategy was to change the format of the meetings and make them less formal. If it looks like a "meeting," smells like a "meeting," and/or if the number of "professionals" greatly outnumber her, Ronda will let people know through her behaviors that she does not want to be present or participate. We now give Ronda the choice of meeting at her workplace or at a restaurant, where we can casually review progress and ask Ronda if she is happy with the services she is receiving and if she wants them to continue. We have also minimized the number of people who participate in these meetings down to three (including Ronda). This has helped to minimize behaviors while increasing Ronda's overall willingness to participate and speak out for herself. This is one of the first antecedent changes we made once we got to know her and understood that one of her triggering events was being with lots of people in professional-looking meetings that focused on her. We believe that much of her behavior may be attributed to her associations with prior meetings that focused on her negative behaviors and things she "needs to work on," which most people would perceive as embarrassing situations to be in. We also feel that we need to respect Ronda's aversion to large meetings that focus on her by minimizing them and making meetings that are "required" by funding sources more pleasant and accommodating to Ronda and her needs. Ronda has also taught us that when we plan future goals and supports, it is best to have individual, personal discussions. With the intent of making meetings casual, we have found it to be helpful to hold "meetings" at a restaurant, at her jobsite after work, or in another casual setting (other than her apartment or a business office setting), while using a napkin or our memory to take notes, as opposed to using tablets or "official" note-taking equipment. These accommodations have helped Ronda be more comfortable attending any "required" professional meetings about her, and her aggressive behaviors have been nonexistent over the past 5 years during these meetings.

Having Ronda Hear Recommendations and Feedback Directly from the Person in Charge

As shared previously, when there are recommendations that relate to her health and safety, Ronda's medical providers should speak directly to her, rather than have staff act as their agents. Similarly, if there are work issues, Ronda is more receptive when she receives feedback directly from her supervisor. If this type of direct contact is not possible, the discussion should be held between Ronda and the people that she knows and trusts best.

Limiting Number of Support Staff

Ronda has historically been adamant about not having more support staff, other than me and Jill (who is Ronda's support coordinator and also Ronda's favorite staff person), even though she gets lonely and calls frequently. We have found that when Ronda meets potential team members casually at community meetings and/or while visiting other people who receive support from our agency, she is more likely to be open to the possibility of having them spend time supporting her. Over time, when Ronda requests support for errands and other activities, we mention to her that those people are available if she would like to have us train them with her. She is more likely to agree to a new staff if she has met them while they are supporting someone else she knows.

Consequence–Change Strategies

It is also important to change consequences in the development of any support plan. We want to minimize any positive or negative reinforcement that is maintaining challenging behaviors, while trying to ensure that we find ways to support "natural" consequences that are in place for other community members in similar situations.

One recent challenge for Ronda involved her missing her morning Access Services ride

to work as a result of some compulsive behaviors that lengthened her morning routine and prevented her from getting outside on time. The team thought it would be appropriate to look more closely at Ronda's morning routines by recording ABC data to identify patterns on the antecedents and consequences related to Ronda's missing her access ride.

Regarding consequences, we found that when she first began to miss her Access ride, Ronda would call her job coach and scream for her to come pick her up and take her to work so she wouldn't be late. After picking up Ronda a few times, we all agreed that the job coach should not bail her out but that Ronda should have the natural consequence of being late or missing work, resulting in a smaller paycheck. As Ronda's supported living agency, we offered Ronda the option of having someone come over in the mornings before work to give her some support to get ready on time, but she adamantly refused to have additional supports come in the mornings. This led to Ronda problem solving and finding natural supports on her own, such as her neighbors and the apartment manager, who would take her to work. Over time, however, this was not a sustainable option, as it became untenable for the apartment managers to continue to drop what they were doing to take Ronda to work.

With coaching from us, her apartment managers sat down with Ronda and told her that they were no longer able to take the time away from their management duties to drive her to work. At this point, Ronda agreed to allow staff to come in and support her in the mornings before work. Ronda now agrees to have support in the mornings to assist her to get ready in time for her ride to work. This has been working well, as she has had less incidents of missing her ride to work and continues to arrive to work without being late or missing workdays.

A similar challenge emerged for Ronda in the workplace itself. Ronda works as a file clerk at the Regional Center—a position she has held for over 5 years (see Figure 28.1). Near the end of her work shift, she would continue to file while ignoring prompts from

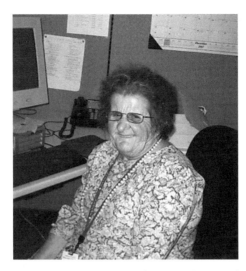

Figure 28.1. Ronda works as a file clerk at the Regional Center.

her supervisor and job coach to begin to get ready to leave. It would take Ronda at least 15 minutes to tidy up all the things on her desk before shutting down her computer and clocking out, which resulted in her clocking out 15 minutes late and missing her Access Services ride home. At first, her employer let the behavior go with only a few warnings, but Ronda's behavior continued to increase. Consistent with her preferences at home, Ronda did not accept feedback from her job coach, who was coming in at the end of the day to help her to clean up and clock out on time. We set up a small, informal meeting that included Ronda, her job coach, me, and her boss, who we all agreed she would most likely respond to. Ronda's boss told her that she needed to start packing up for the day 15 minutes early and that she needed to listen to her job coach. Her boss also let her know that if she was unable to clock out on time or listen to her coaches when they gave her reminders, she would be suspended from work for a day. Once Ronda heard this directive from her boss, Ronda listened and began her new routine of stopping work 15 minutes early, while allowing her job coach to provide her with feedback and reminders as needed.

Ronda's fierce need to be "independent" sparks many of the confrontations that she

has with us (her supported living agency). Many confrontations occur when medical professionals and/or her team determine that she needs additional support due to aging or progressive medical needs and Ronda refuses to allow increased supports or changes in her independence.

QUALITY OF LIFE ENHANCEMENT CHANGES

Reflections on the Importance of Working

Only 11% of parents of adults with disabilities report their child is employed full time and 19% part time. This number is quite staggering when compared with parents of adults without disabilities, who report that 48% of their children are employed full time and 24% part time (Easter Seals, 2010). Labor force statistics for December 2010 indicate that 28% of working-age adults with disabilities are employed, compared with 70% of people without disabilities (Butterworth et. al, 2011).

Working has always been very important to Ronda. During times when she has been unable to work (due to surgeries or medical issues), her behavior reflected her irritability and frustration. Our worst memories of supporting Ronda are these times of unemployment. Here is an excerpt from Ronda's presentation that relates to her passion about working:

Q: What do you think about working?

Ronda: I love to work!

Q: What places have you worked?

Ronda: I worked at Six Flags, Magic Mountain, in food service; at McDonald's, Maria's Italian Kitchen, Red Lobster, and the Avenues office doing filing. But they didn't have enough work for me to do!

Q: Then you had to be out of work for a while.

Ronda: For too long!

Q: What happened?

Ronda: Surgeries.

Q: Let's see, you had two hip replacements, carpal tunnel surgery, two rotator cuff problems, a pacemaker needed to be put in, you broke a finger, and you had a tumor removed from your calf.

Ronda: Yuck, yuck, yuck!

Q: Where did you get a job after your doctors said it was okay to work again?

Ronda: The Regional Center. It was about time!

Q: What do you do?

Ronda: I'm a file clerk.

Q: How long have you worked there?

Ronda: Five years!

Q: Do you like it?

Ronda: I love it! I want to work more hours, but I can't until the (state) budget gets better.

Q: When do you plan to retire?

Ronda: Never! I'm going to work forever. I love to keep busy. I have more energy than most people younger than me. I'm going to keep working! I love to work!

Ronda's words underscore the importance of work to her. Currently, she works in an office environment where she gets to dress up, and she takes great pride in that. Those of us who know her well agree that she will never retire until she is physically unable to work, and hopefully that will never occur. Without work, Ronda feels miserable and finds it difficult to treat others around her with dignity and respect. Work helps Ronda feel whole and take pride in herself, and it fulfills an important purpose for her.

As educators and service providers, we need to raise the expectations for people with intellectual and developmental disabilities and provide them with work-based learning opportunities (real jobs) to assist them to learn skills and determine what type(s) of work they are interested in doing. While supporting people with intellectual and developmental disabilities for more than 30 years, I recognize how important it is for everyone to identify and engage in one or more valued roles in their communities. This can include work (paid or volunteer), attending classes at a local community college, or even supporting an elderly family member. Without valued roles where people have opportunities to contribute, they are more likely to show signs of depression, irritability, and behavior challenges.

Reflections on Relationships Across Time

Relationships are also a critical factor in PBS, especially for adults (Koegel, Koegel, & Dunlap, 1996). Ronda is very involved in her church, which she attends with friends every weekend and some weeknights when dinners and meetings are scheduled. While we initially assisted with rides and support at church activities, we have facilitated the development of natural supports and friends at church, who pick Ronda up each weekend.

Church has been an important part of Ronda's life for over 20 years. Ronda also participates in Bible study and is always the first person to get a "get well," "happy birthday," or anniversary card for fellow worshipers, as well as for her neighbors, family, and friends. Ronda has an amazing gift of remembering special occasions in the lives of her friends, family, and those around her. Ronda's friends frequently joke that she has done all she can to keep the Hallmark store in business! As her memory lapses progress, this is an area that we try to support Ronda with so that she can continue her tradition of handing out cards to loved ones and friends. For example, Ronda's support staff remind and support her to record pertinent birthday and anniversary information into her pocket calendar every year so that she has the visual reminder and cues she needs to continue this tradition.

Over the past 10 years, Ronda has lost three of her close friends and family—Barbara, who helped her move from LARC Ranch to the group home; her younger brother Jay; and Marcella, her best friend of 20 years. Jay and Marcella passed away from cancer, a disease that Ronda detests with a passion. As a result, Ronda is an active donor to the American Cancer Society, and she regularly attends a local Relay for Life Cancer Walk in memory of Jay and Marcella, where she makes a memorial bag and candle for each of them (see Figure 28.2). The loss of her best friend a year and a half ago has been particularly difficult for Ronda, as they spent quite a bit of time together and lived in the same apartment complex. Ronda had done a lot of Marcella's shopping and laundry, and not having those daily routines to do any longer are a painful reminder of her passing.

When Ronda's brother passed away 3 years ago, it became obvious to those around her that she was grieving not only him but also her parents, who had died more than 25 years earlier. Sadly, Ronda was never given the opportunity to grieve at the time of her parents' deaths because she was not immediately told of their passing and was not able to attend their funerals. Too frequently, professionals try to "protect" adults (and youth) with intellectual and developmental disabilities by barring them from participating in the grieving process and attending funerals and graveside services—sometimes even not notifying them when a family member passes away. This tends to lead to more confusion, frustration, and at times depression (Hollins, 1995).

Unlike her experience years earlier with her parents, when Ronda's brother died, she had seen him the week before, was informed right away when he died, and attended his memorial when it was held a few months later. When her best friend Marcella was put into hospice due to her cancer, Ronda went to visit her. Ronda often asked Marcella's sister if she could attend the funeral, even before her friend died. The sister found this question strange and disconcerting, but Ronda just didn't want to be excluded. Ronda has also continued to visit Marcella's apartment building, which is next to hers, many times since her passing. Some neighbors and friends have been uncomfortable with this. It is merely Ronda going through her own grieving process of visiting where her friend used to live. We all need to be allowed to have our grieving process, which includes saying good-bye and attending services and memorials.

Reflections on Community Inclusion

Many seniors have lived lives characterized by isolation; seclusion; separation by location, activities, and schedule; loneliness; negative reputations; labels; limited voice; no power; and low expectations. Our goal is to work with these individuals to establish daily experiences leading to relationships, dignity, choice, real contribution, and inclusion in community life. O'Brien (1989), in his guide for the development of a personal vision, suggested five questions to help us assist people to develop their own personal vision of how they wish to be included within their community:

1. *Community presence:* How can we increase the presence of a person in local community life?

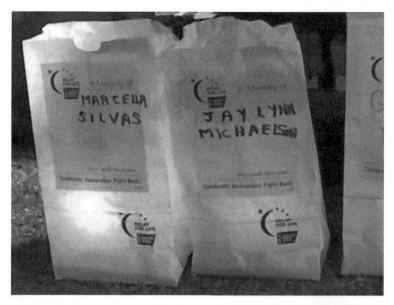

Figure 28.2.   Ronda makes a memorial bag and candle in memory of Jay and Marcella.

2. *Community participation:* How can we expand and deepen people's relationships?

3. *Encouraging valued social roles:* How can we enhance the reputation people have and increase the number of valued ways people can contribute?

4. *Promoting choice:* How can we help people have more control and choice in life?

5. *Supporting contribution:* How can we assist people to develop more competencies?

It is usually not enough to simply get someone an apartment, cross your fingers, and hope that they assimilate and connect with their community. It takes planning and facilitation for most people with intellectual and developmental disabilities to build community connections; identify, choose, and take on valued social roles; and find ways to use and be recognized for their unique gifts and talents.

Using Access Services (Door-to-Door Transportation Service) and/or Staff Rides as Opposed to Using Regular Public Transportation (Bus) Services Ronda had taken the bus independently since 1990, when she first moved out of LARC Ranch

into Barbara's transition skills group home. Ronda had always viewed her ability to take the bus as key to her independence. Unfortunately, once she began to use a cane and ultimately a walker following her hip replacements and the removal of a tumor behind her knee, her access to some of her usual community routines was impaired. As a team, we spoke with Ronda's physical therapist, a person she is willing to take direction from, to request that he be the one to tell Ronda that it was not safe for her to take the bus any longer. Ronda was determined to prove us wrong and insisted that she could still take the bus to run her errands. Instead of telling her she was wrong, we agreed to have her go on the bus with me and show me if she could get on and off the bus safely with all her "stuff." Ronda made a valiant effort, but the exercise helped her to determine that she couldn't take the bus and carry all her stuff the way she used to, especially now that she had a walker. Ronda now accepts rides from her support staff and uses a door-to-door transportation service to get to and from work, see her friends at bowling on the weekend, and attend other outings where she doesn't need a staff member.

Medical Issues and Aging

As all people age, our bodies need more and more attention. Ronda has a high threshold for pain, however, and doesn't always notice (or does not want to notice) when she needs medical care. Eight years ago, we didn't realize that Ronda had appendicitis until several days after it had burst, when she finally complained about some discomfort. We have learned to recognize that whenever Ronda complains about any type of pain, it must be taken seriously.

Years before we ever met Ronda, she had two eye surgeries and several foot operations. We are not sure if these operations left her physical situation better or worse. In 1994, Ronda was hit by a car walking to work, which resulted in a head injury and injuries to her pelvis, elbow, and both legs. Her neurologist believes that this incident precipitated the onset of Alzheimer's disease and Ronda's subsequent memory loss over the years. Ronda currently takes medications to help stop this progression. Ronda has also had operations on a foot due to arthritis and on her right wrist for carpel tunnel syndrome, following a job where she rolled silverware at a restaurant for 5 years. Further surgery was done on her wrist 2 years later, which included the installation of a metal plate in the wrist area. Ronda has had her appendix removed and a pacemaker installed. She has had cataracts removed. Seven years ago, she had a benign tumor the size of a lemon removed from behind her left knee. She has an upper denture, as she has lost her teeth due to nighttime teeth grinding. Through all Ronda's medical and physical ordeals, she makes the best of what physical abilities she has, while she constantly reminds us, "I don't feel my age. I have more energy than anyone I know!"

Ten years following her first hip replacement surgery, Ronda was experiencing a high level of pain in her hip where the replacement had been done. As we shared earlier, Ronda has a high pain threshold, so when Ronda reports that she is in pain, it must be really painful, and we take her reports seriously.

When she went in to see her orthopedic surgeon, however, he was unable to diagnose her pain, got frustrated with Ronda's visits, and sent her home, basically telling her that the pain was "just something she would need to live with." We reminded him that when he did the hip surgery 10 years earlier, he said that it should last about 10 years and that maybe the insert had worn out. The orthopedist didn't think that was the problem and told us that after all Ronda was "older" and that "older people sometimes have pain." Ronda ended up firing him, and we helped her find another orthopedic surgeon who believed her when she talked about the pain she was experiencing. This new surgeon performed her second right hip replacement surgery (successfully) by replacing the old hardware from the first surgery.

When Ronda was in her late 50s she experienced symptoms of menopause, but her doctor considered these symptoms of her disability and referred Ronda to a psychiatrist. It took the advocacy of Ronda's staff to help her doctor understand that these symptoms were indicative of menopause (similar to other people her age) and not simply focus on her disability label when making a diagnosis. When Ronda needed her cataracts removed, we visited five ophthalmologists before a doctor agreed to remove them. We were told, "She won't sit still. She won't follow the directions. It just won't work with her." Basically, the first four ophthalmologists felt that it was okay to simply let Ronda live with increasing visual difficulties due to her cataracts, as she was challenging for them to deal with. Once we found the right professional who had a bit more patience and was willing to get to know Ronda on her terms, the operations were done on both her eyes without complications. This is one of the luxuries about living in a suburban area close to a large urban area; we can generally assist people in getting a second opinions for medical related issues (or, in this case, a fifth opinion).

It has been necessary for Ronda to miss time at her jobs following many of her injuries and surgeries. These times have tended to be the "lows" in Ronda's life, as she is so passionate about working, and these non-work periods were also associated with a higher display of challenging behavior. As retirement is "not an option" for Ronda, we help Ronda express her need to continue working for as long as possible whenever discussion delves into the possibility of retirement. In all our dealings with medical professionals, we have worked to include the people we support as an integral part of the team, always discussing what the options are and then deciding together on the best course of action. Disability or dementia have never stopped that team process.

RONDA'S FUTURE: REFLECTIONS ON AGING AND DEMENTIA

While the life expectancy for people with intellectual and developmental disabilities used to be much lower than the general population, their life expectancy is increasing and is rapidly approaching that of the general population. Variables that may contribute to this increase in life expectancy are the decrease in the incidence of institutionalization and the increase in access to health care more closely resembling those without disabilities. It should be noted that individuals with Down syndrome now have a life expectancy of 55 years, with many individuals living into their 60s and 70s (National Association for Down Syndrome, 2012), while just a few decades ago, most individuals with Down syndrome weren't expected to live past their 40s. As with the general population, as adults with intellectual and developmental disabilities live longer, they are also at an increased risk of developing dementia. Studies now show the prevalence of dementia among people with intellectual disability to be about the same as the general population (about 5% of people age 65 and older). The exception is the prevalence among adults with Down syndrome, which is about 25% for those who are 40 years and older and about 65% for those individuals age 60 and older (Janicki & Dalton, 2000; Strydom et al., 2009).

When Ronda reached the age of 62, we began to notice some increases in obsessive compulsive behaviors (getting stuck on repetitive routines in the morning and throughout her day, leading her to be late for rides and appointments) and some challenges with short-term memory loss. Ronda was diagnosed as having early onset of Alzheimer's disease and dementia, which her neurologist attributed in part to the head injury she sustained in a traffic accident in 1994. Ronda's most significant disability at this time is her progressive memory loss associated with Alzheimer's and dementia. We continue to work with Ronda to learn new nonintrusive support strategies that allow her to maintain her independence sustaining routines as much as possible.

Like other seniors, Ronda needs some additional supports due to her memory loss and decreased ambulation. The supports that are provided are much the same as those utilized by other seniors who do not have disabilities. Some of the supports we have developed to assist Ronda with her memory and dementia symptoms are described in the following sections.

Use of Visual Prompts

Ronda is visual and learns by routine, and for years, she had used a system of lining up all her daily medications and vitamins on the counter in her kitchen. This worked well for her until she began to forget her evening routine of taking her meds. As Ronda lives alone, we were able to determine that she was missing some of her evening doses by counting her pills weekly. Over the past year, Ronda has reluctantly agreed to use a medication box, which is also visual and more clearly shows the permanent product of whether or not she has taken her nighttime or morning meds on a given day. Ronda also has the new routine of calling her support coordinator every night when she takes her meds so that we know she has taken them. If we haven't heard from Ronda by a certain time, we then call her to double check. This new routine allows Ronda to continue to exert her independence by initiating the call to us and helps Ronda be as independent as she can while implementing a system to double check that her meds are indeed taken.

We have also encouraged Ronda to use her large calendar in her home to write down important dates and appointments in her schedule, as she has been forgetting to use her pocket calendar like she used to. This strategy also helps her staff, who can help her check the large calendar to see if she has written down her upcoming appointments. It was becoming too intrusive to ask Ronda if we could look in her pocket calendar daily to check on things, as she is comfortable sharing that information with her favorite staff member but not others.

Ronda sees a neurologist who monitors the progression of her memory loss and prescribes medication meant to slow the onset of the disease. The medications that she takes are the same as other seniors who do not have disabilities.

End-of-Life Planning

Our hope with Ronda is to continue to provide necessary supports in her own home and adapting (and increasing) supports as needed over time in response to Ronda's evolving needs related to aging, dementia, and other medical challenges. We are confident that we will be able to provide, access, and coordinate all needed supports that Ronda will need throughout the rest of her life within her existing home, which is what Ronda's wishes are at this time.

End-of-life planning is something we now include in all our individual service plans when we meet annually for program planning with the Regional Center. We feel that before people are sick or dying, we should find out what their final wishes are: whether they would prefer to be buried or cremated, have hospice services at home or in a nursing home, have a DNR (do not resuscitate) order, and so forth. When it is explained that this way "you can die the way you would like," nearly everyone is willing to participate and share his or her final wishes. We use the "Five Wishes" form, a legal document and planning guide for end-of-life planning through Aging with Dignity, or at a minimum, we assist people to

develop their own advance directive. In some cases, we assist families to work on Power of Attorney. People's wishes can also change across time due to life's circumstances, as Ronda herself indicated. This is a discussion that shouldn't end even after everything is supposedly finished being discussed.

Sometimes families are uncomfortable, and we may need to help them by being the ones to ask the end-of-life questions. Regardless, life and death issues are always handled so the person we are supporting has his or her say and is allowed to live and die with dignity.

CONCLUSION

While Ronda and many other adults with intellectual and developmental disabilities live in their own homes or in group living facilities, the majority of adults with intellectual and developmental disabilities live with their aging parents. More than 75% of people with intellectual and developmental disabilities live with their families. More than 25% of family care providers are over the age of 60 years and another 38% are between 41 and 59 years (Braddock, Hemp, & Rizzolo, 2008). Despite the fact that research-based practices documenting the success of supported living and other person-centered services is increasing, there continues to be an urgent need for aging adults with intellectual and developmental disabilities and their families to have access to quality community living supports and services that address their age-related health and social needs. Not all states have a mandate for support for adults with intellectual and developmental disabilities and their families, so many families receive few support services and often face long residential services waiting lists, estimated at roughly 115,000 families nationally (Lakin, Larson, Salmi, & Scott, 2009).

As the life span of individuals with disabilities continues to increase, planning for the future of these individuals is critical; otherwise, when their aging parents pass away without having detailed plans in place for the care of their dependent adult children, emergency placements may occur that do not adequately match or meet the needs of these individuals. When this occurs (as it too often does), depression, segregation, isolation, and chemical restraint (overmedication) are more likely to occur, especially for individuals who display behavior challenges. PCP (e.g., the McGill Action Planning System [MAPS], Planning Alternative Tomorrows with Hope [PATH], personal futures planning, essential lifestyle planning) and other person-centered approaches such as PBS are recommended for use by professionals seeking to assist families with the planning process for their adult children with intellectual and developmental disabilities (O'Brien & Pearpoint 2007; Smull & Sanderson, 2009).

Ronda and I sincerely hope that others who are supporting aging family members and/or seniors with intellectual and developmental disabilities will learn from and possibly be inspired by Ronda's story. I have certainly learned much from Ronda about how to listen to the needs of people and not simply assume that I know what is best for them. Ronda's wonderful sense of humor has helped us get through some challenging times when neither one of us wanted to back down from what we wanted to achieve, bumping heads at the time. We have learned to work together, as that is the only way that our relationship is able to continue and grow. We also hope that Ronda's story demonstrates that PBS is not a strategy that is applied to address specific problem behaviors but is a way of supporting people to live satisfying and productive lives.

For more information on community and supported living, check out these web sites:

CIRCL: Connections for Information and Resources on Community Living: http://www.allenshea.com/CIRCL/CIRCL.html

"Community for All" Tool Kit: Resources for Supporting Community Living Through the Center on Human Policy, Syracuse University (August 2004): http://thechp.syr.edu/toolkit/

Aging with Dignity: 5 Wishes Template for End-of-Life Planning: http://www.agingwithdignity.org/five-wishes.php

REFERENCES

Association for Positive Behavior Support (APBS). (2007). *Positive behavior support standards of practice: Individual level.* Retrieved from http://www.apbs.org/files/apbs_standards_of_practice_2013_format.pdf

Braddock, D., Hemp, R., & Rizzolo, M.C. (2008). *The state of the states in developmental disabilities: 2008.* Washington, DC: American Association on Intellectual and Developmental Disabilities.

Butterworth, J., Smith, F.A., Hall, A.C., Migliore, A., Winsor, J., Domin, D., & Timmons, J.C. (2011). The national report on employment services and outcomes. Boston: University of Massachusetts.

Charlton, J.I. (1998). *Nothing about us without us: Disability, oppression and empowerment.* Berkeley, CA: University of California Press.

Easter Seals. (2010). *Living with disabilities study.* Retrieved from http://www.westglen.com/online/easter_seals.htm

Education for All Handicapped Children Act of 1975, PL 94-142, 20 U.S.C. §§ 1400 *et seq.*

Hollins, S.C. (1995). Managing grief better: People with intellectual disabilities. *Habilitative Mental Health-care Newsletter, 14*(3).

Individuals with Disabilities Education Act Amendments of 1991, PL 102-119, 20 U.S.C. §§ 1400 *et seq.*

Janicki, M.P., & Dalton, A.J. (2000). Prevalence of dementia and impact on disability services. *Mental Retardation, 38,* 377–389.

Koegel, L.K., Koegel, R.L., & Dunlap, G. (1996). *Positive behavioral support: Including people with difficult behavior in the community.* Baltimore, MD: Paul H. Brookes Publishing Co.

Lakin, K.C., Larson, S., Salmi, P., & Scott, N. (2009). *Residential services for persons with developmental disabilities: Status and trends through 2008.* Minneapolis, MN: Research and Training Center on Community Living, Institute on Community Integration, University of Minnesota.

O'Brien, J. (1989). *What's worth working for? Leadership for better quality human services.* Lithonia, GA: Responsive Systems Associates.

O'Brien, J. (1993). *Supported living: What's the difference?* Lithonia, GA: Responsive Systems Associates.

O'Brien, J., & Pearpoint, J. (2007) *Person-centered planning with MAPS and PATH: A workbook for facilitators.* Toronto, ON: Inclusion Press.

Smull, M.W., & Sanderson, H. (2009). *Essential lifestyle planning for everyone.* Annapolis, MD: The Learning Community.

Strydom, A., Lee, L.A., Jokinen, N., Shooshtari, S., Raykar, V., Torr, J., . . . Maaskant, M.A. (2009). *Report on the state of science on dementia in people with intellectual disabilities.* IASSID Special Interest Research Group on Aging and Intellectual Disabilities. Retrieved from https://iassid.org/images/documents/Aging/state%20of%20the%20science%20dementia%202009.pdf

U.S. Department of Education, Office of Special Education and Rehabilitative Services. (2010). *Thirty-five years of progress in educating children with disabilities through IDEA.* Washington, DC: Author.

Taking Positive Behavior Interventions and Supports into the Future

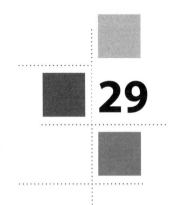

29

Allyson Satter, Nikki Wolf, and Wayne Sailor

The purpose of this chapter is to describe emerging applications and suggest future directions of individual positive behavior interventions and supports (PBIS).[1] PBIS applies the principles of applied behavior analysis to address problem behaviors (Horner, 2000) and is applicable to a variety of school, family, and community settings, as well as perhaps yet conceptualized settings. In this chapter, we provide examples of applications across school, family, and community settings and specific recommendations for sustaining PBIS across settings at the individual level.

For PBIS to be sustained over time, there must be an emphasis placed on conceptualizing PBIS not as a program or even as a philosophy but instead as a problem-solving framework that incorporates research-supported practices to prevent problem behaviors. Therefore, even if the participants, applications, and practices change over time, the fundamental components remain stable and identifiable. It is essential to bear these fundamental components in mind when considering future directions and applications of PBIS. As new applications and directions of PBIS emerge, we must reconfirm what makes PBIS successful and which practices are supported by research. In other words, the future direction of PBIS is not about developing a new framework but rather about clearly defining and refining our current use of data, systems, and practices while remaining connected to the established core components of PBIS.

---

[1] The early 1980s literature on positive behavior support used the descriptor PBS. Later, following legal concerns expressed by the Public Broadcasting System, the descriptor became PBIS. With the advent of whole school applications of innovative practices, the term SWPBIS emerged in the literature of school applications. We use that descriptor throughout this chapter when referring to school applications of PBIS.

In this chapter, we begin by describing emerging applications of PBIS across school, family, and community settings. Then we look beyond emerging applications and provide recommendations for expansion and sustainability based on lessons learned through application of PBIS. Finally, we consider the role of the Association for Positive Behavior Support (APBS) standards of practice in guiding implementation across settings and into the future.

EMERGING APPLICATIONS

Schools

The scientific underpinnings of individual PBIS have remained fairly consistent over the past 30 years with the primary areas of growth taking place in the development of systems (Sugai & Simonsen, 2012). Initially, PBIS was used to help improve student behaviors at the individual level, then as the need to establish systems became apparent, the establishment of School-Wide PBIS (SWPBIS) evolved (Sugai & Simonsen, 2012). Now there are nearly 20,000 schools in the United States implementing SWPBIS with international efforts underway as well (R. Horner, personal communication, April 9, 2013).

Although the initial research and implementation of SWPBIS began in schools at the elementary and middle levels, it is now implemented in many high schools. Across all school levels, it is used with increasing frequency to target specific areas of concern, such as bully prevention (Ross & Horner, 2009; Waasdorp, Bradshaw, & Leaf, 2012). Examining how the individualized tier of SWPBIS is currently being implemented across different school environments enables us to begin to identify future directions and applications of individual SWPBIS in school settings.

School-Wide Positive Behavior Intervention and Support (SWPBIS) in High School Settings

Although the essential elements of SWPBIS are the same across high schools, elementary schools, preschools, or middle schools, implementation varies greatly across these school environments. For example, high schools are usually more complex organizations with more students, more demands, and different behavioral expectations than elementary schools (Sugai, Flannery, & Bohanon-Edmonson, 2004). Therefore, SWPBIS practices, developed and researched at elementary and middle schools, require modification before being applied in high school settings (Bohanon et al., 2006). It is unwise to take the same practices that occur in elementary schools and transfer them to different populations. However, it is important to identify which features of PBIS are essential and should occur at all levels, because if some key elements are neglected, sustainability and generalization will suffer (Flannery & Sugai, 2009). As Bohanon et al. (2006) explain, regardless of the age or setting, we should remember the essential elements of SWPBIS and "model the principles as much as possible to build on strengths and circumvent barriers" (p. 143).

Sugai, Flannery, and Bohanon-Edmonson (2004) warn that implementation at the high school level is more difficult than at the elementary level; therefore, more research is needed to determine which features are feasible and essential (Flannery, Sugai, & Anderson, 2009). They identified key features of SWPBIS across schools, surveyed existing high school teams, and used the results to provide guidelines for high schools. The survey results indicated that the top priorities for schools were schoolwide discipline and obtaining staff buy-in, but few schools focused on classroom level or individualized levels of support.

Establishing and researching individualized supports available in high school settings is particularly important for the sustainability of SWPBIS (Swain-Bradway & Malloy, 2009). Little is known about the differences between secondary and tertiary supports in high schools (Swain-Bradway & Malloy, 2009). Because initial research in high school settings show most efforts occur at the universal level (Bohanon, Fenning, Eber, & Flannery, 2007), future research should examine how to most effectively establish targeted and individualized supports in high schools (Bohanon et al., 2006; Swain-Bradway & Malloy, 2009). Implementing SWPBIS supports at the individual level is difficult due to the time, effort, training, and resources required to do it effectively (Crimmins & Farrell, 2006). However, it is particularly important to address this concern in high schools, because students who exhibit a pattern of behavior problems that indicate a need for tertiary supports are at a higher risk for negative outcomes, such as dropping out of school (Swain-Bradway & Malloy, 2009). Swain-Bradway and Malloy (2009) described the elements high schools should have in place to efficiently and effectively implement secondary and tertiary supports, such as establishing team structures and communication systems, identifying available resources, delegating administrative roles, and determining guides for how to use and collect data. For the tertiary level, they recommended having a unique team for each student, ideally led by the student, to monitor the data, progress, and supports available across multiple settings so that the focus remains on student goals and quality of life.

The student's voice is especially essential in high schools as students approach the end of their school-age years and begin to consider postschool outcomes (Bohanon et al., 2007). If teams make plans that students do not value and do not contribute to the student's quality of life outside of school, there is little hope that the student will become engaged in the process and have success. Therefore, self-determination skills must be taught, valued, and nurtured, so the student's voice truly guides tertiary supports. Pierson, Carter, Lane, and Glaeser (2008) define self-determination as the "ability to take primary control of one's own life and do so in personally meaningful ways" (p.115). Learning the

skills necessary to become self-determined is important because the self-determination of students with disabilities is linked to better outcomes beyond school, such as employment and independent living (Wehmeyer & Palmer, 2003). To learn self-determination, the student must have opportunities to make meaningful decisions and plans for their own lives. Involving students in person-centered transition planning is one way to help develop and utilize self-determination skills (Bohanon, Fenning, Borgmeier, Flannery, & Malloy, 2009; Bohanon et al., 2007; O'Brien & Lovett, 1993).

According to Bohanon, "one of the most comprehensive and intense levels of support at the tertiary level is the wraparound process" (Bohanon et al., 2007, p. 44). Wraparound utilizes a person-centered, team problem-solving process to effectively integrate family, community, and school resources (Eber et al., 2009). One of the defining characteristics of the wraparound process is that the process is driven by the voices of the student and family. Although wraparound teams consist of members across school and community agencies, the goals, strengths, and needs of the student and family are foremost considerations when developing wraparound plans. Wraparound teams, guided by the student and family, utilize functional behavioral assessment (FBA) data to develop comprehensive plans aimed at accessing the resources needed to improve student outcomes (Eber, Hyde, & Suter, 2011; Scott & Eber, 2003).

The rehabilitation, empowerment, natural supports, education, and work (RENEW) model is an example of a transition planning process that supports adolescents who require intensive, individualized supports to remain in school and prepare for positive postschool outcomes (Bohanon et al., 2009; Swain-Bradway & Malloy, 2009). As with the wraparound process, the RENEW planning process includes teams of support staff and mentors from the school, family, and community, helping the individual student set goals and action steps that are desirable to the student. The person-centered planning (PCP) process is focused on utilizing the student's strengths and identifying the available resources needed to help the student achieve his or her personal goals.

Malloy, Sundar, Hagner, Pierias, and Viet (2010) implemented RENEW as a Tier-3 PBIS at a large high school in New Hampshire. They described the following features of RENEW:

> The RENEW model is designed to create a context within which trusting and reciprocal relationships, self-determined behaviors, and career-related plans and activities can be developed using eight strategies: (a) personal futures planning, (b) individualized team development and wraparound services, (c) individualized resource development, (d) flexible education programming, (e) individualized school-to-career planning, (f) employment, (g) mentoring, and (h) connections to community-based resources and networks. Personal futures planning is the lynchpin of the process, helping to elicit the youth's perspective on his or her history, current network of people and supports, strengths, dislikes, dreams, and concerns. The facilitator then help(s) each youth to develop a detailed plan in the context of the young person's desired educational, employment, and adult life goals. (Malloy et al., 2010, p. 21)

After implementing RENEW with 20 students at this high school, Malloy et al. (2010) found significant decreases in "functional impairments in school/work behavior, home behavior, moods and emotions, and self-harmful behavior" (p. 22).

School-Wide Positive Behavior Intervention and Support (SWPBIS) for Bully Prevention in Schools

One new application of the SWPBIS prevention framework is addressing the national concern of bullying. Considering the long-term negative prognosis for both the victims of bullying and the perpetrators (U.S. Department of Education, 2011), this is a problem that schools cannot afford to

ignore. Victims of bullying are more prone to physical and emotional disorders, depression, and suicide (Vanderbilt & Augustyn, 2010), whereas bullies themselves are more prone to drug abuse, convictions for violent crimes, dropping out of school, and other negative life outcomes, such as unemployment and relationship problems (Farrington & Ttofi, 2011; Vanderbilt & Augustyn, 2010). With the spotlight on these dismal outcomes, it is not surprising so much attention is being given to identifying ways to prevent bullying in schools.

Evidence suggests SWPBIS may serve as an effective tool for bully prevention (Waasdorp et al., 2012). Because school climate is related to bullying behavior (Gendron, Williams, & Guerra, 2011) and research shows SWPBIS improves school climate (Bradshaw, Koth, Thornton, & Leaf, 2009) and also reduces behavior problems (Bradshaw, Mitchell, & Leaf, 2010), the implementation of SWPBIS in schools can indirectly affect bullying behavior. The universal level of SWPBIS involves implementing evidence-based practices for all students. In their meta-analysis, Ttofi and Farrington (2010) identified evidence-based practices to reduce bullying, including better playground supervision and targeting factors outside of the school, such as training families about bullying issues. At the tertiary level, SWPBIS targets behaviors that may include the externalizing or internalizing behaviors of bullies, their victims, or both by discouraging the function of the behavior and involving decision makers outside the school, such as families. Because bullying behavior is usually defined as repeated incidents of oppressive attacks over time (Ttofi & Farrington, 2010), students exhibiting bullying behavior should be receiving individualized behavior support within a SWPBIS model.

Ross and Horner (2009) investigated a schoolwide approach to target bullying behavior, which they called bully prevention in PBIS (BPPBIS). They considered BPPBIS a secondary tier of support, even though it was used to teach all students skills for how to "be respectful" and how to respond to bully-ing behavior. In BPPBIS, students who do not respond to this level of intervention would be provided individual function-driven PBIS support. After implementing the second-ary tier of BPPBIS with three elementary schools, results indicated a decrease in the problem behavior of six students that were targeted because of high levels of physical or verbal aggression toward peers. Also, results showed an increase in appropriate responses by victims and bystanders. The results of this study demonstrate the potential that SWP-BIS has for preventing bullying behaviors by empowering and supporting victims, while teaching appropriate social skills to students who bully.

Families

In school settings utilizing a SWPBIS framework, school personnel collaborate with families to provide the appropriate individualized supports for students at risk and with significant behavioral challenges. Early childhood SWPBIS models recognize the essential role families play in support-ing children with challenging behaviors. In community-based and preschool settings at the early childhood level, families not only collaborate in the support process but also become recipients of supports and resources that contribute to their child's development. Research also shows how PBIS implementa-tion can occur within the home (Binnendyk & Lucyshyn, 2009). Examining how individ-ualized PBIS supports can be extended to home settings with families, through early intervention services and home-based ser-vices, we can begin to identify future direc-tions and applications of individual PBIS for families.

Early Intervention (Birth to Age 3): Engaging Families

To prevent and decrease the behavior prob-lems of children, providing early interven-tion services within the family context is critical (Reinke, Splett, Robeson, & Offutt,

2009). Therefore, IDEA (EHA Amendments of 1986, 42 U.S.C., Section 671[a]) requires early intervention services to be delivered by developing an individualized family ser-vice plan, which includes supports for the family, such as home visits (Bruder, 2010). Bruder (2010) identifies three reasons early intervention services are essential: 1) early identification of needs increases the effec-tiveness of interventions, 2) families receive supports that can help prevent developmen-tal delays, and 3) early intervention better prepares children for school, thus reduc-ing the cost once children become school age. Early intervention services that occur before children reach school-age years are dependent on family involvement because the family context is where the infant or young child's learning primarily occurs. Bruder (2010) argues that early intervention should involve a family centered approach that occurs in natural settings, treats fam-ilies respectfully, and seeks family input to determine what supports they need and value. Furthermore, Bruder (2010) and Reinke et al. (2009) recommend implement-ing multitiered systems of support (MTSS), such as SWPBIS, as a method for responding early to all children's needs while providing intensive interventions for individuals, such as those eligible for services through IDEA.

School-Wide Positive Behavior Intervention and Support in Early Childhood (Ages 3–5)

Because PBIS is a prevention framework, it is not surprising that it is being adapted to reach children attending early child-hood programs, especially considering early behavior problems are likely to con-tinue into school-age years (Dunlap & Fox, 2009; Fox & Hemmeter, 2009). One prom-ising early childhood application of SWP-BIS is the teaching pyramid model (Fox & Hemmeter, 2009). The teaching pyramid model provides increasing levels of support and evidence-based interventions; how-ever, the kinds of supports needed differ in early childhood settings with a greater focus placed on caregiver relationships and environments outside of the school setting. The teaching pyramid model also provides individual interventions when children are unresponsive to efforts such as the general instruction of social skills. Individualized positive behavior support at the early childhood level mirrors the same essential elements of tertiary level SWPBIS in elementary and secondary school settings, including team-based decision making, functional assessment of behavior, and development of a comprehensive behavior support plan. In addition, at the early childhood level, significant emphasis is placed on including families in the process and developing plans that address home, community, and school settings (Fox, Carta, Strain, Dunlap, & Hemmeter, 2010; Fox & Hemmeter, 2009; McCart et al., 2010).

Blair, Fox, and Lentini (2010) examined the effects of individualized PBIS on three children in community based early childhood programs. The behaviors of the children in the study included aggression (hitting, biting, pushing, scratching), off-task behaviors, and yelling. Procedures involved conducting FBAs and developing behavior support plans that featured prevention strategies, teaching strategies, and response strategies that were associated with the identified function of the behavior. The results showed decreases in problem behaviors and increases in child engagement for all three students. Wood, Ferro, Umbreit, and Liaupsin (2011) also found a function-based intervention applied with three children in an early intervention preschool setting was effective for improving problem behaviors. The children in the study had the following types of disabilities: severe language delay, Down syndrome, and autism. After conducting FBAs and applying a function-based intervention decision model, function-based interventions were developed that resulted in increases in on-task behavior and decreases in disruptive behavior. Applying the principles of individual PBIS for young

children and their families has emerged as an effective means of intervening early to decrease problem behaviors of children in preschool settings.

McCart et al. (2010) described how integrated SWPBIS can be adapted for use with young children and their families. These researchers identified the essential role families play in shaping the outcomes of young children. Furthermore, they contended that if MTSS are to be effective in early childhood settings, program personnel need to be taught how to engage parents and partner with them throughout the tiered intervention process. For early childhood, at the individual level, both children and their families receive contextually appropriate targeted interventions aimed at helping families access the resources they need to support their child's development.

For early intervention and prevention of behavior problems, Reinke, Splett, Robeson, and Offutt (2009) recommended integrating SWPBIS interventions in schools with a multitiered family support model, the "family check-up" (FCU). They acknowledged that family involvement is strongest at the tertiary tier of SWPBIS, where families collaborate with SWPBIS teams to develop behavior support plans. However, they suggest family involvement should extend beyond just collaboration, offering FCU supports for the families of children at the individual level who have intensive needs. They state that data collected through SWPBIS should be used to identify families who could benefit from individual FCU supports. At the individual level of the FCU model, "families are offered direct support or family intervention such as brief interventions, parenting groups, family therapy, child and/or school involvement, and case management, which vary based on the needs of the family" (p. 38) and can occur at school or community mental health agencies. Integrating the SWPBIS model with a multitiered family support model such as FCU further helps "prevent behavior problems of young children in multiple settings" (Reinke et al., 2009, p. 40).

Family-Centered Positive Behavior Intervention and Support in the Home

Research also shows the potential results of implementing family-centered positive behavior support in home settings for children and families who require intensive supports. For example, Boettcher, Koegel, McNerney, and Koegel (2003) implemented a family-centered PBIS approach with a family while the mother of a child with autism was undergoing intensive surgery. The authors described how the preventive approach was used to support the family during this challenging time. A preventive plan was put in place to prepare the children and caregivers of the family for the changes that would occur while the mother of the family was hospitalized and recovering. The comprehensive plan considered previous functional assessments of how unpredictable events affected the child with autism's behavior and included incentives for appropriate behaviors. The family-centered support plan resulted in improved behaviors of the student with autism and positive reports from family members. This study indicates the potential positive effects of implementing individualized PBIS supports with families in a home setting.

Binnendyk and Lucyshyn (2009) evaluated the effectiveness of family-centered PBIS for a child with autism who would not eat. They implemented a PBIS approach with the child's family in the home setting. The approach consisted of collaborating with the child's family to develop a contextually appropriate plan that met the family's needs and extinguished the child's refusal behavior. To develop the plan, they conducted a functional assessment of the child's behavior and assessed the family environment. Then they trained the family to implement the intervention in the home. The intervention consisted of conducting a comprehensive functional assessment of the behavior and then developing a PBIS behavior support plan with the family. The plan included strategies such as establishing set eating routines, gradually increasing the portion size of food, using pictures to teach the routine, and using a preferred toy or activity to reinforce the desired behavior. Implementation of the plan was first introduced through intensive training with a therapist, and then the plan was done with the mother and subsequently generalized to other foods and with the father. Data were collected to measure the intervention's effectiveness at eliminating the child's target behavior and to determine the effect of the support plan on the family's overall quality of life. The results showed the family-centered PBIS approach improved the child's eating behaviors and the family's overall quality of life.

Communities

In addition to intensive, individualized supports in home and school settings, some individuals will benefit from community based supports. Therefore, services provided by community based organizations, such as mental health agencies, often play a vital role in meeting the needs of individuals who require tertiary supports in the PBIS framework. Furthermore, research is being conducted to identify the effectiveness of implementing PBIS in community settings (Gagnon, Rockwell, & Scott, 2008; McCart, Wolf, Sweeney, & Choi, 2009; Nelson, Jolivette, Leone, & Mathur, 2010). One example is using PBIS in juvenile correction facilities. Youth who are incarcerated in these facilities often have complex needs and require significant supports from teams of comprehensive service providers. The PBIS framework serves as a potential model for how to prevent problem behaviors within these facilities and how to organize the array of individual supports that may be necessary to promote positive outcomes for youth when they return to the community (Nelson et al., 2010). Research has also examined how PBIS can be applied to community mental health agencies (McCart et al., 2009). By examining how individualized supports are being implemented in community settings, such as juvenile correction facilities and community mental health agencies, we can better begin to identify future directions and applications of individual PBIS within these settings.

Positive Behavior Intervention and Support in Juvenile Correction Facilities

Juvenile justice settings serve a population of children and adolescents with significant needs. An alarming proportion of youth incarcerated in juvenile detention centers have disabilities—primarily emotional and learning disabilities (Gagnon & Barber, 2010; Hagner, Malloy, Mazzone, & Cornier, 2008; Quinn, Rutherford, Leone, Osher, & Poirier, 2005). The results of a national survey showed an overrepresentation of students with disabilities in juvenile correction facilities, with 33.4% more students receiving special education services than in public schools (Quinn et al., 2005). Furthermore, the prognosis for these youth after they leave the juvenile correction facilities is dismal, with most released youth reoffending and few returning to finish school (Bohanon et al., 2007; Hagner et al., 2008; Jolivette & Nelson, 2010). PBIS may seem like an unlikely fit for a system that is driven by punishment, but recidivism rates suggest an alternate approach may be warranted (Hagner et al., 2008). Research shows PBIS can be an effective strategy for improving behaviors in these settings and has the potential for improving long-term outcomes of students after they leave the juvenile correction facilities (Gagnon & Barber, 2010; Jolivette & Nelson, 2010). However, overcoming the long-held notion that these kids need to be punished, regardless of whether it is an effective rehabilitation measure, creates considerable challenges when implementing positive, preventive measures (Nelson,

Scott, Gagnon, Jolivette, & Sprague, 2008). Despite these challenges, PBIS is emerging as one of the few interventions that could be used to improve the outcomes of students in juvenile correction facilities (Gagnon et al., 2008; Jolivette & Nelson, 2010) by "reversing the negative trajectory of incarcerated youth" (Nelson et al., 2010, p. 73).

Although all students in juvenile justice facilities have complex needs, facility-wide PBIS (FWPBIS) does not solely occur at the individual level (Sprague, Baus, & Tedder, 2011). Even though the majority of students in these facilities require comprehensive supports, problem behaviors often mimic typical school settings; therefore, by implementing primary and secondary interventions, minor behaviors are likely to be minimized so that emphasis can be placed on appropriately matching individual supports to those with intensive needs (Jolivette & Nelson, 2010; Nelson et al., 2008). Much like SWPBIS, FWPBIS in juvenile correction facilities requires the establishment of a leadership team, staff training, data-based monitoring and action planning, staff buy-in, facility-wide establishment and instruction of behavioral expectations, and reinforcement protocols (Jolivette & Nelson, 2010; Sprague et al., 2011). At the individual level, as in the SWPBIS model, functional assessment data should be used to develop behavior support plans for youth who require intensive individual interventions. Comprehensive teams represented by all relevant service providers, family members, and the target individual should collaborate to develop and implement a plan that is centered on the individual's goals and desires, aimed at improving the individual's quality of life. The RENEW model is one example of a tertiary intervention that can be implemented at the individual level in juvenile correction facilities (Hagner et al., 2008).

Impressive results from the implementation of FWPBIS at the Illinois Youth Center at the Harrisburg Boy's Prison (IYC) and the Iowa Juvenile Home (IJH) demonstrate the potential role PBIS can play in reducing problem behaviors in juvenile correction facilities (Nelson et al., 2008). Implementation at IYC included a ticket exchange reinforcement system at the universal level, a mentoring program at the secondary level, and development of individual plans at the tertiary level. The results of putting these interventions into practice were significant decreases in problem behaviors, where "physical altercations among students declined from 32 per month to zero in three years" (Gagnon et al., 2008, p. 11). At IJH, after implementing FWPBIS, instances of seclusion and restraint decreased by 73% (Gagnon et al., 2008; Nelson et al., 2008). Because preliminary data show the potential of PBIS to be effective in juvenile correction facilities, further implementation and research should occur that seeks to better understand the effectiveness of PBIS with incarcerated youth and determine how best to adapt FWPBIS for these settings.

Community Mental Health Agencies

Less than 40% of youth in special education for emotional or behavioral disorders receive mental health services along with their special education services, despite poor outcomes such as high dropout rates, high percentages of suspension and expulsion, and poor grades (Atkins, Hoagwood, Kutash, & Seidman, 2010). Community mental health professionals and agencies can provide much needed supports to individuals with intense emotional and behavioral needs, although the services they provide are often separate from schools and therefore not easily accessible to individuals and their families, especially in areas affected by poverty (Capella, Frazier, Atkins, Schoenwald, & Glisson, 2008). Researchers envisioned how community mental health services could be provided within a PBIS framework in home, school, and community settings (Atkins et al., 2010; Bradshaw et al., 2012; Capella et al., 2008). Capella et al. (2008) describe how mental health providers can be utilized across the tiers in low-income

schools. For example, at the individual level, community mental health providers could work with schools to provide direct services to students with significant mental health needs (Atkins et al., 2010; Capella et al., 2008). Furthermore, Bradshaw et al. (2012) explain how school and mental health community organizations can partner together to provide services in schools. They describe a collaborative effort among a state department of education, a nonprofit mental health organization, and a university to widely and effectively disseminate PBIS, targeting behavioral and mental health problems in schools across the state.

MTSS, such as PBIS, can also be used as a framework for delivering services to families through community based agencies. McCart et al. (2009) utilized a tiered system, based on response to intervention (RTI) and PBIS frameworks, to support families in an early Head Start setting through a community based agency. For this study, they envisioned the tiers as the level of support families needed. The universal intervention consisted of group training of all parent participants. The targeted intervention consisted of training provided to service coordinators who conducted home visits. Service coordinators, agency management staff, and researchers provided individualized interventions for family members and their children and continued home visits to family participants whom service coordinators identified as needing more support. In addition, the tertiary-level interventions included developing an individualized behavior support plan and identifying specific services needed to address participants' needs. Results showed satisfaction with the training sessions among parent participants and a reduction in stress levels among 12 out of 20 parents who consistently attended training sessions. These results indicate the value of integrating school, home, and community mental health supports and also show that MTSS may be beneficial for envisioning how services are provided through community based agencies.

Adults

The principles of PBIS are not unique to children and adolescents. They can also be used in community settings with adults with problem behavior. According to Gordham (2010), efforts have begun to "bring elements of PBS to long term care, that is, assisted living, enhanced care, skilled nursing, adult foster care, and in-home supports for our aging citizens" (p. 2). For example, LeBlanc (2010) describes a program that uses multidisciplinary teams to provide comprehensive supports for adults with dementia and behavior problems. The prevention model program involved increased engagement of individuals and functional analysis of problem behaviors. Freeman et al. (2005) explains how features of SWPBIS can be applied to community organizations that support adults with disabilities, such as organizations that provide residential support. They provide examples of universal, targeted, and individualized interventions that could occur at each level in such an organization. At the individual level, they recommend developing the capacity of teams within these organizations by including team members with behavioral expertise.

RECOMMENDATION FOR SUSTAINABILITY AND EXPANSION

To sustain PBIS into the future, we must reflect on common features that contribute to its effectiveness across various applications. First, we recommend applying sustainability practices learned through SWPBIS to other settings. Next, in schools, we recommend integrating SWPBIS into the broader framework of MTSS, so as to engage behavior along with academics in a common school-reform format. In nonschool settings, we also recommend providing services in an MTSS format, so as to increase the level of supports provided according to the needs of the individuals receiving services. Then we recommend collaborating with service providers across school and nonschool settings, as is done with wraparound, so that individuals can more easily access a wide array of resources. Finally, we suggest using the APBS standards of practice as a guide for implementation across settings and into the future.

Sustainability of School-Wide Positive Behavior Intervention and Support

Researchers have examined the sustainability features of SWPBIS and individualized PBIS (Bambara, Nonnemacher, & Kern, 2009; Coffey & Horner, 2012). As PBIS expands across settings, it is important to consider what has been learned about sustainability through applications in school settings. Coffey and Horner (2012) conducted a literature review and collected survey data to identify sustainability features associated with implementation of SWPBIS. They concluded administrative support, data-based decision making, and communication were associated with sustainability. Similarly, Bambara et al. (2009) conducted a qualitative study to uncover features associated with the sustainability of individualized PBIS. They discovered school culture, administrative support, professional development, time allotment, and family/student involvement all were related to participants' perceptions of what contributed to effective individualized PBIS implementation. We believe these findings are relevant across settings and should be examined further in future applications of PBIS. PBIS can be implemented with children, youth, or adults in schools, homes, or community settings; in any case, support from leaders and stakeholders, using data to guide decisions, and collaborative communication among key players must occur with fidelity for PBIS to be effective.

Creating Multitiered Systems of Support

Individuals who have complex needs usually require supports from various service providers. Unfortunately, even service providers who work with the same individual may plan and provide services separately from each other. Different teams or departments often plan for different areas without considering how they can work together to offer comprehensive supports. Therefore, we recommend embedding PBIS practices targeted at individuals within an overarching MTSS aimed at targeting the needs of the whole individual.

For example, SWPBIS can be embedded within an MTSS framework aimed at simultaneously targeting academic and behavioral outcomes (Algozzine et al., 2012; Sailor, Doolittle, Bradley, & Danielson, 2009).[2] Although there is considerable evidence showing a correlation between behavior and academic outcomes (Horner et al., 2009; Lassen, Steele, & Sailor, 2006; McIntosh, Flannery, Sugai, Braun, & Cochrane, 2008), often behavioral and academic interventions are viewed as separate practices with different value placed on them, usually with academic interventions taking precedence over emotional/social supports. However, a call for integrated MTSS that incorporate SWPBIS and academic interventions at three tiers has emerged in the literature (Sailor, 2009).

Across grades and settings, effective instruction and effective behavior support follow the same principles: data-based decision making, clearly defined and communicated expectations, and appropriate supports for the individual's level of need (Lewis, 2009). Therefore, by applying an MTSS like SWPBIS to both behavior and academics, schools are able to meet the multiple needs of their students more effectively and efficiently. Academics and behavior are two sides of the same coin: To improve academic outcomes, practitioners must address behaviors so students will be less distracted and more prepared to learn, whereas to improve behaviors, teachers must fully engage students in learning and match instructional practices to students' skill levels (Colvin, Sugai, Good, & Lee, 1997; Sailor et al., 2009). The MTSS framework can also be applied to community settings. For

example, McCart et al. (2009) applied a MTSS framework to the level of support provided to families by a community based agency. Applying the principles of effective instruction and behavior support with differing levels of intensity to match different individuals' needs can occur across schools and agencies, with children and adults alike.

At the individual level of SWPBIS support, teams must consider how behaviors and academic skills affect one another. For example, if SWPBIS teams are making decisions about behavior without considering whether academic needs are related to the function of behavior, their efforts may be futile; similarly, if academic teams are making decisions without fully understanding a student's social and emotional needs, true progress may not occur at the individual level. Therefore, schools must integrate academic and behavioral teams in MTSS with the common goal of matching appropriate services to all areas of student need (Satter & Dunn, 2012). Likewise, community based agencies should also consider the diverse needs of the individuals they serve. For example, in order to meet the academic needs of adolescents in juvenile justice settings, teams must consider how to also address social, emotional, and behavioral needs. Rather than addressing areas of concern in isolation, teams of service providers in various settings must consider the holistic needs of the individuals they serve.

Several examples exist of how schools are integrating MTSS for both academics and behavior. The schoolwide applications model (SAM) integrates SWPBIS and three tiers of academic interventions within the broader framework of MTSS (including RTI for special education identification) as part of a comprehensive school reform model that matches interventions and supports to meet the needs of all students in integrated settings rather than segregating services for special

_____

[2] We use the term *MTSS* to refer to three tiers of academic and behavioral interventions applied through team problem-solving processes in a comprehensive context of school reform. The term *RTI* is typically reserved for "standard protocol," evidence-based, academic interventions applied to determine the eligibility of students for special education services and supports.

education and general education (Sailor, 2009; Sailor, Wolf, Choi, & Roger, 2009; Sailor et al., 2006). In the Ravenswood, California, school district, improvements in language arts and math, as measured by state assessments, significantly correlated with fidelity implementation of the SAM model (Sailor et al., 2006).

Sadler and Sugai (2009) describe one district's experiences over 10 years of implementing academic and behavioral MTSS. In their model, schools used SWPBIS to provide a continuum of behavior supports in conjunction with a multitiered model for literacy instruction. School leadership teams were organized for the purpose of monitoring the effectiveness of the interventions, making data-based decisions accordingly, implementing function-based behavior intervention plans when students did not respond to primary and secondary supports. Watson, Gable, and Greenwood (2011) argued that just as FBAs are used to assess students' challenging behaviors at the individual level, an ecobehavioral approach could be used to assess classroom instruction when considering the best instructional practices for individual students.

Integrate Services Across Settings

Because individuals have complex needs, it is important to consider how home, school, and community agencies can work collaboratively together to best meet those needs for children as well as adults. Combining resources from different agencies can potentially provide more effective supports for individuals than can be provided by each agency separately. For example, when community mental health agencies and schools create partnerships to provide mental health services in schools, students can more readily access these services (Atkins et al., 2010). Previously, we described how wraparound planning is utilized at the high school level to connect home and community supports to school implementation of PBIS. We believe this should occur not just in high schools but across all ages and in homes and community agencies as well to ensure resources are used

more efficiently. For example, Nelson et al. (2010) describe the problem with segregated services that occur in juvenile justice settings:

> Many incarcerated youth are or have been clients of multiple systems. It is not unusual for an incarcerated youth to have at least a mental health treatment plan and an IEP. Yet seldom are these plans integrated in any meaningful way . . . Furthermore, the isolation of intervention strategies often results in wasteful duplication of services, services that effectively cancel out one another; and services that are far more costly and have substantially less impact than if they were integrated. (p. 75).

The wraparound process should be used across settings to connect families, school personnel, and community members together in PCP teams that are pursuing the same goal of improving the individual's quality of life.

Identify Essential Features

Because PBIS procedures are emerging across different disciplines and being implemented in various ways, it is important to focus on which elements uniquely define PBIS and should serve as a guide for taking PBIS into the future while ensuring its sustainability and effectiveness. The APBS standards of practice were developed to identify "those concepts and methods essential to implementation of positive behavior supports on the individual level; that is, with individuals who engage in problem behaviors" (APBS, 2007).

We recommend using the APBS standards of practice as a guide for clarifying PBIS when applied in new settings. The established effectiveness of PBIS at improving behaviors in different home, school, and community settings indicates it has the potential to influence behavior in unrealized and not yet researched areas. As we look to the future, we would do well to consider what should occur to ensure the fundamental components of PBIS remain intact despite how and where they are applied. To accomplish this, we need explicit standards of what defines PBIS across the tiers. At the individual level, the APBS standards of practice can serve as that guide. Although the practices, data, and systems require flexibility and may change according to the setting in which the supports reside, the essential defining elements of individual PBIS, as outlined in the APBS standards of practice, should be consistent across settings. These essential features must be present and implemented with fidelity for individual PBIS to effectively expand into the future.

CONCLUSION

Applications of the PBIS framework should serve as a guide for the future direction of individual PBIS. The science of individualized PBIS has evolved over time into a framework for providing supports and services that meet a variety of needs. Examining how both the science and framework are applied across individuals and settings leads to a better understanding of where PBIS is headed, while also illuminating areas that need additional research.

Applications of PBIS across school, home, and community settings demonstrate the versatility of the PBIS framework. These examples show how the systems, practices, and use of data associated with the PBIS framework are applicable to children, adults, and families with a variety of needs. From these applications, we can learn how systems and practices can be used to enhance the quality of life of individuals, from an adult with Alzheimer's to an adolescent in the juvenile justice system. We also can learn from these applications how service providers can work together across settings to collectively meet the needs of children, families, and adults.

Although it is important to focus on the systems that need to be in place to facilitate PBIS implementation and integration of resources across providers and settings, developing these systems should not be at the expense of researching and improving individual interventions that are needed for those with the most intensive needs (Crimmins & Farrell, 2006). Researchers and implementers must find a balance between developing primary and secondary systems of support across settings and continuing to ensure that individual supports are firmly in place. Future research should focus on how to effectively allocate resources to serve individuals with the most intensive needs, because this level of individualized PBIS is the most time intensive and requires the highest level of expertise to implement.

Finally, the future of PBIS is perhaps coming most sharply into focus in the schools through its rapidly evolving position in the standards-based reform movement. Sailor, Stowe, Turnbull, and Kleinhammer-Tramill (2007) argued for adding a social and behavioral standard to standards-based education with SWPBIS as its basis. The latest iteration of their movement, Common Core State Standards, moves closer to this position but leaves open the particular nature of behavior interventions in schools. The national center on schoolwide inclusive school reform, called the Center on a Schoolwide Integrated Framework for Transformation, funded by the Office of Special Education Programs, embeds SWPBIS in its overall MTSS framework for providing technical assistance to 64 schools within 16 school districts across 5 states, beginning in 2013 and ending in 2017 (http://www.swiftschools.org). The intent of the center is to assist these schools to engage a fully integrated system of supports and services to benefit all students, with MTSS as the primary driver for successfully installing and implementing Common Core instruction.

The future of PBIS expansion and sustainability lies in public policy. It has, as a field, clearly moved from being a "brand" of behavior management to becoming a full-blown movement with wide application across a broad spectrum of social systems. As of this writing, there are several bills before the U.S. Congress with language specific to PBIS. Passage of any one of these will signal the beginning of the emergence of PBIS as "business as usual" in social services systems such as the nation's public schools.

REFERENCES

Algozzine, B., Wang, C., White, R., Cooke, N., Harr, M.B., Algozzine, K.M., . . . Duran, G.Z. (2012). *Effects of Multi-Tier Academic and Behavior Instruction on Difficult to Teach Students*, 79(1), 45–64.

Association for Positive Behavior Support (APBS), (2007). *Positive behavior support standards of practice: Individual level.* Retrieved from http://www.apbs.org/files/apbs_standards_of_practice _2013_format.pdf

Atkins, M.S., Hoagwood, K., Kutash, K., & Seidman, E. (2010). Toward the integration of education and mental health in schools. *Administration and Policy in Mental Health and Mental Health Services Research*, 37(1–2), 40–47.

Bambara, L.M., Nonnemacher, S., & Kern, L. (2009). Sustaining school-based individualized positive behavior support: Perceived barriers and enablers. *Journal of Positive Behavior Interventions*, 11(3), 161–176.

Binnendyk, L., & Lucyshyn, J. (2009). A family-centered positive behavior support approach to the amelioration of food refusal behavior. *Journal of Positive Behavior Interventions*, 11(1), 47–62.

Blair, K.-S.C., Fox, L., & Lentini, R. (2010). Use of positive behavior support to address the challenging behavior of young children within a community early childhood program. *Topics in Early Childhood Special Education*, 30(2), 68–79.

Boettcher, M., Koegel, R.L., McNerney, E.K., & Koegel, L.K. (2003). A family-centered prevention approach to PBS in a time of crisis. *Journal of Positive Behavior Interventions*, 5(1), 55–59.

Bohanon, H., Fenning, P., Borgmeier, C., Flannery, B., & Malloy, J. (2009). Finding a direction for high school positive behavior support. In W. Sailor, G. Dunlap, G. Sugai, & R. Horner (Eds.), *Handbook of positive behavior support* (pp. 581–601). New York, NY: Springer.

Bohanon, H., Fenning, P., Carney, K.L., Minnis-Kim, M.J., Anderson-Harriss, S., Moroz, K.B., . . . Pigott, T.D. (2006). Schoolwide application of positive behavior support in an urban high school: A case study. *Journal of Positive Behavior Interventions*, 8(3), 131–145.

Bohanon, H., Fenning, P., Eber, L., & Flannery, B. (2007). Identifying a roadmap of support for secondary students in school-wide positive behavior support applications. *International Journal of Special Education*, 22, 39–53.

Bradshaw, C.P., Koth, C.W., Thornton, L.A., & Leaf, P.J. (2009). Altering school climate through schoolwide positive behavioral interventions and supports: Findings from a group-randomized effectiveness trial. *Prevention Science*, 10, 100–115.

Bradshaw, C.P., Mitchell, M.M., & Leaf, P.J. (2010). Examining the effects of schoolwide positive behavioral interventions and supports on student outcomes: Results from a randomized controlled effectiveness trial in elementary schools. *Journal of Positive Behavior Interventions*, 12(3), 133–148.

Bradshaw, C.P., Pas, E.T., Bloom, J., Barrett, S., Hershfeldt, P., Alexander, A., . . . Leaf, P. (2012). A statewide collaboration to promote safe and supportive schools: The PBIS Maryland Initiative. *Administration and Policy in Mental Health and Mental Health Services Research*, 39(4), 225–237. doi:10.1007/s10488 -011-0384-6

Bruder, M.B. (2010). Early childhood intervention: A promise to children and families for their future. *Exceptional Children*, 76(3), 339–355.

Capella, E., Frazier, S., Atkins, M.S., Schoenwald, S.K., & Glisson, C. (2008). Enhancing schools' capacity to support children in poverty: An ecological model of school-based mental health services. *Administration and Policy in Mental Health*, 35, 395–409.

Coffey, J.H., & Horner, R. (2012). The sustainability of schoolwide positive behavior interventions and support. *Council for Exceptional Children*, 78(4), 407–422.

Colvin, G., Sugai, G., Good, R.H., & Lee, Y. (1997). Using active supervision and precorrection to improve transition behaviors in an elementary school. *School Psychology Quarterly*, 12(4), 344–363.

Crimmins, D., & Farrell, A.F. (2006). Individualize behavioral supports at 15 years: It's still lonely at the top. *Research and Practice for Persons with Severe Disabilities*, 31(1), 31–45.

Dunlap, G., & Fox, L. (2009). Positive behavior support and early intervention. In W. Sailor, G. Dunlap, G. Sugai, & R.H. Horner (Eds.), *Handbook of positive behavior support* (pp.177–202). New York, NY: Springer.

Eber, L., Hyde, K., Rose, J., Breen, K., McDonald, D., & Lewandowski, H. (2009). Completing the continuum of schoolwide positive behavior support: Wraparound as a tertiary-level intervention. In W. Sailor, G. Dunlap, G. Sugai, & R. Horner (Eds.), *Handbook of positive behavior support* (pp.671–703). New York, NY: Springer.

Eber, L., Hyde, K., & Suter, J.C. (2011). Integrating wraparound into a schoolwide system of positive behavior supports. *Journal of Child and Family Studies*, 20, 78–790.

Farrington, D.P., & Ttofi, M.M. (2011). Bullying as a predictor of offending violence and later life outcomes. *Criminal Behavior and Mental Health*, 21, 90–98.

Flannery, K.B., & Sugai, G. (2009). Introduction to the monograph on high school SWPBS implementation. In K.B. Flannery & G. Sugai (Eds.), *PBS implementation in high schools: Current practices and future directions* (pp. 7–22). Eugene, OR: University of Oregon.

Flannery, K.B., Sugai, G., & Anderson, C. (2009). Schoolwide positive behavior support in high school. *Journal of Positive Behavior Interventions*, 11(3), 177–185.

Fox, L., Carta, J., Strain, P., Dunlap, G., & Hemmeter, M.L. (2010). Response to intervention and the pyramid model. *Infant and Young Children*, 23(1), 3–13.

Fox, L., & Hemmeter, M.L. (2009). A program-wide model for supporting social emotional development and addressing challenging behavior in early childhood settings. In W. Sailor, G. Dunlap, G. Sugai, & R.H. Horner (Eds.), *Handbook of positive behavior support* (pp. 177–202). New York, NY: Springer.

Freeman, R., Smith, C., Zarcone, J., Kimbrough, P., Tieghi-Benet, M., Wickham, D., . . . Hine, K. (2005). Building a statewide plan for embedding positive behavior support in human service organizations. *Journal of Positive Behavior Interventions, 7*(2), 109–119.

Gagnon, J.C., & Barber, B. (2010). Characteristics of and services provided to youth in secure care facilities. *Behavioral Disorders, 16*(1), 7–19.

Gagnon, J.C., Rockwell, S.B., & Scott, T.M. (2008). Positive behavior supports in exclusionary schools: A practical approach based on what we know. *Focus on Exceptional Children, 41*(1), 1–20.

Gendron, B.P., Williams, K.R., & Guerra, N.G. (2011). An analysis of bullying among students within schools: Estimating the effects of individual normative beliefs, self-esteem, and school climate. *Journal of School Violence, 10,* 150–164.

Gordham, K.M. (2010). PBS in other community settings: Quality of life issues in memory care. *Association for Positive Behavior Support Newsletter, 7*(4), 1–4.

Hagner, D., Malloy, J.M., Mazzone, M.W., & Cornier, G.M. (2008). Youth with disabilities in the criminal justice system: Considerations for transition and rehabilitation planning. *Journal of Emotional and Behavior Disorders, 16*(4), 240–247.

Horner, R.H. (2000). Positive behavior supports. *Focus on Autism and Other Developmental Disabilities, 15*(2), 97–105.

Horner, R.H., Sugai, G., Smolkowski, K., Eber, L., Nakasato, J., Todd, A., & Esperanza, J. (2009). A randomized, wait-list controlled effectiveness trial assessing school-wide positive behavior support in elementary schools. *Journal of Positive Behavior Interventions, 11*(3), 133.

Jolivette, K., & Nelson, M.C. (2010). Adapting positive behavioral interventions and supports for secure juvenile justice settings: Improving facility-wide behavior. *Behavioral Disorders, 36*(1), 28–42.

Lassen, S., Steele, M., & Sailor, W. (2006). The relationship of school-wide positive behavior support to academic achievement in an urban middle school. *Psychology in the Schools, 43*(6), 701.

LeBlanc, L.A. (2010). Integrating behavioral psychology services into adult day programming for individuals with dementia. *Behavior Modification, 34*(5), 443–458.

Lewis, T.J. (2009). Connecting school-wide positive behavior support to the academic curriculum in PBIS high schools. In B. Flannery & G. Sugai (Eds.), *SWPBS implementation in high schools: Current practice and future directions* (pp. 57–80). Eugene, OR: University of Oregon.

Malloy, J., Sundar, V., Hagner, D., Pierias, L., & Viet, T. (2010). The efficacy of the RENEW model: Individualized school-to-career services for youth at risk of school dropout. *Journal of at Risk Issues, 15*(2), 17–25.

McCart, A., Lee, J., Frey, A.J., Wolf, N., Choi, J.-H., & Haynes, H. (2010). Response to intervention in early childhood centers: A multi-tiered approach promoting family engagement. *Early Childhood Services, 4*(2), 87–104.

McCart, A., Wolf, N., Sweeney, H., & Choi, J. (2009). The application of a family-based multi-tiered system of support. *National Head Start Association Dialog, 12*(2), 122–132.

McIntosh, K., Flannery, K.B., Sugai, G., Braun, D.H., & Cochrane, K.L. (2008). Relationships between academic and problem behavior in the transition from middle school to high school. *Journal of Positive Behavior Interventions, 10*(4), 243–255.

Nelson, C.M., Jolivette, K., Leone, P.E., & Mathur, S.R. (2010). Meeting the needs of at-risk and adjudicated youth with behavioral challenges: The promise of juvenile justice. *Behavioral Disorders, 36*(1), 70–80.

Nelson, C.M., Scott, T.M., Gagnon, J.C., Jolivette, K., & Sprague, J. (2008). Positive behavior support in the juvenile justice system. *PBIS Newsletter 4*(3). Retrieved September 14, 2012, from http://www.pbis.org/pbis_newsletter/volume_4/issue3.aspx

O'Brien, J., & Lovett, H. (1993). *Finding a way toward everyday lives: The contribution of person centered planning.* Syracuse, NY: Syracuse University, Center on Human Policy.

Pierson, M.R., Carter, E.W., Lane, K.L., & Glaeser, B.C. (2008). Factors influencing the self-determination of transition-age youth with high incidence disabilities. *Career Development for Exceptional Individuals, 31*(2), 115–125.

Quinn, M.M., Rutherford, R.B., Leone, P.E., Osher, D.M., & Poirier, J.M. (2005). Youth with disabilities in juvenile corrections: A national survey. *Council for Exceptional Children, 71*(3), 339–345.

Reinke, W.M., Splett, J.D., Robeson, E.N., & Offutt, C.A. (2009). Combining school and family interventions for the prevention and early intervention of disruptive behavior problems in children: A public health perspective. *Psychology in the Schools, 46*(1), 33–43.

Ross, S.W., & Horner, R.H. (2009). Bully prevention in positive behavior support. *Journal of Applied Behavior Analysis, 42*(42), 747–759.

Sadler, C., & Sugai, G. (2009). Effective behavior and instructional support: A district model for early identification and prevention of reading and behavior problems. *Journal of Positive Behavior Interventions, 11*(1), 35–46.

Sailor, W. (2009). *Making RTI work: How smart schools are reforming education through school-wide response-to-intervention.* San Francisco, CA: Jossey-Bass.

Sailor, W., Doolittle, J., Bradley, R., & Danielson, L. (2009). Response to intervention and positive behavior support. In W. Sailor, G. Dunlap, G. Sugai, & R. Horner (Eds.), *Handbook of positive behavior support* (pp. 729–753). New York, NY: Springer.

Sailor, W., Stowe, M.J., Turnbull, H.R., & Kleinhammer-Tramill, J. (2007). A case for adding a social/behavioral standard to standards-based education with school-wide positive behavior support as its basis. *Remedial and Special Education, 28*(6), 266–276.

Sailor, W., Wolf, N., Choi, H., & Roger, B. (2009). Sustaining positive behavior support in a context of comprehensive school reform. In W. Sailor, G. Dunlap, G. Sugai, & R. Horner (Eds.), *Handbook of positive behavior support* (pp. 639–640). New York, NY: Springer.

Sailor, W., Zuna, N., Choi, J.-H., Thomas, J., McCart, A., & Roger, B. (2006). Anchoring schoolwide positive behavior support in structural school reform.

Research and Practice for Persons with Severe Disabilities, 31(1), 18–30.

Satter, A., & Dunn, J. (2012). A policy analysis of response to intervention. *The Journal of Education Policy, Planning and Administration, 2*(1), 4–23.

Scott, T.M., & Eber, L. (2003). Functional assessment and wraparound as systemic school processes: Primary, secondary, and tertiary system examples. *Journal of Positive Behavior Interventions, 5*(3), 131–143.

Sprague, J., Baus, A., & Tedder, J. (2011). *Positive behavioral interventions and supports within juvenile justice settings: What it looks like and feedback from leadership teams.* Paper presented at the Positive Behavioral Interventions and Supports (PBIS) National Forum, Chicago, IL.

Sugai, G., Flannery, K.B., & Bohanon-Edmonson, H. (2004). *School-wide positive behavior supports in high schools: What will it take?* Eugene, OR: University of Oregon.

Sugai, G., & Simonsen, B. (2012). *Positive behavioral interventions and supports: History, defining features, and misconceptions.* Retrieved September 21, 2012, from http://www.pbis.org/common/pbis resources/publications/PBIS_revisited_June19r_2012 .pdf

Swain-Bradway, J., & Malloy, J. (2009). Secondary and tertiary tier supports in PBIS high schools. In K.B. Flannery & G. Sugai (Eds.), *SWPBS implementation in high schools: Current practice and future directions* (pp. 115–144). Eugene: University of Oregon.

Ttofi, M.M., & Farrington, D.P. (2010). Effectiveness of school-based programs to reduce bullying: A systematic and meta-analytic review. *Journal of Experimental Criminology, 7,* 27–56.

U.S. Department of Education. (2006). *26th Annual report to Congress on the implementation of the Individuals with Disabilities Education Act, 2004* (Vol. 2). Washington, DC: Author.

U.S. Department of Education, Office of Planning, Evaluation, and Policy Development, Policy and Program Studies Service. (2011). *Analysis of state bullying laws and policies.* Washington, DC: Author.

Vanderbilt, D., & Augustyn, M. (2010). The effects of bullying. *Pediatrics and Child Health, 20*(7), 315–320.

Waasdorp, T.E., Bradshaw, C.P., & Leaf, P.J. (2012). The impact of schoolwide positive behavioral interventions and supports on bullying and peer rejection: A randomized controlled effectiveness trial. *Archives of Pediatrics & Adolescent Medicine, 166*(2), 149–156.

Watson, S.M.R., Gable, R.A., & Greenwood, C.R. (2011). Combining ecobehavioral assessment, functional assessment, and response to intervention to promote more effective classroom instruction. *Remedial and Special Education, 32*(4), 334–344.

Wehmeyer, M., & Palmer, S.B. (2003). Adult outcomes for students with cognitive disabilities three-years after high school: The impact of self-determination. *Education and Training in Developmental Disabilities, 38*(2), 131–144.

Wood, B.K., Ferro, J.B., Umbreit, J., & Liaupsin, C. (2011). Addressing the challenging behavior of young children through systematic function-based intervention. *Topics in Early Childhood Special Education, 30*(4), 221–232.

Association for Positive Behavior Support Standards of Practice

Individual Level (SOP-I)

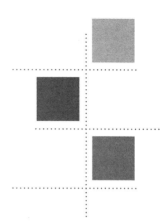

I. FOUNDATIONS OF POSITIVE BEHAVIOR SUPPORT

A. Practitioners of positive behavior support have a historical perspective on the evolution of PBS and its relationship to applied behavior analysis and movements in the disability field.

1. History of applied behavior analysis and the relationship to positive behavior support (PBS)
2. Similarities and unique features of PBS and applied behavior analysis (ABA)
3. Movements in the field of serving people with disabilities that influenced the emergence of PBS practices
   a. Deinstitutionalization
   b. Normalization and social role valorization
   c. Community participation
   d. Supported employment
   e. Least restrictive environment and inclusive schooling
   f. Self-determination

B. Practitioners applying positive behavior support with individuals adhere to a number of basic assumptions about behavior.

1. Problem behavior serves a function.
2. Positive strategies are effective for addressing the most challenging behavior.
3. When positive behavior intervention strategies fail, additional functional assessment strategies are required to develop more effective PBS strategies.
4. Features of the environmental context affect behavior.
5. Reduction of problem behavior is an important (but not the sole) outcome of successful intervention; effective PBS results in improvements

in quality of life, acquisition of valued skills, and access to valued activities.

C. Practitioners applying positive behavior support with individuals include at least 11 key elements in the development of positive behavior support supports.

1. Collaborative team-based decision making
2. Person-centered decision making
3. Self-determination
4. Functional assessment of behavior and functionally derived interventions
5. Identification of outcomes that enhance quality of life and are valued by the individual, their families, and the community
6. Strategies that are acceptable in inclusive community settings
7. Strategies that teach useful and valued skills
8. Strategies that are evidence based and socially and empirically valid to achieve desired outcomes that are at least as effective and efficient as the problem behavior
9. Techniques that do not cause pain or humiliation or deprive the individual of basic needs
10. Constructive and respectful multicomponent intervention plans that emphasize antecedent interventions, instruction in prosocial behaviors, and environmental modification
11. Ongoing measurement of impact

D. Practitioners applying positive behavior support with individuals commit themselves to ongoing and rigorous professional development.

1. Pursue continuing education and in-service training, and consult peer-reviewed journals and current publications to stay abreast of

549

emerging research, trends, and national models of support.

2. Attend national, regional, state, and local conferences.

3. Seek out collaboration, support, and/or assistance when faced with challenges outside of one's expertise.

4. Seek out collaboration, support, and/or assistance when intended outcomes are not achieved in a timely manner.

5. Seek out knowledge from a variety of relevant empirically based fields. These fields include education, behavioral and social sciences, and the biomedical sciences.

E. Practitioners of positive behavior support understand the legal and regulatory requirements related to assessment and intervention regarding challenging behavior and behavioral change strategies.

1. Requirements of IDEA with respect to PBS

2. The purpose of human rights organizations and other oversight committees regarding behavior change

3. State/school/agency regulations and requirements

II. COLLABORATION AND TEAM BUILDING

A. Practitioners of positive behavior support understand the importance of and use strategies to work collaboratively with other professionals, individuals with disabilities, and their families.

1. Understands and respects the importance of collaboration in providing effective PBS services

2. Uses skills needed for successful collaboration, including the ability to:
   a. Communicate clearly
   b. Establish rapport
   c. Be flexible and open
   d. Support the viewpoints of others
   e. Learn from others
   f. Incorporate new ideas within personal framework
   g. Manage conflict

B. Practitioners of positive behavior support understand the importance of and use strategies to support development and effectiveness of collaborative teams.

1. Includes the critical members of a PBS team for the individual considering the age, setting, and types of abilities and disabilities of the individual

2. Evaluates team composition considering the needs of the individual and assists the team in recruiting additional team members to address needed areas of expertise

3. Uses essential team skills, including:
   a. Facilitation
   b. Coaching
   c. Mediation
   d. Consensus building
   e. Meeting management
   f. Team roles and responsibilities

4. Uses strategies and processes to demonstrate sensitivity to and respect for all team members, and diverse opinions and perspectives

5. Facilitates the inclusion of and respect for the values and priorities of families and all team members

6. Supports and participates in advocacy necessary to access supports to carry out team decisions

III. BASIC PRINCIPLES OF BEHAVIOR

A. Practitioners of positive behavior support utilize behavioral assessment and support methods that are based on operant learning.

1. The antecedent behavior consequence model as the basis for all voluntary behavior

2. Operational definitions of behavior

3. Stimulus control, including discriminative stimuli and S-deltas

4. The influence of setting events (or establishing operations), on behavior

5. Antecedent influences on behavior

6. Precursor behaviors

7. Consequences to increase or decrease behavior

B. Practitioners of positive behavior support understand and use antecedent manipulations to influence behavior, such as:

1. Curricular modifications

2. Instructional modifications

3. Behavioral precursors as signals

4. Modification of routines

5. Opportunities for choice/control throughout the day

6. Clear expectations

7. Precorrection

8. Errorless learning

C. Practitioners of positive behavior support understand and use consequence manipulations to increase behavior.

1. Primary reinforcers, and conditions under which primary reinforcers are used

2. Types of secondary reinforcers and their use

3. Approaches to identify effective reinforcers, including:
   a. Functional assessment data
   b. Observation

c. Reinforcer surveys

d. Reinforcer sampling

4. Premack principle

5. Positive reinforcement

6. Negative reinforcement

7. Ratio, interval, and natural schedules of reinforcement

8. Pairing of reinforcers

D. Practitioners of positive behavior support understand consequence manipulations to decrease behavior.

1. The use of punishment, including characteristics, ethical use of punishment, and potential side effects of punishment procedures. (*Any use of punishment, including strategies that are found within integrated natural settings, must be within the parameters of the 11 key elements Identified above in IC, with particular attention to IC9 "techniques that do not cause pain or humiliation or deprive the individual of basic needs."*)

2. Differential reinforcement, including:

   a. Differential reinforcement of alternative behavior

   b. Differential reinforcement of incompatible behavior

   c. Differential reinforcement of zero rates of behavior

   d. Differential reinforcement of lower rates of behavior

3. Extinction, including:

   a. Characteristics of extinction interventions

   b. How to use extinction

   c. Using extinction in combination with interventions to develop replacement behaviors

4. Response cost, including:

   a. Cautions associated with use of response cost

   b. Using response cost with interventions to develop replacement behaviors

5. Time-out, including:

   a. Types of time-out applications

   b. How to implement

   c. Cautions associated with use of time-out

   d. Using time-out with interventions to develop replacement behaviors

E. Practitioners of positive behavior support understand and use methods for facilitating generalization and maintenance of skills.

1. Forms of generalization, including:

   a. Stimulus generalization

   b. Response generalization

   c. Generalization across subjects

2. Maintenance of behaviors across time

IV. DATA-BASED DECISION MAKING

A. Practitioners of positive behavior support understand that data based decision making is a fundamental element of PBS, and that behavioral assessment and support planning begins with defining behavior.

1. Using operational definitions to describe target behaviors

2. Writing behavioral objectives that include:

   a. Conditions under which the behavior should occur

   b. Operational definition of behavior

   c. Criteria for achieving the objective

B. Practitioners of positive behavior support understand that data based decision making is a fundamental element of positive behavior support, and that measuring behavior is a critical component of behavioral assessment and support.

1. Using data systems that are appropriate for target behaviors, including:

   a. Frequency

   b. Duration

   c. Latency

   d. Interval recording

   e. Time sampling

   f. Permanent product recording

2. Developing data collection plans that include:

   a. The measurement system to be used

   b. Schedule for measuring behavior during relevant times and contexts, including baseline data

   c. Manageable strategies for sampling behavior for measurement purposes

   d. How, when, and if the interobserver agreement checks will be conducted

   e. How and when procedural integrity checks will be conducted

   f. Data collection recording forms

   g. How raw data will be converted to a standardized format (e.g., rate, percentage)

   h. Use of criterion to determine when to make changes in the instructional phase

C. Practitioners of positive behavior support use graphic displays of data to support decision making during the assessment, program development, and evaluation stages of behavior support.

1. Converting raw data in standardized format

2. Following graphing conventions, including:

   a. Clearly labeled axes

   b. Increment scales that allow for meaningful and accurate

3. Representation of the data
   a. Phase change lines
   b. Clearly labeled phase change descriptions
   c. Criterion lines

D. Practitioners of positive behavior support use data based strategies to monitor progress.

1. Using graphed data to identify trends and intervention effects
2. Evaluating data regularly and frequently
3. Sharing data with team members for team-based, person-centered decision making
4. Using data to make decisions regarding program revisions to maintain or improve behavioral progress, including decisions relating to maintaining, modifying, or terminating interventions
5. Using data to determine if additional collaborations, support and/or assistance is needed to achieve intended outcomes

V. COMPREHENSIVE PERSON-CENTERED AND FUNCTIONAL BEHAVIOR ASSESSMENTS

A. Practitioners understand the importance of multielement assessments including:

1. Person Centered Planning
2. Quality of Life
3. Environmental/ecology
4. Setting events
5. Antecedents and consequences
6. Social skills/communication/social networks
7. Curricular/instructional needs (e.g., learning style)
8. Health/biophysical

B. Comprehensive assessments result in information about the focus individual in at least the following areas:

1. Lifestyle
2. Preferences and interests
3. Communication/social abilities & needs
4. Ecology
5. Health and safety
6. Problem routines
7. Variables promoting and reinforcing problem behavior:
   a. Preferences/reinforcers
   b. Antecedents
   c. Setting events
   d. Potential replacement behavior
8. Function(s) of behavior
9. Potential replacement behaviors

C. Practitioners who apply positive behavior support conduct Person-Centered Assessments that provide a picture of the life of the individual including:

1. Indicators of quality of life comparable to same age individuals without disabilities (e.g., self-determination, inclusion, friends, fun, variety, access to belongings)
2. The strengths and gifts of the individual
3. The variety and roles of people with whom they interact (e.g., family, friends, neighbors, support providers) and the nature, frequency and duration of such interactions
4. The environments & activities in which they spend time including the level of acceptance and meaningful participation, problematic and successful routines, preferred settings/activities, the rate of reinforcement and/or corrective feedback, and the age appropriateness of settings, activities & materials
5. The level of independence and support needs of the individual including workplace, curricular & instructional modifications, augmentative communication and other assistive technology supports, and assistance with personal management and hygiene
6. The health and medical/biophysical needs of the individual
7. The dreams and goals of the individual and their circle of support
8. Barriers to achieving the dreams and goals
9. The influence of the above information on problem behavior

D. Positive behavior support practitioners conduct Functional Behavioral Assessments that result in:

1. Operationally defined problem behavior
2. The context in which problem behavior occurs most often
3. Identification of setting events that promote the potential for problem behavior
4. Identification of antecedents that set the occasion for problem behavior
5. Identification of consequences maintaining problem behavior
6. A thorough description of the antecedent behavior consequence relationship
7. An interpretation of the function(s) of behavior
8. Identification of potential replacement behavior

E. Positive behavior support practitioners conduct indirect and direct assessment strategies.

1. Indirect assessments include file reviews, structured interviews (e.g., person-centered

planning), checklists, and rating scales (e.g., MAS)

2. Direct assessments include such strategies as scatterplots, anecdotal recording, ABC data, and time/activity analyses

3. Summarize data in graphic and narrative formats

F. Positive behavior support practitioners work collaboratively with the team to develop hypotheses that are supported by assessment data.

1. All assessment information is synthesized and analyzed to determine the possible influence of the following on the occurrence or nonoccurrence of problem behavior:
   a. setting events (or establishing operations)
   b. antecedents/triggers
   c. consequences for both desired and challenging behaviors
   d. ecological variables
   e. lifestyle issues
   f. medical/biophysical problems

2. Hypotheses statements are developed that address:
   a. setting events
   b. antecedents
   c. consequences for both desired and challenging behaviors
   d. function(s) problem behavior serves for the individual

G. Positive behavior support practitioners utilize Functional Analysis of Behavior as necessary on the basis of an understanding of:

1. The differences between functional assessment and functional analysis

2. The advantages & disadvantages of functional analysis

3. The conditions under which each approach may be conducted

VI. DEVELOPMENT AND IMPLEMENTATION OF COMPREHENSIVE, MULTIELEMENT BEHAVIOR SUPPORT PLANS

A. Positive behavior support practitioners apply the following considerations/foundations across all elements of a positive behavior support plan:

1. Behavior support plans are developed in collaboration with the individual and his or her team

2. Behavior support plans are driven by the results of person-centered and functional behavior assessments

3. Behavior support plans facilitate the individual's preferred lifestyle

4. Behavior support plans are designed for contextual fit, specifically in relation to:
   a. The values and goals of the team
   b. The current and desired routines within the various settings in which the individual participates
   c. The skills and buy-in of those who will be implementing the plan
   d. Administrative support

5. Behavior support plans include strategies for evaluating each component plan of the plan

B. Behavior support plans include interventions to improve/support quality of life in at least the following areas:

1. Achieving the individual's dreams

2. The individual's health and physiological needs

3. Promote all aspects of self determination

4. Improvement in individual's active, successful participation in inclusive school, work, home and community settings

5. Promotion of social interactions, relationships, and enhanced social networks

6. Increased fun and success in the individual's life

7. Improved leisure, relaxation, and recreational activities for the individual throughout the day

C. Positive behavior support practitioners develop behavior support plans that include antecedent interventions to prevent the need for problem behavior using the following strategies:

1. Alter or eliminate setting events to preclude the need for problem behavior

2. Modify specific antecedent triggers/circumstances based on the FBA

3. Identify and address behaviors using precursors (i.e., individual's signal that a problem behavior is likely to occur)

4. Make the individual's environment/routines predictable (e.g., personal schedule in format the individual can understand)

5. Build opportunities for choice/control throughout the day that are age appropriate and contextually appropriate

6. Create clear expectations

7. Modify curriculum/job demands so the individual can successfully complete tasks

D. Positive behavior support plans address effective instructional intervention strategies that may include the following:

1. Match instructional strategies to the individual's learning style

2. Provide instruction in the context in which the problem behaviors occur and the use of

alternative skills, including instruction in skills such as:

   a.   Communication skills

   b.   Social skills

   c.   Self-management/monitoring skills

   d.   Other adaptive behaviors as indicated by the FBA and continued evaluation of progress data (e.g., relaxation techniques)

3.   Teach replacement behavior(s) based on competing behavior analysis

4.   Select and teach replacement behaviors that can be as or more effective than the problem behavior

5.   Utilize instructional methods of addressing a problem behavior proactively (including preinstruction; modeling; rehearsal; social stories; incidental teaching; use of peer buddies; meeting sensory needs; direct instruction; verbal, physical, and/or visual prompting)

E. Positive behavior support practitioners employ consequence intervention strategies that consider the following:

1.   Reinforcement strategies are function based and rely on naturally occurring reinforcers as much as possible.

2.   Use the least intrusive behavior reduction strategy (e.g., error correction, extinction, differential reinforcement).

3.   Emergency intervention strategies are used only where safety of the individual or others must be assured.

4.   Plans for avoiding power struggles and provocation

5.   Plan for potential natural consequences. Consider when these should happen and when there should be attempts to avoid them. Although some natural consequences are helpful to the individual (e.g., losing money, missing a bus), others can be detrimental and provide no meaningful experience (e.g., being hit by a car, admission to psychiatric unit).

F. Positive behavior support practitioners develop plans for successful implementation of positive behavior support plans that include:

1.   Action plans for implementation of all components of the intervention including:

   a.   Activities, dates and documentation describing who is responsible for completing each task

   b.   Materials, training and support needed for those doing intervention

   c.   How data will be collected and analyzed to address both impact and fidelity of intervention

   d.   Time lines for meetings, data analysis and targeted outcomes

   e.   Training, supports and time needed for plan implementation

   f.   Criteria for team meetings for immediate modification of PBS plan

   g.   Plans for review of contextual fit. function based interventions, and lifestyle enhancements

2.   Strategies to address systems change needed for implementation of PBS plans that may include:

   a.   Modifying policies/regulations

   b.   Support and training for personnel & families

   c.   Accessing needed resources (financial & personnel)

   d.   Increasing flexibility in routines, & staffing schedules

   e.   Recruiting additional individuals to be team members (e.g., bus driver, peers, neighbors, extended family)

   f.   Interagency collaboration

G. Positive behavior support practitioners evaluate plan implementation and use data to make needed modifications.

1.   Implement plan, evaluate and monitor progress according to time lines

2.   Collect data identified for each component of PBS plan

3.   Analyze data on regular basis to determine needed adjustments

4.   Evaluate progress on Person-Centered Plans (e.g., quality of life, social networks, personal preferences, upcoming transitions)

5.   Modify each element of the PBS plan as indicated by evaluation data

From Association for Positive Behavior Support. (2013). Positive behavior support standards of practice: Individual level. Bloomsburg, PA: Author; reprinted by permission

Index

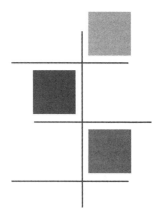

Tables, figures, and footnotes are indicated by *t*, *f*, and *n*, respectively.

Positive punishment, behavior reduction interventions, 157–158
Positive reinforcement
  applied behavior analysis and, 112–114, 112*f*
  consequence-based strategies and, 146–147, 150–155
Poverty, positive behavior support challenges and, 433–445
Power and control, support versus, 505
Power cards, in teaching interventions, 355–357, 356*f*
Precorrection, target behaviors, 120
Preference assessment, functional analysis in outpatient settings, 300–301
"Prepare for Your Day" activities, school-wide positive behavior support plans and, 471–474, 472*f*
Prevention-oriented interventions
  applied behavior analysis, 119
  consequence-based strategies, 148–150
  problem behavior, 89
  target behaviors, 120
Prevent-teach-reinforce model (PTR)
  applied behavior analysis, 119
  generalization and maintenance and, 176–177
  progress in PBS and, 429
  school-wide positive behavior support, 17–18
Primary interventions, applied behavior analysis and, 117–121
Prioritization of behavior challenges
  positive behavior support plans, 426
  team-based strategies for, 59–68
Problem behavior
  absence of, in outpatient functional analysis, 301–302
  antecedent strategies and, 126–127, 132*t*
  choice-making and reduction of, 335–337
  cultural diversity and, 448–449
  identification of, 505–506
  integrated wraparound, PCP, and PSB planning and, 247
  interference in quality of life and, 493–495
  interventions in, 38–39
  lack of control and, 334
  in older adults, 519–521
  personalization of, 53
  positive behavior support research and, 31–35
  reduction of, 34–35
  relevant information in FBA and variability in, 281–282
  teaming strategies and attribution of, 51–52
Problem Behavior Questionnaire (PBQ), 271
Problem solving approaches
  collaborative problem solving, 60–64
  integrated PCP, wraparound, and PBS systems and, 251–255
  post-plan implementation data analysis, 67–68
  self-management plans and, 341–342
Procedural drift
  single-case design structure, 203
  see also Fidelity-of-implementation strategies
Process monitoring, positive behavior support plans, 425–427
Progress monitoring, instructional scaffolding and, 378
Progressive time delay, systematic instruction, 224*f*, 225
Prompting, systematic instruction, 224–229
Prosocial behaviors, interventions using, 38–39
Proximal antecedents
  defined, 125
  developmental disabilities research, 13
PTR, *see* Prevent-teach-reinforce model
Public applied behavior analysis, 115
Punishment

applied behavior analysis, 111–112, 112*f*
behavior reduction interventions, 157–158
consequence interventions and, 146–147
effective use of, 158–159
in functional communication training, 387–388
Purpose and goal of teams, 54, 58

Qualitative studies, developmental disabilities research, 13
Quality of life (QOL) improvements
  basic principles of, 488–489
  best practices for, 241–256
  case studies in, 486–488
  importance of working and, 525–526
  integrated wraparound, PCP, and PSB planning, 247
  life outcomes through integrated system, 251–255, 252*f*
  listening skills and, 504–505
  person-centered planning, 244, 245*t*
  positive behavior support and, 35–36, 484–510
  problem behaviors as barrier to, 493–495
  relationships and, 501–503
  relevant information in FBA and variability in, 282
  respect in, 503–504
  sustainability of, 509–510
Quality-of-life outcomes
  case study in, 513–532
  person-centered planning, 249
  in person-centered planning, 84–85
  person-centered planning and, 490–493
Questionnaires, functional behavioral assessment, 271, 272*t*

Rapport, generalization and maintenance strategies, 174–175
Rate of behavior
  defined, 186
  recording of, 188
Rating scales, functional behavioral assessment, 271, 272*t*
Reactivity, observer reliability and, 195–196
Readiness assessment, systemic change of challenging behaviors, 96
Real-time data analysis, single-case designs, 214–218
Reflexivity, in positive behavior support, 508
Reframing techniques, for challenging beliefs, 61–64
Rehabilitation, empowerment, natural supports, education, and work (RENEW), 535–536
Reinforcement
  applications of, 154–155
  applied behavior analysis, 111–112, 112*f*, 119
  complex scheduling, 171–172, 171*t*
  consequence interventions and, 146–147, 150–155
  continuous versus intermittent, 168
  defined, 168
  extinction and, 156–157
  functional communication training, 387
  maintenance facilitation and failure management, 168
  natural communities for, FCT and, 389–390
  self-recruited reinforcement, 339–340
  simple scheduling, 168–171, 169*t*–170*t*
  of systemic change, 89
  tolerance for delay in, 175
Reinforcer sampling, consequence-based intervention, 151
Relatedness, 334
  positive behavior support and, 501–503